Springer Proceedings in Mathematics & Statistics

Volume 208

Springer Proceedings in Mathematics & Statistics

This book series features volumes composed of selected contributions from workshops and conferences in all areas of current research in mathematics and statistics, including operation research and optimization. In addition to an overall evaluation of the interest, scientific quality, and timeliness of each proposal at the hands of the publisher, individual contributions are all refereed to the high quality standards of leading journals in the field. Thus, this series provides the research community with well-edited, authoritative reports on developments in the most exciting areas of mathematical and statistical research today.

More information about this series at http://www.springer.com/series/10533

Vladimir Panov
Editor

Modern Problems of Stochastic Analysis and Statistics

Selected Contributions
in Honor of Valentin Konakov

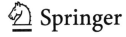 Springer

Editor
Vladimir Panov
Department of Statistics and Data Analysis
Higher School of Economics
Moscow
Russia

ISSN 2194-1009   ISSN 2194-1017   (electronic)
Springer Proceedings in Mathematics & Statistics
ISBN 978-3-319-87997-0   ISBN 978-3-319-65313-6   (eBook)
DOI 10.1007/978-3-319-65313-6

Mathematics Subject Classification (2010): 60Hxx, 60Fxx, 60Jxx, 62Gxx, 62Mxx

Printed on acid-free paper

This Springer imprint is published by Springer Nature
The registered company is Springer International Publishing AG
The registered company address is: Gewerbestrasse 11, 6330 Cham, Switzerland

Preface

This volume brings together latest results in the area of stochastic analysis and statistics. The individual chapters cover a wide range of topics from limit theorems, Markov processes, nonparametric methods, actuarial science, population dynamics, and many others. The volume is dedicated to Valentin Konakov, professor at the Higher School of Economics and the Lomonosov Moscow State University.

Professor Konakov made significant contributions to several areas of stochastics, including discretization and approximation of the stochastic differential equations, nonparametric functional estimation, local limit theorems, extreme value analysis, theory of Gaussian processes. Some of his research findings have become classics. For instance, the parametrix method for diffusions and Markov chains proposed by Valentin Konakov in joint articles with Enno Mammen (Heidelberg University), is now referred to as a classical approach for the analysis of these models. His results were published in top-tier journals like Bernoulli, Probability Theory and Related Fields, Stochastic Processes and their applications, Annales de l'Institut Henri Poincaré (B): Probability and Statistics, and many others.

Valentin Konakov supervised a lot of international projects, e.g., for 12 years he was a head of Russian-German projects jointly funded by RFBR (Russian Foundation of Basic Research) and DFG (Deutsche Forschungsgemeinschaft). From 1994 to 2010, Valentin Konakov worked as an invited professor in the leading universities of Germany and France.

In February 2014, the Higher School of Economics has founded a new international laboratory of Stochastic Analysis and its Applications under the direction of Prof. Konakov (https://lsa.hse.ru/). The team of the laboratory includes scientists from Russia, USA, Germany, France, United Kingdom, which are yet to be linked by close research interests. It is important to note that this team was created on the basis of a long collaboration between Valentin Konakov and his colleagues from foreign universities, namely Stanislav Molchanov (UNC Charlotte, USA), Enno Mammen (Heidelberg University, Germany), and Stéphane Menozzi (University of Evry, France). Nowadays, the Laboratory of Stochastic Analysis and its Applications plays an important role in the scientific community in Moscow.

In view of his professional achievements, Prof. Konakov got the status of tenured (ordinary) professor of the Higher School in Economics. This status is conferred only to outstanding professors, who made a significant contribution to science and development of the university.

On the occasion of Valentin Konakov's 70th birthday, the members of his laboratory organized the international conference "Modern problems of stochastic analysis and statistics" (May 29–June 2, 2016). Many of his coauthors and colleagues came to Moscow to celebrate his anniversary and to present recent results related to his research interests. This volume is mostly prepared by the participants of the conference and is dedicated to Valentin's work and his mathematical heritage. We hope that the book offers a valuable reference for researchers and graduate students interested in modern stochastics.

Moscow, Russia   Vladimir Panov

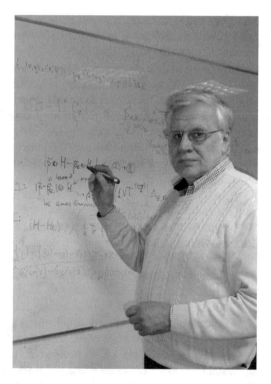

Fig. 1 Valentin Konakov at work. May 2016

Contents

Part X   Ergodic Markov Processes

Contributors

Aurélien Alfonsi Université Paris-Est, Marne La Vallée, France

Pierre Bellec Rutgers University, Piscataway, NJ, USA

Denis Belomestny Duisburg-Essen University, Essen, Germany; National Research University Higher School of Economics, Moscow, Russia

Ekaterina Bulinskaya Lomonosov Moscow State University, Moscow, Russia

Gennaro Cibelli Università di Modena e Reggio Emilia, Modena, Italy

Youri Davydov Saint Petersburg State University, Saint Petersburg, Russia

Bernard Derrida Collège de France, Paris, France

Roberto Garra "Sapienza" Università di Roma, Rome, Italy

Ion Grama Université de Bretagne Sud, Vannes, France

Alexander Gushchin Steklov Mathematical Institute, Moscow, Russia; Laboratory of Stochastic Analysis and its Applications, National Research University Higher School of Economics, Moscow, Russia

Dan Han University of North Carolina at Charlotte, Charlotte, NC, USA

Masafumi Hayashi University of the Ryukyus, Okinawa, Japan

Stefan Häfner PricewaterhouseCoopers GmbH, Frankfurt, Germany

Arturo Kohatsu-Higa Ritsumeikan University, Shiga, Japan

Valentin Konakov National Research University Higher School of Economics, Moscow, Russia

Émile Le Page Université de Bretagne Sud, Vannes, France

Alexander Lykov Lomonosov Moscow State University, Moscow, Russia

Vadim Malyshev Lomonosov Moscow State University, Moscow, Russia

Enno Mammen Heidelberg University, Heidelberg, Germany

Yuliya Mishura Taras Shevchenko National University, Kyiv, Ukraine

Stanislav Molchanov University of North Carolina at Charlotte, Charlotte, USA; National Research University Higher School of Economics, Moscow, Russian Federation

Enzo Orsingher "Sapienza" Università di Roma, Rome, Italy

Sergio Polidoro Università di Modena e Reggio Emilia, Modena, Italy

Kostiantyn Ralchenko Taras Shevchenko National University, Kyiv, Ukraine

Alexandre Richard INRIA, Sophia-Antipolis, France

Zhan Shi Université Pierre et Marie Curie, Paris, France

Denis Talay INRIA, Sophia-Antipolis, France

Alexandre Tsybakov ENSAE ParisTech, Malakoff Cedex, France

Mikhail Urusov Duisburg-Essen University, Essen, Germany

Esko Valkeila Aalto University, Aalto, Finland

Alexander Veretennikov University of Leeds, Leeds, UK; National Research University Higher School of Economics, Moscow, Russian Federation; Institute for Information Transmission Problems, Moscow, Russian Federation

Joseph Whitmeyer University of North Carolina at Charlotte, Charlotte, NC, USA

Part I
Random motions

Random Walks in Nonhomogeneous Poisson Environment

Youri Davydov and Valentin Konakov

Abstract In the first part of the paper, we consider a "random flight" process in R^d and obtain the weak limits under different transformations of the Poissonian switching times. In the second part, we construct diffusion approximations for this process and investigate their accuracy. To prove the weak convergence result, we use the approach of [15]. We consider more general model which may be called "random walk over ellipsoids in R^d". For this model, we establish the Edgeworth-type expansion. The main tool in this part is the parametrix method [5, 7].

Keywords Random walks · Random flights
Random nonhomogeneous environment · Diffusion approximation
Parametrix method

1 Introduction

We consider the moving particle process in R^d which is defined in the following way. There are two independent sequences (T_k) and (ε_k) of random variables.

The variables T_k are nonnegative and $\forall k \quad T_k \leq T_{k+1}$, while variables ε_k form an i.i.d sequence with common distribution concentrated on the unit sphere S^{d-1}.

The values ε_k are interpreted as the directions, and T_k as the moments of change of directions.

A particle starts from zero and moves in the direction ε_1 up to the moment T_1. It then changes direction to ε_2 and moves on within the time interval of length $T_2 - T_1$,

For the second author, this work has been funded by the Russian Academic Excellence Project '5–100'.

Y. Davydov
Saint Petersburg State University, Saint Petersburg, Russia

V. Konakov (✉)
National Research University Higher School of Economics, Moscow, Russia
e-mail: vkonakov@hse.ru

© Springer International Publishing AG 2017
V. Panov (ed.), *Modern Problems of Stochastic Analysis and Statistics*,
Springer Proceedings in Mathematics & Statistics 208,
DOI 10.1007/978-3-319-65313-6_1

3

etc. The speed is constant at all sites. The position of the particle at time t is denoted by $X(t)$.

The study of the processes of this type has a long history. The first work dates back probably to [13] and continued by [6, 14]. In [8] the case was considered where the increments $T_n - T_{n-1}$ form i.i.d. sequence with the common law having a heavy tail. The term "Levy flights" later changed to "Random flights".

To date, a large number of works were accumulated, devoted to the study of such processes, we mention here only articles by [4, 9, 11, 12] which contain an extensive bibliography and where for different assumptions on (T_k) and (ε_k) the exact formulas for the distribution of $X(t)$ were derived.

Our goals are different.

First, we are interested in the global behavior of the process $X = \{X(t), \ t \in R_+\}$, namely, we are looking for conditions under which the processes $\{Y_T, \ T > 0\}$,

$$Y_T(t) = \frac{1}{B(T)} X(tT), \quad t \in [0, 1],$$

weakly converges in $C[0, 1]$: $Y_T \Longrightarrow Y, \ B_T \longrightarrow \infty, \ T \longrightarrow \infty.$

From now on, we suppose that the points (T_k), $T_k \le T_{k+1}$, form a Poisson point process in R_+ denoted by $\mathbf{T}$.

It is clear that in the homogeneous case the process $X(t)$ is a conventional random walk because the spacings $T_{k+1} - T_k$ are independent, and then the limit process is Brownian motion.

In the nonhomogeneous case, the situation is more complicated as these spacings are not independent. Nevertheless, it was possible to distinguish three modes that determine different types of limiting processes.

For a more precise description of the results, it is convenient to assume that $T_k = f(\Gamma_k)$, where $\mathbf{\Pi} = (\Gamma_k)$ is a standard homogeneous Poisson point process on R_+ with intensity 1. In this case,

$$(\Gamma_k) \overset{\mathcal{L}}{=} (\gamma_1 + \gamma_2 + \cdots + \gamma_k),$$

where (γ_k) are i.i.d standard exponential random variables.

If the function f has power growth,

$$f(t) = t^\alpha, \ \alpha > 1/2,$$

the behavior of the process is analogous to the uniform case and then in the limit we obtain a Gaussian process which is a linearly transformed Brownian motion

$$Y(t) = \int_0^t K_\alpha(s) dW(s),$$

where W is a process of Brownian motion, for which the covariance matrix of $W(1)$ coincides with the covariance matrix of ε_1 and $K_\alpha(s)$ is a nonrandom kernel, and its exact expression is given below.

In the case of exponential growth,

$$f(t) = e^{t\beta}, \ \beta > 0,$$

the limiting process is piecewise linear with an infinite number of units, but $\forall \epsilon > 0$ the number of units in the interval $[\varepsilon, 1]$ will be a.s. finite.

Finally, with the super exponential growth of f, the process degenerates: its trajectories are linear functions:

$$Y(t) = \varepsilon t, \ t \in [0, 1], \ \varepsilon \overset{Law}{=} \varepsilon_1.$$

In the second part of the paper, the process $X(t)$ is assumed to be a Markov chain. We construct diffusion approximations for this process and investigate their accuracy. To prove the weak convergence, we use the approach of [15]. Under our assumptions the diffusion coefficients a and b have the property that for each $x \in R^d$ the martingale problem for a and b has exactly one solution P_x starting from x (that is well posed). It remains to check the conditions from [15] which imply the weak convergence of our sequence of Markov chains to this unique solution P_x. We consider also the more general model which may be called as "random walk over ellipsoids in R^d". For this model, we establish the convergence of the transition densities and obtain the Edgeworth-type expansion up to the order $n^{-3/2}$, where n is a number of switching. The main tool in this part is the parametrix method [5, 7].

2 Random Flights in Poissonian Environment

The reader is reminded that we suppose $T_k = f(\Gamma_k)$, where (Γ_k) is a standard homogeneous Poisson point process on R_+. Assume also that $E\varepsilon_1 = 0$.

It is more convenient to consider at first the behavior of the processes

$$Z_n(t) = Y_{T_n}(t),$$

as for $T = T_n$ the paths of Z_n have an integer number of full segments on the interval $[0,1]$. The typical path of $\{Z_n(t), t \in [0, 1]\}$ is a continuous broken line with vertices $\{(t_{n,k}, \frac{S_k}{B_n}), \ k = 0, 1, \ldots, n\}$, where $t_{n,k} = \frac{T_k}{T_n}, \ T_0 = 0, \ B_n = B(T_n), \ S_k = \sum_1^k \varepsilon_i (T_i - T_{i-1})$.

Theorem 1 *Under the previous assumptions*

(1) If the function f has power growth: $f(t) = t^\alpha$, $\alpha > 1/2$, we take $B(T) = T^{\frac{2\alpha-1}{2\alpha}}$.

Then $Z_n \Longrightarrow Y$, where Y is a Gaussian process

$$Y(t) = \sqrt{2\alpha} \int_0^t s^{\frac{\alpha-1}{2\alpha}} \, dW(s),$$

and W is a process of Brownian motion, for which the covariance matrix of $W(1)$ coincides with the covariance matrix of ε_1.

(2) *If the function f has exponential growth: $f(t) = e^{t\beta}$, $\beta > 0$, we take $B(T) = T$.*

Then $Z_n \Longrightarrow Y$, where Y is a continuous piecewise linear process with the vertices at the points $(t_k, Y(t_k))$,

$$t_k = e^{-\beta \Gamma_{k-1}}, \quad \Gamma_0 = 0,$$

$$Y(t_k) = \sum_{i=k}^{\infty} \varepsilon_k (e^{-\beta \Gamma_{i-1}} - e^{-\beta \Gamma_i}), \quad Y(0) = 0.$$

(3) *In the super exponential case, suppose that f is increasing absolutely continuous and such that*

$$\lim_{t \to \infty} \frac{f'(t)}{f(t)} = +\infty.$$

We take $B(T) = T$.

Then $\frac{T_n}{T_{n+1}} \to 0$ in probability, and $Z_n \Longrightarrow Y$, where the limiting process Y degenerates:

$$Y(t) = \varepsilon_1 t, \quad t \in [0, 1].$$

Remark 1 In the case of power growth, the limiting process admits the following representation:

$$Y(t) \overset{\mathcal{L}}{=} \alpha \sqrt{\frac{2}{2\alpha - 1}} W(t^{\frac{2\alpha-1}{\alpha}}),$$

where, as before, W is a Brownian motion, for which the covariance matrix of $W(1)$ coincides with the covariance matrix of ε_1.

It is clear that we can also express Y in another way:

$$Y(t) \overset{\mathcal{L}}{=} \alpha \sqrt{\frac{2}{2\alpha - 1}} K^{\frac{1}{2}} w(t^{\frac{2\alpha-1}{\alpha}}),$$

where w is a standard Brownian motion and K is the covariance matrix of ε_1.

Remark 2 In the case of exponential growth, it is possible to describe the limiting process Y in the following way:

We take a Poisson point process $\mathbf{T} = (t_k)$, $t_k = e^{-\beta \Gamma_{k-1}}$, defined on $(0, 1]$, and define a step process $\{Z(t), t \in (0, 1]\}$,

$$Z(t) = \varepsilon_k \quad \text{for} \ \ t \in (t_{k+1}, t_k].$$

Then

$$Y(t) = \int_0^t Z(s) \, ds.$$

3 Diffusion Approximation

In this section, first we consider a model of random flight which is equivalent to the study of random broken lines $\{X_n(t), \ t \in [0,1]\}$ with the vertices $(\frac{k}{n}, \ X_n(\frac{k}{n}))$, and such that $(h = \frac{1}{n})$

$$X_n\,((k+1)h) = X_n(kh) + hb(X_n(kh)) + \sqrt{h}\,\xi_k(X(kh)),$$

$$X_n(0) = x_0, \quad \xi_k(X_n(kh)) = \rho_k \sigma(X_n(kh))\varepsilon_k, \tag{1}$$

where $\{\varepsilon_k\}$ and $\{\rho_k\}$ are two independent sequences and
$\{\varepsilon_k\}$ are i.i.d. r. v. uniformly distributed on the unit sphere S^{d-1};
$\{\rho_k\}$ are i.i.d. r. v. having an absolutely continuous distribution, $\rho_k \geq 0$, $E\rho_k^2 = d$;
$b: R^d \longrightarrow R^d$ is a bounded measurable function and $\sigma : R^d \longrightarrow R^d \times R^d$ is a bounded measurable matrix function.

Theorem 2 *Let $X = \{X(t), \ t \in [0,1]\}$ be a solution of stochastic equation*

$$X(t) = x_0 + \int_0^t b(X(s))ds + \int_0^t \sigma(X(s))dw(s).$$

Suppose that b and σ are continuous functions satisfying the Lipschitz condition

$$|b(t) - b(s)| + |\sigma(t) - \sigma(s)| \leq K|t - s|.$$

Moreover, it is supposed that $b(x)$ and $\frac{1}{\det(\sigma(x))}$ are bounded.
    Then,

$$X_n \Longrightarrow X \quad in \quad \mathbb{C}[0,1].$$

Our next result is about the approximation of the transition density. We consider now more general models given by a triplet $(b(x), \sigma(x), f(r; \theta))$, $x \in R^d$, $r \geq 0$, $\theta \in R^+$, where $b(x)$ is a vector field, $\sigma(x)$ is a $d \times d$ matrix, $a(x) := \sigma\sigma^T(x) > \delta I$, $\delta > 0$, and $f(r; \theta)$ is a radial density depending on a parameter θ controlling the frequency of changes of directions, namely, the frequency increases when θ decreases. Suppose $X(0) = x_0$. The vector $b(x_0)$ acts by shifting a particle from x_0 to $x_0 + \Delta(\theta)b(x_0)$, where $\Delta(\theta) = c_d\theta^2$, $c_d > 0$. Several examples of such functions $\Delta(\theta)$ for different models will be given below. Define

$$\mathcal{E}_{x_0}(r) := \{x : \left|a^{-1/2}(x_0)(x - x_0 - \Delta(\theta)b(x_0))\right|^2 = r^2\},$$

$$\mathcal{S}^d_{x_0}(r) := \{y : |y - x_0 - \Delta(\theta)b(x_0)|^2 = r^2\}.$$

The initial direction is defined by a random variable ξ_0, and the law of ξ_0 is a pushforward of the spherical measure on $\mathcal{S}^d_{x_0}(1)$ under affine change of variables

$$x - x_0 - \Delta(\theta)b(x_0) = a^{1/2}(x_0)(y - x_0 - \Delta(\theta)b(x_0)).$$

Then particle moves along the ray l_{x_0} corresponding to the directional unit vector

$$\varepsilon_0 := \frac{\xi_0 - x_0 - \Delta(\theta)b(x_0)}{|\xi_0 - x_0 - \Delta(\theta)b(x_0)|},$$

and changes the direction in $(r, r + dr)$ with probability

$$\det\left(a^{-1/2}(x_0)\right) \cdot f\left(r \left|a^{-1/2}(x_0)e_0\right|\right) dr. \tag{2}$$

Let ρ_0 be a random variable independent of ξ_0 and distributed on l_{x_0} with the radial density (2). We consider the point $x_1 = x_0 + \Delta(\theta)b(x_0) + \rho_0\varepsilon_0$. Let (ε_k, ρ_k) be independent copies of (ε_0, ρ_0). Starting from x_1, we repeat the previous construction to obtain $x_2 = x_1 + \Delta(\theta)b(x_1) + \rho_1\varepsilon_1$. After n switches, we arrive at the point x_n,

$$x_n = x_{n-1} + \Delta(\theta)b(x_{n-1}) + \rho_{n-1}\varepsilon_{n-1}.$$

To obtain the one-step characteristic function $\Psi_1(t)$, we make use of formula (6) from [17] (see also the proof of Theorem 2.1 in [10]):

$$\Psi_1(t) = E e^{i\langle t, \rho_0\varepsilon_0\rangle} = \int_0^\infty \int_{\mathcal{E}_{x_0}(r)} e^{i\langle t, a^{1/2}(x_0)a^{-1/2}(x_0)\xi\rangle} \mu_{\mathcal{E}_{x_0}(r)}(d\xi) d\Phi_{\mathcal{E}}(r) =$$

$$= \int_0^\infty \int_{\mathcal{S}^d_{x_0}(r)} e^{i\langle a^{1/2}(x_0)t, y\rangle} \lambda_r^d(dy) f(r; \theta) dr =$$

$$= 2^{\frac{d-2}{2}} \Gamma\left(\frac{d}{2}\right) \int_0^\infty \frac{J_{\frac{d-2}{2}}\left(r \left|a^{1/2}(x_0)t\right|\right)}{\left(r \left|a^{1/2}(x_0)t\right|\right)^{\frac{d-2}{2}}} f(r; \theta) dr, \tag{3}$$

where $J_\nu(z)$ is the Bessel function, $d\Phi_{\mathcal{E}}(r)$ is the F-measure of the layer between $\mathcal{E}_{x_0}(r)$ and $\mathcal{E}_{x_0}(r+dr)$, and F is the law of $\rho_0\varepsilon_0$. Now we make our main assumption about the radial density:

(A1) The function $f(r; \theta)$ is homogeneous of degree -1, that is

$$f(\lambda r; \lambda\theta) = \lambda^{-1} f(r; \theta), \quad \forall\lambda \neq 0.$$

Denote by $p_{\mathcal{E}}(n, x, y)$ the transition density after n switches in the RF model described above. To obtain the one-step transition density $p_{\mathcal{E}}(1, x, y)$ (we write (x, y) instead of (x_0, x_1)), we use the inverse Fourier transform, (3) and **(A1)**. We have

$$p_{\mathcal{E}}(1, x, y) = \Delta^{-d/2}(\theta) q_x \left(\frac{y - x - \Delta(\theta) b(x)}{\sqrt{\Delta(\theta)}} \right), \tag{4}$$

where

$$q_x(z) = \frac{2^{\frac{d-2}{2}} \Gamma\left(\frac{d}{2}\right)}{(2\pi)^d} \int_{R^d} \cos \langle \tau, z \rangle \left[\int_0^\infty \frac{J_{\frac{d-2}{2}}\left(\rho \left|a^{1/2}(x)\tau\right|\right)}{\left(\rho \left|a^{1/2}(x)\tau\right|\right)^{\frac{d-2}{2}}} f(\rho; c_d) d\rho \right] d\tau. \tag{5}$$

Consider two examples.

Example 1 We put $\Delta(\theta) = (d + 1)^2 \theta^2$ and

$$f(r; \theta) = \frac{1}{\Gamma(d)} r^{-1} \left(\frac{r}{\theta}\right)^d \exp\left(-\frac{r}{\theta}\right).$$

Using (3), formula 6.623 (2) on p. 694 from [3], and the doubling formula for the Gamma function, we obtain

$$p_{\mathcal{E}}(1, x, y) = \Delta^{-d/2}(\theta) q_x \left(\frac{y - x - \Delta(\theta) b(x)}{\sqrt{\Delta(\theta)}} \right),$$

where

$$q_x(z) = \frac{(d + 1)^{d/2}}{2^d \pi^{(d-1)/2} \Gamma\left(\frac{d+1}{2}\right) \left|\det a^{1/2}(x)\right|} e^{-\sqrt{d+1}\left|a^{-1/2}(x)z\right|}.$$

It is easy to check that

$$\int z_i q_x(z) = 0, \quad \int z_i z_j q_x(z) dz = a_{ij}(x).$$

Example 2 We put $\Delta(\theta) = \theta^2/2$ and

$$f(r; \theta) = C_d r^{-1} \left(\frac{r}{\theta}\right)^d \exp\left(-\frac{r^2}{\theta^2}\right),$$

where $C_d = \frac{2^{(d+1)/2}}{(d-2)!!\sqrt{\pi}}$ if d is odd, and $C_d = \frac{2}{[(d-2)/2]!}$ if d is even. From (3) and formula 6.631 (4) on p. 698 of [3], we obtain

$$p_{\mathcal{E}}(1, x, y) = \Delta^{-d/2}(\theta) \phi_x \left(\frac{y - x - \Delta(\theta) b(x)}{\sqrt{\Delta(\theta)}} \right),$$

where

$$\phi_x(z) = \frac{1}{(2\pi)^{d/2}\sqrt{\det a(x)}}\exp\left(-\frac{1}{2}\langle a^{-1}(x)z,z\rangle\right).$$

It is easy to see that the transition density (4) corresponds to the one-step transition density in the following Markov chain model:

$$X_{(k+1)\Delta(\theta)} = X_{k\Delta(\theta)} + \Delta(\theta)\,b(X_{k\Delta(\theta)}) + \sqrt{\Delta(\theta)}\xi_{(k+1)\Delta(\theta)},$$

where the conditional density (under $X_{k\Delta(\theta)} = x$) of the innovations $\xi_{(k+1)\Delta(\theta)}$ is equal to $q_x(\cdot)$. If we put $\theta = \theta_n = \sqrt{\frac{2}{n}}$, then $\Delta(\theta_n) = \frac{1}{n}$ and we obtain a sequence of Markov chains defined on an equidistant grid

$$X_{\frac{k+1}{n}} = X_{\frac{k}{n}} + \frac{1}{n}b(X_{\frac{k}{n}}) + \frac{1}{\sqrt{n}}\xi_{\frac{k+1}{n}}, \quad X_0 = x_0. \tag{6}$$

Note that the triplet $(b(x), \sigma(x), f(r;\theta))$, $x \in R^d$, $r \geq 0$, $\theta \in R^+$, of Example 2 corresponds to the classical Euler scheme for the d-dimensional SDE

$$dX(t) = b(X_t)dt + \sigma(X_t)dW(t), \quad X(0) = x_0. \tag{7}$$

Let $p(1, x, y)$ be transition density from 0 to 1 in the model (7). We make the following assumptions.

(A2) The function $a(x) = \sigma\sigma^T(x)$ is uniformly elliptic.

(A3) The functions $b(x)$ and $\sigma(x)$ and their derivatives up to the sixth order are continuous and bounded uniformly in x. The sixth derivative is globally Lipschitz.

Theorem 3 *Under the assumptions (A2) and (A3,) we have the following expansion: for any positive integer S as $n \to \infty$*

$$\sup_{x,y\in R^d}\left(1+|y-x|^S\right)\cdot\left|p_\varepsilon(n,x,y) - p(1,x,y) - \frac{1}{2n}p\otimes\left(L_*^2 - L^2\right)p(1,x,y)\right| = O(n^{-3/2}),$$
$$\tag{8}$$

where

$$L = \frac{1}{2}\sum_{i,j=1}^d a_{ij}(x)\partial^2_{x_ix_j} + \sum_{i=1}^d b_i(x)\partial_{x_i}. \tag{9}$$

The operator L_* in (8) is the same operator as in (9) but with coefficients "frozen" at x. It means that when calculating degrees of the operator we do not differentiate coefficients and we consider them as constants, taking them out of the derivative.

Clearly, $L = L_*$ but, in general, $L^2 \neq L_*^2$. The convolution-type binary operation $\otimes$ is defined for functions f and g in the following way:

$$(f \otimes g)(t,x,y) = \int_0^t ds \int_{R^d} f(s,x,z)g(t-s,z,y)dz.$$

Proof It follows immediately from Theorem 1 of [7].

4 Proof of Theorem 1

4.1 Asymptotic Behavior in Case (3)

We have, by taking $B_n = B(T_n) = T_n$:

$$\sup_{t \in \left[0, \frac{T_{n-1}}{T_n}\right]} \|X_n(t)\|_\infty \leq \sum_{k=1}^{n-1} \frac{T_k - T_{k-1}}{T_n} = \frac{T_{n-1}}{T_n} \xrightarrow[n \to \infty]{} 0 \text{ a.s.}$$

At the same time,

$$X_n(1) = \frac{S_{n-1} + \varepsilon_n(T_n - T_{n-1})}{T_n} = \varepsilon_n + o(1) \Rightarrow \mathcal{P}_{\varepsilon_1}$$

Therefore, the process X_n converges weakly to the process $\{Y(t)\}$, $Y(t) = \varepsilon_1 t$, $t \in [0, 1]$.

This process is in some sense degenerate. Hence, this case is not very interesting.

4.2 Asymptotic Behavior in Case (2)

Take $B_n = T_n$ and show that the limit process Y is not trivial. For simplicity fix $\beta = 1$. We have now $t_{n,k} := \frac{T_k}{T_n} = e^{-(\Gamma_n - \Gamma_k)} = e^{-(\gamma_{k+1} + \cdots + \gamma_n)}$, and

$$X_n\left(t_{n,k}\right) = \sum_{i=1}^{k} \varepsilon_i (e^{-(\gamma_{i+1} + \cdots + \gamma_n)} - e^{-(\gamma_i + \cdots + \gamma_n)}), \quad k = 1, \ldots, n.$$

The process X_n is completely defined by two independent vectors $(\varepsilon_1, \ldots, \varepsilon_n)$ and $(\gamma_1, \ldots, \gamma_n)$. Hence, its distribution will be the same if we replace these vectors by $(\varepsilon_n, \ldots, \varepsilon_1)$ and $(\gamma_n, \ldots, \gamma_1)$. In another words, the process $(X_n(\cdot)) \overset{\mathcal{L}}{=} (Y_n(\cdot))$, where $Y_n(\cdot)$ is a broken line with vertices $(\tau_{n,k}, Y_n(\tau_{n,k}))$, $(\tau_{n,k}) \downarrow$, $\tau_{n,1} = 1$, $\tau_{n,k} = e^{-(\gamma_1 + \cdots + \gamma_{k-1})}$, $k = 2, \ldots, n$, and

$$Y_n(\tau_{n,k}) = \sum_{i=k}^{n-1} \varepsilon_i \left(e^{-(\gamma_1 + \cdots + \gamma_{i-1})} - e^{-(\gamma_1 + \cdots + \gamma_i)}\right) + \varepsilon_n e^{-(\gamma_1 + \cdots + \gamma_{n-1})};$$

$Y_n(0) = 0$, and $\gamma_0 := 0$.

Using the notation $\Gamma_k = \gamma_1 + \cdots + \gamma_k$, we get the more compact formula:

$$Y_n(\tau_{n,k}) = \sum_{i=k}^{n-1} \varepsilon_i \left(e^{-\Gamma_{i-1}} - e^{-\Gamma_i} \right) + \varepsilon_n e^{-\Gamma_{n-1}}.$$

Consider now the process $\{Y(t), t \in [0, 1]\}$ defined as follows:

$$Y(0) = 0, \quad Y(t_k) = \sum_{i=k}^{\infty} \varepsilon_i \left(e^{-\Gamma_{i-1}} - e^{-\Gamma_i} \right), \tag{10}$$

where $t_k = e^{-\Gamma_{k-1}}$, $k = 2, 3, \ldots, t_1 = 1$; for $t \in [t_{k+1}, t_k]$, $Y(t)$ is defined by linear interpolation. The paths of Y are continuous broken lines, starting at 0 and having an infinite number of segments in the neighborhood of zero.

The evident estimation

$$\sup_{t \in [0,1]} |Y(t) - Y_n(t)| \le \left| \sum_{i=n}^{\infty} \varepsilon_i \left(e^{-\Gamma_{i-1}} - e^{-\Gamma_i} \right) \right| + e^{-\Gamma_{n-1}} \le$$

$$\le \sum_{i=n}^{\infty} \left(e^{-\Gamma_{i-1}} - e^{-\Gamma_i} \right) + e^{-\Gamma_{n-1}} = 2e^{-\Gamma_{n-1}} \longrightarrow 0 \quad \text{a.s.}$$

shows that a.s. $Y_n(\cdot) \xrightarrow{\mathbb{C}[0,1]} Y(\cdot)$.

Conclusion: In case (2), the process X_n converges weakly to $Y(\cdot)$.

Remark 3 In the case where $\beta \ne 1$, it is simply necessary to replace $e^{-\Gamma_k}$ by $e^{-\frac{\Gamma_k}{\beta}}$.

Remark 4 It seems that the last result could be expanded by considering more general sequences (ε_k).

Interpretation: $\frac{\varepsilon_k}{|\varepsilon_k|}$ defines the direction and $|\varepsilon_k|$ defines the velocity of displacement in this direction on the step S_k.

4.3 Asymptotic Behavior in Case of Power Growth

In this case, $T_k = \Gamma_k^\alpha$, $\alpha > 1/2$, $t_{n,k} = \frac{T_k}{T_n} = \left(\frac{\Gamma_k}{\Gamma_n} \right)^\alpha$, and

$$X_n(t_{n,k}) = \frac{1}{B_n} \sum_{i=1}^{k} \varepsilon_i (\Gamma_i^\alpha - \Gamma_{i-1}^\alpha); \quad \Gamma_0 = 0, \ k = 0, 1, \ldots, n. \tag{11}$$

Let $x \in \mathbb{R}^d$ be such that $|x| = 1$. We will show below that

$$\mathrm{Var}\left(\sum_{i=1}^{n} \langle \varepsilon_i, x \rangle (\Gamma_i^\alpha - \Gamma_{i-1}^\alpha) \right) = E\langle \varepsilon_i, x \rangle^2 \sum_{i=1}^{n} E(\Gamma_i^\alpha - \Gamma_{i-1}^\alpha)^2 \sim C(x) n^{2\alpha-1}, \ n \to \infty,$$

where $C(x) = \frac{2\alpha^2}{2\alpha-1} E\langle \varepsilon_1, x \rangle^2$. Therefore it is natural to take $B_n^2 = n^{2\alpha-1}$.

We proceed in five steps:

Step 1: Lemmas

Step 2: We compare $X_n(\cdot)$ with $Z_n(\cdot)$ where $Z_n(t_{n,k}) = \frac{\alpha}{B_n} \sum_{i=1}^{k} \varepsilon_i \gamma_i \Gamma_{i-1}^{\alpha-1}$ and show that $\|X_n - Z_n\|_\infty \xrightarrow{\mathbb{P}} 0$.

Step 3: We compare $Z_n(\cdot)$ with $W_n(\cdot)$ where $W_n(t_{n,k}) = \frac{\alpha}{B_n} \sum_{i=1}^{k} \varepsilon_i \gamma_i (i-1)^{\alpha-1}$ and state that $\|Z_n - W_n\|_\infty \xrightarrow{\mathbb{P}} 0$.

Step 4: We show that process $U_n(\cdot)$,

$$U_n\left(\left(\frac{k}{n}\right)^\alpha\right) = \frac{\alpha}{B_n} \sum_{i=1}^{k} \varepsilon_i \gamma_i (i-1)^{\alpha-1},$$

converges weakly to the limiting process

$$Y(t) = \sqrt{2\alpha} \int_0^t s^{\frac{\alpha-1}{2\alpha}} \, dW(s);$$

here $W(\cdot)$ is a process of Brownian motion, for which the covariance matrix of $W(1)$ coincides with the covariance matrix of ε_1.

Step 5: We show that the convergence $W_n \Rightarrow Y$ follows from the convergence $U_n \Rightarrow Y$.

Finally: We get the convergence $X_n \Rightarrow Y$.

4.3.1   Step 1

This section contains several technical lemmas necessary for realization of subsequent steps.

Lemma 1 *Let $\alpha > 0$ and $m \geq 1$. Then $\forall x > 0,\ h > 0$*

$$(x+h)^\alpha - x^\alpha = \sum_{k=1}^{m} a_k h^k x^{\alpha-k} + R(x,h), \tag{12}$$

where

$$a_k = \frac{\alpha(\alpha-1)\dots(\alpha-k+1)}{k!},$$

and

$$|R(x,h)| \leq |a_{m+1}| h^{m+1} \max\{x^{\alpha-(m+1)}, (x+h)^{\alpha-(m+1)}\}. \tag{13}$$

Proof By the formula of Taylor–Lagrange, we have (12) with

$$|R(x, y)| \leq \frac{1}{(m+1)!} h^{m+1} \sup_{x \leq t \leq x+h} |f^{(m+1)}(t)|,$$

where $f(t) = t^\alpha$. As $f^{(m+1)}(t) = \alpha(\alpha - 1) \ldots (\alpha - m)t^{\alpha-(m+1)}$, we get the claimed result. □

Lemma 2 *For $\alpha \geq 0$ and $k \to \infty$*

$$\left(1 + \frac{\alpha}{k}\right)^k = e^\alpha + O\left(\frac{1}{k}\right). \tag{14}$$

Proof It follows from the inequalities:

$$0 \leq e^\alpha - \left(1 + \frac{\alpha}{k}\right)^k \leq \frac{e^\alpha \alpha^2}{k}. \qquad \qquad □$$

Lemma 3 *Let Γ be the Gamma function. Then as $k \to \infty$*

$$\frac{\Gamma(k + \alpha)}{\Gamma(k)} = k^\alpha + O(k^{\alpha-1}).$$

Proof It follows from Lemma 2 and well-known asymptotic (see a.e. [16], v. 2, 12.33)

$$\Gamma(t) = t^{t-\frac{1}{2}} e^{-t} \sqrt{2\pi} \left(1 + \frac{1}{12t} + O\left(\frac{1}{t^2}\right)\right), \quad t \to \infty.$$

Lemma 4 *For any real β, we have as $k \to \infty$*

$$E(\Gamma_k^\beta) = k^\beta + O(k^{\beta-1}).$$

Proof The result follows from the well-known fact that

$$E(\Gamma_k^\beta) = \frac{\Gamma(k + \beta)}{\Gamma(k)}$$

and Lemma 3.

Lemma 5 *Let $\alpha \geq 0$. The following relations take place as $k \to \infty$:*

$$\Gamma_{k+1}^\alpha - \Gamma_k^\alpha = \alpha \gamma_{k+1} \Gamma_k^{\alpha-1} + \rho_k, \tag{15}$$

where $|\rho_k| = O(k^{\alpha-2})$ in probability;

$$E|\Gamma_{k+1}^\alpha - \Gamma_k^\alpha|^2 = 2\alpha^2 k^{2\alpha-2} + O(k^{2\alpha-3}); \tag{16}$$

$$E|\Gamma_{k+1}^\alpha - \Gamma_k^\alpha - \alpha \gamma_{k+1} \Gamma_k^{\alpha-1}|^2 = O(k^{2\alpha-4}). \tag{17}$$

Proof of Lemma 5 We find, by applying Lemma 1,

$$\Gamma_{k+1}^\alpha - \Gamma_k^\alpha = \alpha \gamma_{k+1} \Gamma_k^{\alpha-1} + R(\Gamma_k, \gamma_{k+1}), \tag{18}$$

where

$$R(\Gamma_k, \gamma_{k+1}) \le \frac{1}{2}\gamma_{k+1}^2 \max_{\Gamma_k \le s \le \Gamma_{k+1}} |\alpha(\alpha-1)|s^{\alpha-2} \le \frac{|\alpha(\alpha-1)|}{2}\gamma_{k+1}^2 \max\{\Gamma_{k+1}^{\alpha-2}, \Gamma_k^{\alpha-2}\}. \tag{19}$$

As $\Gamma_k \sim k$ a.s. when $k \to \infty$, we get (15).
The proofs of (16) and (17) follow directly from (18), (19) and Lemma 4. $\quad\square$

We deduce immediately from (16) the following relation.

Corollary 1 *We have*

$$\sum_1^{n-1} E|\Gamma_{k+1}^\alpha - \Gamma_k^\alpha|^2 = \frac{2\alpha^2}{2\alpha-1}n^{2\alpha-1} + O(n^{2\alpha-2}).$$

4.3.2 Step 2

We show that $\|X_n - Z_n\|_\infty \xrightarrow{\mathbb{P}} 0$, where

$$Z_n(t_{n,k}) = \frac{\alpha}{B_n} \sum_{i=1}^k \varepsilon_i \gamma_i \Gamma_{i-1}^{\alpha-1}.$$

It is clear that

$$\delta_n := \|X_n - Z_n\|_\infty = \sup_{t\in[0,1]} |X_n(t) - Z_n(t)| = \max_{k\le n} |X(t_{n,k}) - Z_n(t_{n,k})| = \max_{k\le n} |r_k|,$$

where

$$r_k = \frac{1}{B_n} \sum_{i=1}^k \varepsilon_i \left[\Gamma_i^\alpha - \Gamma_{i-1}^\alpha - \alpha\gamma_i \Gamma_{i-1}^{\alpha-1}\right] = \sum_{i=1}^k \varepsilon_i \xi_i,$$

and

$$\xi_i = \left(\Gamma_i^\alpha - \Gamma_{i-1}^\alpha - \alpha\gamma_i \Gamma_{i-1}^{\alpha-1}\right) \frac{1}{B_n}.$$

Let $\mathfrak{M} = \sigma(\xi_1, \xi_2, \ldots, \xi_n) = \sigma(\gamma_1, \gamma_2, \ldots, \gamma_n)$. Under condition $\mathfrak{M}$, the sequence (r_k) is the sequence of sums of independent random variables with mean zero. By Kolmogorov's inequality,

$$\mathbb{P}\{\max_{k\leq n}|r_k|\geq t\} = \mathrm{E}\{\mathbb{P}\{\max_{k\leq n}|r_k|\geq t\mid \mathfrak{M}\}\} \leq \mathrm{E}\left(\frac{1}{t^2}\sum_{j=1}^n \xi_j^2\right) = \frac{1}{t^2}\sum_{j=1}^n \mathrm{E}\xi_j^2.$$

(20)

By Lemma 5, $\mathrm{E}\xi_j^2 = O(j^{-3})$. Therefore,

$$\sum_{j=1}^n \mathrm{E}\xi_j^2 = O(n^{-2}).$$

Finally, we get from (20): $\forall t > 0$

$$\mathbb{P}\{\delta_n \geq t\} \xrightarrow[n\to\infty]{} 0,$$

which gives the convergence $\|X_n - Z_n\|_\infty \xrightarrow{\mathbb{P}} 0$.

4.3.3   Step 3

We show now that $\|Z_n - W_n\|_\infty \xrightarrow[n\to\infty]{\mathbb{P}} 0$; where $W_n(t_{n,k}) = \frac{\alpha}{B_n}\sum_{i=1}^k \varepsilon_i\gamma_i(i-1)^{\alpha-1}$.
We have

$$\Delta_n = \sup_{t\in[0,1]}|Z_n(t) - W_n(t)| = \max_{k\leq n}|Z_n(t_{n,k}) - W_n(t_{n,k})| = \max_{k\leq n}\{|\beta_k|\},$$

where $\beta_k = \frac{\alpha}{B_n}\sum_{i=1}^k \varepsilon_i\gamma_i\left(\Gamma_{i-1}^{\alpha-1} - (i-1)^{\alpha-1}\right)$.

Similar to the previous case, (β_k) under condition $\mathfrak{M}$ is the sequence of sums of independent random variables with mean zero. Therefore,

$$\mathbb{P}\{\max_{k\leq n}\{|\beta_k|\}\geq t\} = \mathrm{E}\left(\mathbb{P}\{\max_{k\leq n}\{|\beta_k|\}\geq t\mid \mathfrak{M}\}\right) \leq \frac{1}{t^2}\sum_{j=1}^n \mathrm{E}\eta_j^2,$$

where $\eta_j = \frac{\alpha}{B_n}\gamma_j\left(\Gamma_{j-1}^{\alpha-1} - (j-1)^{\alpha-1}\right)$.

Estimation of $\mathrm{E}\eta_j^2$.

By independence of γ_j and Γ_{j-1}

$$\mathrm{E}\eta_j^2 = \frac{2\alpha^2}{B_n^2}\mathrm{E}\left(\Gamma_{j-1}^{\alpha-1} - (j-1)^{\alpha-1}\right)^2.$$

Let us change $j-1$ to k

$$
\mathrm{E}\left(\Gamma_k^{\alpha-1} - k^{\alpha-1}\right)^2 = \mathrm{E}\left(\Gamma_k^{2\alpha-2}\right) + k^{2\alpha-2} - 2k^{\alpha-1}\mathrm{E}\left(\Gamma_k^{\alpha-1}\right) =
$$

$$
= \frac{\Gamma(k+2\alpha-2)}{\Gamma(k)} + k^{2\alpha-2} - 2k^{\alpha-1}\frac{\Gamma(k+\alpha-1)}{\Gamma(k)} = (\text{by Lemma 3}) =
$$

$$
= \left[k^{2\alpha-2} + O(k^{2\alpha-3}) + k^{2\alpha-2} - 2k^{2\alpha-2}\right] = O(k^{2\alpha-3}).
$$

Hence,

$$
\mathrm{E}\eta_j^2 \le C\frac{j^{2\alpha-3}}{n^{2\alpha-1}}.
$$

It follows from this estimation that
  for $\alpha > 1$

$$
\sum_{j=1}^{n} \mathrm{E}\eta_j^2 \le \frac{C}{n};
$$

for $\alpha = 1$

$$
\sum_{j=1}^{n} \mathrm{E}\eta_j^2 \le \frac{\log n}{n};
$$

and for $1/2 < \alpha < 1$

$$
\sum_{j=1}^{n} \mathrm{E}\eta_j^2 \le \frac{C}{n^{2\alpha-1}}.
$$

We have finally $\mathbb{P}\{\max_{k\le n}|\beta_k| \ge t\} \to 0,\ n \to \infty$, which gives the convergence
$\|W_n - Z_n\| \xrightarrow{\mathbb{P}} 0$.

4.3.4 Step 4

Let U_n be the process defined at the points $\frac{k}{n}$ by

$$
U_n\left(\left(\frac{k}{n}\right)^\alpha\right) = \frac{\alpha}{B_n}\sum_{i=1}^{k} \varepsilon_i \gamma_i (i-1)^{\alpha-1}, \quad k = 1, 2, \ldots, n,
$$

and by linear interpolation on the intervals $[\frac{k}{n}, \frac{k+1}{n}]$, $k = 0, \ldots, n-1$. We now state
the weak convergence of the processes U_n to the process Y,

$$
Y(t) = \sqrt{2\alpha}\int_0^t s^{\frac{\alpha-1}{2\alpha}}\,\mathrm{d}W(s),
$$

W is a Brownian motion, for which the covariance matrix of $W(1)$ coincides with
the covariance matrix of ε_1.

The proof is standard because $U_n(\cdot)$ represents a (more or less) usual broken line constructed by the consecutive sums of independent (nonidentically distributed) random variables. One could apply Prokhorov's theorem (see [2], Chap. IX, Sect. 3, Theorem 1).

Only one thing must be checked: the Lindeberg condition.

Let $\varepsilon > 0$. We have

$$\Lambda_n(\varepsilon) := \frac{1}{B_n^2} \sum_1^n E\left\{\|\varepsilon_i \gamma_i (i-1)^{\alpha-1}\|^2 \mathbf{1}_{\{\|\varepsilon_i \gamma_i (i-1)^{\alpha-1}\| \geq \varepsilon B_n\}}\right\} =$$

$$= \frac{1}{n^{2\alpha-1}} \sum_2^n (i-1)^{2\alpha-2} E\left\{\gamma_1^2 \mathbf{1}_{\{|\gamma_1|(i-1)^{\alpha-1}\| \geq \varepsilon n^{\alpha-1/2}\}}\right\}.$$

As

$$\{|\gamma_1|(i-1)^{\alpha-1}\| \geq \varepsilon n^{\alpha-1/2}\} \subset \{|\gamma_1| \geq \varepsilon\sqrt{n}\}$$

for $2 \leq i \leq n$, we get

$$\Lambda_n(\varepsilon) \leq \frac{1}{2\alpha-1} E\gamma_1^2 \mathbf{1}_{\{|\gamma_1| \geq \varepsilon\sqrt{n}\}} \to 0,$$

as $n \to \infty$.

It means that the Lindeberg condition is fulfilled, and by the above-mentioned Prokhorov's theorem the process U_n is weakly converging. To identify the limiting process with Y, it is sufficient to state that for any $0 < s < t \leq 1$, and for any $x \in \mathbb{R}^d$, $|x| = 1$, we have the convergence $\langle U_n(t) - U_n(s), x \rangle \Longrightarrow \langle Y(t) - Y(s), x \rangle$.

It is clear that

$$[U_n(t) - U_n(s)] - \left[U_n\left(\left(\frac{k}{n}\right)^\alpha\right) - U_n\left(\left(\frac{l}{n}\right)^\alpha\right)\right] \xrightarrow{P} 0,$$

if $\left(\frac{k}{n}\right)^\alpha \to t$, $\left(\frac{l}{n}\right)^\alpha \to s$.

Let $l < k$. As

$$\left\langle U_n\left(\left(\frac{k}{n}\right)^\alpha\right) - U_n\left(\left(\frac{l}{n}\right)^\alpha\right), x \right\rangle = \frac{\alpha}{B_n} \sum_{i=l+1}^k \langle \varepsilon_i, x \rangle \gamma_i (i-1)^{\alpha-1},$$

by the theorem of Lindeberg–Feller, it is sufficient to state the convergence of variances.

We have

$$\mathrm{Var}\left\langle U_n\left(\left(\frac{k}{n}\right)^\alpha\right) - U_n\left(\left(\frac{l}{n}\right)^\alpha\right), x \right\rangle =$$

$$= \frac{2\alpha^2}{n^{2\alpha-1}} E \langle \varepsilon_1, x \rangle^2 \sum_{i=l+1}^{k} (i-1)^{2\alpha-2} \xrightarrow[n \to \infty]{} \frac{2\alpha^2}{2\alpha-1} E \langle \varepsilon_1, x \rangle^2 [t^{\frac{2\alpha-1}{\alpha}} - s^{\frac{2\alpha-1}{\alpha}}],$$

and

$$\mathrm{Var} \langle Y(t) - Y(s), x \rangle = 2\alpha E \langle \varepsilon_1, x \rangle^2 \int_s^t u^{\frac{\alpha-1}{\alpha}} \, du = \frac{2\alpha^2}{2\alpha-1} E \langle \varepsilon_1, x \rangle^2 [t^{\frac{2\alpha-1}{\alpha}} - s^{\frac{2\alpha-1}{\alpha}}],$$

which are the same. Therefore, indeed $U_n \Rightarrow Y$.

4.3.5 Step 5: Convergence $X_n \Rightarrow Y$.

Due to the steps 2 and 3, it is sufficient to show that $W_n \Rightarrow Y$.

Let $f_n : [0, 1] \to [0, 1]$, be a piecewise linear continuous function such that $f_n(t_{n,k}) = \left(\frac{k}{n}\right)^\alpha; t_{n,k} = \left(\frac{\Gamma_k}{\Gamma_n}\right)^\alpha; k = 0, 1, \dots, n$.

By definition of W_n and U_n, we have

$$W_n(t) = U_n(f_n(t)), \ t \in [0, 1].$$

By the corollary to Lemma 6 (see below), the function f_n converges in probability uniformly to f, $f(t) = t$, and by previous step $U_n \Rightarrow Y$.

It means that we can apply Lemma 7 which gives the necessary convergence.

Lemma 6 *Let*

$$M_n = \max_{k \le n} \left\{ \left| \frac{\Gamma_k}{\Gamma_n} - \frac{k}{n} \right| \right\}.$$

Then $M_n \xrightarrow{\mathrm{P}} 0, \ n \to \infty$.

Proof of Lemma 6 We have

$$\mathbb{P}\{M_n > \varepsilon\} = \mathrm{E} \left\{ \mathbb{P} \left\{ \max_{k \le n} \left| \frac{\Gamma_k}{\Gamma_n} - \frac{k}{n} \right| > \varepsilon \mid \Gamma_n \right\} \right\} =$$

$$= \int_0^\infty \mathbb{P} \left\{ \max_{k \le n} \left| \frac{\Gamma_k}{\Gamma_n} - \frac{k}{n} \right| > \varepsilon \mid \Gamma_n = t \right\} \mathcal{P}_{\Gamma_n}(dt) = \tag{21}$$

$$= \int_0^\infty \mathbb{P} \left\{ \max_{k \le n} \left| \xi_{n,k} - \frac{k}{n} \right| > \varepsilon \right\} \mathcal{P}_{\Gamma_n}(dt) = \mathbb{P} \left\{ \max_{k \le n} \left| \xi_{n,k} - \frac{k}{n} \right| > \varepsilon \right\},$$

where $(\xi_{n,k})_{k=1,\dots,n}$ are the order statistics from $[0, 1]$-uniform distribution.

Let $\delta_n := \max_{k \le n} |\xi_{n,k} - \frac{k}{n}|$. Evidently, $\delta_n \le \sup_{[0,1]} |F_n^*(x) - x|$, where F_n^* is the uniform empirical distribution function. By Glivenko–Cantelli theorem, $\sup_{[0,1]} |F_n^*(x) - x| \to 0$ a.s, which gives the convergence $M_n \to 0$ in probability. $\qquad\square$

Corollary 2 $M_n^{(1)} = \max_{k \leq n} \left| \left(\frac{\Gamma_k}{\Gamma_n} \right)^{\alpha} - \left(\frac{k}{n} \right)^{\alpha} \right| \xrightarrow{\mathbb{P}} 0, \ n \to \infty.$

The proof follows directly from Lemma 6 due to the uniform continuity of the function $h(x) = x^{\alpha}, \ x \in [0, 1].$

Lemma 7 *Let $\{U_n\}$ be a sequence of continuous processes on $[0, 1]$ weakly convergent to some limit process U. Let $\{f_n\}$ be a sequence of random continuous bijections $[0, 1]$ on $[0, 1]$ which in probability uniformly converges to the identity function $f(t) \equiv t$. Then the process W_n, $W_n(t) = U_n(f_n(t))$, $t \in [0, 1]$, will converge weakly to U.*

Proof of Lemma 7 By theorem 4.4 from [1], we have the weak convergence in $\mathbb{M} := \mathbb{C}[0, 1] \times \mathbb{C}[0, 1]$

$$(U_n, f_n) \Longrightarrow (U, f).$$

By Skorohod representation theorem, we can find random elements $(\tilde{U}_n, \tilde{f}_n)$ and $(\tilde{U}, \tilde{f})$ of $\mathbb{M}$ (defined probably on a new probability space) such that

$$(U_n, f_n) \overset{\mathcal{L}}{=} (\tilde{U}_n, \tilde{f}_n), \quad (U, f) \overset{\mathcal{L}}{=} (\tilde{U}, \tilde{f}),$$

and $(\tilde{U}_n, \tilde{f}_n) \to (\tilde{U}, \tilde{f})$ a.s. in $\mathbb{M}$.

As the last convergence implies evidently the a.s. uniform convergence of $\tilde{U}_n(\tilde{f}_n(t))$ to $\tilde{U}(\tilde{f}(t))$, we get the convergence in distribution of $U(f_n(\cdot))$ to $U(f(\cdot)) = U(\cdot)$. $\qquad \qquad \square$

5 Proof of Theorem 2

Proof of Theorem 2. We need some facts from [15]. Consider $(\Omega, \mathcal{M})$, where $\Omega = \mathbb{C}([0, \infty); R^d)$ be the space of continuous trajectories from $[0, \infty)$ into R^d. Given $t \geq 0$ and $\omega \in \Omega$ let $x(t, \omega)$ denote the position of ω in R^d at time t. If we put

$$D(\omega, \omega') = \sum_{n=1}^{\infty} \frac{1}{2^n} \frac{\sup_{0 \leq t \leq n} \left| x(t, \omega) - x(t, \omega') \right|}{1 + \sup_{0 \leq t \leq n} \left| x(t, \omega) - x(t, \omega') \right|}$$

then it is well known that D is a metric on Ω and (Ω, D) is a Polish space. The convergence induced by D is the uniform convergence on bounded t-intervals. For simplicity, we will omit ω in the future and we will be assuming that all our processes are homogeneous in time. Analogous results for time-inhomogeneous processes may be obtained by simply considering the time-space processes.

We will use $\mathcal{M}$ to denote the Borel σ-field of subsets of (Ω, D), $\mathcal{M} = \sigma[x(t) : t \geq 0]$. We also will consider an increasing family of σ-algebras $\mathcal{M}_t = \sigma[x(s) : 0 \leq s \leq t]$. The classical approach to the construction of diffusion processes corresponding to given coefficients a and b involves a transition probability function

$P(s, x; t, \cdot)$ which allows to construct for each $x \in R^d$, a probability measure P_x on $\Omega = \mathbb{C}([0, \infty); R^d)$ with the properties that

$$P_x(x(0) = x) = 1$$

and

$$P_x(x(t_2) \in \Gamma \,|\mathcal{M}_{t_1}) = P(t_1, x(t_1); t_2, \Gamma) \, a.s. \, P_x$$

for all $0 \le t_1 < t_2$ and $\Gamma \in \mathcal{B}_{R^d}$ (the Borel σ-algebra in R^d). It appears that this measure is a martingale measure for a special martingale related with the second-order differential operator

$$L = \frac{1}{2} \sum_{i,j=1}^{d} a^{ij}(\cdot) \frac{\partial^2}{\partial x_i \partial x_j} + \sum_{i=1}^{d} b^i(\cdot) \frac{\partial}{\partial x_i},$$

namely, for all $f \in \mathbb{C}_0^\infty(R^d)$

$$P_x(x(0) = x) = 1,$$

$$\left(f(x(t)) - \int_0^t Lf(x(u))du, \, \mathcal{M}_t, \, P_x \right) \tag{22}$$

is a martingale. We will say that the martingale problem for a and b is *well posed* if, for each x, there is exactly one solution to that martingale problem starting from x. We will be working with the following setup. For each $h > 0$, let $\Pi_h(x, \cdot)$ be a transition function on R^d. Given $x \in R^d$, let P_x^h be the probability measure on Ω characterized by the properties that

$$(i) \quad P_x^h(x(0) = x) = 1, \tag{23}$$

$$(ii) \quad P_x^h\left\{ x(t) = \frac{(k+1)h - t}{h} x(kh) + \frac{t - kh}{h} x((k+1)h), \quad kh \le t < (k+1)h \right\} = 1 \tag{24}$$

$$\text{for all } k \ge 0,$$

$$(iii) \quad P_x^h(x((k+1)h) \in \Gamma \mid \mathcal{M}_{kh}) = \Pi_h(x(kh), \Gamma), \quad P_x^h - a.s.$$

$$\text{for all } k \ge 0 \text{ and } \Gamma \in \mathcal{B}_{R^d}. \tag{25}$$

Define

$$a_h^{ij}(x) = \frac{1}{h} \int_{|y - x| \le 1} (y_i - x_i)(y_j - x_j) \Pi_h(x, dy), \tag{26}$$

$$b_h^i(x) = \frac{1}{h} \int_{|y-x|\le 1} (y_i - x_i)\Pi_h(x, dy), \tag{27}$$

and

$$\Delta_h^\varepsilon(x) = \frac{1}{h}\Pi_h(x, R^d \setminus B(x, \varepsilon)), \tag{28}$$

where $B(x, \varepsilon)$ is the open ball with center x and radius ε. What we are going to assume is that for all $R > 0$

$$\lim_{h \searrow 0} \sup_{|x| \le R} \|a_h(x) - a(x)\| = 0, \tag{29}$$

$$\lim_{h \searrow 0} \sup_{|x| \le R} |b_h(x) - b(x)| = 0, \tag{30}$$

$$\sup_{h > 0} \sup_{x \in R^d} (\|a_h(x)\| + |b_h(x)|) < \infty, \tag{31}$$

$$\lim_{h \searrow 0} \sup_{x \in R^d} \Delta_h^\varepsilon(x) = 0. \tag{32}$$

Theorem A. ([15], p. 272, Theorem 11.2.3). *Assume that in addition to (29)–(32) the coefficients a and b are continuous and have the property that for each $x \in R^d$ the martingale problem for a and b has exactly one solution P_x starting from x (that is well posed). Then P_x^h converges weakly to P_x uniformly in x on compact subsets of R^d.*

Sufficient conditions for the well posedness are given by the following theorem. Let S_d be the set of symmetric nonnegative definite $d \times d$ real matrices.

Theorem B. ([15], p. 152, Theorem 6.3.4). *Let $a : R^d \longrightarrow S_d$ and $b : R^d \longrightarrow R^d$ be bounded measurable functions and suppose that $\sigma : R^d \longrightarrow R^d \times R^d$ is a bounded measurable function such that $a = \sigma\sigma^*$. Assume that there is an A such that*

$$\|\sigma(x) - \sigma(y)\| + |b(x) - b(y)| \le A|x - y| \tag{33}$$

for all $x, y \in R^d$. Then the martingale problem for a and b is well posed and the corresponding family of solutions $\{P_x : x \in R^d\}$ is Feller continuous (that is $P_{x_n} \to P_x$ weakly if $x_n \to x$).

Note that (33) and uniform ellipticity of $a(x)$ imply the existence of the transition density $p(s, x; t, y)$ ([15], Theorem 3.2.1, p. 71).

Consider the model

$$X((k+1)h) = X(kh) + hb(X(kh)) + \sqrt{h}\xi(X(kh)),$$

$$\xi(X(kh)) = \rho_k \sigma(X(kh))\varepsilon_k, \tag{34}$$

where $\{\varepsilon_k\}$ are i.i.d. random vectors uniformly distributed on the unit sphere S^{d-1}, and $\{\rho_k\}$ are i.i.d. random variables having a density, $\rho_k \geq 0$, $E\rho_k^2 = d$. Let us check the conditions (29)–(32). It is easy to see that

$$\Pi_h(x, dy) = p_h^x(y)dy, \quad \text{where} \quad p_h^x(y) = h^{-d/2} f_\xi \left(\frac{y - x - hb(x)}{\sqrt{h}} \right). \qquad (35)$$

Here, f_ξ denotes the density of the random vector ξ. Let us check (32). Note that $E\xi = 0$ and the covariance matrix of the vector ξ is equal to

$$Cov(\xi, \xi^T) = E(\rho_k^2 \sigma(x)\varepsilon_k \varepsilon_k^T \sigma^T(x)) = a(x). \qquad (36)$$

We have

$$h\Delta_h^\varepsilon(x) = \Pi_h(x, R^d \setminus B(x, \varepsilon)) = \int_{R^d \setminus B(x,\varepsilon)} p_h^x(y)dy =$$

$$= \int_{v + \sqrt{h}b(x) \in R^d \setminus B(0, \frac{\varepsilon}{\sqrt{h}})} f_\xi(v)dv = P\left\{ \xi \in \overline{B\left(0, \frac{\varepsilon}{\sqrt{h}}\right)} - \sqrt{h}b(x)) \right\} \leq$$

$$\leq P\left\{ |\xi|^2 \geq \frac{\varepsilon^2}{4h} \right\} = o(h). \qquad (37)$$

The last equality is a consequence of the Markov inequality. The equality (36), the uniform ellipticity of $a(x)$ and (37) imply (32). To prove (29), note that by (33)

$$a_h^{ij}(x) = \frac{1}{h} \int_{|y-x| \leq 1} (y_i - x_i)(y_j - x_j) p_h^x(y)dy =$$

$$= \int_{|v + \sqrt{h}b(x)| \leq \frac{1}{\sqrt{h}}} (v_i + \sqrt{h}b^i(x))(v_j + \sqrt{h}b^j(x)) f_\xi(v)dv =$$

$$= \int_{|v + \sqrt{h}b(x)| \leq \frac{1}{\sqrt{h}}} v_i v_j f_\xi(v)dv + o(\sqrt{h}) = a(x) + o(1). \qquad (38)$$

To check (30), note that

$$b_h^i(x) = \frac{1}{h} \int_{|y-x| \leq 1} (y_i - x_i) p_h^x(y)dy =$$

$$= \frac{1}{\sqrt{h}} \int_{|v + \sqrt{h}b(x)| \leq \frac{1}{\sqrt{h}}} (v_i + \sqrt{h}b^i(x)) f_\xi(v)dv =$$

$$= b^i(x) \int_{|v+\sqrt{h}b(x)| \le \frac{1}{\sqrt{h}}} f_\xi(v) dv - \frac{1}{\sqrt{h}} \int_{|v+\sqrt{h}b(x)| > \frac{1}{\sqrt{h}}} v_i f_\xi(v) dv. \quad (39)$$

To estimate the second integral in (39), we apply the Cauchy–Schwarz inequality

$$\frac{1}{\sqrt{h}} \int_{|v+\sqrt{h}b(x)| > \frac{1}{\sqrt{h}}} |v| f_\xi(v) dv \le \frac{1}{\sqrt{h}} \left(\int |v|^2 f_\xi(v) dv \right)^{1/2} \left(P(|\xi|^2 \ge \frac{1}{4h}) \right)^{1/2} = o(1),$$

$$(40)$$

and (39), (40) imply (30). Finally, (31) follows from our calculations and assumptions of Theorem B. Weak convergence P_x^h to P_x follows now from Theorems A and B cited above. $\qquad \square$

Acknowledgements Sincere thanks are due to the referees whose suggestions and comments have helped us to revise the article.

References

1. Billingsley, P.: Convergence of Probability Measures. John Wiley and Sons, New York (1968)
2. Gikhman, I.I., Skorohod, A.V..: Introduction to the Theory of Random Processes. Dover Publications (1996)
3. Gradshtein, I., Ryzhik, I.: Table of Integrals, Series and Products, 6th edn. Academic Press (2000)
4. Kolesnik, A.D. The explicit probability distribution of a six-dimensional random flight, Theory Stoch. Process **15**(30), 1, 33–39 (2009)
5. Konakov, V.: Metod parametriksa dlya diffusii i cepei Markova, Preprint (in Russian), Izdatel'stvo popechitel'skogo soveta mehaniko-matematiceskogo fakul'teta MGU, Seriya WP BRP "STI". (2012)
6. Kluyver, J.C.: A local probability problem. In: Proceedings of the Section of Sciences, Koninklijke Akademie van Wetenschappen te Amsterdam, vol. 8, pp. 341–350 (1905)
7. Konakov, V., Mammen, E.: Small time Edgeworth-type expansions for weakly convergent non homogenious Markov chains. PTRF **143**, 137–176 (2009)
8. Mandelbrot, B.: The Fractal Geometry of Nature, New York (1982)
9. Orsingher, E., De Gregorio, A.: Reflecting random flights. J. Stat. Phys. **160**(6), 1483–1506 (2015)
10. Orsingher, De Gregorio: Random flights in higher spaces. J. Theor. Probab. **20**(4), 769–806 (2007)
11. Orsingher, E., Garra, R.: Random flights governed by Klein-Gordon type partial differential equations. Stoch. Proc. Appl. **124**, 2171–2187 (2014)
12. Orsingher, E., De Gregorio, A.: Flying randomly in R^d with Dirichlet displacements. Stoch. Proc. Appl. **122**, 676–713 (2012)
13. Pearson, K.: The problem of the Random Walk. Nature **72**(1865), 294 (1905)
14. Rayleigh, L.: On the problem of the random flights and of random vibrations in one, two and three dimensions. Philos. Mag. **37**, 321–347 (1919)
15. Stroock, D.W., Varadhan, S.R.S.: Multidimensional Diffusion Processes. Springer, Berlin (1979)
16. Whittaker, E.T., Watson, G.N.: A Course of Modern Analysis, 4th edn., Cambridge (1927)
17. Yadrenko, M.I.: Spectral Theory of Random Fields. Springer, Berlin (1983)

Random Motions with Space-Varying Velocities

Roberto Garra and Enzo Orsingher

Abstract Random motions on the line and on the plane with space-varying velocities are considered and analyzed in this paper. On the line we investigate symmetric and asymmetric telegraph processes with space-dependent velocities and we are able to present the explicit distribution of the position $\mathcal{T}(t)$, $t > 0$, of the moving particle. Also the case of a nonhomogeneous Poisson process (with rate $\lambda = \lambda(t)$) governing the changes of direction is analyzed in three specific cases. For the special case $\lambda(t) = \alpha/t$, we obtain a random motion related to the Euler–Poisson–Darboux (EPD) equation which generalizes the well-known case treated, e.g., in (Foong, S.K., Van Kolck, U.: Poisson random walk for solving wave equations. Prog. Theor. Phys. **87**(2), 285–292, 1992, [6], Garra, R., Orsingher, E.: Random flights related to the Euler-Poisson-Darboux equation. Markov Process. Relat. Fields **22**, 87–110, 2016, [8], Rosencrans, S.I.: Diffusion transforms. J. Differ. Equ. **13**, 457–467, 1973, [16]). A EPD-type fractional equation is also considered and a parabolic solution (which in dimension $d = 1$ has the structure of a probability density) is obtained. Planar random motions with space-varying velocities and infinite directions are finally analyzed in Sect. 5. We are able to present their explicit distributions, and for polynomial-type velocity structures we obtain the hyper- and hypoelliptic form of their support (of which we provide a picture).

Keywords Planar random motions · Damped wave equations · Euler–Poisson–Darboux fractional equation

MSC 2010 60G60 · 35R11

R. Garra · E. Orsingher (✉)
"Sapienza" Università di Roma, Rome, Italy
e-mail: enzo.orsingher@uniroma1.it

R. Garra
e-mail: roberto.garra@sbai.uniroma1.it

© Springer International Publishing AG 2017

V. Panov (ed.), *Modern Problems of Stochastic Analysis and Statistics*,
Springer Proceedings in Mathematics & Statistics 208,
DOI 10.1007/978-3-319-65313-6_2

1 Introduction

The telegraph process represents a simple prototype of finite velocity random motions on the line, whose probability law is governed by a hyperbolic partial differential equation that is the classical telegraph equation, widely used in mathematical physics both in problems of electromagnetism and heat conduction (see for example [2]). In [13], the authors studied a generalization of the classical telegraph process with space-time-varying propagation speed. Within this framework, the probabilistic model is based on the limit of a persistent random walk on a nonuniform lattice. The consequence of the assumption of a space-time-depending velocity $c(x, t)$ is that the probability law of the corresponding finite velocity random motion is governed by the following telegraph equation with variable coefficients

$$\frac{\partial}{\partial t}\left[\frac{1}{c(x,t)}\frac{\partial p}{\partial t}\right] + 2\lambda \frac{1}{c(x,t)}\frac{\partial p}{\partial t} = \frac{\partial}{\partial x}\left[c(x,t)\frac{\partial p}{\partial x}\right]. \qquad (1.1)$$

In some cases, it is possible to find the explicit form of the probability law of this generalization of the telegraph process, by solving equation (1.1) subject to suitable initial conditions. In particular, we focus our attention on the case of space-depending velocity, where (1.1) becomes

$$\frac{\partial^2 p}{\partial t^2} + 2\lambda \frac{\partial p}{\partial t} = c(x)\frac{\partial}{\partial x}\left[c(x)\frac{\partial p}{\partial x}\right]. \qquad (1.2)$$

The function $c(x) \in C^1(\mathbb{R})$ represents the velocity of a particle running through point x and thus must be $c(x) \geq 0$. The transformation

$$y = \begin{cases} \displaystyle\int_0^x \frac{dw}{c(w)}, & x > 0 \\ \displaystyle -\int_x^0 \frac{dw}{c(w)}, & x < 0 \end{cases} \qquad (1.3)$$

implies that

$$\frac{\partial}{\partial x} = \frac{1}{c(x)}\frac{\partial}{\partial y} \qquad (1.4)$$

and converts (1.2) into the classical telegraph equation. Provided that

$$\int_{\min\{0,x\}}^{\max\{0,x\}} \frac{dw}{c(w)} < +\infty, \qquad (1.5)$$

we take $y = 0$ for $x = 0$. These conditions on $c = c(x)$ must hold in all parts of the paper, suitably adapted to the specific cases.

In principle, the transformation (1.3) is sufficient for converting (1.2) into the telegraph equation with constant velocity in the frame (y, t) but we need also (1.3) for the necessary changes of the probability distributions. For the case where $c(x) \notin C^1(\mathbb{R})$ in some isolated points, we can replace it with a suitable smoothed version $c_\epsilon(x)$ and then apply the procedure just described and finally take $\epsilon \to 0$.

A possible example of velocity function is $c(x) = |x|^\alpha$ which for $0 < \alpha < 1$ denotes a moderately increasing velocity and for $\alpha < 0$ has fading off effect on motions. Of course for $\alpha \geq 1$, the particle undergoes an accelerating process and looses the character of a finite velocity motion.

In this paper, we consider the asymmetric telegraph process with space-varying velocity and also the symmetric telegraph process with a nonhomogeneous Poisson process governing the changes of space-dependent velocities.

A section is devoted to a fractional Euler–Poisson–Darboux-type equation and to the discussion of a special class of nonnegative solutions.

While the telegraph process on the line is essentially a persistent random walk with only two possible directions, the picture of finite velocity random motions on the plane and in the space is more complicated and gives rise to the studies of random flights (see for example [3–5, 15]). An interesting result, in this context, was proved by Kolesnik and Orsingher in [12], where the connection between planar random motions with an infinite number of possible directions and the damped wave equation was discussed. In their model, the motion is described by a particle taking directions θ_j, $j = 1, 2, \ldots$, uniformly distributed in $[0; 2\pi)$ at Poisson paced times. The orientations θ_j are i.i.d. r.v.'s independent from the homogeneous Poisson process $N(t)$ of rate λ governing the changes of direction. The particle starts off at time $t = 0$ from the origin and moves with constant velocity c. At the epochs of the Poisson process, the particle takes new directions (uniformly distributed in $[0, 2\pi)$), independent from its previous evolution. Under these assumptions, it is possible to prove that the explicit probability law of the current position $(X(t), Y(t))$ of the randomly moving particle is a solution of the damped wave equation

$$\frac{\partial^2 p}{\partial t^2} + 2\lambda \frac{\partial p}{\partial t} = c^2 \left[\frac{\partial^2 p}{\partial x^2} + \frac{\partial^2 p}{\partial y^2} \right]. \tag{1.6}$$

In the last part of this paper, we consider the effect of a space-varying speed of propagation on the model of planar random motions with infinite possible directions, leading to the equation

$$\frac{\partial^2 p}{\partial t^2} + 2\lambda \frac{\partial p}{\partial t} = c_1(x) \frac{\partial}{\partial x} \left(c_1(x) \frac{\partial p}{\partial x} \right) + c_2(y) \frac{\partial}{\partial y} \left(c_2(y) \frac{\partial p}{\partial y} \right). \tag{1.7}$$

We show the consequence of assuming space-varying velocities on the form of the support $\mathcal{D}$ of the distribution of $(X(t), Y(t))$. By means of the transformation (suitably extended as in the one-dimensional case)

$$u = \int_0^x \frac{dw}{c_1(w)}$$

$$v = \int_0^y \frac{dz}{c_2(z)},$$

The Eq. (1.7) is reduced to the form (1.6) and thus we can obtain the explicit distribution $p(x, y, t)$ of $(X(t), Y(t))$. We then examine the form of the support of $p = p(x, y, t)$ and analyze its dependence on the space-varying velocity.

In the special case where $c_1(x) = |x|^\gamma / c_1$, $c_2(y) = |y|^\beta / c_2$, $\gamma, \beta < 1$, we obtain that the boundary of $\mathcal{D}$ is hyperelliptic for $\gamma = \beta < 0$ and hypoelliptic for $1 > \gamma = \beta > 0$ and elliptic for $\gamma = \beta = 0$.

2 Telegraph Process with Drift and Space-Varying Velocity

In this section, we consider a generalization of the telegraph process with drift considered by Beghin et al. (see Ref. [1]) in the case where the velocity is assumed to be space-varying. In particular, here we consider the random motion of a particle moving on the line and switching from the space-varying (positive) velocity $c(x)$ to $-c(x)$ after an exponentially distributed time with rate λ_1 and from $-c(x)$ to $c(x)$ after an exponential time with a different rate λ_2. For the description of the random position of the particle $X(t)$ at time $t > 0$, we use the following probability densities:

$$\begin{cases} f(x, t)dx = P\{X(t) \in dx, V(t) = c(x)\} \\ b(x, t)dx = P\{X(t) \in dx, V(t) = -c(x)\}, \end{cases} \tag{2.1}$$

satisfying the system of partial differential equations (see [14] for a detailed probabilistic derivation)

$$\begin{cases} \dfrac{\partial f}{\partial t} = -c(x)\dfrac{\partial f}{\partial x} - \lambda_1 f + \lambda_2 b \\ \dfrac{\partial b}{\partial t} = c(x)\dfrac{\partial b}{\partial x} + \lambda_1 f - \lambda_2 b. \end{cases} \tag{2.2}$$

Defining

$$p(x, t) = f + b, \quad w = f - b, \tag{2.3}$$

we have the following system of equations

$$\begin{cases} \dfrac{\partial p}{\partial t} = -c(x)\dfrac{\partial w}{\partial x} \\ \dfrac{\partial w}{\partial t} = -c(x)\dfrac{\partial p}{\partial x} + \lambda_2(p - w) - \lambda_1(p + w). \end{cases} \tag{2.4}$$

Therefore, the probability law $p(x, t)$ is governed by the following telegraph-type equation with space-varying velocity and drift

$$\frac{\partial^2 p}{\partial t^2} + (\lambda_1 + \lambda_2)\frac{\partial p}{\partial t} = c(x)\frac{\partial}{\partial x}(c(x)\frac{\partial p}{\partial x}) + c(x)(\lambda_1 - \lambda_2)\frac{\partial p}{\partial x}. \tag{2.5}$$

In order to eliminate the drift term and to find the explicit form of the probability law, we now introduce the following Lorentz-type transformation of variables:

$$\begin{cases} x' = A\int_0^x \frac{dw}{c(w)} + Bt \\ t' = C\int_0^x \frac{dw}{c(w)} + Dt. \end{cases} \tag{2.6}$$

By means of some calculation we obtain that, by taking the following choice of the coefficients appearing in (2.6)

$$A = D = 1, \quad B = C = \frac{\lambda_1 - \lambda_2}{\lambda_1 + \lambda_2}, \tag{2.7}$$

equation (2.5) becomes the classical telegraph equation

$$\frac{\partial^2 p}{\partial t'^2} + (\lambda_1 + \lambda_2)\frac{\partial p}{\partial t'} = \frac{\partial^2 p}{\partial x'^2} \tag{2.8}$$

and we can therefore find the following explicit probability law, starting from that of the classical telegraph process (with $\lambda = \frac{\lambda_1 + \lambda_2}{2}$)

$$p(x,t) = \frac{e^{-\lambda t}}{2}\left\{\delta\left(t - \left|\int_0^x \frac{dx'}{c(x')}\right|\right) + \delta\left(t + \left|\int_0^x \frac{dx'}{c(x')}\right|\right)\right\}$$
$$+ \frac{e^{-\lambda t}}{2c(x)}\left[\lambda I_0\left(\lambda\sqrt{t^2 - \left|\int_0^x \frac{dx'}{c(x')}\right|^2}\right) + \frac{\partial}{\partial t}I_0\left(\lambda\sqrt{t^2 - \left|\int_0^x \frac{dx'}{c(x')}\right|^2}\right)\right] \times \mathbf{1}_D(x)\right\},$$

where $\mathbf{1}_D$ is the characteristic function of the set

$$D := \left\{x \in \mathbb{R} : \left|\left(\int_0^x \frac{dx'}{c(x')}\right)\right| < t\right\}$$

and $I_0(\cdot)$ is the modified Bessel function of order zero.

3 Nonhomogeneous Telegraph Processes with Space-Varying Velocities

Let us recall that a telegraph process $\mathcal{T}(t), t > 0$, where changes of direction are paced by a nonhomogeneous Poisson process, denoted by $\mathcal{N}(t)$, with time-dependent rate $\lambda(t), t > 0$, has distribution $p(x,t)$ satisfying the Cauchy problem (see e.g., [10]):

$$\begin{cases} \dfrac{\partial^2 p}{\partial t^2} + 2\lambda(t)\dfrac{\partial p}{\partial t} = c^2\dfrac{\partial^2 p}{\partial x^2}, \\[4mm] p(x,0) = \delta(x), \quad \dfrac{\partial p}{\partial t}(x,t)\Big|_{t=0} = 0. \end{cases} \tag{3.1}$$

In order to obtain explicit distributions in some specific cases, we observe that the transformation

$$p(x,t) = e^{-\int_\epsilon^t \lambda(s)\,ds} v(x,t), \tag{3.2}$$

converts (3.1) into

$$\frac{\partial^2 v}{\partial t^2} - [\lambda'(t) + \lambda^2(t)]v = c^2\frac{\partial^2 v}{\partial x^2}. \tag{3.3}$$

In (3.2), we exclude the initial time instant (which, however, does not play any role in the subsequent differential transformations) in order to avoid pathologies at $t = 0$. Functions of the form $\lambda(t) = \alpha/t$ and $\lambda(t) = \lambda \coth \lambda t$, for $t > 0$, display an initial high-valued intensity of the Poisson events which hinder the particle to reach the endpoints of the support interval. Then, in order to find the explicit probability law of $\mathcal{T}(t)$ from (3.1), a mathematical trick is to solve the following Riccati equation emerging from (3.3) (see [8, 9]):

$$\lambda'(t) + \lambda^2(t) = const. \tag{3.4}$$

In this way, it is possible to find, in particular, the following probability laws with absolutely continuous components given by

$$P\left\{ Y(t) \in dx \right\}/dx = \frac{1}{2c \cosh \lambda t}\frac{\partial}{\partial t} I_0\left(\frac{\lambda}{c}\sqrt{c^2 t^2 - x^2} \right), \quad |x| < ct, \tag{3.5}$$

and

$$P\left\{ X(t) \in dx \right\}/dx = \frac{\lambda I_0\left(\frac{\lambda}{c}\sqrt{c^2 t^2 - x^2} \right)}{2c \sinh \lambda t}, \quad |x| < ct, \tag{3.6}$$

corresponding to the cases

$$\begin{cases} \lambda(t) = \lambda \tanh \lambda t, \\ \lambda(t) = \lambda \coth \lambda t, \end{cases}$$

respectively. We observe that the process $Y(t)$ has a discrete component of the distribution concentrated at $x = \pm ct$ (see [9]), while $X(t)$ has only an absolutely continuous distribution (see [8]).

Starting from (3.5) and (3.6), we can clearly build other families of explicit probability laws of the form

$$
\left\{
\begin{aligned}
&P\left\{Y(t)\in dx\right\}/dx = \frac{1}{2c(x)\cosh\lambda t}\frac{\partial}{\partial t} I_0\left(\lambda\sqrt{t^2 - \left|\int_0^x \frac{dx'}{c(x')}\right|^2}\right),\\[2mm]
&P\left\{X(t)\in dx\right\}/dx = \frac{\lambda}{2c(x)\sinh\lambda t} I_0\left(\lambda\sqrt{t^2 - \left|\int_0^x \frac{dx'}{c(x')}\right|^2}\right),\\[2mm]
&\qquad\qquad\text{for }\left\{x:\left|\int_0^x \frac{dx'}{c(x')}\right| < t\right\},
\end{aligned}
\right.
\tag{3.7}
$$

which depend on the particular choice of $c(x) > 0$ (s.t. condition (1.5) is fullfilled for all x). These probability laws are clearly related to the following partial differential equations:

$$
\begin{cases}
\dfrac{\partial^2 p}{\partial t^2} + 2\lambda\tanh\lambda t\,\dfrac{\partial p}{\partial t} = c(x)\dfrac{\partial}{\partial x}c(x)\dfrac{\partial p}{\partial x},\\[3mm]
\dfrac{\partial^2 p}{\partial t^2} + 2\lambda\coth\lambda t\,\dfrac{\partial p}{\partial t} = c(x)\dfrac{\partial}{\partial x}c(x)\dfrac{\partial p}{\partial x},
\end{cases}
\tag{3.8}
$$

respectively.

Another interesting case is $\lambda(t) = \frac{\alpha}{t}$, which converts Eq. (3.1) into the classical Euler–Poisson–Darboux equation

$$
\frac{\partial^2 u}{\partial t^2} + \frac{2\alpha}{t}\frac{\partial u}{\partial t} = \frac{\partial^2 u}{\partial x^2}, \quad x\in\mathbb{R}, t > 0.
\tag{3.9}
$$

The first probabilistic interpretation of the fundamental solution of the EPD equation was given by Rosencrans in [16] and some of its generalizations have been considered in [8]. In the spirit of the previous observations, we have that the solution of the Cauchy problem

$$
\begin{cases}
\dfrac{\partial^2 v}{\partial t^2} + \dfrac{2\alpha}{t}\dfrac{\partial v}{\partial t} = c(x)\dfrac{\partial}{\partial x}c(x)\dfrac{\partial v}{\partial x},\\[3mm]
v(x,0) = \delta(x),\\[3mm]
\left.\dfrac{\partial v}{\partial t}\right|_{t=0} = 0
\end{cases}
\tag{3.10}
$$

can be written as

$$
v(x,t) = \frac{1}{B(\alpha,\frac{1}{2})\,c(x)t}\left(1 - \frac{\left|\int_0^x \frac{dx'}{c(x')}\right|^2}{t^2}\right)^{\alpha-1}, \quad\text{for }\left\{x:\left|\int_0^x \frac{dw}{c(w)}\right| < t\right\}.
\tag{3.11}
$$

We finally observe that it is possible to consider other cases of nonhomogeneous telegraph processes with space-dependent velocities according to the following simple steps:

• Consider the equation

$$\frac{\partial^2 p}{\partial t^2} + 2\lambda(t)\frac{\partial p}{\partial t} = c(x)\frac{\partial}{\partial x}c(x)\frac{\partial p}{\partial x}, \tag{3.12}$$

governing a telegraph process on the line, where the changes of direction are given by a nonhomogeneous Poisson process with a deterministic time-dependent rate $\lambda(t)$ and with space-dependent velocity $c(x)$.
• Define the new variables $x' = \int_0^x \frac{du}{c(u)}$ and $t' = \int_0^t \gamma(s)ds$, where $\gamma(t)$ is a $C^1[0, +\infty)$ function that will be defined in the next step;
• In the new variables, we have that $p(x', t')$ satisfies the equation

$$\gamma^2(t')\frac{\partial^2 p}{\partial t'^2} + (\gamma' + 2\lambda\gamma)\frac{\partial p}{\partial t'} = \frac{\partial^2 p}{\partial x'^2}; \tag{3.13}$$

• Take $\gamma(t)$ such that $\frac{\gamma'}{\gamma} = -2\lambda(t)$. Then the problem is finally reduced to the following D'Alembert equation with a time-depending coefficient

$$\frac{\partial^2 p}{\partial t'^2} = \frac{1}{\gamma^2(t')}\frac{\partial^2 p}{\partial x'^2}. \tag{3.14}$$

• By taking the further change of variable $(x', t') \rightarrow (\gamma(t')x', t')$ and calling $x'' = \gamma(t')x'$ we finally reduce Eq. (3.14) to the classical D'Alembert equation in the variables (x'', t')

$$\frac{\partial^2 u}{\partial t'^2} = \frac{\partial^2 u}{\partial x''^2}. \tag{3.15}$$

Thus an observer in the framework (x'', t') sees the original random motion transformed into a deterministic one governed by the classical D'Alembert equation.

4   Time-Fractional Euler–Poisson–Darboux Equation with Variable Velocity

We here provide some new results about the Euler–Poisson–Darboux equation involving time-fractional derivatives in the sense of Riemann–Liouville (see [11]) and with space-varying velocity. It is well known that the EPD equation governs a telegraph process with time-dependent rate $\lambda(t) = \alpha/t$. As far as we know this is the first investigation about the time-fractional EPD equation.

Theorem 4.1 *The d-dimensional time-fractional EPD-type equation*

$$\left(\frac{\partial^{2\nu}}{\partial t^{2\nu}} + \frac{C_1}{t^{\nu}} \frac{\partial^{\nu}}{\partial t^{\nu}} \right) u = \Delta u, \tag{4.1}$$

with $\nu \in (0, 1) \setminus \{\frac{1}{2}, \frac{1}{3}, \frac{1}{4}, \frac{1}{5}\}$ *and*

$$C_1 = -\frac{\Gamma(1 - 4\nu)}{\Gamma(1 - 5\nu)}, \tag{4.2}$$

admits the following nonnegative solution:
for $C_2 > 0$

$$u(\mathbf{x}_d, t) = \begin{cases} \frac{1}{t^{\nu}} \left[1 - C_2 \frac{\|\mathbf{x}_d\|^2}{t^{2\nu}} \right], & \|\mathbf{x}_d\| < \frac{t^{\nu}}{C_2^{1/2}}, \\ 0 & elsewhere, \end{cases} \tag{4.3}$$

while for $C_2 < 0$

$$u(\mathbf{x}_d, t) = \frac{1}{t^{\nu}} \left[1 - C_2 \frac{\|\mathbf{x}_d\|^2}{t^{2\nu}} \right], \quad \forall \, \mathbf{x}_d \in \mathbb{R}^d \tag{4.4}$$

where $\mathbf{x}_d = (x_1, x_2, \ldots, x_d), d \in \mathbb{N}$ *and*

$$C_2 = -\frac{1}{2d} \left[\frac{\Gamma(1 - \nu)}{\Gamma(1 - 3\nu)} - \frac{\Gamma(1 - 4\nu)}{\Gamma(1 - 5\nu)} \frac{\Gamma(1 - \nu)}{\Gamma(1 - 2\nu)} \right]$$

Proof By considering that (4.1) has the structure of an EPD equation, we determine a parabolic-type solution. By using the well-known fact that (see [11], p. 71)

$$\frac{\partial^{\alpha} t^{\beta}}{\partial t^{\alpha}} = \frac{\Gamma(\beta + 1) t^{\beta - \alpha}}{\Gamma(\beta + 1 - \alpha)}, \quad \text{for } \alpha > 0 \text{ and } \beta > -1, \tag{4.5}$$

we can calculate the exact form of the coefficient C_2 such that (4.3) is a solution of (4.1). We assume that $\nu \neq \frac{1}{2}, \frac{1}{3}, \frac{1}{4}, \frac{1}{5}$ in order to avoid the singularities in the coefficients appearing in C_1 and C_2. □

Remark 4.2 It is possible to construct a probability law with compact support, starting from the general Theorem 4.1 in the one-dimensional case, assuming that ν is such that C_2 is positive. In this case, we have that the probability law

$$p(x, t) = \frac{N}{t^{\nu}} \left[1 - C_2 \frac{|x|^2}{t^{2\nu}} \right], \quad |x| < \frac{t^{\nu}}{C_2^{1/2}}, \tag{4.6}$$

with

$$C_2 = -\frac{1}{2}\left[\frac{\Gamma(1-\nu)}{\Gamma(1-3\nu)} - \frac{\Gamma(1-4\nu)}{\Gamma(1-5\nu)}\frac{\Gamma(1-\nu)}{\Gamma(1-2\nu)}\right]$$

and $N = \frac{3}{4}\sqrt{C_2}$ the normalizing constant satisfies the one-dimensional time-fractional EPD-type Eq. (4.1).

We remark that it is not a trivial matter to find the explicit values of $\nu \in (0, 1)$ such that the coefficient $C_2 > 0$.

Notice that it is extremely hard to ascertain that functions of the form

$$u(x, t) = \frac{N}{t^\beta}\left(1 - \frac{\|\mathbf{x}_d\|^2}{t^\alpha}\right)^\gamma \tag{4.7}$$

are solutions of (4.1) for $\gamma \neq 1$ and suitable β and α.

We can also observe, with the following Proposition, that we are able to find a solution for a time-fractional EPD-type equation of higher order.

Proposition 4.3 *The d-dimensional time-fractional EPD-type equation*

$$\left(\frac{\partial^{2\nu}}{\partial t^{2\nu}} + \frac{C_1}{t^\nu}\frac{\partial^\nu}{\partial t^\nu}\right)u = \sum_{j=1}^{d}\frac{\partial^{2n}u}{\partial x_j^{2n}}, \quad n \in \mathbb{N}, \tag{4.8}$$

with $\nu \in (0, 1) \setminus \{\frac{1}{2}, \frac{1}{3}, \frac{1}{4}, \frac{1}{5}\}$ and

$$C_1 = -\frac{\Gamma(1-4\nu)}{\Gamma(1-5\nu)}, \tag{4.9}$$

admits the following nonnegative solution:
for $C_2 > 0$

$$u(x_1, \ldots, x_d, t) = \begin{cases} \frac{1}{t^\nu}\left[1 - C_2\frac{\sum_{j=1}^{d}x_j^{2n}}{t^{2\nu}}\right], & \sum_{j=1}^{d}x_j^{2n} < \frac{t^{2\nu}}{C_2}, \\ 0 & elsewhere \end{cases} \tag{4.10}$$

and for $C_2 < 0$

$$u(x_1, \ldots, x_d, t) = \frac{1}{t^\nu}\left[1 - C_2\frac{\sum_{j=1}^{d}x_j^{2n}}{t^{2\nu}}\right], \quad \forall \mathbf{x}_d \in \mathbb{R}^d \tag{4.11}$$

where $d \in \mathbb{N}$ and

$$C_2 = -\frac{1}{(2n)!d}\left[\frac{\Gamma(1-\nu)}{\Gamma(1-3\nu)} - \frac{\Gamma(1-4\nu)}{\Gamma(1-5\nu)}\frac{\Gamma(1-\nu)}{\Gamma(1-2\nu)}\right].$$

Starting from (4.6), we have the following corollary.

Corollary 4.4 *Taking $\nu \in (0, 1)$ such that $C_2 > 0$, the probability law*

$$p(x, t) = \frac{N}{c(x)t^\nu} \left[1 - C_2 \frac{\left| \int_0^x \frac{dx'}{c(x')} \right|^2}{t^{2\nu}} \right], \quad for \left\{ x : \left| \int_0^x \frac{dx'}{c(x')} \right| < \frac{t^\nu}{C_2^{1/2}} \right\},$$

(4.12)

with $N = \frac{3}{4}\sqrt{C_2}$ and

$$C_2 = -\frac{1}{2} \left[\frac{\Gamma(1-\nu)}{\Gamma(1-3\nu)} - \frac{\Gamma(1-4\nu)}{\Gamma(1-5\nu)} \frac{\Gamma(1-\nu)}{\Gamma(1-2\nu)} \right],$$

satisfies the time-fractional EPD-type equation with nonconstant coefficients

$$\left(\frac{\partial^{2\nu}}{\partial t^{2\nu}} + \frac{C_1}{t^\nu} \frac{\partial^\nu}{\partial t^\nu} \right) p = c(x) \frac{\partial}{\partial x} c(x) \frac{\partial p}{\partial x},$$

(4.13)

with

$$C_1 = -\frac{\Gamma(1-4\nu)}{\Gamma(1-5\nu)}.$$

5   Planar Random Motions with Space-Varying Velocity

We start our analysis from the damped wave equation with space-depending velocities as follows:

$$\frac{\partial^2 p}{\partial t^2} + 2\lambda \frac{\partial p}{\partial t} = c_1(x) \frac{\partial}{\partial x} c_1(x) \frac{\partial p}{\partial x} + c_2(y) \frac{\partial}{\partial y} c_2(y) \frac{\partial p}{\partial y}.$$

(5.1)

By taking the change of variables

$$\begin{cases} z = \int_0^x \frac{dx'}{c_1(x')} \\ w = \int_0^y \frac{dy'}{c_2(y')}, \end{cases} \quad (x, y) \in \mathbb{R}^2,$$

(5.2)

we obtain

$$\frac{\partial^2 p}{\partial t^2} + 2\lambda \frac{\partial p}{\partial t} = \frac{\partial^2 p}{\partial z^2} + \frac{\partial^2 p}{\partial w^2}.$$

(5.3)

The transformation (5.2) must be extended on the whole plane $(x, y) \in \mathbb{R}^2$ by suitably adapting the considerations discussed in the introduction. The absolutely continuous component of the distribution of the position $(X(t), Y(t))$ of the moving particle performing the planar motion described in the introduction satisfies (5.3) (see [12]). Therefore, returning to the original variables (x, y), we are able to understand the role played by the variable velocity on the model considered in [12]. The absolutely continuous component of the probability law is given by

$$p(x, y, t) = \frac{\lambda}{2\pi c_1(x) c_2(y)} \frac{\exp\left\{ -\lambda t + \lambda \sqrt{t^2 - \left| \int_0^x \frac{dx'}{c_1(x')} \right|^2 - \left| \int_0^y \frac{dy'}{c_2(y')} \right|^2} \right\}}{\sqrt{t^2 - \left| \int_0^x \frac{dx'}{c_1(x')} \right|^2 - \left| \int_0^y \frac{dy'}{c_2(y')} \right|^2}},$$

(5.4)

provided that both $c_1(x)$ and $c_2(y)$ are positive and such that $\int_{\min\{0,x\}}^{\max\{0,x\}} \frac{dx'}{c_1(x')} < \infty$

for all $x \in \mathbb{R}$ and $\int_{\min\{0,y\}}^{\max\{0,y\}} \frac{dy'}{c_2(y')} < \infty$ for all $y \in \mathbb{R}$, respectively.

Therefore, the support of $p(x, y, t)$ is given by the set

$$\mathcal{D} := \left\{ (x, y) : \left| \int_0^x \frac{dx'}{c_1(x')} \right|^2 + \left| \int_0^y \frac{dy'}{c_2(y')} \right|^2 < t^2 \right\}.$$

(5.5)

The set $\mathcal{D}$ is therefore a *deformation* of the circle representing the support of $(X(t), Y(t))$ in the case of constant velocity. From formula (5.4), we can extract the conditional distribution of this class of generalized planar random motions. Since

$$P\{X(t) \in dx, Y(t) \in dy\} = \sum_{n=0}^{\infty} P\{X(t) \in dx, Y(t) \in dy | N(t) = n\} P\{N(t) = n\} dx dy, \quad (5.6)$$

where $P\{N(t) = n\}$ is the homogeneous Poisson distribution of rate λ, we have that the conditional distribution is obviously given by

$$P\{X(t) \in dx, Y(t) \in dy | N(t) = n\}$$

$$= \frac{n}{2\pi t^n} \left[t^2 - \left| \int_0^x \frac{dx'}{c_1(x')} \right|^2 - \left| \int_0^y \frac{dy'}{c_2(y')} \right|^2 \right]^{\frac{n}{2}-1} \frac{dx dy}{c_1(x) c_2(y)}.$$

(5.7)

The planar motion with space-varying velocity after n changes of direction can be described as

$$\begin{cases} X(t) = \sum_{j=1}^{n+1} \left(\int_{t_{j-1}}^{t_j} c_1(X(s)) ds \right) \cos \theta_j \\ Y(t) = \sum_{j=1}^{n+1} \left(\int_{t_{j-1}}^{t_j} c_2(Y(s)) ds \right) \sin \theta_j, \end{cases}$$

(5.8)

where $0 = t_0 < t_1 < \cdots < t_j < \cdots < t_n < t_{n+1} = t$ are the epochs of the Poisson process and θ_j are the directions of motion assumed at times t_j. The reader can ascertain that (5.8) coincides with equation (12) of [12] in the case $c_1 = c_2 = const.$.

The intuitive idea underlying (5.8) is that at Poisson times t_j the particle chooses its direction randomly and the displacement performed is determined by the local velocity field. During $(s, s + ds)$, for example, the x-coordinate makes a step of length $c_1(X(s))ds$ depending on the position occupied at time s.

We also observe that we can arrive at (5.7) by expanding (5.4) and then using (5.6).

In order to understand the role of considering different velocities on both axes, we consider a general domain that includes some interesting cases. It corresponds to taking the space-dependent velocities of the form $c_1(x) = \frac{|x|^\gamma}{c_1}$ and $c_2(y) = \frac{|y|^\beta}{c_2}$, with $\gamma, \beta < 1$ and $c_1, c_2 > 0$. The functions $c_1(x)$ and $c_2(x)$ considered here can be regarded as the limit of approximating smooth functions excluding $x = y = 0$. With this choice, we obtain a family of probability laws concentrated inside domains of the form

$$\mathcal{D}_{\gamma,\beta} := \left\{ (x, y) : \left(\frac{c_1|x|^{1-\gamma}}{1-\gamma} \right)^2 + \left(\frac{c_2|y|^{1-\beta}}{1-\beta} \right)^2 < t^2 \right\}. \tag{5.9}$$

This means that the boundary of the support of this family of probability laws is given by a superellipse, also known as a Lamé curves including a wide class of geometrical figures like hypoellipses (for $\gamma = \beta < 0$) and hyperellipses (for $\gamma = \beta > 0$). We consider, in particular, two interesting cases.

The first one is the case in which $c_1(x) = c_1$ and $c_2(y) = c_2$ and $c_1 \neq c_2 \neq 0$. In this case, the support of the probability law is clearly given by the ellipse:

$$\mathcal{D}_{0,0} : \left\{ (x, y) : c_1^2|x|^2 + c_2^2|y|^2 < t^2 \right\}. \tag{5.10}$$

The second interesting case is given by the choice $c_1(x) = c_1|x|^{2/3}$ and $c_2(y) = c_2|y|^{2/3}$, leading to the compact support

$$\mathcal{D}_{2/3,2/3} : \left\{ (x, y) : 9c_1^2|x|^{2/3} + 9c_2^2|y|^{2/3} < t^2 \right\}. \tag{5.11}$$

For $c_1 = c_2 = 1/3$, we obtain as boundary of $\mathcal{D}_{2/3,2/3}$ the astroid (see Fig. 1). For $c_1 \neq c_2 \neq 1$, we have instead a squeezed astroid, possibly on both axes.

Another interesting class of d-dimensional random motions at finite velocities is related to the EPD equation

$$\frac{\partial^2 v}{\partial t^2} + \frac{2\alpha + d - 1}{t} \frac{\partial v}{\partial t} = \sum_{j=1}^{d} c_j(x_j) \frac{\partial}{\partial x_j} c_j(x_j) \frac{\partial v}{\partial x_j}. \tag{5.12}$$

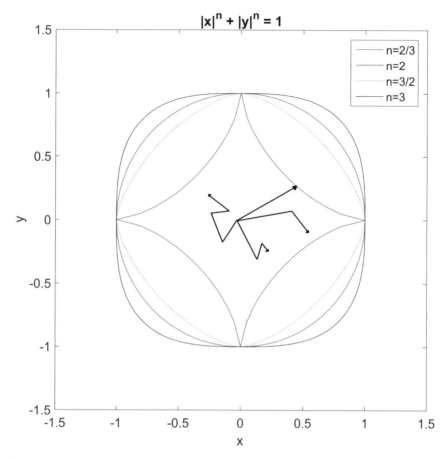

Fig. 1 We represent the boundary of the compact support $\mathcal{D}_{\gamma,\beta}$ of the family of probability laws (5.4), in the hypoelliptic ($n = 2/3$ leading to the astroid and $n = 3/2$), elliptic ($n = 2$), and hyperelliptic case ($n = 3$). Here, we assume that $c_1 = c_2 = 1$ and $n = 2(1 - \gamma) = 2(1 - \beta)$. We show, as an example, four sample paths with zero, two, three, and four changes of direction, in the case when the random motion takes place in the astroid

In this case, the probability law $p(x_1, x_2, \ldots, x_d, t)$ of the particle moving in the d-dimensional space has the form

$$p(x_1, x_2, \ldots, x_d, t) = \frac{1}{\prod_{j=1}^{d} c_j(x_j)} \frac{\Gamma(\alpha + \frac{d}{2})}{\pi^{d/2}\Gamma(\alpha)t^{d+2\alpha-2}} \left(t^2 - \sum_{j=1}^{d} \left| \int_0^{x_j} \frac{du_j}{c_j(u_j)} \right|^2 \right)^{\alpha-1},$$

(5.13)

for $\displaystyle\sum_{j=1}^{d} \left| \int_0^{x_j} \frac{du_j}{c_j(u_j)} \right|^2 < t^2$

and represents a solution of (5.12). The projection on the axes $x_1, \ldots, x_d$ of the probability law (5.13) coincides with the one-dimensional motion dealt with in Sect. 3.

A more general random motion in $\mathbb{R}^d$ with space-varying velocities leads to equation

$$\frac{\partial^2 p}{\partial t^2} + 2\lambda(t)\frac{\partial p}{\partial t} = \sum_{j=1}^{d} c_j(x_1, \ldots x_j, \ldots, x_d)\frac{\partial}{\partial x_j}c_j(x_1, \ldots x_j, \ldots, x_d)\frac{\partial}{\partial x_j}p.$$

(5.14)

This can be object of future research.

Acknowledgements We are very greatful to both referees for their suggestions and comments.

References

1. Beghin, L., Nieddu, L., Orsingher, E.: Probabilistic analysis of the telegrapher's process with drift by means of relativistic transformations. Int. J. Stoch. Anal. **14**(1), 11–25 (2001)
2. Cattaneo, C.R.: Sur une forme de l' équation de la chaleur éliminant le paradoxe d'une propagation instantanée. Comptes Rendus **247**(4), 431–433 (1958)
3. De Gregorio, A.: Transport processes with random jump rate. Stat. Probab. Lett. **118**, 127–134 (2016)
4. De Gregorio, A., Orsingher, E.: Flying randomly in $\mathbb{R}^d$ with dirichlet displacements. Stoch. Process. Appl. **122**(2), 676–713 (2012)
5. D'Ovidio, M., Orsingher, E., Toaldo, B.: Time-changed processes governed by space-time fractional telegraph equations. Stoch. Anal. Appl. **32**(6), 1009–1045 (2014)
6. Foong, S.K., Van Kolck, U.: Poisson random walk for solving wave equations. Prog. Theor. Phys. **87**(2), 285–292 (1992)
7. Garra, R., Orsingher, E., Polito, F.: Fractional Klein-Gordon equations and related stochastic processes. J. Stat. Phys. **155**(4), 777–809 (2014)
8. Garra, R., Orsingher, E.: Random flights related to the Euler-Poisson-Darboux equation. Markov Process. Relat. Fields **22**, 87–110 (2016)
9. Iacus, S.M.: Statistical analysis of the inhomogeneous telegrapher's process. Stat. Probab. Lett. **55**, 83–88 (2001)
10. Kaplan, S.: Differential equations in which the poisson process plays a role. Bull. Am. Math. Soc. **70**(2), 264–268 (1964)
11. Kilbas, A.A., Srivastava, H.M., Trujillo, J.J.: Theory and Applications of Fractional Differential Equations, vol. 204. Elsevier Science Limited, Amsterdam (2006)
12. Kolesnik, A.D., Orsingher, E.: A planar random motion with an infinite number of directions controlled by the damped wave equation. J. Appl. Probab. **42**(4), 1168–1182 (2005)
13. Masoliver, J., Weiss, G.H.: Telegraphers equations with variable propagation speeds. Phys. Rev. E. **49**(5), 3852–3854 (1994)
14. Orsingher, E.: Probability law, flow function, maximum distribution of wave-governed random motions and their connections with Kirchoff's laws. Stoch. Process. Appl. **34**(1), 49–66 (1990)
15. Pogorui, A.A., Rodríguez-Dagnino, R.M.: Random motion with uniformly distributed directions and random velocity. J. Stat. Phys. **147**(6), 1216–1225 (2012)
16. Rosencrans, S.I.: Diffusion transforms. J. Differ. Equ. **13**, 457–467 (1973)

Part II
Parametrix and Heat Kernel Estimates

Parametrix Methods for One-Dimensional Reflected SDEs

Aurélien Alfonsi, Masafumi Hayashi and Arturo Kohatsu-Higa

Abstract In this article, we revisit in a didactic manner the forward and backward approaches of the parametrix method for one-dimensional reflected stochastic differential equations on the half line. We give probabilistic expressions for the expectation of functionals of its solution and we also discuss properties of the associated density.

Keywords Reflected SDEs · Parametrix method · Probabilistic representation

1 Introduction

Reflected stochastic differential equations appear naturally in various applications due to the natural restrictions one has to impose to the solution of a stochastic differential equation (SDE). From the point of view of partial differential equations, this corresponds to the solution of parabolic differential equations with Neumann-type conditions.

Aurélien Alfonsi—This research benefited from the support of the "Chaire Risques Financiers", Fondation du Risque and of Labex Bézout.
Masafumi Hayashi—This research was supported by KAKENHI grant 26800061.
Arturo Kohatsu-Higa—This research was supported by KAKENHI grant 2434002.

A. Alfonsi
Université Paris-Est, 6 Et 8 Avenue Blaise Pascal, 77455 Marne La Vallée,
Cedex 2, France
e-mail: aurelien.alfonsi@enpc.fr

M. Hayashi
University of the Ryukyus, Nishihara-cho, Okinawa 903-0213, Japan
e-mail: hayashim6@gmail.com

A. Kohatsu-Higa (✉)
Ritsumeikan University, 1-1-1 Nojihigashi, Kusatsu, Shiga 525-8577, Japan
e-mail: khts00@fc.ritsumei.ac.jp; arturokohatsu@gmail.com

© Springer International Publishing AG 2017
V. Panov (ed.), *Modern Problems of Stochastic Analysis and Statistics*,
Springer Proceedings in Mathematics & Statistics 208,
DOI 10.1007/978-3-319-65313-6_3

43

In this article, we base our discussion on the following one-dimensional stochastic differential equation reflected on $D = (0, \infty)$ of the type[1]

$$X_t(x) = x + \int_0^t \sigma(X_s(x)) \, dW_s + L_t(x). \tag{1}$$

Here, $x \in \bar{D} = [0, \infty)$ and W is a one-dimensional Wiener process on $(\Omega, \mathcal{F}, P)$ with the natural filtration $(\mathcal{F}_t)_{t \geq 0}$.

We say that $\{(X_t(x), L_t(x))\}_{t \geq 0} \equiv \{(X_t, L_t)\}_{t \geq 0}$ is a solution to (1) if it satisfies the following conditions:

L1. Both X_t and L_t are nonnegative, continuous, and $\mathcal{F}_t$-adapted processes satisfying (1).

L2. $L_0 = 0$ and $t \to L_t$ is increasing P-a.s.

L3. The support of the measure dL_s is carried by $\partial D = \{0\}$ in the following sense:

$$L_t = \int_0^t \mathbf{1}(X_s = 0) \, dL_s.$$

We will give an alternative probabilistic representation for $E[f(X_t)]$ which is based on the parametrix methodology used to prove the existence and uniqueness of fundamental solutions for parabolic partial differential equations (for a general reference on this method, see [6]).

This method provides a Taylor like expansion for the fundamental solution of a parabolic partial differential equation. It has been used in order to solve a variety of problems in partial differential equations. In particular, it has been used by Valentin Konakov and his collaborators in the past years in order to study the properties of the Euler scheme between other Markov chain-type diffusion approximations (see [13–15]).

One of the possible applications of a probabilistic representation is to use it for Monte Carlo simulations. This probabilistic representation was introduced in [2][2] for the case of diffusions, although recently we have also found similar expressions ubiquitously in other fields of probability and its applications (see, e.g., [4, 9, 21]).

This methodology produces a simulation method without bias using the reflected Euler–Maruyama scheme for Hölder-type coefficients. This method is related with the so-called random multilevel Monte Carlo method as described in [8] (for the basic description of this method, see [7]) which applies it to Lipschitz coefficients in the non-reflected case. It is also related with the so-called exact simulation methods which only applies in one dimension as described in [5] (for the basic description of this method, see [3]).

---

[1] We consider the reflected SDE without drift just to simplify the discussion. For a general case scenario, see [20].

[2] See also, the typo-corrected version with comments on the webpage of the second author.

On the other hand, this method may give a large variance except for particular situations. Therefore, variance reduction methods have to be studied. Such study in the case of diffusions without reflection has been performed in [1].

The study of reflected stochastic differential equations using the parametrix method has been done in [20] using what we call the backward parametrix method[3] The goal of this article is to give a simple introduction to these methods in the reflecting SDE case. In particular, we will obtain the backward method which can be used when coefficients are bounded and Hölder continuous. Based on this, we will also provide the forward parametrix method.

In order to keep the article within a minimal simplicity, we have decided not to consider multidimensional reflected SDEs. Standard modifications through boundary parametrization could be applied in order to consider some classes of smooth boundaries in the multidimensional case. We also do not discuss the oblique reflection or sticky boundary case.

Notations: The space of measurable bounded functions $f: \bar{D} = [0, \infty) \to \mathbb{R}$ is denoted by $\mathcal{M}_b(\bar{D})$. We will denote the partial derivatives of a function f with respect to its i-th variable by $\partial_i f$. The sup-norm of the function f will be denoted by $\|f\|_\infty$. The space $C_b^k(\bar{D})$ consists of all bounded functions with k bounded continuous derivatives on $\bar{D}$ where the derivatives and the continuity at 0 are understood with the right limits at 0 only. For $k \in (0, 1)$, $C_b^k(\bar{D})$ denotes the class of bounded functions which are k-Hölder continuous with a bounded Hölder constant.

As usual, constants are denoted by the letters K or C and, in the proofs of upper bounds, they may change value from one line to the next. Indicator functions may be denoted indifferently using $\mathbf{1}_A(x)$ or $\mathbf{1}(x \in A)$. We also remark that in each section a different approximation process is used and although the same symbol $\bar{X}$ maybe used, this may denote a different approximation which is clearly stated at the beginning of each section.

2   Reflected SDEs and its Approximation Process

In this section, we start with a general review of reflected stochastic differential equations and their approximations.

Let $\{W_t\}_{t \geq 0}$ be a one-dimensional standard Brownian motion on the canonical filtered probability space $(\Omega, \mathcal{F}, \{\mathcal{F}_t\}_{t \geq 0}, P)$.

---

[3]The reason for the use of "backward" on this terminology is that one uses an Euler scheme which runs backward in time. Researchers in parabolic partial differential equation prefer the terminology forward because the method corresponds to the application of the forward Kolmogorov equation to the density of X. As the current article deals with approximations using the Euler scheme, we will keep using the former terminology. The forward method was known as early as [11]. See [10] for a translation (see also the historical references there). The backward method appeared in [19]. Thanks to Valentin for these references. The essential idea for the method was first introduced for elliptic equations and is due to [17].

We assume that the coefficients of the SDE (1) satisfy the following hypotheses:

(H) $a := \sigma^2$ is uniformly elliptic and bounded:

$$0 < \underline{a} := \inf_{x \in \bar{D}} a(x) \leq \sup_{x \in \bar{D}} a(x) =: \bar{a}.$$

(Hf) $\sigma: \bar{D} \to \mathbb{R}$ is such that $\sigma \in C_b^2(\bar{D})$.
(Hb) $\sigma: \bar{D} \to \mathbb{R}$ is such that $a \in C_b^\alpha(\bar{D})$.

The hypothesis (H) will always be in force. Hypothesis (Hf) will be assumed in the forward method and the Hypothesis (Hb) will be used in the backward formulation.

For standard results on the existence and uniqueness of solutions for reflected SDEs and their properties, we refer the reader to, e.g., Lions–Sznitman [18] under (H) and Tsuchiya [20] under (Hb).

We define

$$P_t f(x) = E[f(X_t(x))]. \tag{2}$$

Then P_t is a Feller semigroup and its generator, denoted by $\mathscr{L}$, can be described for $f \in \mathscr{D} := \{f \in C_b^2(\bar{D}): f'(0) = 0\}$ as

$$\mathscr{L}f(x) = \frac{1}{2}a(x)\partial_x^2 f(x)1_D(x). \tag{3}$$

For more details, see Lemma 2.2. We recall that the main result in [20] implies that for any measurable and bounded function $f: \bar{D} \to \mathbb{R}$ then $P_t f \in C_b^2(\bar{D})$ for any $t \in (0, T]$ and $(P_t f)'(0) = 0$. That is, $P_t f \in \mathscr{D}$.

These results may seem difficult to digest for a probability audience without much training on analysis. Therefore, this article only uses as a basis the results in [18] and we will reprove the statements in [20] under the present simplified setting using an argument which has a probabilistic flavor.

Before introducing the reader to the parametrix method, we will first discuss an approximation process which is usually called the parametrix. The approximation process to be used will be the reflected Brownian motion.

Let $x, z \in \bar{D}$ be fixed, and we consider the following SDE with frozen coefficients and with reflecting boundary conditions:

$$\bar{X}_t^{(z)}(x) = x + \sigma(z) \cdot W_t + \bar{L}_t^{(z)}(x). \tag{4}$$

We say that $(\bar{X}_t^{(z)}(x), \bar{L}_t^{(z)}(x))$ is a solution to (4) if $(\bar{X}_t^{(z)}(x), \bar{L}_t^{(z)}(x))$ satisfies the following conditions:

A1. $\bar{X}_t^{(z)}(x) \geq 0$ and $\bar{L}_t^{(z)}(x)$ are continuous progressively measurable processes satisfying (4);

A2. $\bar{L}_0^{(z)}(x) = 0$ and $t \to \bar{L}_t^{(z)}(x)$ is increasing P-a.s.;

A3.   the measure $d\bar{L}_s^{(z)}$ is carried by ∂D:

$$\bar{L}_t^{(z)}(x) = \int_0^t \mathbf{1}\left(\bar{X}_s^{(z)}(x) = 0\right) d\bar{L}_s^{(z)}(x).$$

It is known (see e.g., Lemma 6.14 in Chap. 3 of Karatzas and Shreve [12]) that there is a unique pathwise solution to (4), which is given by

$$\bar{L}_t^{(z)}(x) = \max\{0, \max_{0\le s\le t} \{-(x + \sigma(z)W_s)\}\}. \tag{5}$$

For a Brownian motion B, Tanaka's formula yields that $|x + \sigma(z)B_t| = x + \sigma(z)\int_0^t \mathrm{sgn}(x + \sigma(z)B_s)\,dB_s + K_t$, where K is an increasing process supported by the set $\{s; x + \sigma(z)B_s = 0\}$. By Lévy's theorem, the martingale $\int_0^t \mathrm{sgn}(x + \sigma(z)B_s)\,dB_s$ is a Brownian motion. Thus, $(|x + \sigma(z)B|, K)$ also satisfies (4) and has the same law as $(\bar{X}^{(z)}(x), \bar{L}^{(z)}(x))$. In particular, we get that $\bar{X}_t^{(z)}$ admits the density

$$P(\bar{X}_t^{(z)}(x) \in A) = \int_A \bar{\pi}_t^{(z)}(x, x')\,dx',$$

where for $x, x' \ge 0$

$$\bar{\pi}_t^{(z)}(x, x') = \tilde{H}_0(x' - x, a(z)t) + \tilde{H}_0(x' + x, a(z)t). \tag{6}$$

Here, we use the following notation for Hermite-type functions

$$\tilde{H}_n(x, a) = \left(\frac{d}{dx}\right)^n \left[\frac{1}{\sqrt{2\pi a}} \exp(-\frac{x^2}{2a})\right]. \tag{7}$$

Using this notation, one has for $x, x' \ge 0$ and $i \in \mathbb{N}$ the following general formulas for the derivatives[4] of the density function $\bar{\pi}^{(z)}$:

$$\partial_{x'}^i \partial_x^j \bar{\pi}_t^{(z)}(x, x') = (-1)^j \tilde{H}_{i+j}(x' - x, a(z)t) + \tilde{H}_{i+j}(x' + x, a(z)t), \tag{8}$$
$$\partial_t^i \bar{\pi}_t^{(z)}(x, x') = 2^{-i} a(z)^i \partial_{x'}^{2i} \bar{\pi}_t^{(z)}(x, x') = 2^{-i} a(z)^i \partial_x^{2i} \bar{\pi}_t^{(z)}(x, x').$$

By using Hypothesis (H) and the following lemma is also known as the space-time inequality Lemma 2.1 below, we get the upper bound

$$\left|\partial_{x'}^i \partial_x^j \bar{\pi}_t^{(z)}(x, x')\right| \le C t^{-(i+j)/2} \left(\tilde{H}_0(x' - x, 2\bar{a}t) + \tilde{H}_0(x' + x, 2\bar{a}t)\right), \tag{9}$$

where $C > 0$ depends on $i, j, \bar{a}$, and $\underline{a}$ but is independent of t.

---

[4]By these properties, it may appear at first that the symmetry of the density $\bar{\pi}_t^{(z)}(x, x')$ with respect to the variables (x, x') is important, but in fact this is not the case. This can be seen if one considers the general case including a drift coefficient like in [20].

Lemma 2.1 *Let $n \in \mathbb{N}$ and $k \geq 0$ then there exists universal constants $C_{n,k}$ that do not depend on a such that for all $x \in \mathbb{R}$ and any $a > 0$,*

$$|x|^k |\tilde{H}_n(x, a)| \leq C_{n,k} a^{(k-n)/2} \tilde{H}_0(x, 2a). \tag{10}$$

Proof Let $\varphi(x) = e^{-x^2/2}$. We have $\tilde{H}_n(x, a) = \frac{1}{\sqrt{2\pi a} a^{n/2}} \varphi^{(n)}(\frac{x}{\sqrt{a}})$ and thus (10) with $C_{n,k} = \sqrt{2} \sup_{x \in \mathbb{R}} \left\{ |x|^k |\varphi^{(n)}(x)| \exp(\frac{x^2}{4}) \right\} < \infty$. $\square$

We define the approximating semigroup as

$$\bar{P}_t^{(z)} f(x) = E[f(\bar{X}_t^{(z)}(x))], \tag{11}$$

and denote by $\bar{\mathscr{L}}^{(z)} = \frac{a(z)}{2} \partial_x^2$ its generator. Recall that $\mathscr{D} = \{f \in C_b^2(\bar{D}): f'(0) = 0\}$. Note that the condition $f'(0) = 0$ is related to the Neumann condition of the partial differential equation associated to (1).

Lemma 2.2 *For $t > 0$, $z \geq 0$ we have that $\bar{\pi}_t^{(z)}(\cdot, \cdot) \in C_b^\infty(\bar{D} \times \bar{D})$ and $\partial_x \bar{\pi}_t^{(z)}(0, x') = 0$. For any bounded measurable function f, we have that $\bar{P}_t^{(z)} f \in \mathscr{D}$. Furthermore, for $f \in \mathscr{D}$, we have for $x \in \bar{D}$, $t > 0$,*

$$\lim_{h \to 0^+} \frac{1}{h} (\bar{P}_h^{(z)} f(x) - f(x)) = \bar{\mathscr{L}}^{(z)} f(x),$$

$$\partial_t \bar{P}_t^{(z)} f(x) = \bar{P}_t^{(z)} \bar{\mathscr{L}}^{(z)} f(x) = \bar{\mathscr{L}}^{(z)} \bar{P}_t^{(z)} f(x),$$

$$\lim_{h \to 0^+} \frac{1}{h} (P_h f(x) - f(x)) = \mathscr{L} f(x), \ \partial_t P_t f(x) = P_t \mathscr{L} f(x).$$

Proof The proof of the first part of the above statement follows from (8) by direct calculation.

Let $t \geq 0$, $h > 0$. Itô's formula for semimartingales yields that for $f \in \mathscr{D}$

$$f(X_{t+h}(x)) - f(X_t(x)) = \int_t^{t+h} \frac{a(X_s(x))}{2} f''(X_s(x)) ds + \int_t^{t+h} f'(X_s(x)) dL_s(x)$$

$$+ \int_t^{t+h} f'(X_s(x)) dW_s.$$

From $f'(0) = 0$ and (L3), we get $\int_t^{t+h} f'(X_s(x)) dL_s(x) = 0$. By taking the expectation, we get $P_{t+h} f(x) = P_t f(x) + \int_t^{t+h} P_s \mathscr{L} f(x) ds$, which gives the desired result since $s \mapsto P_s \mathscr{L} f(x) = \frac{1}{2} E[a(X_s(x)) f''(X_s(x))]$ is continuous. $\square$

3 The Backward Method

Through this section, we will assume that hypotheses (H) and (Hb) hold.

3.1 Presentation of the Backward Method

To start describing the backward method, we define the operator

$$\mathcal{P}_t f(x) = \int f(x') \bar{\pi}_t^{(x')}(x, x') dx'. \tag{12}$$

For $f \in M_b$, the function $x \mapsto \mathcal{P}_t f(x)$ is well defined and finite, and we have from (H) and (6) that $\|\mathcal{P}_t f\|_\infty \le \sqrt{\bar{a}/\underline{a}} \|f\|_\infty$. Besides, from (9) and Lebesgue's theorem, the partial derivatives $\partial_t^k \partial_x^l \mathcal{P}_t f(x) = \int f(x') \partial_t^k \partial_x^l \bar{\pi}_t^{(x')}(x, x') dx'$ are well defined and satisfy $|\partial_t^k \partial_x^l \mathcal{P}_t f(x)| \le Ct^{-(k+l/2)} \|f\|_\infty$, where $C > 0$ is a constant depending on $k, l, \bar{a}$, and $\underline{a}$. Using (8), we have

$$\forall t > 0, \mathcal{P}_t f \in \mathcal{D} \text{ and } \partial_t \mathcal{P}_t f(x) = \int f(x') \bar{\mathscr{L}}^{(x')} \bar{\pi}_t^{(x')}(\cdot, x')(x) dx'. \tag{13}$$

The operator $\mathcal{P}$ may look strange at first sight, and in general $x' \mapsto \bar{\pi}_t^{(x')}(x, x')$ is not a density function. However, one may interpret it as a "reversed" transition operator[5] and we have for f, g continuous with bounded support the duality formula:

$$\int g(x) \mathcal{P}_t f(x) dx = \int \bar{P}_t^{(x')} g(x') f(x') dx'.$$

Now we will define the operator which will measure the distance between the marginal law of the approximation and the marginal law of the solution of the reflected SDE. That is, we define

$$\mathcal{S}_t(f)(x) := (\mathscr{L} - \partial_t) \mathcal{P}_t f(x)$$

$$= \int f(x') (\mathscr{L} - \bar{\mathscr{L}}^{(x')}) \bar{\pi}_t^{(x')}(\cdot, x')(x) dx'.$$

In the formula above, we see that one applies the difference of the generators of the processes X and $\bar{X}_t^{(x')}$ to the "density" of the "reversed" approximating reflected SDE. Then one has that

$$\mathcal{S}_t(f)(x) = \int_0^\infty f(x') \theta_t^*(x, x') \bar{\pi}_t^{(x')}(x, x') dx' \tag{14}$$

$$\theta_t^*(x, x') = \frac{1}{2}(a(x) - a(x')) \partial_x^2 \bar{\pi}_t^{(x')}(x, x') (\bar{\pi}_t^{(x')}(x, x'))^{-1}, \quad \text{for } x, x' \ge 0.$$

Lemma 3.1 Let $f \in C_b^0(\bar{D})$ then $\lim_{t \downarrow 0} \mathcal{P}_t f(x) = f(x)$, $x \ge 0$.

---

[5]That is, through a proper renormalization one may say that $\bar{\pi}_t^{(x')}(x, x')$ is proportional to the density of a reflected Brownian motion at the point $x \ge 0$ which starts at x' with diffusion coefficient $\sigma(x')$.

Proof We will discuss the case $x > 0$, the case $x = 0$ follows similarly. From (6), we have

$$
\begin{aligned}
\mathcal{P}_t f(x) &= \int_0^\infty \frac{f(x')}{\sqrt{2\pi a(x')t}} \left[e^{-\frac{(x'-x)^2}{2a(x')t}} + e^{-\frac{(x'+x)^2}{2a(x')t}} \right] dx' \\
&= \int_{-\infty}^\infty \mathbf{1}(\xi \geq \frac{-x}{\sqrt{a(x)t}}) \frac{f(x(t,\xi))\sqrt{a(x)}}{\sqrt{2\pi a(x(t,\xi))}} \left[e^{-\frac{a(x)\xi^2}{2a(x(t,\xi))}} + e^{-\frac{(x(t,\xi)+x)^2}{2a(x(t,\xi))t}} \right] d\xi,
\end{aligned}
$$

by using the change of variable $x' = x + \sqrt{a(x)t}\xi =: x(t, \xi)$. The integrand is dominated by $2 \frac{\|f\|_\infty \sqrt{\bar{a}}}{\sqrt{2\pi \underline{a}}} e^{-\frac{\underline{a}\xi^2}{2\bar{a}}}$, which gives the claim by Lebesgue's theorem. □

The idea of the parametrix method is to obtain a Taylor expansion. As in the classical Taylor formula a first step toward obtaining it is the mean value theorem or the first-order Taylor formula with residue.

Lemma 3.2 *Let $f : \bar{D} \to \mathbb{R}$ be a measurable and bounded function. Then for any $0 < s < t < T$ we have that*

$$
E[\mathcal{P}_{T-t} f(X_t)] - E[\mathcal{P}_{T-s} f(X_s)] = \int_s^t E[\mathcal{S}_{T-u} f(X_u)] du. \tag{15}
$$

Proof Since $\mathcal{P}_t f(x) \in C^{1,2}((0, T] \times \bar{D})$, we can apply Itô's formula. The stochastic integral has a null expectation since $\partial_x \mathcal{P}_{T-u} f$ is bounded for $u \in [s, t]$, and we obtain (15) by using (13). □

Now we are getting close to the first-order expansion. In fact, for $t \uparrow T$, we have that $E[\mathcal{P}_{T-t} f(X_t)] \to E[f(X_T)]$ and for $s \downarrow 0$, we have that $E[\mathcal{P}_{T-s} f(X_s)] \to \mathcal{P}_T f(x)$ which is the approximation. Therefore, the right side of (15) represents the residue of first order for the Taylor formula.

In order for this argument to work, we need to repeat the previous arguments in order to show uniform integrability as $s \downarrow 0$ and $t \uparrow T$ of the integrand on the right side of (15). This will lead to obtain a linear relation which can be iterated as is the case in Taylor expansions.

Theorem 3.1 *Let (H) and (Hb) hold. Then, for $f \in M_b$ and $u > 0$, there exists a positive universal constant C independent of u, f, and x such that*

$$
|\mathcal{S}_u f(x)| \leq \frac{C\|f\|_\infty}{u^{1-\alpha/2}}. \tag{16}
$$

In particular, when $f \in C_b^0$, $|E[f(X_T)] - \mathcal{P}_T f(x)| \leq C\|f\|_\infty T^{\alpha/2}$ and we have

$$
E[f(X_T)] - \mathcal{P}_T f(x) = \int_0^T E[\mathcal{S}_{T-u} f(X_u)] du. \tag{17}
$$

Proof For $x, x' \geq 0$, we have

$$\left|(\mathscr{L} - \bar{\mathscr{L}}^{(x')})\bar{\pi}_u^{(x')}(\cdot, x')(x)\right| = \left|\frac{1}{2}(a(x) - a(x'))\left(\tilde{H}_2(x' - x, a(x')u) + \tilde{H}_2(x' + x, a(x')u)\right)\right|$$

$$\leq C|x - x'|^\alpha \left(\left|\tilde{H}_2(x' - x, a(x')u)\right| + \left|\tilde{H}_2(x' + x, a(x')u)\right|\right)$$

$$\leq \frac{C}{u^{1-\alpha/2}}\left(\tilde{H}_0(x' - x, 2\bar{a}u) + \tilde{H}_0(x' + x, 2\bar{a}u)\right), \tag{18}$$

by using Lemma 2.1 for the last inequality. This gives (16). Then, we use Lemma 3.1 to take limits on (15) when $s \downarrow 0$ and $t \uparrow T$ and get (17). □

Remark 1 We note that the above argument does not use the continuity of the operator P_t in $L^2(\bar{D})$ directly which is important if one wants to define the dual operator. This point is essential when using semigroup theory arguments. In fact, one may define $P_t: C_c^\infty(\bar{D}_K) \subseteq L^2(\bar{D}_K) \to L^2(\bar{D}_K)$ for $\bar{D}_K = \bar{D} \cap [0, K]$ with $P_t f(x) := E[f(X_t(x))]$. This assertion follows as $\int_{\bar{D}} g(x) P_t f(x) dx \leq \|f\|_\infty \|g\|_{L^1(\bar{D}_K)}$. Then the dual operator of P_t can be defined as an unbounded operator as well as its generator. Still, the actions of these operators on $C_c^\infty(\bar{D}_K)$ are well understood, and therefore proofs can be carried out. Once the proofs are obtained as in [2], then one may take the limit as $K \uparrow \infty$.

As stated previously, formula (15) is a first-order Taylor formula and now our goal is to iterate and eventually obtain an infinite-order Taylor expansion. In order to do this, there are two issues to tackle. The first is to prove that $\mathcal{S}_{T-u} f \in C_b^0$ in order to iterate the formula using the same procedure. Second, we need to obtain a bound for the iterations in order to be able to prove that the infinite sums converge and that the residue converges to zero. We do all this in the next lemma, for which we introduce the following notation:

- for (possibly non-commutative) operators A_j, $j = 1, \ldots, n$, we use the shorthand notation $\prod_{j=1}^n A_j := A_n \ldots A_1$,
- we denote by $\mathcal{E}_{\alpha,\beta}(z)$ the Mittag–Leffler function:

$$\mathcal{E}_{\alpha,\beta}(z) := \sum_{k=0}^\infty \frac{z^k}{\Gamma(\beta + \alpha k)}, \quad z \in \mathbb{C}, \ \alpha, \beta > 0,$$

- for $f: \bar{D} \to \mathbb{R}$ bounded measurable and $T > 0$, we define

$$\mathcal{I}_T^n f(x) = \int_0^T \cdots \int_0^{v_2} \mathcal{P}_{v_{n+1}-v_n} \prod_{j=0}^{n-1} \mathcal{S}_{v_{j+1}-v_j} f(x) dv_1 \ldots dv_n,$$

where $v_0 = 0$ and $v_{n+1} = T$.

Lemma 3.3 *For $f \in C_b^0(\bar{D})$, we have*

$$E[f(X_T)] = \sum_{i=0}^{\infty} \mathcal{I}_T^i f(x),$$

where the sum converges uniformly on $x \geq 0$ and on compact sets for T.

Proof Let $u_1 \in [0, T)$. The function $f_{T-u_1}^1 := \mathcal{S}_{T-u_1} f$ is bounded by Theorem 3.1 and continuous by (13) and (Hb). We can thus use the second result of Theorem 3.1 and get

$$E[f_{T-u_1}^1 (X_{u_1})] - \mathcal{P}_{u_1} f_{T-u_1}^1 (x) = \int_0^{u_1} E[\mathcal{S}_{u_1-u_2} f_{T-u_1}^1 (X_{u_2})] du_2.$$

Furthermore, the bounds obtained in Theorem 3.1 give

$$\left| \mathcal{S}_{u_1-u_2} f_{T-u_1}^1 (X_{u_2}) \right| \leq \frac{C \|f_{T-u_1}^1\|_\infty}{(u_1 - u_2)^{1-\alpha/2}} \leq \frac{C^2 \|f\|_\infty}{((T-u_1)(u_1-u_2))^{1-\alpha/2}}.$$

We therefore obtain from Theorem 3.1 that

$$E[f(X_T)] - \mathcal{P}_T f(x) = \int_0^T \mathcal{P}_{u_1} \mathcal{S}_{T-u_1} f(x) du_1$$

$$+ \int_0^T \int_0^{u_1} E[\mathcal{S}_{u_1-u_2} \mathcal{S}_{T-u_1} f(X_{u_2})] du_2 du_1.$$

This is a second-order Taylor expansion and the integrability of the second order is assured. The residue is bounded by

$$\int_0^T \int_0^u \frac{C^2 \|f\|_\infty}{((T-u_1)(u_1-u_2))^{1-\alpha/2}} du_2 du_1 = \frac{2C^2}{\alpha} \|f\|_\infty \int_0^T \frac{u^{\alpha/2}}{(T-u)^{1-\alpha/2}} du$$

$$= \frac{2C^2}{\alpha} \|f\|_\infty T^\alpha B(1 + \alpha/2, \alpha/2),$$

where $B(a, b) := \int_0^1 u^{a-1}(1-u)^{b-1} du = \frac{\Gamma(a)\Gamma(b)}{\Gamma(a+b)}$ denotes the Beta function. By repeating the argument iteratively and by using the change of variables $v_i = T - u_i$, we get that

$$E[f(X_T)] = \sum_{i=0}^{n-1} \mathcal{I}_T^i f(x) + R_n(T, x)$$

$$R_n(T, x) := \int_0^T \cdots \int_0^{u_{n-1}} E\left[\prod_{j=0}^{n-1} \mathcal{S}_{u_j-u_{j+1}} f(X_{u_n}) \right] du_n \dots du_1.$$

Furthermore, the following estimates are satisfied for $n = 1, \ldots$

$$|\mathcal{I}_T^n f(x)| + |R_n f(T, x)| \leq \frac{C^n \|f\|_\infty T^{n\alpha/2}}{\Gamma(1 + n\alpha/2)}. \tag{19}$$

We get $\sum_{i=0}^\infty \|\mathcal{I}_T^i f\|_\infty \leq \|f\|_\infty \mathcal{E}_{\alpha/2,1}(CT^{\alpha/2})$, which gives the claim. $\qquad \square$

Before continuing into the main theoretical results, we will give now the probabilistic representation.

The interpretation of the argument presented here should be clear. In fact, when proving a first-order Taylor expansion formula for a smooth function f, one usually defines $g(\alpha) = f(x + \alpha(y - x))$, $\alpha \in [0, 1]$, then one obtains

$$f(y) - f(x) = g(1) - g(0) = \int_0^1 g'(s)ds = \int_0^1 f'(x + \alpha(y - x))(y - x)ds.$$

The same heuristic argument has been applied before. In fact, formula (15) is the equivalent to the above formula. The derivative concept above now becomes $\mathcal{L} - \bar{\mathcal{L}}^{(x')}$ in the definition of the difference operator S which at the same time measures the distance between the reflected stochastic differential equation and its approximation.

3.2 The Backward Simulation Method

To clarify how the probabilistic representation will be obtained, let us do first the representation for $\mathcal{I}^1$. We have

$$\mathcal{I}_t^1(f)(x) = \int_0^t du_1 \mathcal{P}_{u_1} \mathcal{S}_{t-u_1}(f)(x)$$

$$= \int_0^t du_1 \int f(y_2) \theta_{t-u_1}^*(y, y_2) \bar{\pi}_{t-u_1}^{(y_2)}(y_2, y) \bar{\pi}_{u_1}^{(y)}(y, x) dy dy_2.$$

Note that in the above expression, we have used the symmetry of the density $\bar{\pi}^{(z)}$ in the space arguments. Now suppose for simplicity that f is a density function. Then the probabilistic kernels $f(y_2)\bar{\pi}_{t-u_1}^{(y_2)}(y_2, y)\bar{\pi}_{u_1}^{(y)}(y, x)dy_2dy$ can be interpreted as a Markov chain which starts from a point $\overline{X}_0$ randomly chosen using the density f and whose transitions are obtained following the density $y_2 \to \bar{\pi}_{t-u_1}^{(y_2)}(y_2, \overline{X}_0)$ which is finally evaluated at the function $y \to \bar{\pi}_{u_1}^{(y)}(y, x)$.[6] Adding a Poisson process N with parameter λ and the random jump times τ_j, $j \in \mathbb{N}$, gives the following simulation

---

[6] When f is not a density function, one has to draw the initial point according to some density funtion q_0 and then multiply by the well-defined weight $\frac{f(y_2)}{q_0(y_2)}$. That is, we apply an importance sampling method.

method. Let $\Theta^*(t, x, y) = \theta_t^*(x, y)$ as in (14) and let us suppose that f is a density function. Therefore, we have the following result.

Theorem 3.2 *Let $f \colon \bar{D} \to \mathbb{R}_+$ be a continuous and bounded density function. Suppose that the assumptions (H) and (Hb) are satisfied. Then*

$$E[f(X_T(x))] = E\left[\bar{\pi}_{T-\tau_{N_T}}^{\bar{X}_{\tau_{N_T}}}(x, \bar{X}_{\tau_{N_T}})M_T\right], \tag{20}$$

$$M_T := e^{\lambda T} \lambda^{-N_T} \prod_{j=0}^{N_T-1} \Theta^*(\tau_{j+1} - \tau_j, \bar{X}_{\tau_{j+1}}, \bar{X}_{\tau_j}). \tag{21}$$

The above product is interpreted as being equal to 1 if $N_T = 0$. Furthermore, $E[|M_T|] < \infty$.

The result on the finiteness of the first moment of M_T can be achieved using the space-time inequalities like it was done in the proof of Lemma 3.3. In fact, $E[|M_T|] = \sum_{i=0}^{\infty} |\mathcal{I}_T^i g(x)|$ with $g = 1$, which is smaller than $\mathcal{E}_{\alpha/2,1}(CT^{\alpha/2})$ by using the bound just after (19).

From the above interpretation, one sees that the simulation method goes backward with respect to the dynamics of X.

Simulation method

1. Let $\tau_0 = 0$, $\Lambda_0 = 1$, and $\bar{X}_0$ be a random variable with density function f.
   For $i = 0, 1, \ldots$, perform the following steps:
2. Simulate an exponential random variable E_{i+1} with parameter λ and set $\tau_{i+1} = \tau_i + E_{i+1}$.
3. If $\tau_{i+1} > T$, go to step 6. Otherwise continue with 4.
4. Compute $\bar{X}_{\tau_{i+1}} = Z_{\tau_{i+1}-\tau_i}^{i+1}(\bar{X}_{\tau_i})$ where Z^{i+1} is computed using the simulation method given in Lépingle [16]. That is,

$$Z_{\tau_{i+1}-\tau_i}^{i+1}(\bar{X}_{\tau_i}) = \bar{X}_{\tau_i} + \sigma(\bar{X}_{\tau_i})G_{i+1}\sqrt{\tau_{i+1} - \tau_i} + \max\{0, -\bar{X}_{\tau_i} + Y_i\}$$

$$Y_i = \frac{1}{2}\left\{-\sigma(\bar{X}_{\tau_i})G_{i+1}\sqrt{\tau_{i+1} - \tau_i} + \left(a(\bar{X}_{\tau_i})V_{i+1} + a(\bar{X}_{\tau_i})G_{i+1}^2(\tau_{i+1} - \tau_i)\right)^{1/2}\right\}.$$

Here G_{i+1} is a standard Gaussian random variable and V_{i+1} is an exponential random variable with parameter $(2(\tau_{i+1} - \tau_i))^{-1}$.

5. Next one computes $\Lambda_{i+1} = \Lambda_i \Theta^*(\tau_{i+1} - \tau_i, \bar{X}_{\tau_{i+1}}, \bar{X}_{\tau_i})$. Go back to 2.
6. The final simulation value is

$$S = e^{\lambda T} \lambda^{-N_T} \bar{\pi}_{T-\tau_{N_T}}^{\bar{X}_{\tau_{N_T}}}(x, \bar{X}_{\tau_{N_T}})\Lambda_{N_T}.$$

Here, $N_T = \max\{i; \tau_i < T\}$. Finally, repeat steps 1–6 as many times as the Monte Carlo simulation requires and take the average.

Remark 2 The simulation method based on (20) assumes that f is a density function which generates the random starting point of the reflected Euler scheme. Heuristically, the appearance of the kernel function $\bar{\pi}_{T-\tau_{N_T}}^{\overline{X}_{\tau_{N_T}}}(x, \overline{X}_{\tau_{N_T}})$ measures how close is the final point of the simulation to the starting point x of the reflected stochastic differential equation X. In this sense, this method uses an approximation to a reflected diffusion bridge. For this reason, its performance may strongly depend on the point x.

Finally, we can take limits in the above formula to obtain the final result for this section, which completes the backward formulation.

Theorem 3.3 *Let $f \in \mathcal{M}_b(\bar{D})$ then*

$$E[f(X_T)] = \sum_{i=0}^{\infty} \mathcal{I}_T^i f(x). \tag{22}$$

Furthermore, $P_T f \in \mathcal{D}$, $\partial_t P_t f(x) = \mathcal{L} P_t f(x)$, and the density of X_T, denoted by $p_T(x, y)$, exists and it belongs to the space $C^{0,2}((0, T] \times \bar{D})$ as a function of (T, x). Besides, it satisfies the boundary condition $\partial_x p_T(0, y) = 0$. Its probabilistic representation for its density $p_T(x, y)$ is given by (20) for $\bar{X}_0 = y$. In analytical terms, one has

$$p_T(x, y) = \bar{\pi}_T^{(y)}(x, y) + \sum_{i=1}^{\infty} \mathcal{I}_T^i \delta_y(x) \tag{23}$$

$$\mathcal{I}_T^n \delta_y(x) := \int_0^T \cdots \int_0^{v_2} \mathcal{P}_{v_{n+1}-v_n} \prod_{j=0}^{n-1} \mathcal{S}_{v_{j+1}-v_j} \delta_y(x) dv_1 ... dv_n,$$

$$S_t(\delta_y)(x) := \theta_t^*(x, y) \bar{\pi}_t^{(y)}(x, y). \tag{24}$$

In the above definition of $\mathcal{I}_T^n \delta_y(x)$, we use δ_y to make it reminiscent of the Dirac delta distribution function. For the unexperienced reader, $\mathcal{I}_T^n \delta_y(x)$ should just be interpreted as the definition of a function which depends on (T, x, y) and the parameter n. A similar remark applies for $S_t(\delta_y)(x)$.

Note that in particular, the above results imply that $\partial_t P_t f(x) = \mathcal{L} P_t f(x)$ which complements the results in Lemma 3.1. Furthermore, the simulation method previously described can also be generalized for $f \in \mathcal{M}_b(\bar{D})$.

Proof The extension to functions $f \in \mathcal{M}_b(\bar{D})$ is obtained by a direct application of the functional monotone theorem.

The result on the density is a particular case of Theorem 3.3 of [20] (see Friedman [6], Chap. 1 for a general description of the parametrix method). Here, we just give a brief idea of its proof. First one shows that the expansion (23) holds. To do so, we consider the transition density $\hat{\pi}_t(x, y) = \tilde{H}_0(y - x, 2\bar{a}t) + \tilde{H}_0(y + x, 2\bar{a}t)$, for $x, y \geq 0$, and show by induction on n that[7]

---

[7]Note that the operator $\mathcal{L} - \tilde{\mathcal{L}}$ is applied to the variable x.

$$|(\mathscr{L} - \bar{\mathscr{L}})\mathcal{I}_T^n \delta_y(\cdot)(x)| \leq \frac{C^{n+1}\Gamma(\alpha/2)^{(n+1)}T^{(n+1)\alpha/2-1}}{\Gamma((n+1)\alpha/2)}\hat{\pi}_T(x, y),$$

$$(\mathscr{L} - \bar{\mathscr{L}})\mathcal{I}_T^n \delta_y(\cdot)(x) := \int_0^T \cdots \int_0^{v_2} \mathcal{S}_{v_{n+1}-v_n} \prod_{j=0}^{n-1} \mathcal{S}_{v_{j+1}-v_j}\delta_y(x)dv_1 \ldots dv_n.$$

Note that for $n = 0$, we have $|(\mathscr{L} - \bar{\mathscr{L}}^{(y)})\bar{\pi}_T^{(y)}(\cdot, y)(x)| \leq CT^{\alpha/2-1}\hat{\pi}_T(x, y)$ from (18) for a constant C depending on $\underline{a}$ and $\bar{a}$, α and the Hölder constant of a. Now, we suppose that the induction hypothesis is true for $n - 1$, and we use the formula

$$\mathcal{I}_T^n \delta_y(x) = \int_0^T \int_0^\infty (\mathscr{L} - \bar{\mathscr{L}})\mathcal{I}_v^{n-1}\delta_y(\cdot)(z)\bar{\pi}_{T-v}^{(z)}(x, z)dzdv \qquad (25)$$

which gives

$$(\mathscr{L} - \bar{\mathscr{L}})\mathcal{I}_T^n \delta_y(\cdot)(x) = \int_0^T \int_0^\infty (\mathscr{L} - \bar{\mathscr{L}})\mathcal{I}_v^{n-1}\delta_y(\cdot)(z)\frac{1}{2}(a(x) - a(z))\partial_x^2\bar{\pi}_{T-v}^{(z)}(x, z)dzdv.$$

This yields

$$|(\mathscr{L} - \bar{\mathscr{L}})\mathcal{I}_T^n \delta_y(\cdot)(x)| \leq \int_0^T \int_0^\infty \frac{C^n\Gamma(\alpha/2)^n v^{n\alpha/2-1}}{\Gamma(n\alpha/2)}\hat{\pi}_v(z, y)Cv^{\alpha/2-1}\hat{\pi}_{T-v}(x, z)dzdx$$

$$= \frac{C^{n+1}\Gamma(\alpha/2)^{(n+1)}T^{(n+1)\alpha/2-1}}{\Gamma((n+1)\alpha/2)}\hat{\pi}_T(x, y).$$

From (25) and $|\bar{\pi}_t^{(y)}(x, y)| \leq C\hat{\pi}_t(x, y)$, we deduce for $n \geq 1$

$$|\mathcal{I}_T^n \delta_y(x)| \leq C\frac{C^n\Gamma(\alpha/2)^n T^{n\alpha/2}}{\Gamma(n\alpha/2)n\alpha/2}\hat{\pi}_T(x, y).$$

Therefore, the series (23) converges absolutely and therefore it corresponds to the density of the random variable in (22) by exchange of summations and integral. Proving that $P_T f \in \mathscr{D}$ and that $p_T(x, y)$ is differentiable with respect to (T, x) has many points in common and it follows the same arguments as in [6]. The argument being long, we do not detail it here. We just remark that the proof of existence of the first derivative in x is done by differentiating each term $\mathcal{I}_T^n \delta_y(x)$ and proving the uniform convergence of the infinite sum which gives explicit upper bounds for the density derivatives which prove the boundedness of $\partial_x P_t f(x)$. For the second derivative, one has to use the Hölder property of the function $\left((\mathscr{L} - \bar{\mathscr{L}}) \prod_{j=2}^n P_{v_{j+1}-v_j}(\mathscr{L} - \bar{\mathscr{L}})\right)\bar{\pi}_{v_1}^{(y)}(\cdot, y)(\cdot)$ and one obtains similar results as for the first derivatives. Note that the fact that $\partial_x \mathcal{I}_T^n \delta_y(0) = 0$ follows readily from a similar property satisfied by $\partial_x \bar{\pi}_{T-v}^{(z)}(x, z)|_{x=0} = 0$.

Finally, note that $\lim_{h\to 0+} \frac{P_h(P_t f)(x) - P_t f(x)}{h} = \mathcal{L}P_t f(x)$, followed by Lemma 2.2 as $P_t f \in \mathscr{D}$. $\qquad \square$

Note that one can also prove that corresponding heat equation $\partial_t p_t(x, y) = \frac{1}{2}a(x)\partial_x^2 p_t(x, y)$ for $(t, x) \in (0, T] \times \bar{D}$ with $\lim_{t \to 0^+} p_t(x, \cdot) = \delta_x(\cdot)$ is satisfied but we do not discuss this here.

4 The Forward Method

Throughout this section, we will assume that hypotheses (Hf) and (H) hold.

4.1 Presentation of the Forward Method

We define the approximating semigroup as

$$\bar{P}_t^{(x)} f(x) = E[f(\bar{X}_t^{(x)}(x))], \tag{26}$$

and note that $\bar{\mathscr{L}}^{(x)}$ is its generator.

We remark that Theorem 3.3 proves that for any $t > 0$ and $f \in \mathcal{M}_b$ then $P_t f \in \mathscr{D}$. Therefore, $\partial_t P_t f(x) = \mathscr{L} P_t f(x)$ and $\partial_t \bar{P}_t^{(z)} f(x) = \bar{\mathscr{L}}^{(z)} \bar{P}_t^{(z)} f(x)$ are also satisfied for $f \in \mathcal{M}_b$. This will be used in what follows. Now, we present the arguments in order to expand $P_T f(x)$ using the parametrix method. We will use the following shorthand notation

$$\bar{\pi}_t(x, x') \equiv \bar{\pi}_t^{(x)}(x, x') \text{ and } \bar{P}_t f(x) = \bar{P}_t^{(x)} f(x).$$

We will proceed in a series of steps in order to make clear to the reader the problems involved in developing the parametrix method.

Lemma 4.1 *Let $f \in \mathcal{M}_b(\bar{D})$ then we have*

$$P_T f(x) - \bar{P}_T^{(x)} f(x) = \int_0^T \int_{\bar{D}} P_{T-s} f(x')(\theta_s(x, x')\bar{\pi}_s(x, x')dx' + \hat{\theta}_s(x)\delta_0(dx'))ds, \tag{27}$$

where $\delta_0(dx')$ denotes the point mass measure at zero and the functions $\theta_t: \bar{D}^2 \to \mathbb{R}$ and $\hat{\theta}_t: \bar{D} \to \mathbb{R}$, $t > 0$ are defined by

$$\theta_t(x, x')\bar{\pi}_t(x, x') = \frac{1}{2}\partial_{x'}^2\left(\bar{\pi}_t(x, x')[a(x') - a(x)]\right),$$

$$\hat{\theta}_t(x) = \bar{\pi}_t(x, 0)\frac{a'(0)}{2}.$$

Furthermore, the following estimates are satisfied for $x, x' \in \bar{D}$ $t > 0$

$$|\theta_t(x, x')|\bar{\pi}_t(x, x') \le C \left\{ 1 + \frac{1}{\sqrt{t}} \right\} \tilde{H}_0(x - x', 2\bar{a}t), \tag{28}$$

$$|\hat{\theta}_t(x)| \le C\bar{\pi}_t(x, 0). \tag{29}$$

Here, C is a constant which depends on the upper and lower bounds for a and its first derivative at $x = 0$.

As the similar result in the backward case (see Lemma 3.2), this result can be heuristically interpreted as a first-order Taylor expansion. To explain this, note that the left side of (27) measures the difference between the semigroup $P_t f(x) = E[f(X_t(x))]$ and its parametrix (or approximation) $\bar{P}_t^{(x)} f(x) = E[f(\bar{X}_t^{(x)}(x))]$. The right-hand side of (27) is the residue of first order (or mean value theorem) which is a "middle" point between these two semigroups. The weight functions θ and $\hat{\theta}$ represent the derivatives in the Taylor expansion.

Proof The proof follows the same arguments as in [2] except that in this case one has boundary terms. In fact, first note that due to the results in Lemma 2.2 and Theorem 3.3, we have $-\partial_t (\bar{P}_t^{(x)} P_{T-t} f)(x) = \bar{P}_t^{(x)} (\mathscr{L} - \bar{\mathscr{L}}^{(x)}) P_{T-t} f(x)$ for $t \in [0, T)$. In fact, this follows because the generators of P and $\bar{P}^{(x)}$ are well defined on $\mathscr{D}$ and $P_{T-t} f \in \mathscr{D}$ (see Theorem 3.3). Next, by the definition of $\bar{P}^{(x)}$ and (6), we have that

$$\bar{P}_t^{(x)} (\mathscr{L} - \bar{\mathscr{L}}^{(x)}) P_{T-t} f(x) = \frac{1}{2} \int_0^\infty \bar{\pi}_t(x, x')(a(x') - a(x))\partial_{x'}^2 P_{T-t} f(x')dx'.$$

Using Lemma 2.2, we apply the integration by parts formula twice and using the fact that $\partial_{x'} P_t f(0) = \partial_{x'} \bar{\pi}_t(x, 0) = 0$ and (8) for $i = 1, 2$, $j = 0$ we obtain

$$\bar{P}_t^{(x)} (\mathscr{L} - \bar{\mathscr{L}}^{(x)}) P_{T-t} f(x) = \frac{1}{2} \bar{\pi}_t(x, x')(a(x') - a(x))\partial_{x'} P_{T-t} f(x')\Big|_{x'=0}^\infty$$

$$- \frac{1}{2} \int_{\bar{D}} \partial_{x'}(\bar{\pi}_t(x, x')(a(x') - a(x)))\partial_{x'} P_{T-t} f(x')dx'$$

$$= -\frac{1}{2} \partial_{x'}(\bar{\pi}_t(x, x')(a(x') - a(x))) P_{T-t} f(x')\Big|_{x'=0}^\infty$$

$$+ \int_{\bar{D}} P_{T-t} f(x')\theta_t(x, x')\bar{\pi}_t(x, x')dx'.$$

This finally gives

$$\bar{P}_t^{(x)} (\mathscr{L} - \bar{\mathscr{L}}^{(x)}) P_{T-t} f(x) = \int_{\bar{D}} P_{T-t} f(x')(\theta_t(x, x')\bar{\pi}_t(x, x')dx' + \hat{\theta}_t(x)\delta_0(dx')). \tag{30}$$

In order to finish the proof, one needs to use that

$$P_T f(x) - \bar{P}_T^{(x)} f(x) = \int_0^T -\partial_t (\bar{P}_t^{(x)} P_{T-t} f)(x) dt.$$

In order for the above to be satisfied, one needs to prove the integrability of the integrand. In fact, the integrand (30) is continuous and bounded for $t \in (\epsilon, T]$ for any fixed $\epsilon \in (0, T)$. The main problem is when ϵ tends to zero. Therefore, we need to find upper bounds for the integrand in (30). These are stated in (28) and (29) which we prove next.

The bound (29) is obvious, so we focus on proving (28). To do so, we need to bound each of the following terms:

$$\theta_t(x, x') \bar{\pi}_t(x, x') = \frac{1}{2} \partial_{x'}^2 \bar{\pi}_t(x, x') [a(x') - a(x)] + \partial_{x'} \bar{\pi}_t(x, x') a'(x') + \frac{1}{2} \bar{\pi}_t(x, x') a''(x').$$
(31)

We explain how to treat the first term in detail. Using (8) for $i = 0$, $j = 1, 2$, (Hf), the inequality $|x' - x| \le x + x'$ for $x, x' \in \bar{D}$, and the space-time inequality, we have

$$|\partial_{x'}^2 \bar{\pi}_t(x, x') [a(x') - a(x)]| \tag{32}$$
$$\le \|a'\|_\infty |x' - x| (|\tilde{H}_2(x - x', a(x)t)| + |\tilde{H}_2(x + x', a(x)t)|) \tag{33}$$
$$\le \|a'\|_\infty (|x' - x| |\tilde{H}_2(x - x', a(x)t)| + (x + x') |\tilde{H}_2(x + x', a(x)t)|)$$
$$\le C \frac{\|a'\|_\infty}{\sqrt{t a(x)}} \tilde{H}_0(x - x', 2a(x)t) \le \frac{C}{\sqrt{t}} \tilde{H}_0(x - x', 2\bar{a}t).$$

The two other terms in (31) can be handled similarly, which yields (28).

With this estimate, we see that the degeneration of the integrand on the right-hand side of (30) is of the order $O(t^{-1/2})$ as $t \downarrow 0$ which is therefore integrable.

In a final note, one also needs to prove that $\lim_{\epsilon \to 0} \bar{P}_{T-\epsilon}^{(x)} P_\epsilon f(x) = \bar{P}_T^{(x)} f(x)$. This is done using Fubini's theorem. The other convergence $\lim_{\epsilon \to 0} \bar{P}_\epsilon^{(x)} P_{T-\epsilon} f(x) = P_T f(x)$ is also proved easily. $\qquad \square$

Remark 3 Note that the rate $O(t^{-1/2})$ follows from the fact that a is a Lipschitz bounded function.

In order to obtain a higher order expansion and eventually an infinite-order expansion, we need to introduce the operator S_t, $t > 0$ for any measurable and bounded function $g: \bar{D} \to \mathbb{R}$ by

$$S_t g(x) = \int_{\bar{D}} g(x') (\theta_t(x, x') \bar{\pi}_t(x, x') dx' + \hat{\theta}_t(x) \delta_0(dx')).$$

With this definition, we can write the first-order expansion of $P_T f$ as

$$P_T f(x) = \bar{P}_T^{(x)} f(x) + \int_0^T S_t P_{T-t} f(x) dt. \tag{34}$$

The iteration of this formula gives the main result for the forward parametrix approach.

Theorem 4.1 *For $f \in M_b(\bar{D})$, define for $x \in \bar{D}$, $t > 0$*

$$I_t^0(f)(x) = \bar{P}_t^{(x)} f(x)$$

and recursively for $n \geq 1$

$$I_t^n(f)(x) = \int_0^t S_s I_{t-s}^{n-1}(f)(x) \, ds.$$

Then we have

$$P_t f(x) = \sum_{n=0}^{\infty} I_t^n(f)(x),$$

where the sum converges uniformly for $x \geq 0$ and t in compact intervals in $\mathbb{R}_+$.

Proof Using (28) and (29), we have

$$\exists C > 0, \forall t > 0, \ \|S_t g\|_\infty \leq C \frac{\|g\|_\infty}{\sqrt{t}} \tag{35}$$

for any function $g \in M_b(\bar{D})$. Here, the constant C is independent of t and g. With all these estimates one obtains the finiteness of the integral in (34) and therefore (34) is satisfied.

Note that the above terms are integrable due to (35). Now, we repeat the arguments already used in [2] (see Sect. 3: A functional linear equation). In fact, from the iteration of (34), one obtains

$$P_t f(x) = \bar{P}_t f(x) + \int_0^t S_{t-s_1} P_{s_1} f(x) \, ds_1$$

$$= I_t^0(f)(x) + \int_0^t S_{t-s_1} \left(\bar{P}_{s_1} f(x) + \int_0^{s_1} S_{s_1-s_2} P_{s_2} f(x) \, ds_2 \right) ds_1$$

$$= I_t^0(f)(x) + \int_0^t S_{t-s_1} I_{s_1}^0(f)(x) \, ds_1 + \int_0^t \int_0^{s_1} S_{t-s_1} S_{s_1-s_2} P_{s_2} f(x) \, ds_2 \, ds_1.$$

By repeating this procedure, we obtain

$$P_t f(x) = \sum_{n=0}^{N} I_t^n(f)(x) + R_t^N(f)(x),$$

with

$$R_t^N(f)(x) = \int_0^t \int_0^{s_1} \cdots \int_0^{s_N} \left(\prod_{j=0}^{N} S_{s_{N-j}-s_{N-j+1}} \right) P_{s_{N+1}} f(x) ds_{N+1} \ldots ds_1.$$

All we have to do is to show that

$$\lim_{N \to \infty} \| R_t^N(f)(\cdot) \|_\infty = 0.$$

By (35), we have

$$\| R_t^{N-1}(f) \|_\infty \leq \int_0^t \int_0^{s_1} \cdots \int_0^{s_{N-1}} \left\| \left(\prod_{j=1}^{N} S_{s_{N-j}-s_{N-j+1}} \right) P_{s_N} f(\cdot) \right\|_\infty ds_N \cdots ds_1$$

$$\leq C \int_0^t \int_0^{s_1} \cdots \int_0^{s_{N-1}} (t-s_1)^{-\frac{1}{2}} \left\| \left(\prod_{j=1}^{N-1} S_{s_{N-j}-s_{N-j+1}} \right) P_{s_N} f(\cdot) \right\|_\infty ds_N \cdots ds_1$$

$$\vdots$$

$$\leq C^N \int_0^t \int_0^{s_1} \cdots \int_0^{s_{N-1}} \prod_{i=0}^{N-1} (s_i - s_{i+1})^{-\frac{1}{2}} \| P_{s_N} f \|_\infty ds_N \cdots ds_1$$

$$\leq C^N \| f \|_\infty \int_0^t \int_0^{s_1} \cdots \int_0^{s_{N-1}} \prod_{i=0}^{N-1} (s_i - s_{i+1})^{-\frac{1}{2}} ds_N \cdots ds_1,$$

where we put $s_0 = t$ and we have used that $\| P_t f \|_\infty \leq \| f \|_\infty$. Using the result (its proof can be carried out by induction on N), we obtain for $N \in \mathbb{N}$

$$\int_0^t \int_0^{s_1} \cdots \int_0^{s_{N-1}} \prod_{i=0}^{N-1} (s_i - s_{i+1})^{-\frac{1}{2}} ds_N \cdots ds_1 = t^{\frac{N}{2}} \frac{\Gamma^N(\frac{1}{2})}{\Gamma(\frac{N+2}{2})},$$

which yields to $\| R_t^N(f) \|_\infty \to 0$ for any $t > 0$.

Remark 4 Note that we have the following bound for I^n:

$$\| I_t^n(f) \|_\infty \leq C^n \frac{\| f \|_\infty t^{n/2}}{\Gamma(n/2 + 1)}, \quad t > 0.$$

Again, this bound is reminiscent of the bounds for Taylor expansions.

4.2 The Forward Simulation Method

In this section, we will give a probabilistic representation formula for $I_T^n(f)$ which may be used for simulation.

We first have $I_T^0(f)(x) = \bar{P}_T f(x) = E[f(\bar{X}_T^{(x)}(x))]$. To understand the procedure we will follow, we give now the interpretation for $n = 1$ in detail. In order to do this, we introduce the general flow notation for the reflected approximation for $t \geq s$

$$Z_t(s, x) := x + \sigma(x) \cdot (B_t - B_s) + \bar{L}_t(s, x).$$

Define U_i as a sequence of i.i.d. random variables with Bernoulli law of parameter $p \in (0, 1)$ independent of B. We let $\overline{X}_0 = x$ and we define $\overline{X}_{t_1} := U_1 Z_{t_1}(0, \overline{X}_0)$. The additional random variables to be used in the probabilistic representation are defined as

$$\Theta_i(t, x, x') := (1 - p)^{-1} \hat{\theta}_t(x)(1 - U_{i+1}) + p^{-1} \theta_t(x, x') U_{i+1} \mathbf{1}_{x' > 0}.$$

Then one can check that for $f : \bar{D} \to \mathbb{R}$, measurable and bounded,

$$E[\Theta_0(t_1, x, \overline{X}_{t_1}) f(\overline{X}_{t_1})]$$
$$= \int_{\bar{D}} f(x_1) \left(\theta_{t_1}(x, x_1) \bar{\pi}_{t_1}(x, x_1) dx_1 + \hat{\theta}_{t_1}(x) \delta_0(dx_1) \right)$$
$$= S_{t_1} f(x).$$

To obtain the probabilistic representation for $I_T^1 f(\overline{X}_0)$, we define $\overline{X}_T = Z_T(t_1, \overline{X}_{t_1})$. Then

$$E[\Theta_0(t_1, x, \overline{X}_{t_1}) f(\overline{X}_T)] = E[\Theta_0(t_1, x, \overline{X}_{t_1}) \bar{P}_{T-t_1} f(\overline{X}_{t_1})] = S_{t_1} \bar{P}_{T-t_1} f(x). \quad (36)$$

Note that the estimates in (28) and (29) give the integrability of the random variable $\Theta_0(t_1, x, \overline{X}_{t_1}) f(\overline{X}_T)$ for any bounded measurable function f and $t \in (0, T]$. If τ_1 denotes a uniform random variable on the interval $[0, T]$ which is independent of all previously defined random variables and processes, then we have that

$$E[\Theta_0(\tau_1, x, \overline{X}_{\tau_1}) f(\overline{X}_T)] = T^{-1} I_T^1 f(\overline{X}_0).$$

One can further link the r.v. τ_1 with a Poisson process if one notes that if a Poisson process has jumped only once in the interval $[0, T]$ then the jump time is distributed as a uniform r.v. in $[0, T]$. We will use this in the general case.

Now to deal with the general case for $n \geq 1$, we have $I_T^n(f) = \int_0^T S_{T-u_n} I_{u_n}^{n-1}$ $(f) du_n$, which gives

$$I_T^n(f) = \int_{0 < u_1 < \cdots < u_n < T} S_{T-u_n} \cdots S_{u_2 - u_1} \bar{P}_{u_1} f \, du_1 \ldots du_n$$

$$= \int_{0 < t_1 < \cdots < t_n < T} S_{t_1} \cdots S_{t_n - t_{n-1}} \bar{P}_{T - t_n} f \, dt_1 \ldots dt_n, \tag{37}$$

by setting $t_i = T - u_{n+1-i}$, and observing that $0 < u_1 < \cdots < u_n < T$ if and only if $0 < t_1 < \cdots < t_n < T$.

Define the partition $\Delta : 0 = t_0 < t_1 < \cdots < t_n < t_{n+1} = T$. Generalizing the previous definitions, we have that for $n \in \mathbb{N}^*$, one defines the random variables $\overline{X}_{t_{i+1}} := U_{i+1} Z_{t_{i+1}}(t_i, \overline{X}_{t_i})$ for $i \in \{1, \ldots, n\}$ and $\overline{X}_T := Z_{t_{n+1}}(t_n, \overline{X}_{t_n})$. With these definitions, we get from (36) the following probabilistic representation:

$$\left(\prod_{j=1}^{n} S_{t_{n-j+1} - t_{n-j}} \right) \bar{P}_{T - t_n} f(x) = E \left[f(\overline{X}_T) \prod_{j=0}^{n-1} \Theta_j (t_{j+1} - t_j, \overline{X}_{t_j}, \overline{X}_{t_{j+1}}) \right]. \tag{38}$$

In order to interpret the time integrals in (37), let us consider a Poisson process $\{N_t; t \in [0, T]\}$ of parameter λ with jump times given by $\{0 = \tau_0 < \cdots < \tau_{N_T} \leq T\}$ independent of all previously defined random variables and stochastic processes. Then, we define $\overline{X}_{\tau_{i+1}} := U_{i+1} Z_{\tau_{i+1}}(\tau_i, \overline{X}_{\tau_i})$ for $0 \leq i \leq n - 1$ and $\overline{X}_T := Z_T(\tau_{N_T}, \overline{X}_{\tau_{N_T}})$. Then we have the following lemma.

Theorem 4.2 *Let $f : \bar{D} \to \mathbb{R}$ be a measurable and bounded function. Suppose that the assumptions (Hf) and (H) are satisfied. Then*

$$E[f(X_T)] = E \left[f(\overline{X}_T) M_T \right], \tag{39}$$

$$M_T := e^{\lambda T} \lambda^{-N_T} \prod_{j=0}^{N_T - 1} \Theta_j (\tau_{j+1} - \tau_j, \overline{X}_{\tau_j}, \overline{X}_{\tau_{j+1}}). \tag{40}$$

The above product is interpreted as being equal to 1 if $N_T = 0$. Furthermore, $E[M_T] = 1$ and $E[|M_T|] < \infty$.

Proof The claim is a consequence of (37), (38) and Theorem 4.1, since we have

$$E \left[f(\overline{X}_T) \lambda^{-N_T} \prod_{j=0}^{N_T - 1} \Theta_j (\tau_{j+1} - \tau_j, \overline{X}_{\tau_j}, \overline{X}_{\tau_{j+1}}) \,\middle|\, N_T = n \right]$$

$$= \frac{n!}{(\lambda T)^n} \int_{0 < t_1 < \cdots < t_n < T} \left(\prod_{j=1}^{n} S_{t_{n-j+1} - t_{n-j}} \right) \bar{P}_{T - t_n} f(x) dt_1 \ldots dt_n = \frac{n!}{(\lambda T)^n} I_T^n(f).$$

Note that we have used the fact that given $N_T = n$ then the jump times $\tau_1, \ldots, \tau_n$ are distributed as the order statistics of a sequence of n independent uniform random variables on the interval $[0, T]$. Therefore, their joint density is given by $\frac{n!}{T^n} \mathbf{1}_{0 < t_1 < \cdots < t_n < T} dt_1 \ldots dt_n$. Furthermore, the estimate (35) gives the integrability of the expectation on the right side of (39).

We now give a brief description of the Monte Carlo simulation method with sample size N.

Monte Carlo simulation method

Set $S = 0$. Repeat the following steps M times ($M \in \mathbb{N}^*$ represents the number of simulations to be used in the sample average)

1. Let $X_0 = x$, $\tau_0 = 0$, $\Lambda_0 = 1$

For $i = 0, 1, \ldots$, perform the following steps

2. Simulate an exponential random variable E_{i+1} of parameter λ and set $\tau_{i+1} = \tau_i + E_{i+1}$.

3. If $\tau_{i+1} > T$, go to step 6 with $N_T = i$. Otherwise, continue with step 4.

4. Compute for a p-Bernoulli random variable U_{i+1}, $\overline{X}_{\tau_{i+1}} = U_{i+1} Z_{\tau_{i+1}}(\tau_i, \overline{X}_{\tau_i})$ where Z is computed using the simulation method given in Lépingle [16]. That is,

$$Z_{\tau_{i+1}}(\tau_i, \overline{X}_{\tau_i}) = \overline{X}_{\tau_i} + \sigma(\overline{X}_{\tau_i}) G_{i+1} \sqrt{\tau_{i+1} - \tau_i} + \max\{0, -\overline{X}_{\tau_i} + Y_i\} \tag{41}$$

$$Y_i = \frac{1}{2} \left\{ -\sigma(\overline{X}_{\tau_i}) G_{i+1} \sqrt{\tau_{i+1} - \tau_i} + \left(a(\overline{X}_{\tau_i}) V_{i+1} + a(\overline{X}_{\tau_i}) G_{i+1}^2 (\tau_{i+1} - \tau_i) \right)^{1/2} \right\}.$$

Here G_{i+1} is a standard Gaussian random variable and V_{i+1} is an exponential random variable with parameter $(2(\tau_{i+1} - \tau_i))^{-1}$.

5. Next one computes $\Lambda_{i+1} = \Lambda_i \Theta_i(\tau_{i+1} - \tau_i, \overline{X}_{\tau_i}, \overline{X}_{\tau_{i+1}})$. Go back to 2.

6. Finalize by computing $\overline{X}_T = Z_T(\tau_{N_T}, \overline{X}_{\tau_{N_T}})$ using (41).

For each simulation, add to S the value $e^{\lambda T} \lambda^{-N_T} f(\overline{X}_T) \Lambda_{N_T}$. Finally, compute S/M.

When programming the above Monte Carlo simulation method, formulas (8) for $i = 0, 1, 2$ and $j = 0$, and

$$\theta_t(x, x') = \left(\frac{a''(x')}{2} + \frac{\partial_{x'} \bar{\pi}_t(x, x')}{\bar{\pi}_t(x, x')} a'(x') + \frac{\partial_{x'}^2 \bar{\pi}_t(x, x')}{\bar{\pi}_t(x, x')} \frac{[a(x') - a(x)]}{2} \right)$$

are useful.

Remark 5 As discussed in [1], one may use importance of sampling on the jump times of the Poisson process. In fact, one just needs to consider a renewal process $R_t = \sum_{j=1}^{\infty} \mathbf{1}_{\tau_j \leq t}$ where $\tau_j = \sum_{i=1}^{j} \zeta_i$ and $\{\zeta_i\}$ is a sequence of independent positive random variables with common density ξ. Then one performs importance sampling using the factor $p_n(t_1, \ldots, t_n; t) := \prod_{i=1}^{n} \xi(t_i - t_{i-1}) P(\zeta_{n+1} > t - t_n) P(R_t = n)^{-1}$ within each integral of order n. Here $t_0 = 0$. Then the simulation method and its probabilistic representation is given by

$$E[f(X_T)] = E \left[\frac{f(\overline{X}_T)}{p_n(\tau_1, \ldots, \tau_n; T)} \prod_{j=0}^{R_T - 1} \Theta_j(\tau_{j+1} - \tau_j, \overline{X}_{\tau_j}, \overline{X}_{\tau_{j+1}}) \right].$$

A wise choice of ξ leads to a Monte Carlo simulation method with finite variance. For more details, see [1].

Table 1 Calculation of $E[e^{-X_T}]$ with $T = 1$, $X_0 = 1/2$, $\sigma(x) = \frac{1}{2} + \frac{1}{4}\cos(x)$. We have used $M = 10^6$ samples and $\bar{N} = 10$ time steps for the discretization schemes and $\lambda = 1$, $p = 0.9$ for both parametrix methods

	Scheme 1	Scheme 2	Forward	Backward
Mean	0.544456	0.54441	0.545028	0.543441
Precision (95%)	4.62×10^{-4}	4.62×10^{-4}	3.9×10^{-3}	4.06×10^{-3}

To test numerically the method, we compare it with the standard Monte Carlo method with discretization schemes for the reflected SDE (1). We will use two discretization schemes on the regular time grid with $\bar{N}$ steps.

- Scheme 1 or Reflected Euler scheme:

$$\hat{X}_{(k+1)\frac{T}{N}} = \left| \hat{X}_{(k+1)\frac{T}{N}} + \sigma(\hat{X}_{(k+1)\frac{T}{N}})(W_{(k+1)\frac{T}{N}} - W_{k\frac{T}{N}}) \right|$$

$$\hat{L}_{(k+1)\frac{T}{N}} = \hat{L}_{k\frac{T}{N}} + 2\left(\hat{X}_{(k+1)\frac{T}{N}} + \sigma(\hat{X}_{(k+1)\frac{T}{N}})(W_{(k+1)\frac{T}{N}} - W_{k\frac{T}{N}}) \right)^-,$$

with $x^- = \max(-x, 0)$.
- Scheme 2 or Lépingle's scheme: $(\hat{X}_{(k+1)\frac{T}{N}}, \hat{L}_{(k+1)\frac{T}{N}})$ is obtained from $(\hat{X}_{k\frac{T}{N}}, \hat{L}_{k\frac{T}{N}})$ by using Lepingle's scheme with frozen coefficient $\sigma(\hat{X}_{k\frac{T}{N}})$.

We have reported in Table 1 an example of a Monte Carlo evaluation with the discretization scheme, the forward Parametrix method, and the backward Parametrix method presented in the previous sections. The precision indicated in the table is the empirical standard error multiplied by $1.96/\sqrt{M}$. It is worth to mention here that the variance of the estimator given by the Parametrix method may have an infinite variance as indicated in Remark 5. In fact, we observe some fluctuations on the empirical variance between two Monte Carlo runs. This effect becomes enhanced as parameters of the problem become large.

Here, our goal is simply to validate numerically the algorithms of the Parametrix method. We obtain indeed results that are in line with a classical Monte Carlo method with standard discretization schemes. This variance explosion problem needs to be further studied.

References

1. Andersson, P., Kohatsu-Higa, A.: Unbiased simulation of stochastic differential equations using parametrix expansions. To appear in Bernoulli (2016)
2. Bally, V., Kohatsu-Higa, A.: A probabilistic interpretation of the parametrix method. Ann. Appl. Probab. **25**(6), 3095–3138 (2015)
3. Beskos, A., Papaspiliopoulos, O., Roberts, G.O.: Retrospective exact simulation of diffusion sample paths with applications. Bernoulli **12**(6), 1077–1098 (2006)

4. Ermakov, S.M., Nekrutkin, V.V., Sipin, A.S.: Random Processes for Classical Equations of Mathematical Physics. Mathematics and its Applications (Soviet Series), vol. 34. Kluwer Academic Publishers Group, Dordrecht (1989). Translated from the Russian by Ermakov and Nekrutkin
5. Étoré, P., Martinez, M.: Exact simulation for solutions of one-dimensional stochastic differential equations with discontinuous drift. ESAIM: PS **18**, 686–702 (2014)
6. Friedman, A.: Partial Differential Equations of Parabolic Type. Prentice-Hall, Englewood Cliffs (1964)
7. Giles, M.B.: Multilevel Monte Carlo path simulation. Oper. Res. **56**(3), 607–617 (2008)
8. han Rhee, C., Glynn, P.W.: A new approach to unbiased estimation for sde's. In: Simulation Conference (WSC), Proceedings of the 2012 Winter, pp. 1–7 (2012)
9. Hersh, R.: Random evolutions: a survey of results and problems. Rocky Mt. J. Math. **4**(3), 443–478 (1974)
10. Il'in, A.M., Kalashnikov, A.S., Oleĭnik, O.A.: Second-order linear equations of parabolic type. Tr. Semin. im. I. G. Petrovskogo **21**, 9–193, 341 (2001)
11. Il'in, A.M., Kalašnikov, A.S., Oleĭnik, O.A.: Second-order linear equations of parabolic type. Uspehi Mat. Nauk. **17**(3 (105)), 3–146 (1962)
12. Karatzas, I., Shreve, S.E.: Brownian Motion and Stochastic Calculus. Graduate Texts in Mathematics, vol. 113, 2nd edn. Springer, New York (1991)
13. Konakov, V., Mammen, E.: Local limit theorems for transition densities of Markov chains converging to diffusions. Probab. Theory Relat. Fields **117**(4), 551–587 (2000)
14. Konakov, V., Menozzi, S.: Weak error for stable driven stochastic differential equations: expansion of the densities. J. Theor. Probab. **24**(2), 454–478 (2011)
15. Konakov, V., Menozzi, S., Molchanov, S.: Explicit parametrix and local limit theorems for some degenerate diffusion processes. Ann. Inst. Henri Poincaré Probab. Stat. **46**(4), 908–923 (2010)
16. Lépingle, D.: Euler scheme for reflected stochastic differential equations. Math. Comput. Simul. **38**(1–3), 119–126 (1995). Probabilités numériques (Paris, 1992)
17. Levi, E.E.: Sulle equazioni lineari totalmente ellittiche alle derivate parziali. Rendiconti del Circolo Matematico di Palermo (1884–1940) **24**(1), 275–317 (1907)
18. Lions, P.L., Sznitman, A.S.: Stochastic differential equations with reflecting boundary conditions. Commun. Pure Appl. Math. **37**(4), 511–537 (1984)
19. McKean Jr., H.P., Singer, I.M.: Curvature and the eigenvalues of the laplacian. J. Differ. Geom. **1**(1–2), 43–69 (1967)
20. Tsuchiya, M.: On the oblique derivative problem for diffusion processes and diffusion equations with Hölder continuous coefficients. Trans. Am. Math. Soc. **346**(1), 257–281 (1994)
21. Wagner, W.: Unbiased Monte Carlo estimators for functionals of weak solutions of stochastic differential equations. Stochastics Stochastics Rep. **28**(1), 1–20 (1989)

Harnack Inequalities and Bounds for Densities of Stochastic Processes

Gennaro Cibelli and Sergio Polidoro

Dedicated to Valentin Konakov in occasion of his 70th birthday.

Abstract We consider possibly degenerate parabolic operators in the form

$$\mathcal{L} = \sum_{k=1}^{m} X_k^2 + X_0 - \partial_t,$$

that are naturally associated to a suitable family of stochastic differential equations, and satisfying the Hörmander condition. Note that, under this assumption, the operators in the form $\mathcal{L}$ have a smooth fundamental solution that agrees with the density of the corresponding stochastic process. We describe a method based on Harnack inequalities and on the construction of Harnack chains to prove lower bounds for the fundamental solution. We also briefly discuss PDE and SDE methods to prove analogous upper bounds. We eventually give a list of meaningful examples of operators to which the method applies.

Keywords Density of a stochastic process · Kolmogorov equations
Hypoelliptic PDEs · Harnack inequality · Harnack chain · Asymptotic estimates

1 Introduction

Let $(W_t)_{t\geq0}$ denote an m-dimensional Brownian motion, $W_t = (W_t^1, \ldots, W_t^m)$ on some filtered probability space $(\Omega, \mathcal{F}, (\mathcal{F})_{t\geq0}, \mathbb{P})$. We consider a collection of

G. Cibelli · S. Polidoro (✉)
Università di Modena e Reggio Emilia, Via Campi 213/b, 41125 Modena, Italy
e-mail: sergio.polidoro@unimore.it

G. Cibelli
e-mail: gennaro.cibelli@unimore.it

© Springer International Publishing AG 2017
V. Panov (ed.), *Modern Problems of Stochastic Analysis and Statistics*,
Springer Proceedings in Mathematics & Statistics 208,
DOI 10.1007/978-3-319-65313-6_4

space-time functions $(\sigma_{ij})_{(i,j)\in\{1,...,N\}\times\{1,...,m\}}$, $(b_i)_{i\{1,...,N\}}$ such that the following SDE

$$dZ_t^i = \sum_{j=1}^{m} \sigma_{ij}(Z_t,t) \circ dW_t^j + b_i(Z_t,t)dt, \qquad i = 1,\ldots,N, \quad t \geq 0 \qquad (1)$$

is well posed at least in the weak sense. Here "$\circ\, dW_t$" stands for the Stratonovich integral. We denote by $Z_t^{x_0}$ the solution of the SDE (1) with initial condition $Z_0^{x_0} = x_0$. The Eq. (1) is associated to the Kolmogorov operator

$$\mathscr{L} = \sum_{i=1}^{m} X_i^2 + X_0 - \partial_t,$$

where

$$X_i(x,t) = \frac{1}{\sqrt{2}} \sum_{j=1}^{m} \sigma_{ij}(x,t)\partial_{x_j}, \quad i = 1,\ldots,m, \qquad X_0(x,t) = \sum_{i=1}^{N} b_i(x,t)\partial_{x_i}. \quad (2)$$

In this note, we describe a general method to prove upper and lower bounds for the fundamental solution of $\mathscr{L}$. Specifically, we say that a nonnegative function $\Gamma(x,t;y,s)$ defined for $x, y \in \mathbb{R}^N$ and $t > s$, is a fundamental solution for $\mathscr{L}$ if

(i) in the weak sense, $\mathscr{L}\Gamma(\cdot,\cdot;y,s) = 0$ in $]s,+\infty[\times\mathbb{R}^N$ and $\mathscr{L}^*\Gamma(t,x;\cdot,\cdot) = 0$ in $]-\infty,t[\times\mathbb{R}^N$ where $\mathscr{L}^*$ denotes the formal adjoint operator of $\mathscr{L}$;

(ii) for any bounded function $\varphi \in C(\mathbb{R}^N)$ and $x, y \in \mathbb{R}^N$, we have

$$\lim_{(x,t)\to(y,s)} u(x,t) = \varphi(y), \qquad \lim_{(y,s)\to(x,t)} v(y,s) = \varphi(x), \qquad (3)$$

where

$$u(x,t) := \int_{\mathbb{R}^N} \Gamma(x,t;y,s)\varphi(y)dy, \qquad v(y,s) := \int_{\mathbb{R}^N} \Gamma(x,t;y,s)\varphi(x)dx. \qquad (4)$$

Note that the functions in (4) are weak solutions of the following backward and forward Cauchy problems:

$$\begin{cases} \mathscr{L}u(t,x) = 0, & (x,t) \in]s,+\infty[\times\mathbb{R}^N, \\ u(x,s) = \varphi(x), & x \in \mathbb{R}^N, \end{cases} \qquad \begin{cases} \mathscr{L}^*v(y,s) = 0, & (y,s) \in]-\infty,t[\times\mathbb{R}^N, \\ v(y,t) = \varphi(y), & y \in \mathbb{R}^N. \end{cases}$$

We introduce the $N \times N$ matrix $A(x,t) = \big(a_{ij}(x,t)\big)_{i,j=1,...,N}$ whose elements are

$$a_{ij}(x,t) = \frac{1}{2}\sum_{k=1}^{m} \sigma_{ik}(x,t)\sigma_{jk}(x,t), \qquad i,j = 1,\ldots,N,$$

and we note that

$$\langle A(x, t)\xi, \xi \rangle = \tfrac{1}{2}\|\sigma(t, x)\xi\|^2 \geq 0. \quad \text{for every} \quad \xi \in \mathbb{R}^N.$$

If the smallest eigenvalue of $A(t, x)$ is uniformly positive, we say that the operator $\mathscr{L}$ is uniformly parabolic.

A keystone result in the theory of parabolic partial differential equations reads as follows. Assume that there exist two positive constants λ, Λ such that

$$\lambda|\xi|^2 \leq \langle A(x, t)\xi, \xi \rangle \leq \Lambda|\xi|^2, \quad \text{for every } (x, t) \in \mathbb{R}^N \times]0, T[, \text{ and } \xi \in \mathbb{R}^N. \quad (5)$$

If $\Gamma = \Gamma(x, t, \xi, \tau)$ denotes the fundamental solution of the PDE

$$\partial_t u(x, t) = \sum_{i,j=1}^{N} \partial_{x_i} \left(a_{ij}(x, t)\partial_{x_j} u(x, t) \right), \quad (x, t) \in \mathbb{R}^N \times]0, T[, \quad (6)$$

then there exist positive constants c^-, C^-, c^+, C^+ only depending on N, Λ, λ such that

$$\frac{c^-}{(t - \tau)^{N/2}} \exp\left(-C^- \frac{|x - \xi|^2}{t - \tau}\right) \leq \Gamma(x, t; \xi, \tau) \leq \frac{C^+}{(t - \tau)^{N/2}} \exp\left(-c^+ \frac{|x - \xi|^2}{t - \tau}\right),$$

$$(7)$$

for every $(x, t), (\xi, \tau) \in \mathbb{R}^N \times]0, T[$ with $\tau < t$. We emphasize that the constants in (7) do not depend on T. This upper bound has been proved by Aronson [1] for operators with bounded measurable coefficients a_{ij}'s, while the lower bound has been proved by Moser [32, 33]. The results by Aronson and by Moser improve the earliest estimates given by Nash in his seminal work [34]. We also refer to the article of Escauriaza [16] for non-divergence form operators.

The results described above have been extended by several authors to possibly degenerate operators in the form

$$\mathscr{L} := \sum_{k=1}^{m} X_k^2 + Y, \quad Y := X_0 - \partial_t, \quad (8)$$

where $X_0, X_1, \ldots, X_m$ are smooth vector fields on $\mathbb{R}^{N+1}$, that is

$$X_i(x, t) = \sum_{j=1}^{N} c_{i,j}(x, t)\partial_{x_j}, \quad i = 0, \ldots, m. \quad (9)$$

for some smooth functions $c_{i,j}$'s. In particular, upper bounds have been proved by a PDE approach that goes back to Aronson's work [1], or by an approach based on Lyapunov functions (see [30] and the references therein). Several authors prove bounds analogous to (7) in the framework of stochastic processes. We refer to the works of Malliavin [28], Kusuoka and Stroock [27], where a general method to prove upper bounds for density is introduced and to the work of Ben Arous and Léandre [6], where the Malliavin Calculus is further developed. We also refer to the monograph of Nualart [35] for a comprehensive presentation of this subject.

In general, lower bounds have been proved by following the idea introduced by Moser in [32]. In this note, we briefly describe this method for uniformly parabolic partial differential equations, then we give an overview of more recent articles where it has been adapted to the study of degenerate parabolic equations in the form (8). This idea is also used in the works where lower bounds are proved by probabilistic methods. We refer to Kohatsu-Higa [23], Bally [3], Bally and Kohatsu-Higa [4].

We now give a list of examples of operators considered in this note. Each one of them is the prototype of a wide family of differential operators.

- *Heat operator on the Heisenberg group* $\mathscr{L} = X_1^2 + X_2^2 - \partial_t$, where

$$X_1 = \partial_x - \tfrac{1}{2}y\partial_w, \qquad X_2 = \partial_y + \tfrac{1}{2}x\partial_w.$$

Note that $\mathscr{L}$ acts on the variable $(x, y, w, t) \in \mathbb{R}^4$, and writes in the form (8) with $X_0 = 0$. The degenerate elliptic operator $\Delta_{\mathbb{H}} = X_1^2 + X_2^2$ is said *sub-Laplacian* on the Heisenberg group.

- *Kolmogorov Operator* $\mathscr{L} = \partial_{xx} + x\partial_y - \partial_t$, $(x, y, t) \in \mathbb{R}^3$. In this case $\mathscr{L} = X^2 + Y$ with $X = \partial_x$, $Y = x\partial_y - \partial_t$.
- *More Degenerate Kolmogorov Operators* $\mathscr{L} = \partial_{xx} + x^2\partial_y - \partial_t$, $(x, y, t) \in \mathbb{R}^3$. In this case $\mathscr{L} = X^2 + Y$ with $X = \partial_x$, $Y = x^2\partial_y - \partial_t$.
- *Asian Option Operator* $\mathscr{L} = x^2\partial_{xx} + x\partial_x + x\partial_y - \partial_t$, $(x, y, t) \in \mathbb{R}^+ \times \mathbb{R}^2$. In this case, $\mathscr{L} = X^2 + Y$ with $X = x\partial_x$, $Y = x\partial_y - \partial_t$.

All the operators in the above list are strongly degenerate, since the smallest eigenvalue of the characteristic form is zero for all the above examples. In general, operators in the form (8) cannot be uniformly parabolic if $m < N$. On the other hand, all the examples do satisfy the following condition:

HYPOTHESIS [H] $\mathscr{L} = \sum_{k=1}^{m} X_k^2 + Y$ *satisfies the Hörmander condition if*

$$\text{rank } (\text{Lie}\{X_1, \ldots, X_m, Y\}(x, t)) = N + 1, \qquad \text{for every} \quad (x, t) \in \mathbb{R}^{N+1}.$$

In the sequel we only consider operators $\mathscr{L}$ satisfying the Hörmander condition. It is know that, for this family of operators, the law of the stochastic process (1) is absolutely continuous with respect to the Lebesgue measure in $\mathbb{R}^N$, and that its density is smooth. Moreover, for every pairs (ξ, τ), $(x, t) \in \mathbb{R}^N \times [0, T[$ with $\tau > t$, the density $p(\xi, \tau; x, t)$ is linked with the fundamental solution Γ of $\mathscr{L}$. Precisely, if p denotes the density of the process

$$\begin{cases} dZ_s^i = \sum_{i,j=1}^{m} \sigma_{ij}(Z_s, T-s) \circ dW_s^i + b_i(Z_s, T-s)ds, & i = 1, \ldots, N, \quad t < s \leq T; \\ Z_t^i = x_i, & i = 1, \ldots, N, \end{cases}$$

then Γ is defined by the relation

$$\Gamma(x, t; \xi, \tau) = p(\xi, T - \tau; x, T - t).$$

It is known that the regularity properties of the operators satisfying the Hörmander condition are related to a Lie group structure that replaces the usual Euclidean one. In the proof of the lower bounds for positive solutions the geometric aspects of this *non Euclidean* structure will be explicitly used. To make the exposition clear, in Sect. 2 we recall the method used by Moser in [32] to prove the lower bound in (7) for uniformly parabolic operators. In Sect. 3 we describe how the method outlined in Sect. 2 is adapted to the degenerate ones, satisfying the Hörmander condition [H]. The remaining Sects. 4, 5, 6, and 7 are devoted to the examples listed above.

2 Uniformly Parabolic Equations

In this section, we describe the method introduced by Moser [32] to prove the lower bound (7) of the fundamental solution for uniformly parabolic equations. The main ingredient of the method is the *parabolic Harnack inequality*, first proved by Hadamard [18] and, independently, by Pini [36] in 1954 for the heat equation, then by Moser [32, 33] for uniformly parabolic equations in divergence form (6). Its statement requires some notation (see Fig. 1). Let

$$Q_r(x, t) = B(x, r) \times]t - r^2, t[,$$

denote the parabolic cylinder whose upper basis is centered at (x, t). Let $\alpha, \beta, \gamma, \delta \in$ $]0, 1[$ be given constants, with $\alpha < \beta < \gamma < 1$,

$$Q_r^-(x, t) = B(x, \delta r) \times]t - \gamma r^2, t - \beta r^2[\qquad Q_r^+(x, t) = B(x, \delta r) \times]t - \alpha r^2, t[.$$

Theorem 1 (Parabolic Harnack inequality) *Let* $Q_r(x, t) \subset \mathbb{R}^{N+1}$, *and let* $\alpha, \beta, \gamma, \delta$ $\in]0, 1[$ *be given constants, with* $\alpha < \beta < \gamma < 1$. *Then there exists* $C = C(\alpha, \beta, \gamma, \delta,$ $\lambda, \Lambda, N)$ *such that*

$$\sup_{Q_r^-(x,t)} u \leq C \inf_{Q_r^+(x,t)} u$$

Fig. 1 Parabolic Harnack inequality

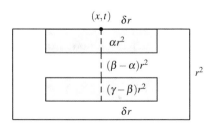

Fig. 2 Parabolic Harnack
inequality

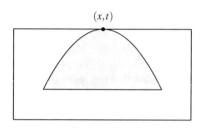

for every u $: Q_r(x, t) \to \mathbb{R}, u \geq 0$, *satisfying* (6). *Here* λ, Λ *are the constants in* (5).

Remark 1 Note that C does not depend on the point (x, t) and on r, then the Harnack inequality is invariant with respect to the *Euclidean translation* $(x, t) \mapsto (x + x_0, t + t_0)$, and to the *parabolic dilation* $(x, t) \mapsto (rx, r^2 t)$. For this reason, the above statement is often referred to as *invariant Harnack inequality*.

In the sequel, we will use the following version of the parabolic Harnack inequality (see Fig. 2). For any given $c \in]0, 1[$ we denote by

$$P_r(x, t) = \big\{ (y, s) \in Q_r(x, t) \mid 0 < t - s \leq cr^2 < t, |y - x|^2 \leq t - s \big\}.$$

Corollary 1 *Let* $Q_r(x, t) \subset \mathbb{R}^{N+1}$, *and let* $c \in]0, 1[$ *be a given constant. Then there exists* $C = C(c, \lambda, \Lambda, N)$ *such that*

$$\sup_{P_r(x,t)} u \leq Cu(x, t)$$

for every u $: Q_r(x, t) \to \mathbb{R}, u \geq 0$, *satisfying* (6). *Here* λ, Λ *are the constants in* (5).

Proof For every positive ρ we denote

$$S_\rho(x, t) = B(x, \rho) \times \{t - \rho^2\}.$$

Let $\alpha, \beta, \gamma \in]0, 1[$ be such that $\alpha < \beta \leq c \leq \gamma < 1$, and let $\delta = \sqrt{c}$. Then, for every $\rho \in [0, r]$ we have that u is a nonnegative solution of (6) in the domain $Q_\rho(x, t)$. Since $S_\rho(x, t) \subset Q_\rho^-(x, t)$, from Theorem 1 we obtain

$$\sup_{S_\rho(x,t)} u \leq \sup_{Q_\rho^-(x,t)} u \leq C \inf_{Q_\rho^+(x,t)} u \leq Cu(x, t),$$

and the conclusion follows from the fact that $P_r(x, t) = \cup_{0 < \rho \leq r} S_\rho(x, t)$. $\square$

With Corollary 1 in hand, we can easily obtain the following *non local* Harnack inequality, first proved by Moser (Theorem 2 in [32]). We also refer to Aronson and Serrin [2] for more general uniformly parabolic differential operators.

Fig. 3 Harnack chain

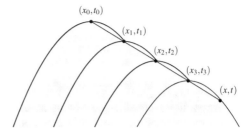

Theorem 2 *Let $u : \mathbb{R}^N \times]0, T[\to \mathbb{R}$ be a nonnegative solution of the parabolic Eq. (6). Then there exists a positive constant $C = C(c, \lambda, \Lambda, N)$ such that*

$$u(x, t) \le C^{1 + \frac{|x_0 - x|^2}{t_0 - t}} u(x_0, t_0),$$

for every $(x_0, t_0), (x, t) \in \mathbb{R}^N \times]0, T[$ with $t_0 - t < c\, t_0$.

Proof Let $(x_0, t_0), (x, t) \in \mathbb{R}^N \times]0, T[$, with $t_0 - t < c t_0$, choose $r = \sqrt{t}$ and note that the cylinder $Q_r(x_0, t_0)$ is contained in $\mathbb{R}^N \times]0, T[$. If $(x, t) \in P_r(x_0, t_0)$ we simply apply Corollary 1 and the proof is complete. If otherwise $(x, t) \notin P_r(x_0, t_0)$, we consider the segment whose end points are (x_0, t_0) and (x, t), and denote by (x_1, t_1) the point where it intersects the boundary of $P_r(x_0, t_0)$. Note that $t_1 \ge t > (1 - c)t_0$, then (x_1, t_1) belongs to the lateral part of the boundary of $P_r(x_0, t_0)$. By Corollary 1 we have

$$u(x_1, t_1) \le C u(x_0, t_0).$$

We then iterate the argument. We define a finite sequence (x_j, t_j), with $j = 2, \ldots, k$ such that (x_j, t_j) belonging to the boundary of $P_r(x_{j-1}, t_{j-1})$ for $j = 2, \ldots, k$, and $(x, t) \in P_r(x_k, t_k)$ (see Fig. 3). By applying k times Corollary 1 we then find

$$u(x, t) \le C u(x_k, t_k) \le C^2 u(x_{k-1}, t_{k-1}) \le \cdots \le C^{k+1} u(x_0, t_0).$$

To conclude the proof it is sufficient to note that the integer k only depends on the slope of the line connecting (x_0, t_0) to (x, t) and that a simple computation gives $k < \frac{|x_0 - x|^2}{t_0 - t}$. $\square$

The set $\{(x_0, t_0), (x_1, t_1), \ldots (x_k, t_k), (x, t)\}$ appearing in the above proof is often referred to as *Harnack chain*. By using the following property of the fundamental solution Γ of the differential operator appearing in (6)

$$\Gamma(0, t) \ge \frac{C}{t^{N/2}}, \qquad \text{for every } t > 0, \tag{10}$$

for some positive constant $C = C(\lambda, \Lambda, N)$. We refer to Nash [34] and to Fabes-Strook [17, Lemma 2.6] for a derivation of (10). By choosing $c = \frac{1}{2}$ in Theorem 2, we conclude that there exist two positive constants C^-, c^- such that

$$\Gamma(x, t, y, s) \geq \frac{C^-}{(t-s)^{N/2}} \exp\left(-c^- \frac{|x-y|^2}{t-s}\right),$$

for every (x, t), $(y, s) \in \mathbb{R}^{N+1}$ with $0 < s < t < T$.

We explicitly note that the method described above also applies to non-divergence uniformly parabolic operators, if we rely on the Harnack inequality proved by Krylov and Safonov [26]. In this setting, the inequality (10) holds for t belonging to any bounded interval $]0, T[$ and the constant C may depend on T. We refer to the manuscript of Konakov [24] for the derivation of (10) by using the a parametrix expansion, to the article of Escauriaza [16] and to the monograph of Bass [5] for uniformly parabolic operators with bounded measurable coefficients.

Remark 2 Before considering degenerate parabolic operators, we point out that the method used in the proof of Theorem 2 only relies on the following two ingredients.

(i) The invariance with respect to the Euclidean translation and to the parabolic dilation $(x, t) \mapsto (x_0 + \rho x, t_0 + \rho^2 t)$ are the properties that allow us to obtain Corollary 1 from Theorem 1.
(ii) Segments are very simple supports for the construction of Harnack chains. In the study of degenerate parabolic operators, a more sophisticated construction will be needed.

3   Degenerate Hypoelliptic Operators

Consider a linear second-order differential operator in the form (8)

$$\mathscr{L} = \sum_{k=1}^{m} X_k^2 + X_0 - \partial_t.$$

satisfying the Hörmander condition [H]. We introduce a definition based on the vector fields $X_1, \ldots, X_m, Y$.

Definition 1 We say that γ is an $\mathscr{L}$-*admissible path* starting from $z_0 \in \mathbb{R}^{N+1}$ if it is an absolutely continuous solution of the following ODE:

$$\dot{\gamma}(\tau) = \sum_{k=1}^{m} \omega_k(\tau) X_k(\gamma(\tau)) + Y(\gamma(\tau))$$

$$\gamma(0) = z_0.$$

with $\omega_1, \ldots, \omega_m \in L^1([0, T])$.

Let Ω be an open subset of $\mathbb{R}^{N+1}$ and $z_0 \in \Omega$. The *attainable set* of z_0 in Ω is

$$\mathscr{A}_{z_0}(\Omega) = \big\{ z \in \Omega \mid \text{there exists an } \mathscr{L}\text{-admissible path } \gamma \text{ such that}$$

$$\gamma(0) = z_0, \ \gamma(T) = z \text{ and } \gamma(\tau) \in \Omega \text{ for } 0 \le \tau \le T \big\}.$$

The following version of the Harnack inequality is based on the definition of attainable set. It has been introduced in [10, 11] and in its general form in [22] for operators in the form (8).

Theorem 3 *Let u be a nonnegative solution of $\mathscr{L}u = 0$ in some bounded open set $\Omega \subset \mathbb{R}^{N+1}$, and let $z_0 \in \Omega$. Suppose that $Int\left(\overline{\mathscr{A}_{z_0}(\Omega)}\right) \ne \emptyset$. Then, for every compact set $K \subset Int\left(\overline{\mathscr{A}_{z_0}(\Omega)}\right)$ there exists a positive constant C_K, only depending on Ω, K, z_0 and $\mathscr{L}$, such that*

$$\sup_K u(z) \le C_K u(z_0).$$

If the operator $\mathscr{L}$ is also invariant with respect to suitable non-Euclidean *translations* and *dilations*, then Theorem 3 restores an *invariant Harnack inequality* useful for the construction of Harnack chains.

HYPOTHESIS [G1] *There exists a Lie group* $\mathbb{G} = \left(\mathbb{R}^{N+1}, \circ\right)$ *such that* $X_1, \ldots, X_m, Y$ *are left invariant on* $\mathbb{G}$, *i.e.: given* $\xi \in \mathbb{R}^{N+1}$ *and denoting by* $\ell_\xi(z) = \xi \circ z$, *the left translation of* $z \in \mathbb{R}^{N+1}$ *it holds*

$$X_i(u(\ell_\xi(z))) = (X_i u)(\ell_\xi(z)), \qquad i = 1, \ldots, m,$$
$$Y(u(\ell_\xi(z))) = (Y u)(\ell_\xi(z)),$$

for every smooth function u.

As we will see in the next sections, all the examples listed in the Introduction do satisfy the above assumption, that replaces the usual invariance with respect to the Euclidean translation. For some operators $\mathscr{L}$ considered in this note, the vector fields $X_1, \ldots, X_m, Y$ are also invariant with respect to a rescaling property $(\delta_\lambda)_{\lambda>0}$ of the Lie group $\mathbb{G}$, which replaces the multiplication by a positive scalar in a vector space.

HYPOTHESIS [G2] *There exists a dilation $(\delta_\lambda)_{\lambda>0}$ on the Lie group $\mathbb{G}$ such that the vector fields $X_1, \ldots, X_m$ are δ_λ-homogeneous of degree one and Y is δ_λ-homogeneous of degree two. i.e.:*

$$X_i(u(\delta_\lambda(z))) = \lambda(X_i u)(\delta_\lambda(z)), \qquad i = 1, \ldots, m,$$
$$Y(u(\delta_\lambda(z))) = \lambda^2(Y u)(\delta_\lambda(z)),$$

for every smooth function u.

When both of assumptions [G1] and [G2] are satisfied, we say that

$$\mathbb{G} = \left(\mathbb{R}^{N+1}, \circ, (\delta_\lambda)_{\lambda>0}\right)$$

is a *homogeneous* Lie group and the operator $\mathscr{L}$ is invariant with respect to the left translations of $\mathbb{G}$, and homogeneous of degree 2 with respect to the dilation of $\mathbb{G}$. In this case, we easily obtain from Theorem 3 an invariant Harnack inequality analogous to Corollary 1. Consider any bounded open set $\Omega \subset \mathbb{R}^{N+1}$ with $0 \in \Omega$ and suppose that it is *star-shaped* with respect to $(\delta_\lambda)_{\lambda > 0}$, that is

$$\delta_r(\Omega) := \{\delta_r(z) \mid z \in \Omega\} \subset \Omega, \qquad \text{for every } r \in]0, 1].$$

If $\text{Int}\left(\overline{\mathscr{A}_0(\Omega)}\right) \neq \emptyset$, we choose any compact set $K \subset \text{Int}\left(\overline{\mathscr{A}_0(\Omega)}\right)$. For every $r > 0$ and $z_0 \in \mathbb{R}^{N+1}$ we set

$$\Omega_r(z_0) = z_0 \circ \delta_r(\Omega) := \{z_0 \circ \delta_r(z) \mid z \in \Omega\}.$$

Note that we also have $z_0 \circ \delta_\rho(K) \subset \text{Int}\left(\overline{\mathscr{A}_{z_0}(\Omega_r(z_0))}\right)$ for every $\rho \in]0, r]$, since Ω is star-shaped. We define

$$\mathscr{P}_r(z_0) = \bigcup_{0 < \rho \leq r} z_0 \circ \delta_\rho(K).$$

Theorem 4 *Let $\mathscr{L}$ be an operator in the form* (8) *satisfying assumptions [G1] and [G2] and let $\Omega_r(z_0)$ as above. Suppose that $\text{Int}\left(\overline{\mathscr{A}_{z_0}(\Omega_r(z_0))}\right) \neq \emptyset$, then*

$$\sup_{\mathscr{P}_r(z_0)} u(x, t) \leq C_K u(z_0)$$

for every positive solution u of $\mathscr{L}u = 0$ in $\Omega_r(z_0)$. Here C_K is the same constant appearing in Theorem 3.

Theorem 4 is the Harnack inequality that replaces Corollary 1 in the non-Euclidean setting that is natural for the study of degenerate operators $\mathscr{L}$. In accordance with Remark 2, this is the first ingredient for the construction of Harnack chains. It turns out that the second ingredient is the $\mathscr{L}$-admissible path, which is the natural substitute of the segment used in the Euclidean setting. To replicate the construction made in the proof of Theorem 2 we only need to choose γ, with $\gamma(0) = (x_0, t_0)$, and $\mathscr{P}_{(x_0, t_0)}$ with the following property:

there exists $s_0 \in]0, t_0 - t[$ such that $\gamma(s) \in \mathscr{P}_{(x_0, t_0)}$ for $s \in]0, s_0]$. \qquad (11)

All the examples in this note satisfy (11). Thus we have what we need to construct a Harnack chain $\{(x_0, t_0), (x_1, t_1), \ldots (x_k, t_k), (x, t)\}$ with starting point at (x_0, t_0) and end point at (x, t).

In order to find an accurate bound of the positive solutions of $\mathscr{L}u = 0$ we need to control the *length* k of the Harnack chain. It is possible to prove that there exists a positive constant h such that, if we construct the Harnack chain by using the $\mathscr{L}$-admissible path γ as in Definition 1, with $z_0 = (x_0, t_0)$ and $z = (x, t)$, then $T = t_0 - t$ and we have

$$k \leq \tfrac{1}{h}\Phi(\omega) + 1, \qquad \Phi(\omega) := \int_0^{t_0-t} \|\omega(s)\|^2 d\,s. \tag{12}$$

In the sequel, we will refer to the integral appearing in (12) as the *cost* of the path γ associated to the *control* $(\omega_1, \ldots, \omega_m)$. We then conclude that there exist three positive constants θ, h and M, with $\theta < 1$ and $M > 1$, only depending on the operator $\mathscr{L}$ such that

$$u(x, t) \leq M^{1+\frac{\Phi(\omega)}{h}} u(x_0, t_0), \tag{13}$$

for every positive solution u of $\mathscr{L}u = 0$, were (x_0, t_0), $(x, t) \in \mathbb{R}^N \times]0, T[$ are such that $0 < t_0 - t < \theta t_0$.

Note that (13) provides us with a bound depending on the choice of the $\mathscr{L}$-admissible path γ steering (x_0, t_0) to (x, t). In order to get the best exponent, we can optimize the choice of γ. With this spirit, we define the *Value function*

$$\Psi(x_0, t_0; x, t) = \inf_{\omega} \{\Phi(\omega)\}, \tag{14}$$

where the *infimum* is taken in the set of all the $\mathscr{L}$-admissible paths γ steering (x_0, t_0) to (x, t), and satisfying (11). We summarize this construction in the following general statement.

Let $\mathscr{L}$ be an operator in the form (8) satisfying conditions [H], [G1], and [G2], and assume that there is a positive r and an open star-shaped set Ω with $0 \in \Omega$ such that $\text{Int}\left(\overline{\mathscr{A}_0(\Omega_r(0))}\right) \neq \emptyset$. Moreover, if all the $\mathscr{L}$-admissible paths γ steering (x_0, t_0) to (x, t) satisfy (11), then there exist three positive constants θ, h and M, with $\theta < 1$ and $M > 1$, only depending on the operator $\mathscr{L}$ such that the following property holds.

Let (x_0, t_0), $(x, t) \in \mathbb{R}^{N+1}$ with $0 < t_0 - t < \theta t_0$. Then, for every positive solution $u : \mathbb{R}^N \times]0, T[$ of $\mathscr{L}u = 0$ it holds

$$u(x, t) \leq M^{1+\frac{1}{h}\Psi(x_0, t_0; x, t)} u(x_0, t_0). \tag{15}$$

Inequality (15) is the main step in the proof of our lower bound for the fundamental solution. All the examples considered in this note satisfy conditions [H], [G1]. Some examples also satisfy [G2], some examples do not. However, in this case, a scale invariant Harnack inequality still holds true, then the method provides us with a lower bound of the fundamental solution.

4 Degenerate Hypoelliptic Operators on Homogeneous Groups

The Heat operator on the Heisenberg group

$$\mathscr{L} = X_1^2 + X_2^2 - \partial_t$$

where

$$X_1 = \partial_x - \tfrac{1}{2}y\partial_w, \qquad X_2 = \partial_y + \tfrac{1}{2}x\partial_w$$

are vector fields acting on the variable $(x, y, w, t) \in \mathbb{R}^4$, is the simplest example of degenerate operator built by a sub-Laplacian on a stratified Lie group. The vector fields X_1, X_2 are invariant with respect to the left translation on the Heisenberg group on $\mathbb{R}^3$, whose operation is defined as

$$(x_0, y_0, w_0) \circ (x, y, w) = \left(x_0 + x, y_0 + y, w_0 + w + \tfrac{1}{2}(x_0 y - y_0 x)\right).$$

The above operation is extended to $\mathbb{R}^4$ by setting

$$(x_0, y_0, w_0, t_0) \circ (x, y, w, t) = \left(x_0 + x, y_0 + y, w_0 + w + \tfrac{1}{2}(x_0 y - y_0 x), t_0 + t\right).$$

Moreover $\mathscr{L}$ is invariant with respect to the following dilation:

$$\delta_r(x, y, w, t) = \left(rx, ry, r^2 w, r^2 t\right),$$

then the hypotheses [G1] and [G2] are fulfilled by $\mathscr{L}$. Furthermore, it satisfies the following property.
[C] *For every $x_0, x \in \mathbb{R}^N$, and for every positive T there exists an absolutely contin-uous path $\gamma_0 : [0, T] \to \mathbb{R}^N$ such that*

$$\dot{\gamma}_0(\tau) = \sum_{k=1}^m \omega_k(\tau) X_k(\gamma_0(\tau)), \quad \gamma_0(0) = x_0, \ \gamma_0(T) = x. \tag{16}$$

Note that, for operators $\mathscr{L}$ in the form (8) with $X_0 = 0$, condition [C] is equivalent to the *strong* Hörmander condition

$$\operatorname{rank} \operatorname{Lie}\{X_1, \dots, X_m\}(x) = N, \qquad \forall x \in \mathbb{R}^N.$$

Moreover, for every $\Omega \subset \mathbb{R}^{N+1}$ and for every $(x_0, t_0) \in \Omega$, there exist a positive ε and a neighborhood U of x_0 such that $U \times]t_0, t_0 - \varepsilon[\subset \mathscr{A}_{(x_0, t_0)}(\Omega)$. This particular geometric property of the attainable set implies that an invariant Harnack inequality analogous to the standard parabolic one holds for this operator. The only difference is that the Euclidean translation and the parabolic dilations are replaced by the oper-ations used to satisfy hypotheses [G1] and [G2]. In conclusion, the hypotheses we need to prove (15) are satisfied by the heat operator on the Heisenberg group. In particular, this method leads us to the lower bound of the following version of (7): there exist positive constants c^-, C^-, c^+, C^+ such that

$$\frac{c^-}{\sqrt{|\mathscr{B}_{t-\tau}(x)|}} \exp\left(-C^- \frac{d_{CC}(x,\xi)^2}{t-\tau}\right) \leq \Gamma(x,t,\xi,\tau) \leq \frac{C^+}{\sqrt{|\mathscr{B}_{t-\tau}(x)|}} \exp\left(-c^+ \frac{d_{CC}(x,\xi)^2}{t-\tau}\right),$$

(17)

where d_{CC} denotes the *Carnot-Caratheodory distance*

$$d_{CC}(x_0, x) = \inf\{\ell(\gamma_0) \mid \gamma_0 \text{ is as in (16)}\}, \quad \ell(\gamma) := \int_0^T \|\omega(s)\| ds.$$

and $|\mathscr{B}_r(x)|$ is the volume of the metric ball with center at x and radius r. To make more precise the analogy between (7) and (17), we recall that if $\mathbb{H}$ is a homogeneous Lie group on $\mathbb{R}^N$, then

$$|\mathscr{B}_r(x)| = r^Q |\mathscr{B}_1(0)|,$$

where Q is an integer called *homogeneous dimension* of $\mathbb{H}$. We recall that the upper bound was proved by Davies in [13], and the upper and lower bounds are due to Jerison and Sánchez-Calle [20] and to Varopoulos, Saloff-Coste and Coulhon [44]. Note that $\Psi(x_0, t_0; x, t) = \frac{d_{CC}(x_0,x)^2}{t_0-t}$. Indeed, if we consider the path $\gamma(s) = (\gamma_0(s), t_0 - s)$ with $0 \leq s \leq t_0 - t$, then by the Cauchy–Schwarz inequality, we obtain $\ell(\gamma_0) \leq \sqrt{\Phi(\omega)}\sqrt{t_0 - t}$. Moreover the equality occurs only if the norm of the control ω is constant, that is

$$\ell(\gamma_0) = \sqrt{\Phi(\omega)}\sqrt{t_0 - t} \iff (\omega_1^2 + \cdots + \omega_m^2)(s) = \frac{\Phi(\omega)}{t_0 - t} \text{ for every } s \in [0, t_0 - t].$$

We refer to the article [8] for the study of a more general class of operator satisfying [G1], [G2] and [C], that includes heat operators on Carnot groups and also operators $\mathscr{L}$ with $X_0 \neq 0$. We also recall that in the article [12] the analogous upper bound has been proved by using a PDE method combined with the Optimal Control Theory.

5 Degenerate Kolmogorov Equations

The simplest degenerate example of degenerate Kolmogorov operator is

$$\mathscr{L} := \partial_x^2 + x\partial_y - \partial_t, \quad (x, y, t) \in \mathbb{R}^2 \times]0, T[,$$

(18)

it writes in the form (8), if the vector fields X, Y are

$$X(x, y, t) = \partial_x \sim \begin{pmatrix} 1 \\ 0 \\ 0 \end{pmatrix}, \qquad Y(x, y, t) = x\partial_y - \partial_t \sim \begin{pmatrix} 0 \\ x \\ -1 \end{pmatrix}.$$

$\mathscr{L}$ is related to the following stochastic process

$$\begin{cases} X_t = x_0 + W_t, \\ Y_t = y_0 + \int_0^t (x_0 + W_s)\, ds. \end{cases} \tag{19}$$

which satisfies the *Langevin equation* $dX_t = dW_t, dY_t = X_t dt$. We recall that this kind of stochastic process appears in several research areas. For instance, in Kinetic Theory, $(X_t)_{t\geq 0}$ describes the velocity of a particle, while $(Y_t)_{t\geq 0}$ is its position. We note that

(i) X and Y are invariant with respect to the left translation of the group defined by the following operation

$$(x_0, y_0, t_0) \circ (x, y, t) = (x + x_0, y + y_0 - t x_0, t + t_0), \qquad (x, y, t), (x_0, y_0, t_0) \in \mathbb{R}^3, \tag{20}$$

(ii) X and Y are homogeneous of degree 1 and 2, respectively, with respect to the dilation

$$(\delta_\rho)_{\rho>0} : (x, y, t) \mapsto (\rho x, \rho^3 y, \rho^2 t) = \mathrm{diag}(\rho, \rho^3, \rho^2) \cdot \begin{pmatrix} x \\ y \\ t \end{pmatrix}. \tag{21}$$

In particular, $\mathscr{L}$ satisfies the Hypotheses [G1] and [G2].

(iii) The $\mathscr{L}$-admissible paths are the solutions $\gamma(s) = (x(s), y(s), t(s))$ of the following equation

$$\begin{cases} \dot{x}(s) = \omega(s), \quad x(0) = x_0, \\ \dot{y}(s) = x(s), \quad y(0) = y_0, \\ \dot{t}(s) = -1, \quad t(0) = t_0. \end{cases}$$

It is easy to check that the attainable set of the point $(0, 0, 0)$ in the open set $\Omega =]-1, 1[^3$ is $A_{(0,0,0)}(\Omega) = \{(x, y, t) \in \Omega \mid t < -|y|\}$, (see Fig. 4).

As the interior of $A_{(0,0,0)}(\Omega)$ is not empty, Theorem 4 gives an invariant Harnack inequality for $\mathscr{L}$, and we can apply (15) to prove lower bounds for positive solutions defined on the domain $\mathbb{R}^2 \times]0, T[$. The Optimal Control Theory provides us with an explicit expression of the value function Ψ_0 for $\mathscr{L}$ in (18)

$$\Psi_0(x, y, t; \xi, \eta, \tau) = \frac{(x - \xi)^2}{t - \tau} + \frac{12}{(t - \tau)^3}\left(y - \eta - (t - \tau)\frac{(x+\xi)}{2}\right)^2. \tag{22}$$

This is a remarkable fact, as it is known that the explicit expression of the fundamental solution of $\mathscr{L}$ was written by [25] and is

Fig. 4 $\mathcal{A}_{(0,0,0)}(\Omega)$

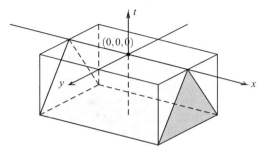

$$\Gamma_0(x, y, t; \xi, \eta, \tau) = \frac{\sqrt{3}}{2\pi(t-\tau)^2} \exp\left(-\frac{(x-\xi)^2}{4(t-\tau)} - \frac{3}{(t-\tau)^3}\left(y - \eta - (t-\tau)\frac{(x+\xi)}{2}\right)^2\right).$$

(23)

We briefly discuss here the anisotropic dilation (21). We first note that the Hörmander condition is satisfied since

$$[X, Y] = XY - YX = \partial_y \sim \begin{pmatrix} 0 \\ 1 \\ 0 \end{pmatrix}$$

and that ∂_y is homogeneous of degree three as XY and YX are both homogeneous of degree three. This explains the exponent 3 appearing in (21). Moreover, since

$$\det\left(\mathrm{diag}(\rho, \rho^3)\right) = \rho^4,$$

then $Q = 4$ is the spatial homogeneous dimension of $\mathbb{R}^2$ with respect to the dilation (21). Furthermore, in view of (19), such dilation has a natural probabilistic meaning as one has $\mathrm{Var}(X_t) = t$ and $\mathrm{Var}(Y_t) = t^3/3$.

The lower bound based on the value function Ψ is useful as we consider Kolmogorov equations in the form

$$\partial_t u(x, t) = \sum_{i,j=1}^{m} a_{ij}(x, t)\partial^2_{x_i x_j} u(x, t) + \sum_{i,j=1}^{N} b_{ij}x_j\partial_{x_i} u(x, t), \qquad (x, t) \in \mathbb{R}^N \times]0, T[,$$

(24)

with bounded Hölder continuous coefficients a_{ij}'s. In the study of this family of operators, we assume that $m < N$, the matrix $\left(a_{ij}(t, x)\right)_{i,j=1,\dots,m}$ is uniformly positive in $\mathbb{R}^m$. Moreover, the Hörmander condition is satisfied for the operator $\mathscr{L}_{(\xi,\tau)}$ *frozen* at some point $(\xi, \tau) \in \mathbb{R}^{N+1}$, that is obtained from the equation in (24) by replacing every function $a_{ij} = a_{ij}(x, t)$ with $a_{ij}(\xi, \tau)$. It turns out that this condition does not depend on the choice of the point (ξ, τ), that $\mathscr{L}_{(\xi,\tau)}$ is invariant with respect to a Lie group $\mathbb{G}$ on $\mathbb{R}^{N+1}$ which does not depend on (ξ, τ). In this case, the *parametrix method* provides us with the existence of a fundamental solution Γ of the operator introduced in (24). The method also gives an upper bound of the form

$$\Gamma(x, t; \xi, \tau) \leq \frac{C^+}{(t-\tau)^{Q/2}} \exp\left(-c^+ \Psi(x, t; \xi, \tau)\right) \quad (\xi, \tau), (x, t) \in \mathbb{R}^N \times]0, T[, \ t > \tau,$$

where Q is the *homogeneous dimension* of the space $\mathbb{R}^N$ with respect to the underlying Lie Group in $\mathbb{R}^{N+1}$, and C^+, c^+ are constants depending on the operator. The method described in this section gives the analogous lower bound for Γ

$$\frac{c^-}{(t-t_0)^{Q/2}} \exp\left(-C^- \Psi(x, t; x_0, t_0)\right) \leq \Gamma(x, t; x_0, t_0) \quad (x_0, t_0), (x, t) \in \mathbb{R}^N \times]0, T[.$$

We conclude this section with a discussion on another meaningful example of operator which writes in the form (24) and is somehow more degenerate than (18). It is

$$\mathscr{L} = \partial_{x_1}^2 + x_1 \partial_{x_2} + \cdots + x_{N-1} \partial_{x_N} - \partial_t, \tag{25}$$

which is related to the following stochastic process:

$$dX_t^1 = dW_t, \quad dX_t^2 = X_t^1 dt, \quad \ldots \quad , dX_t^N = X_t^{N-1} dt, \quad t \geq 0. \tag{26}$$

As the operator defined in (18), the one in (25) can be written as $\mathscr{L} = X^2 + Y$ with

$$X(x, t) = \partial_{x_1} \sim \begin{pmatrix} 1 \\ 0 \\ \vdots \\ 0 \end{pmatrix}, \qquad Y(x, t) = \sum_{j=1}^{N-1} x_j \partial_{x_{j+1}} - \partial_t \sim \begin{pmatrix} 0 \\ x_1 \\ x_2 \\ \vdots \\ -1 \end{pmatrix}.$$

Note that, in this case, $\partial_{x_{j+1}} = [\partial_{x_j}, Y]$ for $j = 1, \ldots, N-1$. As a consequence, $\mathscr{L}$ is invariant with respect to the dilation defined by the following matrix:

$$\mathrm{diag}(\rho, \rho^3, \ldots, \rho^{2N-1}, \rho^2),$$

then its homogeneous dimension Q is equal to N^2. Accordingly, we have that $\mathrm{Var}(X_t^j) = c_j t^{2j-1}$, $j = 1, \ldots, N$, where c_j is a positive constant.

We recall that the parametrix method has been used by several authors for the study of degenerate Kolmogorov equations. We recall the works of Weber [45], Il'In [19], Sonin [42], Polidoro [37, 38], Di Francesco and Polidoro [15]. In particular, the lower bound of the fundamental is proved in [38] and in [15].

More recently, Delarue and Menozzi [14] extended the above bounds to a class of Degenerate Kolmogorov Operator with possibly nonlinear drifts satisfying Hörmander condition, under spatial Hölder continuity assumptions on the coefficients a_{ij}'s. They obtained analogous bounds by combining stochastic control methods with the parametrix representation of the fundamental solution given by McKean and Singer in [29].

6   More Degenerate Equations

In this section, we consider a stochastic process studied By Cinti, Menozzi, and Polidoro in [10]. It is similar to the one considered in Sect. 4, as it writes as follows:

$$\mathscr{L} := \partial_x^2 + x^2 \partial_y - \partial_t, \qquad (x, y, t) \in \mathbb{R}^2 \times (0, T), \tag{27}$$

and is related to the following stochastic differential equation

$$\begin{cases} X_t = x_0 + W_t, \\ Y_t = y_0 + \int_0^t (x_0 + W_s)^2 \, ds. \end{cases} \tag{28}$$

A representation of the density of this process has been obtained from the seminal works of Kac [21] in terms of the Laplace transform of the process $(Y_t)_{t \geq 0}$. We also refer to the monograph of Borodin and Salminen [7] for an expression in terms of special functions. We also quote the works of Smirnov [41] and Tolmatz [43] on the distribution function of the square of the Brownian bridge.

   We give explicit upper and lower bounds for the density of the process $(X_t, Y_t)_{t \geq 0}$ by the approach described in Sect. 3. Note that new difficulties appear in the study of the operator $\mathscr{L}$ defined in (27). Indeed, if we write $\mathscr{L}$ as follows:

$$\mathscr{L} = X^2 + Y, \quad \text{with} \quad X = \partial_x, \; Y = x^2 \partial_y - \partial_t,$$

then the commutator $[X, Y](x, y, t) = 2x\partial_y$ vanishes in the set $\{x = 0\}$, and we need a second commutator $[X, [X, Y]](x, y, t) = 2\partial_y$ to satisfy the Hörmander condition at every point of $\mathbb{R}^3$. As a consequence, a Lie group leaving invariant the equation $\mathscr{L}u = 0$ cannot exist. This problem is overcome by a *lifting procedure* (see Rothshild and Stein [40]). Specifically, we consider the following operator:

$$\widetilde{\mathscr{L}} := \partial_x^2 + x\partial_w + x^2\partial_y - \partial_t, \qquad (x, y, w, t) \in \mathbb{R}^3 \times (0, T),$$

and we consider any solution of $\mathscr{L}u = 0$ as a function that does not depend on w, and that solves the equation $\widetilde{\mathscr{L}}u = 0$. The lifting procedure allows us to rely on the Lie group invariance of $\widetilde{\mathscr{L}}$ in the study of the positive solutions of $\mathscr{L}u = 0$. Indeed, we have

(i) The operator $\widetilde{\mathscr{L}}$ is invariant with respect to the following Lie group operation:

$$(x_0, y_0, w_0, t_0) \circ (x, y, w, t) = (x + x_0, y + y_0 + 2x_0w - tx_0^2, w + w_0 - tx_0, t + t_0),$$

Fig. 5 Projection of $\mathcal{A}_{(0,0,0,0)}(\Omega)$ on the set $\{x = 0\}$

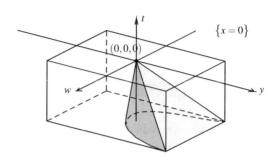

defined for every (x, y, w, t), $(x_0, y_0, w_0, t_0) \in \mathbb{R}^4$. In particular, it holds

$$(\widetilde{\mathscr{L}}u)(z_0 \circ z) = \widetilde{\mathscr{L}}(u(z_0 \circ z)),$$

for every $z_0 = (x_0, y_0, w_0, t_0)$ and $z = (x, y, w, t) \in \mathbb{R}^4$.

(ii) The operator $\mathscr{L}$ is invariant with respect to the following dilation:

$$(\delta_\rho)_{\rho \geq 0} : (x, y, w, t) \mapsto (\rho x, \rho^4 y, \rho^3 w, \rho^2 t).$$

That is, it holds:

$$\rho^2 (\mathscr{L}u)(\rho x, \rho^3 y, \rho^2 t) = \mathscr{L}(u(\rho x, \rho^3 y, \rho^2 t)).$$

(iii) The attainable set of the *origin* in the box $\Omega =]-1, 1[^4$ is

$$\mathcal{A}_{(0,0,0,0)}(\Omega) = \left\{ (x, w, y, t) \in]-1, 1[^4 \mid 0 \leq y \leq -t, w^2 \leq -ty \right\}.$$

Figure 5 describes the projection on the hyperplane $\{x = 0\}$ of the set $\mathcal{A}_{(0,0,0,0)}$

Then, an invariant Harnack inequality needed to construct Harnack chains for the positive solutions of $\mathscr{L}u = 0$ is available. The main result of the article [10] is the following:

Theorem 5 *Let* Γ *denote the fundamental solution of* $\partial_{xx} + x^2 \partial_y - \partial_t$.

- *If* $\eta - y \leq 0$, *then* $\Gamma(x, y, t, \xi, \eta, \tau) = 0$;
- *if* $\frac{\eta - y}{(t - \tau)^2} > \frac{x^2 + \xi^2}{t - \tau} + 1$, *then*

$$\Gamma(x, y, t, \xi, \eta, \tau) \approx \frac{1}{(t - \tau)^{5/2}} \exp\left(-C \left(\frac{(x - \xi)^2}{t - \tau} + \frac{\eta - y}{(t - \tau)^2} \right) \right);$$

- *if* $0 < \frac{\eta - y}{(t - \tau)^2} < \frac{1}{2}$, *then*

$$\Gamma(x, y, t, \xi, \eta, \tau) \approx \frac{1}{(t - \tau)^{5/2}} \exp\left(-C \left(\frac{x^4 + \xi^4 + (t - \tau)^2}{\eta - y} \right) \right).$$

We conclude this section with some remarks. We first note that, because of the particular form of the attainable set $\mathcal{A}_{(0,0,0,0)}(\Omega)$, it is not true that all the $\mathscr{L}$-admissible paths γ steering z_0 to z satisfy (11). For this reason, in the proof of our main result we do not solve any optimal control problem. We prove our lower bound by choosing smart admissible paths. This construction does not guarantee the optimality of the lower bounds. However, the comparison with the upper bound, that has the same asymptotic behavior, shows the optimality of both of them. The diagonal bounds and the upper bounds have been obtained by using probabilistic methods, and Malliavin Calculus in particular.

We eventually recall that more general operators and stochastic processes are studied in [10]. Precisely, we consider for every positive integer k the process $(X_t, Y_t)_{t \geq 0}$, with value in $\mathbb{R}^n \times \mathbb{R}$

$$
\begin{cases}
X_t = x + W_t \\
Y_t = y + \int_0^t \sum_j (x + W_s)_j^k \, ds
\end{cases}
$$

whose Kolmogorov equation is

$$
\mathscr{L} := \tfrac{1}{2} \Delta_x + (x_1^k + \cdots + x_n^k) \partial_y - \partial_t
$$

and

$$
\begin{cases}
X_t = x + W_t, \quad (k \text{ even}) \\
Y_t = y + \int_0^t |x + W_s|^k \, ds
\end{cases}
$$

whose Kolmogorov equation is

$$
\mathscr{L} := \tfrac{1}{2} \Delta_x + |x|^k \partial_y - \partial_t.
$$

We refer to the article [10] for the precise statement of our achievements and for further details.

7 Operators Related to Arithmetic Average Asian Options

In this section, we consider the operator

$$
\mathscr{L} = x^2 \partial_{xx} + x \partial_x + x \partial_y - \partial_t
$$

with $(x, y, t) \in \mathbb{R}^+ \times \mathbb{R} \times (0, T)$. It appears in the Black and Scholes setting when we consider the pricing problem for Arithmetic Average Asian Option. Specifically, we assume that the price of an asset $(X_t)_{t \geq 0}$ is described by a Geometric Brownian Motion and that the option depends on the arithmetic average of $(X_t)_{t \geq 0}$. Then, according to the Black and Scholes theory, the value of the option v is modeled by a function $v = v(t, X_t, Y_t)$ where

$$\begin{cases} X_t = x_0 e^{\sqrt{2}W_t}, \\ Y_t = y_0 + x_0 \int_0^t e^{\sqrt{2}W_s} ds. \end{cases} \tag{29}$$

This system was widely studied by Yor who wrote in [46] its joint density (see equation (6.e) in Sect. 6 of [46])

$$p(x, y, t; x_0, y_0) = \frac{2\sqrt{x_0}}{\sqrt{x}(y - y_0)^2} \frac{e^{\frac{\pi^2}{t}}}{\pi \sqrt{\pi t}} \exp\left(-\frac{x + x_0}{(y - y_0)}\right) \psi\left(\frac{2\sqrt{x x_0}}{y - y_0}, \frac{t}{2}\right), \tag{30}$$

where

$$\psi(z, t) = \int_0^\infty e^{-\frac{\xi^2}{2t}} e^{-z \cosh(\xi)} \sinh(\xi) \sin\left(\frac{\pi \xi}{t}\right) d\xi. \tag{31}$$

As in the previous example, the density of the stochastic process $(X_t, Y_t)_{t \geq 0}$ is not strictly positive in the whole set $\mathbb{R}^+ \times \mathbb{R} \times (0, T)$. In particular, its support is $\mathbb{R}^+ \times (y_0, +\infty) \times (t_0, T)$.

Monti and Pascucci observe in [31] that $\mathscr{L}$ is invariant with respect to the following group operation on $\mathbb{R}^+ \times \mathbb{R}^2$:

$$(x_0, y_0, t_0) \circ (x, y, t) = (x_0 x, y_0 + x_0 y, t_0 + t). \tag{32}$$

Indeed, if we set

$$v(x, y, t) = u(x_0 x, y_0 + x_0 y, t_0 + t), \tag{33}$$

then $\mathscr{L}v = 0$ if, and only if, $\mathscr{L}u = 0$.

Note that $\mathscr{L}$ is not invariant with respect to any dilation group $(\delta_\rho)_{\rho \geq 0}$. On the other hand, as

$$\mathscr{L} = X^2 + Y, \quad \text{with} \quad X(x, y, t) = x \partial_x, \ Y(x, y, t) = x \partial_y - \partial_t,$$

we have that $\mathscr{L}$ can be approximated by the Kolmogorov operator (18) defined in Sect. 5. Indeed, we can consider the coefficient x of the vector field X as a smooth function that is bounded and bounded by below on every compact set $K \subset \mathbb{R}^+ \times \mathbb{R} \times (0, T)$. For this reason, the Harnack inequality introduced in Sect. 5 also applies to $\mathscr{L}$.

The $\mathscr{L}$ admissible paths are the solutions of the following differential equation:

$$\begin{cases} \dot{x}(s) = \omega(s)x(s), & x(0) = x_0, \\ \dot{y}(s) = x(s), & y(0) = y_0, \\ \dot{t}(s) = -1, & t(0) = t_0, \end{cases}$$

and we denote by $\Psi(x_0, y_0, t_0, x, y, t)$ the value function of the relevant optimal control problem with quadratic cost. The main result for the fundamental solution $\Gamma(x, y, t; x_0, y_0, t_0)$ of the operator $\mathcal{L}$ is the following

Theorem 6 *Let Γ be the fundamental solution of $\mathcal{L}$. Then, for every $(x_0, y_0, t_0) \in \mathbb{R}^+ \times \mathbb{R} \times [0, T[$ we have*

$$\Gamma(x, y, t, x_0, y_0, t_0) = 0 \quad \forall\, (x, y, t) \in \mathbb{R}^+ \times \mathbb{R}^2 \setminus \{] - \infty, y_0[\times]t_0, T[\}. \quad (34)$$

Moreover, for arbitrary $\varepsilon \in]0, 1[$, there exist two positive constants $c_\varepsilon^-, C_\varepsilon^+$ depending on ε, on T and on the operator $\mathcal{L}$, and two positive constants C^-, c^+, only depending on the operator $\mathcal{L}$ such that

$$\frac{c_\varepsilon^-}{x_0^2(t - t_0)^2} \exp\left(-C^- \Psi(x, y + x_0\varepsilon(t - t_0), t - \varepsilon(t - t_0); x_0, y_0, t_0)\right) \leq$$

$$\Gamma(x, y, t; x_0, y_0, t_0) \leq \qquad\qquad (35)$$

$$\frac{C_\varepsilon^+}{x_0^2(t - t_0)^2} \exp\left(-c^+ \Psi(x, y - x_0\varepsilon, t + \varepsilon; x_0, y_0, t_0)\right),$$

for every $(x, y, t) \in \mathbb{R}^+ \times] - \infty, y_0 - x_0\varepsilon(t - t_0)[\times]t_0, T[.$

Note that, since the proof of Theorem 6 is based on local estimates of the solution of $\mathcal{L}u = 0$ and $\mathcal{L}$ is *locally* well approximated by the operator introduced in (18), the diagonal bound in (35) agrees with the diagonal term of Γ_0 in (23). Furthermore, the diagonal estimate corresponds to the product of the standard deviations of the random variables X_t and Y_t defined in (29). Indeed,

$$\mathrm{Var}(X_t) = x_0^2 e^{2t}\left(e^{2t} - 1\right) = 2x_0^2 t + o(t), \quad \text{as } t \to 0,$$

$$\mathrm{Var}(Y_t) = x_0^2 \left(\frac{1}{6}\left(e^{4t} - 1\right) - \frac{2}{3}\left(e^t - 1\right) - \left(e^t - 1\right)^2\right) = \frac{2}{3} x_0^2 t^3 + o(t^3), \quad \text{as } t \to 0.$$

Clearly, the knowledge of the asymptotic behavior of the function Ψ is crucial for the application of our Theorem 6. In [9], it is shown that one can write the function Ψ in terms of the function g defined as follows

$$g(r) = \begin{cases} \frac{\sinh(\sqrt{r})}{\sqrt{r}}, & r > 0, \\ 1, & r = 0, \\ \frac{\sin(\sqrt{-r})}{\sqrt{-r}}, & -\pi^2 < r < 0, \end{cases}$$

and it is proven the following proposition:

Proposition 1 *For every $(x, y, t), (x_0, y_0, t_0) \in \mathbb{R}^+ \times \mathbb{R}^2$, with $t_0 < t$ and $y_0 > y$, we have*

$$\begin{cases} \Psi(x_1, y_1, t_1; x_0, y_0, t_0) = E(t_1 - t_0) + \frac{4(x_1 + x_0)}{y_0 - y_1} - 4\sqrt{E + \frac{4x_1 x_0}{(y_0 - y_1)^2}}, \\[2mm] if\ E \geq -\frac{\pi^2}{t_1 - t_0}; \\[2mm] \Psi(x_1, y_1, t_1; x_0, y_0, t_0) = E(t_1 - t_0) + \frac{4(x_1 + x_0)}{y_0 - y_1} + 4\sqrt{E + \frac{4x_1 x_0}{(y_0 - y_1)^2}}, \\[2mm] if\ -\frac{4\pi^2}{t_1 - t_0} < E < -\frac{\pi^2}{t_1 - t_0}. \end{cases}$$

where

$$E = \frac{4}{(t - t_0)^2} g^{-1}\left(\frac{y_0 - y}{(t - t_0)\sqrt{x x_0}}\right).$$

Moreover,

$$\frac{\Psi(x, y, t; x_0, y_0, t_0)}{\frac{4}{(t - t_0)} \log^2\left(\frac{y_0 - y}{(t - t_0)\sqrt{x x_0}}\right) + \frac{4(x_0 + x)}{y_0 - y}} \to 1, \quad as \quad \frac{y_0 - y}{(t - t_0)\sqrt{x_0 x}} \to +\infty;$$

$$\frac{\Psi(x, y, t; x_0, y_0, t_0)}{\frac{4(\sqrt{x} + \sqrt{x_0})^2}{y_0 - y} - \frac{4\pi^2}{(t - t_0)}} \to 1, \quad as \quad \frac{y_0 - y}{(t - t_0)\sqrt{x_0 x}} \to 0.$$

The above expression for the value function Ψ has been obtained by using the Pontryagin Maximum Principle [39], the upper bound in (35) is a consequence of the fact that Ψ satisfies the Hamilton–Jacobi–Bellman equation $Y\Psi + \frac{1}{4}(X\Psi)^2 = 0$.

To our knowledge, it is not easy to compare the integral expression of p in (30) with the estimates given in Proposition 1, then Theorem 6 provides us with an alternative explicit information on the asymptotic behavior of p. Moreover, the method described in this section also applies to the divergence form operator $\widetilde{\mathscr{L}}$ defined as

$$\widetilde{\mathscr{L}} u = x\partial_x (a x \partial_x u) + b x \partial_x u + x \partial_y u - \partial_t u,$$

where a and b are smooth bounded coefficients, with a bounded by below and $x \partial_x a$ bounded. Note that, in this case, an expression of Γ analogous to (30) is not available. A further consequence of (35) is the following result. By applying (35) to Γ and to the fundamental solutions $\Gamma^\pm$ of the operators

$$\mathscr{L}^\pm u = \lambda^\pm x^2 \partial_{xx} u + x \partial_x u + x \partial_y u - \partial_t u, \quad (x, y, t) \in \mathbb{R}^+ \times \mathbb{R} \times]0, T[, \quad (36)$$

we obtain

$$k^- \Gamma^-\left(x, y + \varepsilon(t + 1), t - \varepsilon(t + 1)\right)$$
$$\leq \Gamma(x, y, t)$$
$$\leq k^+ \Gamma^+\left(x, y - \frac{\varepsilon}{1 - \varepsilon}(t + 1), t + \frac{\varepsilon}{1 - \varepsilon}(t + 1)\right),$$

for every $(x, y, t), \in \mathbb{R}^+ \times \mathbb{R} \times]0, T[$ with $y + \varepsilon(t + 1) < 0$ and $t > \varepsilon/(1 - \varepsilon)$. Hence, we obtain lower and upper bounds for the fundamental solution Γ of the *variable coefficients operator* $\widetilde{\mathscr{L}}$ in terms of the fundamental solutions $\Gamma^{\pm}$ of the *constant coefficients operators* $\mathscr{L}^{\pm}$, whose expressions, up to some scaling parameters, agree with the function p in (30). We refer to the article [9] for the precise statement of the results of this section and for further details.

Acknowledgements We thank the anonymous referee for his/her careful reading of our manuscript and for several suggestions that have improved the exposition of our work.

References

1. Aronson, D.G.: Bounds for the fundamental solution of a parabolic equation. Bull. Am. Math. Soc. **73**, 890–896 (1967)
2. Aronson, D.G., Serrin, J.: Local behavior of solutions of quasilinear parabolic equations. Arch. Ration. Mech. Anal. **25**, 81–122 (1967)
3. Bally, V.: Lower bounds for the density of locally elliptic Itô processes. Ann. Probab. **34**, 2406–2440 (2006)
4. Bally, V., Kohatsu-Higa, A.: Lower bounds for densities of Asian type stochastic differential equations. J. Funct. Anal. **258**, 3134–3164 (2010)
5. Bass, R.: Diffusions and elliptic operators. Springer, New York (1998)
6. Ben, G.: Arous and R. Léandre, Décroissance exponentielle du noyau de la chaleur sur la diagonale. Probab. Theory Related Fields **90**, 175–202 (1991)
7. Borodin, A.N., Salminien, P.: Handbook of Brownian motionfacts and formulae, Probability and its Applications, 2nd edn. Birkhauser, Basel (2002)
8. Boscain, U., Polidoro, S.: Gaussian estimates for hypoelliptic operators via optimal control. Rend. Lincei Math. Appl. **18**, 333–342 (2007)
9. Cibelli, G., Polidoro, S., Rossi, F.: Sharp estimates for Geman-Yor Processes and Application to Arithmetic Average Asian Option, Submitted
10. Cinti, C., Menozzi, S., Polidoro, S.: Two-sides bounds for degenerate processes with densities supported in subsets of $\mathbb{R}^n$, Potential Analysis, pp. 1577–1630 (2014)
11. Cinti, C., Nyström, K., Polidoro, S.: A note on Harnack inequalities and propagation sets for a class of hypoelliptic operators. Potential Anal. **33**, 341–354 (2010)
12. Cinti, C., Polidoro, S.: Pointwise local estimates and Gaussian upper bounds for a class of uniformly subelliptic ultraparabolic operators. J. Math. Anal. Appl. **338**, 946–969 (2008)
13. Davies, E.B.: Explicit constants for Gaussian upper bounds on heat kernels. Am. J. Math. **109**, 319–333 (1987)
14. Delarue, F., Menozzi, S.: Density estimates for a random noise propagating through a chain of differential equations. J. Funct. Anal. **259**, 1577–1630 (2010)
15. Di Francesco, M., Polidoro, S.: Schauder estimates, Harnack inequality and Gaussian lower bound for Kolmogorov-type operators in non-divergence form. Adv. Differ. Equ. **11**, 1261–1320 (2006)
16. Escauriaza, L.: Bounds for the fundamental solution of elliptic and parabolic equations in nondivergence form. Comm. Partial Differ. Equ. **25**, 821–845 (2000)
17. Fabes, E.B., Stroock, D.W.: A new proof of Moser's parabolic Harnack inequality using the old ideas of Nash. Arch. Ration. Mech. Anal. **96**, 327–338 (1986)
18. Hadamard, J.: Extension à l' équation de la chaleur d'un théorème de A. Harnack. Rend. Circ. Mat. Palermo **2**(3), 337–346 (1954)
19. Il'in, A.M.: On a class of ultraparabolic equations. Dokl. Akad. Nauk SSSR **159**, 1214–1217 (1964)
20. Jerison, D.S., Sánchez-Calle, A.: Estimates for the heat kernel for a sum of squares of vector fields. Indiana Univ. Math. J. **35**, 835–854 (1986)

21. Kac, M.: On distributions of certain Wiener functionals. Trans. Am. Math. Soc. **65**, 1–13 (1949)
22. Kogoj, A., Polidoro, S.: Harnack Inequality for Hypoelliptic Second Order Partial Differential Operators (to appear on Potential Analysis) (2016)
23. Kohatsu, A.: Higa, Lower bounds for densities of uniformly elliptic random variables on Wiener space. Probab. Theory Related Fields **126**, 421–457 (2003)
24. Konakov, V.: Parametrix method for diffusion and Markov chains, Russian preprint available on https://www.hse.ru/en/org/persons/22565341
25. Kolmogoroff, A.: Zufällige Bewegungen (zur Theorie der Brownschen Bewegung). Ann. of Math. 35(2), 116–117 (1934)
26. Krylov, N.V., Safonov, M.V.: A certain property of solutions of parabolic equations with measurable coefficients. Izv. Akad. Nauk SSSR Ser. Mat. **44**, 161–175 (1980)
27. Kusuoka, S., Stroock, D.: Applications of the Malliavin calculus. III. J. Fac. Sci. Univ. Tokyo Sect. IA Math. **34**, 391–442 (1987)
28. Malliavin, P.: Stochastic calculus of variation and hypoelliptic operators. In: Proceedings of the International Symposium on Stochastic Differential Equations, pp. 195–263. Wiley, New York-Chichester-Brisbane (1978)
29. McKeane Jr., H.P., Singer, I.M.: Curvature and the eigenvalues of t-he Laplacian. J. Differ. Geom. **1**, 43–69 (1967)
30. Metafune, G., Pallara, D., Rhandi, A.: Global properties of invariant measures. J. Funct. Anal. **223**, 396–424 (2005)
31. Monti, L., Pascucci, A.: Obstacle problem for arithmetic Asian options. C.R. Math. Acad. Sci. Paris **347**, 1443–1446 (2009)
32. Moser, J.: A Harnack inequality for parabolic differential equations. Comm. Pure Appl. Math. **17**, 101–134 (1964)
33. Moser, J.: correction to: a Harnack inequality for parabolic differential equations. Comm. Pure Appl. Math. **20**, 231–236 (1967)
34. Nash, J.: Continuity of solutions of parabolic and elliptic equations. Am. J. Math. **80**, 931–954 (1958)
35. Nualart, D.: The Malliavin Calculus and Related Topics. Probability and its Applications. Springer, New York (2000)
36. Pini, B.: Sulla soluzione generalizzata di Wiener per il primo problema di valori al contorno nel caso parabolico. Rend. Sem. Mat. Univ. Padova **23**, 422–434 (1954)
37. Polidoro, S.: On a class of ultraparabolic operators of Kolmogorov-Fokker-Planck type. Matematiche (Catania) **49**, 53–105 (1994)
38. Polidoro, S.: A global lower bound for the fundamental solution of Kolmogorov–Fokker–Planck equations. Arch. Ration. Mech. Anal. **137**, 321–340 (1997)
39. Pontryagin, L.S., Mishchenko, E., Boltyanskii, V., Gamkrelidze, R.: The Mathematical Theory of Optimal Processes. Wiley, New York (1962)
40. Rothschild, L., Stein, E.M.: E, Hypoelliptic differential operators and nilpotent groups. Acta Math **137**, 247–320 (1976)
41. Smirnov, N.: Sur la distribution de 2 (criterium de M. von Mises). C. R. Acad. Sci. Paris **202**, 449–452 (1936)
42. Sonin, I.M.: A class o degerate diffusion processes. Teor. Verojatnost. i Primenen **12**, 540–547 (1967)
43. Tolmatz, L.: Asymptotics of the distribution of the integral of the absolute value of the Brownian bridge for large arguments. Ann. Probab. **28**, 132–139 (2000)
44. Varopoulos, N.T., Saloff-Coste, L., Coulhon, T.: Analysis and Geometry on Groups. Cambridge Tracts in Mathematics, vol. 100. Cambridge University Press, Cambridge (1992)
45. Weber, M.: The fundamental solution of a degenerate partial differential equation of parabolic type. Trans. Am. Math. Soc. **71**, 24–37 (1951)
46. Yor, M.: On some exponential functionals of Brownian motion. Adv. Appl. Probab. **24**, 509–531 (1992)

Part III
Local Limit Theorems

A Survey on Conditioned Limit Theorems for Products of Random Matrices and Affine Random Walks

Ion Grama

Abstract This paper is a survey of results on the asymptotics of the exit time from certain domains and conditioned limit theorems to stay in the same domains for two type of Markov walks studied in Grama et al. (Prob Theory Rel Fields, 2016, [15]) and Grama et al. (Ann I.H.P., 2016, [16]).

Keywords Conditioned Markov walks · General linear group
Affine Markov walk · Limit theorems

1 Introduction and Previous Results

Let $(X_n)_{n \geqslant 1}$ be independent identically distributed random variables. Consider the random walk $S_n = X_1 + \cdots + X_n$. For a starting point $y > 0$ denote by τ_y the exit time of the process $(y + S_n)_{n \geqslant 1}$ from the positive part of the real line. Many authors have investigated the asymptotic behavior of the probability of the event $\tau_y \geqslant n$ and of the conditional law of $y + S_n$ given $\tau_y \geqslant n$ as $n \to +\infty$. There is a waste literature on this subject. We refer the reader to Iglehart [18], Bolthausen [2], Doney [11], Bertoin and Doney [1], Borovkov [3, 4]. Eichelsbacher and Köning [12], Denisov, Vatutin and Wachtel [7], Denisov and Wachtel [8, 10] have considered random walks in $\mathbb{R}^d$ and studied the exit times from the cones. Walks with increments forming a Markov chain have been considered by Presman [21, 22], Varapoulos [23, 24], Dembo [6], Denisov and Wachtel [9]. Varapoulos [23, 24] studied Markov chains with bounded increments and obtained lower and upper bounds for the probabilities of the exit time from cones.

The purpose of this paper is to present some recent results on the asymptotic of the exit time and on the conditioned law for two particular cases of Markov chains. In Sect. 2 we treat products of i.i.d. random matrices which lead to the study of a certain Markov chain. The results of this section have been obtained in collaboration

I. Grama (✉)
Université de Bretagne Sud, 56017 Vannes, France
e-mail: ion.grama@univ-ubs.fr

© Springer International Publishing AG 2017
V. Panov (ed.), *Modern Problems of Stochastic Analysis and Statistics*,
Springer Proceedings in Mathematics & Statistics 208,
DOI 10.1007/978-3-319-65313-6_5

with Émile Le Page and Marc Peigné [15]. The second case deals with a Markov
chain defined by affine transformations on the real line. The results of the Sect. 3
have been obtained in collaboration with Ronan Lauvergnat and Émile Le Page [16].
In both cases our proofs rely upon a strong approximation result for Markov chains
established in [14]. A short sketch of the proofs is given in Sect. 4 based on the results
of [15].

2 Products of i.i.d Random Matrices

Let $\mathbb{G} = GL(d, \mathbb{R})$ be the general linear group of $d \times d$ invertible matrices w.r.t.
ordinary matrix multiplication. If g is an element of of $\mathbb{G}$ by $\|g\|$ we mean the operator
norm and if v is an element of the vector space $\mathbb{V} = \mathbb{R}^d$ the norm $\|v\|$ is Euclidean.
Let μ be a probability measure on $\mathbb{G}$ and suppose that on the probability space
$(\Omega, \mathcal{F}, \mathbf{Pr})$ we are given an i.i.d. sequence $(g_n)_{n \geq 1}$ of $\mathbb{G}$-valued random elements of
the same law $\mathbf{Pr}(g_1 \in dg) = \mu(dg)$. Let $G_n = g_n \ldots g_1$ and $v \in \mathbb{V} \smallsetminus \{0\}$ be a starting point. The object of interest is the size of the vector $G_n v$ which is controlled by
the quantity $\log \|G_n v\|$. It follows from the results of Le Page [19] that, under appro-
priate assumptions, the sequence $(\log \|G_n v\|)_{n \geq 1}$ behaves like a sum of i.i.d. r.v.'s
and satisfies standard classical properties such as the law of large numbers, law of
iterated logarithm and the central limit theorem.

Introduce the following conditions. Let $N(g) = \max\{\|g\|, \|g\|^{-1}\}$, supp$\mu$ be
the support of the measure μ and $\mathbb{P}(\mathbb{V})$ be the projective space of $\mathbb{V}$.

P1. *There exists $\delta_0 > 0$ such that*

$$\int_{\mathbb{G}} N(g)^{\delta_0} \mu(dg) < \infty,$$

The next condition requires, roughly speaking, that the dimension of the support
of suppμ cannot be reduced.

P2 (Strong irreducibility). *The support* suppμ *of* μ *acts strongly irreducibly on*
$\mathbb{V}$*, i.e. no proper union of finite vector subspaces of $\mathbb{V}$ is invariant with respect to all*
elements g of the group generated by suppμ*.*

The sequence $(h_n)_{n \geq 1}$ of elements of $\mathbb{G}$ is said to be contracting for the pro-
jective space $\mathbb{P}(\mathbb{V})$ if $\lim_{n \to \infty} \log \frac{a_1(n)}{a_2(n)} = \infty$, where $a_1(n) \geq \ldots \geq a_d(n)$ are the
eigenvalues of the symmetric matrix $h_n' h_n$ and h_n' is the transpose of h_n.

P3 (Proximality). *The closed semigroup generated by* suppμ *contains a contracting*
sequence for the projective space $\mathbb{P}(\mathbb{V})$.

For example **P3** is satisfied if the closed semigroup generated by suppμ contains
a matrix with a unique simple eigenvalue of maximal modulus. For more details we
refer to Bougerol and Lacroix [5] and to the references therein.

In the sequel for any $v \in V \smallsetminus \{0\}$ we denote by $\overline{v} = \mathbb{R}v \in \mathbb{P}(V)$ its direction and for any direction $\overline{v} \in \mathbb{P}(V)$ we denote by v a vector in $V \smallsetminus \{0\}$ of direction $\overline{v}$. Define the function $\rho : \mathbb{G} \times \mathbb{P}(V) \to \mathbb{R}$ called norm cocycle by setting

$$\rho(g, \overline{v}) := \log \frac{\|gv\|}{\|v\|}, \quad \text{for } (g, \overline{v}) \in \mathbb{G} \times \mathbb{P}(V). \tag{1}$$

It is well known (see Le Page [19] and Bougerol and Lacroix [5]) that under conditions **P1–P3** there exists an unique μ-invariant measure ν on $\mathbb{P}(V)$ such that, for any continuous function φ on $\mathbb{P}(V)$,

$$(\mu * \nu)(\varphi) = \nu(\varphi).$$

Moreover the upper Lyapunov exponent

$$\gamma = \gamma_\mu = \int_{\mathbb{G} \times \mathbb{P}(V)} \rho(g, \overline{v})\, \mu(dg)\, \nu(d\overline{v})$$

is finite and there exists a constant $\sigma > 0$ such that for any $v \in V \smallsetminus \{0\}$ and any $t \in \mathbb{R}$,

$$\lim_{n \to \infty} \mathbf{Pr}\left(\frac{\log \|G_n v\| - n\gamma}{\sigma \sqrt{n}} \le t \right) = \Phi(t),$$

where $\Phi(\cdot)$ is the standard normal distribution.

Denote by $\mathbb{B}$ the closed unit ball in V and by $\mathbb{B}^c$ its complement. For any $v \in \mathbb{B}^c$ define the exit time of the random process $G_n v$ from $\mathbb{B}^c$ by

$$\tau_v = \min\{n \ge 1 : G_n v \in \mathbb{B}\}.$$

In the sequel, we consider that the upper Lyapunov exponent γ is equal to 0. The fact that $\gamma = 0$ does not imply that the events

$$\{\tau_v > n\} = \{G_k v \in \mathbb{B}^c : k = 1, \dots, n\}, \quad n \ge 1$$

occur with positive probability for any $v \in \mathbb{B}^c$. To ensure this we need the following additional condition:

P4. *There exists $\delta > 0$ such that*

$$\inf_{s \in \mathbb{S}^{d-1}} \mu(g : \log \|gs\| > \delta) > 0.$$

Our first result gives the asymptotic of the probability of the exit time.

Theorem 2.1 *Under conditions **P1-P4**, for any $v \in \mathbb{B}^c$,*

$$\mathbf{Pr}\,(\tau_v > n) = \frac{2V\,(v)}{\sigma\sqrt{2\pi n}}\,(1 + o\,(1))\ \ as\ n \to \infty,$$

where V is a positive function on $\mathbb{B}^c$.

Moreover, we prove that the limit law of the quantity $\frac{1}{\sigma\sqrt{n}}\log\|G_n v\|$, given the event $\{\tau_v > n\}$ coincides with the Rayleigh distribution $\Phi^+(t) = 1 - \exp\left(-\frac{t^2}{2}\right)$:

Theorem 2.2 *Under conditions **P1–P4**, for any $v \in \mathbb{B}^c$ and for any $t \geq 0$,*

$$\lim_{n\to\infty}\mathbf{Pr}\left(\frac{\log\|G_n v\|}{\sigma\sqrt{n}} \leq t\,\middle|\,\tau_v > n\right) = \Phi^+(t)\,.$$

The study of the products of random matrices is reduced to the case of a Markov chain in the following way. Consider the homogenous Markov chain $(X_n)_{n\geq 0}$ with values in the product space $\mathbb{X} = \mathbb{G} \times \mathbb{P}\,(\mathbb{V})$ and initial value $X_0 = (g, \overline{v}) \in \mathbb{X}$ by setting $X_1 = (g_1, g \cdot \overline{v})$ and

$$X_{n+1} = (g_{n+1}, g_n \ldots g_1 g \cdot \overline{v})\,,\ n \geq 1.$$

Let $v \in \mathbb{V} \setminus \{0\}$ be a starting vector and $\overline{v}$ be its direction. Iterating the cocycle property $\rho\,(g_2 g_1, \overline{v}) = \rho\,(g_2, g_1 \cdot \overline{v}) + \rho\,(g_1, \overline{v})$ one gets the basic representation

$$\log\|G_n g v\| = y + \sum_{k=1}^{n}\rho\,(X_k)\,,\ n \geq 1,$$

where $y = \log\|gv\|$ determines the "size" of the vector gv. We deal with the random walk $(y + S_n)_{n\geq 0}$ associated to the Markov chain $(X_n)_{n\geq 0}$, where $X_0 = x = (g, \overline{v})$ is an arbitrary element of $\mathbb{X}$, y is any real number and

$$S_0 = 0,\ S_n = \sum_{k=1}^{n}\rho\,(X_k)\,,\ n \geq 1.$$

The results for $\log\|G_n v\|$ stated in this section are obtained by taking $X_0 = x = (I, \overline{v})$ as the initial state of the Markov chain $(X_n)_{n\geq 0}$ and setting $y = \ln\|v\|$ and $V\,(v) = V\,((I, \overline{v}), \ln\|v\|)$. The function V is the harmonic function related to the transition probability of the Markov chain $(X_n, y + S_n)_{n\geq 0}$.

3   Results for Affine Markov Walks

On the probability space $(\Omega, \mathcal{F}, \mathbb{P})$ consider the affine recursion

$$X_{n+1} = a_{n+1}X_n + b_{n+1},\qquad n \geq 0,$$

where (a_i, b_i), $i \geq 1$ is a sequence of independent real random pairs of the same law as the generic random pair (a, b) and $X_0 = x \in \mathbb{R}$ is a starting point. Denote by $\mathbb{E}$ the expectation pertaining to $\mathbb{P}$. Denote by $\mathbb{P}_x$ and $\mathbb{E}_x$ the probability and the corresponding expectation generated by the finite dimensional distributions of $(X_n)_{n \geq 0}$ starting at $X_0 = x$.

We make use of the following conditions:

A1. *1. There exists a constant $\alpha > 2$ such that $\mathbb{E}\left(|a|^{\alpha}\right) < 1$ and $\mathbb{E}\left(|b|^{\alpha}\right) < +\infty$.*

2. The random variable b is non-zero with positive probability, $\mathbb{P}(b \neq 0) > 0$, and centered, $\mathbb{E}(b) = 0$.

A2. *For all $x \in \mathbb{R}$ and $y > 0$,*

$$\mathbb{P}_x\left(\tau_y > 1\right) = \mathbb{P}\left(ax + b > -y\right) > 0.$$

A3. *For any $x \in \mathbb{R}$ and $y > 0$, there exists $p_0 \in (2, \alpha)$ such that for any constant $c > 0$, there exists $n_0 \geq 1$ such that,*

$$\mathbb{P}_x\left(\left(X_{n_0}, y + S_{n_0}\right) \in K_{p_0,c}, \ \tau_y > n_0\right) > 0,$$

where

$$K_{p_0,c} = \left\{(x, y) \in \mathbb{R} \times \mathbb{R}_+^*, \ y \geq c\left(1 + |x|^{p_0}\right)\right\}.$$

Using the techniques from [17] it can be shown that, under condition **A1**, the Markov chain $(X_n)_{n \geq 0}$ has a unique invariant measure **m** and its partial sum S_n satisfies the central limit theorem

$$\mathbb{P}_x\left(\frac{S_n - n\mu}{\sigma\sqrt{n}} \leq t\right) \rightarrow \Phi(t) \quad \text{as} \quad n \rightarrow +\infty,$$

with

$$\mu = \frac{\mathbb{E}(b)}{1 - \mathbb{E}(a)} = 0$$

and

$$\sigma^2 = \frac{\mathbb{E}(b^2)}{1 - \mathbb{E}(a^2)} \frac{1 + \mathbb{E}(a)}{1 - \mathbb{E}(a)} > 0.$$

Moreover, it is easy to see that under **A1** the Markov chain $(X_n)_{n \geq 0}$ has no fixed point: $\mathbb{P}(ax + b = x) < 1$, for any $x \in \mathbb{R}$.

For any $y \in \mathbb{R}$ consider the affine Markov walk $(y + S_n)_{n \geq 0}$ starting at y and define its exit time

$$\tau_y = \min\{k \geq 1, \ y + S_k \leq 0\}.$$

Our first result gives the asymptotic of the probability of the exit time.

Theorem 3.1 *Assume either conditions **A1**, **A2**, **A3** and* $\mathbb{E}(a) \geq 0$, *or Conditions **A1** and **A3**. For any* $x \in \mathbb{R}$ *and* $y > 0$,

$$\mathbb{P}_x\left(\tau_y > n\right) = \frac{2V(x, y)}{\sqrt{2\pi n \sigma}}\left(1 + o\left(1\right)\right) \text{ as } n \to \infty,$$

where V *is a positive function on* $\mathbb{R} \times \mathbb{R}_+^*$.

As in the previous section the function V is the harmonic function related to the transition probability of the two dimensional Markov chain $(X_n, y + S_n)_{n \geq 0}$.

Our second result gives the asymptotic of the law of $(y + S_n)_{n \geq 0}$ conditioned to stay positive.

Theorem 3.2 *Assume either conditions **A1**, **A2**, **A3** and* $\mathbb{E}(a) \geq 0$, *or Conditions **A1** and **A3**. For any* $x \in \mathbb{R}$, $y > 0$ *and* $t > 0$,

$$\mathbb{P}_x\left(\frac{y + S_n}{\sigma\sqrt{n}} \leq t \,\middle|\, \tau_y > n\right) \xrightarrow[n \to +\infty]{} \Phi^+(t),$$

where $\Phi^+(t) = 1 - e^{-\frac{t^2}{2}}$ *is the Rayleigh distribution function.*

4   Sketch of the Proof

We start by giving a sketch of the proof of the results in Sect. 2.

We follow the arguments in [15] (we also refer the reader to the proof in [10] where the case of sums of independent random variables in $\mathbb{R}^d$ is considered). Denote by $\mathbb{P}_x$ the probability measure generated by the finite dimensional distributions of $(X_k)_{k \geq 0}$ starting at $X_0 = x \in \mathbb{X}$ and by $\mathbb{E}_x$ the corresponding expectation. For any $(x, y) \in \mathbb{X} \times \mathbb{R}$ consider the transition kernel

$$\mathbf{Q}_+(x, y, \cdot) = 1_{\mathbb{X} \times \mathbb{R}_+^*}(\cdot)\,\mathbf{Q}(x, y, \cdot),$$

where $\mathbf{Q}\left(x, y, dx' \times dy'\right)$ is the transition probability of the two dimensional Markov chain $(X_n, y + S_n)_{n \geq 0}$ under the measure $\mathbb{P}_x$. A positive $\mathbf{Q}_+$-harmonic function V is any function $V : \mathbb{X} \times \mathbb{R}_+^* \to \mathbb{R}_+^*$ satisfying

$$\mathbf{Q}_+ V = V. \tag{2}$$

Extend V by setting $V(x, y) = 0$ for $(x, y) \in \mathbb{X} \times \mathbb{R}_-$.

We first should prove the existence of a positive $\mathbf{Q}_+$-harmonic function. For any $y > 0$ denote by τ_y the first time when the Markov walk $(y + S_n)_{n \geq 0}$ becomes negative: $\tau_y = \min\{n \geq 1 : y + S_n \leq 0\}$.

Theorem 4.1 *Assume hypotheses **P1–P5**.*
1. For any $x \in \mathbb{X}$ and $y > 0$ the limit

$$V(x, y) = \lim_{n \to +\infty} \mathbb{E}_x \left(y + S_n; \tau_y > n \right)$$

exists and satisfies $V(x, y) > 0$.
2. The function V is $\mathbf{Q}_+$-harmonic, i.e., for any $x \in \mathbb{X}$ and $y > 0$,

$$\mathbb{E}_x \left(V(X_1, y + S_1); \tau_y > 1 \right) = V(x, y).$$

The proof of this theorem is rather lengthy. Skipping the technical details, the main difficulty is to show the integrability of the random variable S_{τ_y}, i.e., that for any $x \in \mathbb{X}$ and $y > 0$ it holds $\mathbb{E}_x \left(|y + S_{\tau_y}| \right) \leq c(1 + y) < +\infty$. The integrability is obtained by using a martingale approximation (see Gordin [13]) $M_n = \sum_{k=1}^{n} (\theta(X_k) - \mathbf{P}\theta(X_{k-1})), n \geq 1$, where θ is the solution of the Poisson equation $\rho = \theta - \mathbf{P}\theta$ and the norm cocycle ρ is defined in (1).

Lemma 4.2 *It holds $\sup_{n \geq 0} |S_n - M_n| \leq a = 2 \|\mathbf{P}\theta\|_\infty$. $\mathbb{P}_x$-a.s. for any $x \in \mathbb{X}$.*

Once integrabilty of S_{τ_y} established, for any $x \in \mathbb{X}$ set

$$V(x, y) = \begin{cases} -\mathbb{E}_x M_{\tau_y} & \text{if } y > 0, \\ 0 & \text{if } y \leq 0. \end{cases}$$

The following proposition presents some properties of the function V.

Proposition 4.3 *The function V satisfies*
1. For any $y > 0$ and $x \in \mathbb{X}$,

$$V(x, y) = \lim_{n \to +\infty} \mathbb{E}_x \left(y + M_n; \tau_y > n \right) = \lim_{n \to +\infty} \mathbb{E}_x \left(y + S_n; \tau_y > n \right).$$

2. For any $y > 0$ and $x \in \mathbb{X}$,

$$0 \vee (y - a) \leq V(x, y) \leq c(1 + y).$$

3. For any $x \in \mathbb{X}$, $\lim_{y \to +\infty} \frac{V(x,y)}{y} = 1$.
4. For any $x \in \mathbb{X}$, the function $V(x, \cdot)$ is increasing.

The harmonicity of V is established in the following way. Let $x \in \mathbb{X}$ and $y > 0$ and set $V_n(x, y) = \mathbb{E}_x \left(y + S_n; \tau_y > n \right)$, for any $n \geq 1$. By the Markov property we have

$$V_{n+1}(x, y) = \mathbb{E}_x \left(y + S_{n+1}; \tau_y > n + 1 \right)$$
$$= \mathbb{E}_x \left((V_n(X_1; y + S_1)); \tau_y > 1 \right).$$

Taking the limit as $n \to +\infty$, by Lebesgue's dominated convergence theorem, we get

$$V(x, y) = \lim_{n \to +\infty} \mathbb{E}_x \left(V_n (X_1; y + S_1); \tau_y > 1 \right)$$
$$= \mathbb{E}_x \left(\lim_{n \to +\infty} V_n (X_1; y + S_1); \tau_y > 1 \right)$$
$$= \mathbb{E}_x V (X_1, y + S_1) 1_{\{\tau_y > 1\}}$$
$$= \mathbf{Q}_+ V (x, y), \tag{3}$$

which proves that V is harmonic. We refer to [15] for all the details.

We now give some hints how to prove Theorem 4.5. From the strong approximation result [14] it follows that without loss of generality we can reconstruct the Markov walk $(S_n)_{n \geq 1}$ on the same probability space with the standard Brownian motion $(B_t)_{t \geq 0}$ such that for any $\varepsilon \in (0, \varepsilon_0)$, $x \in \mathbb{X}$ and $n \geq 1$,

$$\mathbb{P}_x \left(\sup_{0 \leq t \leq 1} \left| S_{[nt]} - \sigma B_{nt} \right| > n^{1/2 - 2\varepsilon} \right) \leq c_\varepsilon n^{-2\varepsilon}, \tag{4}$$

where c_ε depends on ε and $\varepsilon_0 > 0$. Using the strong approximation (4) and the well-known results on the exit time for standard Brownian motion (see Lévy [20]) we establish the following:

Lemma 4.4 *Let $\varepsilon \in (0, \varepsilon_0)$ and $(\theta_n)_{n \geq 1}$ be a sequence of positive numbers such that $\theta_n \to 0$ and $\theta_n n^{\varepsilon/4} \to +\infty$ as $n \to +\infty$. Then*
1. There exists a constant $c > 0$ such that, for n sufficiently large,

$$\sup_{x \in \mathbb{X}, \ y \in [n^{1/2 - \varepsilon}, \theta_n n^{1/2}]} \left| \frac{\mathbb{P}_x (\tau_y > n)}{\frac{2y}{\sqrt{2\pi n}\sigma}} - 1 \right| \leq c\theta_n.$$

2. There exists a constant $c_\varepsilon > 0$ such that for any $n \geq 1$ and $y \geq n^{1/2 - \varepsilon}$,

$$\sup_{x \in \mathbb{X}} \mathbb{P}_x (\tau_y > n) \leq c_\varepsilon \frac{y}{\sqrt{n}}.$$

The previous result holds for y in the interval $[n^{1/2 - \varepsilon}, \theta_n n^{1/2}]$. To extend it to a fixed $y > 0$ consider the first time ν_n when $|y + M_k|$ exceeds $2n^{1/2 - \varepsilon}$:

$$\nu_n = \min \left\{ k \geq 1 : |y + M_k| \geq 2n^{1/2 - \varepsilon} \right\}, \tag{5}$$

where $\varepsilon > 0$ is small enough. Using Markov property and Lemma 4.4 we show that

$$\mathbb{P}_x (\tau_y > n) = \frac{2}{\sqrt{2\pi n}\sigma} \mathbb{E}_x \left(y + S_{\nu_n}; \tau_y > \nu_n, \nu_n \leq n^{1 - \varepsilon} \right)$$

$$+o\left(n^{-1/2}\right).$$

To end the proof one has to prove that for any $x \in \mathbb{X}$ and $y > 0$,

$$\lim_{n \to +\infty} \mathbb{E}_x \left(y + S_{\nu_n}; \tau_y > \nu_n, \nu_n \le n^{1-\varepsilon}\right) = V(x, y). \tag{6}$$

Again, for details, we refer to [15]. Our main result concerning the limit behavior of the exit time τ_y is as follows:

Theorem 4.5 *Assume hypotheses P1–P5. Then, for any $x \in \mathbb{X}$ and $y > 0$,*

$$\mathbb{P}_x \left(\tau_y > n\right) \sim \frac{2V(x, y)}{\sigma\sqrt{2\pi n}} \text{ as } n \to +\infty.$$

Moreover, there exists a constant c such that for any $y > 0$ and $x \in \mathbb{X}$,

$$\sup_{n \ge 1} \sqrt{n}\mathbb{P}_x \left(\tau_y > n\right) \le c \frac{1 + y}{\sigma}.$$

The proof of Theorem 2.2 follows the same line using the following:

Lemma 4.6 *Let $\varepsilon \in (0, \varepsilon_0)$, $t > 0$ and $(\theta_n)_{n \ge 1}$ be a sequence such that $\theta_n \to 0$ and $\theta_n n^{\varepsilon/4} \to +\infty$ as $n \to +\infty$. Then*

$$\lim_{n \to +\infty} \sup \left| \frac{\mathbb{P}_x \left(\tau_y > n - k, \frac{y+S_{n-k}}{\sqrt{n}} \le t\right)}{\frac{2y}{\sqrt{2\pi n}} \frac{1}{\sigma^3} \int_0^t u \exp\left(-\frac{u^2}{2\sigma^2}\right) du} - 1 \right| = 0, \tag{7}$$

where $\sup$ *is taken over* $x \in \mathbb{X}$, $k \le n^{1-\varepsilon}$ *and* $n^{1/2-\varepsilon} \le y \le \theta_n n^{1/2}$.

The results exposed in Sect. 3 are more delicate but can be proved using similar technics which can be found in [16].

References

1. Bertoin, J., Doney, R.A.: On conditioning a random walk to stay nonnegative. Ann. Probab. **22**(4), 2152–2167 (1994)
2. Bolthausen, E.: On a functional central limit theorem for random walks conditioned to stay positive. Ann. Probab. **4**(3), 480–485 (1976)
3. Borovkov, A.A.: On the asymptotic behavior of distributions of first-passage times, I. Math. Notes **75**(1–2), 23–37 (2004)
4. Borovkov, A.A.: On the asymptotic behavior of distributions of first-passage times, II. Math. Notes **75**(3–4), 322–330 (2004)
5. Bougerol, P., Lacroix, J.: Products of Random Matrices with Applications to Schödinger Operators. Birghäuser, Boston-Basel-Stuttgart (1985)

6. Dembo, A., Ding, J., Gao, F.: Persistence of iterated partial sums. Annales de l'Institut Henri Poincaré, Probabilités et Statistiques **49**(3), 873–884 (2013)
7. Denisov, D., Vatutin, V., Wachtel, V.: Local probabilities for random walks with negative drift conditioned to stay nonnegative. Electron. J. Probab. **19**(88), 1–17 (2014)
8. Denisov, D., Wachtel, V.: Conditional limit theorems for ordered random walks. Electron. J. Probab. **15**, 292–322 (2010)
9. Denisov, D., Wachtel, V.: Exit times for integrated random walks. Annales de l'Institut Henri Poincaré, Probabilités et Statistiques **51**(1), 167–193 (2015)
10. Denisov, D., Wachtel, V.: Random walks in cones. Ann. Probab. **43**(3), 992–1044 (2015)
11. Doney, R.A.: Conditional limit theorems for asymptotically stable random walks. Zeitschrift für Wahrscheinlichkeitstheorie und Verwandte Gebiete **70**(3), 351–360 (1985)
12. Eichelsbacher, P., König, W.: Ordered random walks. Electron. J. Probab. **13**, 1307–1336 (2008)
13. Gordin, M.I.: The central limit theorem for stationary processes. Soviet Math. Dokl. **10**, 1174–1176 (1969)
14. Grama, I., Le Page, E., Peigné, M.: On the rate of convergence in the weak invariance principle for dependent random variables with applications to Markov chains. Colloq. Math. **134**, 1–55 (2014)
15. Grama, I., Le Page, E., Peigné, M.: Conditioned limit theorems for products of random matrices. Prob. Theory Rel. Fields **168**(3–4), 601–639 (2017)
16. Grama, I., Lauvergnat, R., Le Page, E.: Limit theorems for affine Markov walks conditioned to stay positive. Ann. I.H.P. (2016). arXiv:1601.02991. (to appear)
17. Guivarc'h, Y., Le Page, E.: On spectral properties of a family of transfer operators and convergence to stable laws for affine random walks. Ergod. Theory Dyn. Syst. **28**(02), 423–446 (2008)
18. Iglehart, D.L.: Functional central limit theorems for random walks conditioned to stay positive. Ann. Probab. **2**(4), 608–619 (1975)
19. Le Page, E.: Théorèmes limites pour les produits de matrices aléatoires. Springer Lecture Notes, vol. 928, pp. 258–303 (1982)
20. Lévy, P.: Théorie de l'addition des variables aléatoires. Gauthier-Villars, Paris (1937)
21. Presman, E.: Boundary problems for sums of lattice random variables, defined on a finite regular Markov chain. Theory Probab. Appl. **12**(2), 323–328 (1967)
22. Presman, E.: Methods of factorization and a boundary problems for sums of random variables defined on a markov chain. Izvestija Akademii Nauk SSSR **33**, 861–990 (1969)
23. Varopoulos, N.Th.: Potential theory in conical domains. Math. Proc. Camb. Philos. Soc. **125**(2), 335–384 (1999)
24. Varopoulos, N.Th.: Potential theory in conical domains. II. Math. Proc. Camb. Philos. Soc. **129**(2), 301–320 (2000)

Bounds in the Local Limit Theorem for a Random Walk Conditioned to Stay Positive

Ion Grama and Émile Le Page

Abstract Let $(X_i)_{i \geq 1}$ be a sequence i.i.d. random variables and $S_n = \sum_{i=1}^{n} X_i$, $n \geq 1$. For any starting point $y > 0$ denote by τ_y the first moment when the random walk $(y + S_k)_{k \geq 1}$ becomes negative. We give some bounds of order $n^{-3/2}$ for the expectations $\mathbb{E}\left(g\left(y + S_n\right); \tau_n > n\right)$, $y \in \mathbb{R}_+^*$ which are valid for a large class of bounded measurable function g with constants depending on some norms of the function g.

Keywords Exit time · Random walk conditioned to stay positive
Local limit theorem

1 Notations and Main Results

Let $(X_i)_{i \geq 1}$ be a sequence of i.i.d. real valued r.v.'s on the probability space $(\Omega, \mathcal{F}, \mathbb{P})$. Assume that $\mathbb{E} X_1 = 0$ and $\mathbb{E} X_1^2 = \sigma^2 \in \mathbb{R}_+^* := (0, \infty)$. Denote

$$S_n := \sum_{i=1}^{n} X_i, \ n \geq 1. \tag{1.1}$$

For any starting point $y > 0$, let τ_y be the first moment when the random walk $(y + S_k)_{k \geq 1}$ becomes non-positive

$$\tau_y := \inf \{k \geq 1 : y + S_k \leq 0\}. \tag{1.2}$$

I. Grama (✉) · É. Le Page
Université de Bretagne Sud, 56017 Vannes, France
e-mail: ion.grama@univ-ubs.fr

É. Le Page
e-mail: emile.le-page@univ-ubs.fr

© Springer International Publishing AG 2017
V. Panov (ed.), *Modern Problems of Stochastic Analysis and Statistics*,
Springer Proceedings in Mathematics & Statistics 208,
DOI 10.1007/978-3-319-65313-6_6

Define the reversals $X_1^* = -X_n$, $X_2^* = -X_{n-1}$, ..., $X_n^* = -X_1$ and

$$S_k^* := \sum_{i=1}^{k} X_i^*, \ k = 1, ..., n.$$

We can easily extend X_k^* and S_k to all $k \geq n$: it is enough to extend X_i for non-positive indices $i = 0, -1, -2, ...$. For any "end" point $z > 0$ set

$$\tau_z^* := \inf \{k \geq 1 : z + S_k^* < 0\}. \tag{1.3}$$

The exact asymptotics for the probabilites $\mathbb{P}(\tau_y > n)$ and $\mathbb{P}(\tau_y^* > n)$ have been studied for many authors. We refer to Spitzer [13], Iglehart [12], Bertoin and Doney [1], Borovkov [2–4], Doney [8], Caravenna [5], Denisov and Wachtel [6, 7], Vatutin and Wachtel [16], Eichelsbacher and König [9]. We state a well-known result for independent random variables in $\mathbb{R}^1$, which gives a bound for the probabilities $\mathbb{P}(\tau_y > n)$ and $\mathbb{P}(\tau_y^* > n)$. We refer to [11], where the case of affine random walks was considered (the i.i.d. random walk in $\mathbb{R}^1$ is a particular case); see also Denisov and Wachtel [7] for the case of random walks in cones in $\mathbb{R}^d$.

Theorem 1.1 *There exists a constant c such that for any $y > 0$ and $n \geq 1$,*

$$\mathbb{P}(\tau_y > n) \leq c\frac{1+y}{\sigma\sqrt{n}} \ \text{ and } \ \mathbb{P}(\tau_y^* > n) \leq c\frac{1+y}{\sigma\sqrt{n}}. \tag{1.4}$$

The goal of the paper is to prove bounds of order $n^{-3/2}$ on the expectation

$$\mathbb{E}(g(y + S_n); \tau_y > n) := \mathbb{E}g(y + S_n) 1_{\{\tau_y > n\}} \tag{1.5}$$

for a large class of function $g : \mathbb{R}_+^* \to \mathbb{R}_+ := [0, \infty)$ and $y > 0$, under the additional assumption that X_1 is strongly non-lattice, i.e., that for any $\varepsilon > 0$ it holds

$$\sup_{|t|>\varepsilon} |\mathbb{E}e^{itX_1}| < 1.$$

An equivalent statement is that the characteristic function of X_1 satisfies Cramer's strong non-lattice condition $\limsup |Ee^{itX_1}| < 1$ as $|t| \to +\infty$.

A specificity of our results is that we do not require that the function g has integrable Fourier transform. Instead, our bound involves a constant depending on some weighted L_1 norm of the function g defined below.

Let $\varepsilon > 0$. For any bounded measurable function $g : \mathbb{R}_+^* \to \mathbb{R}_+$ and any $x \in \mathbb{R}$ set

$$g_\varepsilon(x) := \sup_{u \in [x-\varepsilon, x+\varepsilon] \cap \mathbb{R}_+^*} g(u), \tag{1.6}$$

where $\sup \emptyset = 0$. In the sequel we shall assume without mentioning explicitly at each occurence that the function g is such that g_ε is measurable. For any bounded measurable function $h : \mathbb{R} \to \mathbb{R}_+$ and $p > 0$ define

$$\|h\|_{1,p} := \int_{\mathbb{R}} (1 + |x|)^p h(x) \, dx \quad \text{and} \quad \|h\|_1 := \int_{\mathbb{R}} h(x) \, dx. \qquad (1.7)$$

Our first result gives two bounds of order $1/n$. The first one depends on the initial value y, the second one gives a bound not depending on y.

Theorem 1.2 *Assume that X_1 is strongly non-lattice. Then there exist an absolute constant $c > 0$ and a decreasing sequence of positive numbers $(r_n)_{n \geq 1}$, $r_n \to 0$ as $n \to \infty$, depending only on the law of X_1 such that for any bounded measurable function $g : \mathbb{R}_+^* \to \mathbb{R}_+$, $n \geq 1$ and $y > 0$ it holds*

$$\mathbb{E}\left(g(y + S_n); \tau_y > n\right) \leq c \left\|g_{r_n}\right\|_1 \frac{1+y}{n} \qquad (1.8)$$

and

$$\mathbb{E}\left(g(y + S_n); \tau_y > n\right) \leq c \left\|g_{r_n}\right\|_{1,1} \frac{1}{n}. \qquad (1.9)$$

The following assertion is the main result of the paper.

Theorem 1.3 *Assume that X_1 is strongly non-lattice. Then there exist an absolute constant $c > 0$ and a decreasing sequence of positive numbers $(r_n)_{n \geq 1}$, $r_n \to 0$ as $n \to \infty$, depending only on the law of X_1 such that for any bounded measurable function $g : \mathbb{R}_+^* \to \mathbb{R}_+$, $n \geq 1$ and $y > 0$ it holds*

$$\mathbb{E}\left(g(y + S_n); \tau_y > n\right) \leq c \left\|g_{r_n}\right\|_{1,1} \frac{1+y}{n^{3/2}}. \qquad (1.10)$$

The bounds stated above make sense if the norms $\left\|g_{r_n}\right\|_1$ and $\left\|g_{r_n}\right\|_{1,1}$ of the function g_{r_n} appearing in the r.h.s. of (1.8), (1.9) and (1.10) are finite. The bounds for the expectation $\mathbb{E}\left(g(y + S_n^*); \tau_y^* > n\right)$ are similar and therefore will not be formulated separately.

Bounds of order $n^{3/2}$ for the expectation (1.5) are known in the literature for random walks on lattices, see [6, 7]. They can be extended relatively straightforwardly to the case when X_1 has a density. To the best of our knowledge, in the non-lattice case, bounds of type (1.8), (1.9) and (1.10), with an explicit dependence of the constants for an arbitrary function g, have not been considered in the literature. These type of bounds are useful for finding exact asymptotic in a conditioned local limit theorem for a large class of functions, which, however, is outside the scope of the present paper.

We continue by showing how the norms $\left\|g_{r_n}\right\|_1$ and $\left\|g_{r_n}\right\|_{1,1}$ can be bounded for two particular cases.

Case I. Let $\mathcal{I}$ be the set of indicators $g(x) = 1_{[a,b]}(x)$, $x \in \mathbb{R}$, with $0 < a < b < +\infty$. For any $g \in \mathcal{I}$ and $\varepsilon > 0$ we have $g_\varepsilon = 1_{[a-\varepsilon, b+\varepsilon]}$. Moreover, $\|g_\varepsilon\|_1 = b - a + 2\varepsilon$ and $\|g_\varepsilon\|_{1,1} = (b - a + 4\varepsilon)(a + b)/2$, for ε small enough. From Theorems 1.2 and 1.3 we get

Corollary 1.4 *Assume that X_1 is strongly non-lattice. Then there exist an absolute constant c and a decreasing sequence of positive numbers $(r_n)_{n\geq 1}$, $r_n \to 0$ as $n \to \infty$, depending only on the law of X_1, such that for any $0 < a < b < +\infty$, $y > 0$ and n large enough, it holds*

$$\mathbb{P}\left(y + S_n \in [a, b], \tau_y > n\right) \leq c(b - a + r_n)\frac{1 + y}{n},$$

$$\mathbb{P}\left(y + S_n \in [a, b], \tau_y > n\right) \leq c(b - a + r_n)(a + b)\frac{1}{n},$$

$$\mathbb{P}\left(y + S_n \in [a, b], \tau_y > n\right) \leq c(b - a + r_n)(a + b)\frac{1 + y}{n^{3/2}}.$$

In particular with $b = a + \Delta$ and some $\Delta_0 > 0$ we have the following bounds which hold uniformly in $r_n \leq \Delta \leq \Delta_0$. More precisely, there exist an absolute constant c and a decreasing sequence of positive numbers $(r_n)_{n \geq 1}$, $r_n \to 0$ as $n \to \infty$, depending only on the distribution function of X_1 such that for any $a > 0$, $y > 0$ and n large enough, it holds

$$\sup_{r_n \leq \Delta \leq \Delta_0} \frac{\mathbb{P}\left(y + S_n \in [a, a + \Delta]; \tau_y > n\right)}{\Delta} \leq \frac{c(1 + y)}{n},$$

$$\sup_{r_n \leq \Delta \leq \Delta_0} \frac{\mathbb{P}\left(y + S_n \in [a, a + \Delta]; \tau_y > n\right)}{\Delta} \leq \frac{c(a + \Delta_0)}{n},$$

$$\sup_{r_n \leq \Delta \leq \Delta_0} \frac{\mathbb{P}\left(y + S_n \in [a, a + \Delta]; \tau_y > n\right)}{\Delta} \leq \frac{c(a + \Delta_0)(1 + y)}{n^{3/2}}.$$

Case II. Let $\mathcal{G}_0$ be the set of bounded measurable functions $g : \mathbb{R}_+^* \to \mathbb{R}_+$ for which $\|g\|_{\mathcal{G}_0} = \|g\|_1 + \|\omega_g\|_1 < \infty$, where

$$\omega_g(x) = \sup_{y > 0,\, y \neq x} \frac{|g(x) - g(y)|}{|x - y|}, \quad x > 0.$$

Set $\|g\|_{\mathcal{G}_1} = \|g\|_{1,1} + \|\omega_g\|_{1,1}$. Let $\mathcal{G}_1$ be the set of bounded measurable functions $g : \mathbb{R}_+^* \to \mathbb{R}_+$ for which $\|g\|_{\mathcal{G}_1} < \infty$. Note that for any $g \in \mathcal{G}_0$, $\varepsilon > 0$ and $x > 0$,

$$|g_\varepsilon(x)| \leq |g(x)| + |g(x) - g_\varepsilon(x)| \leq |g(x)| + \varepsilon \omega_g(x), \tag{1.11}$$

which implies

$$\|g_\varepsilon\|_1 \le \|g\|_1 + \varepsilon \|\omega_g\|_1 \le (1 + \varepsilon) \|g\|_{\mathcal{G}_0},$$
$$\|g_\varepsilon\|_{1,1} \le \|g\|_{1,1} + \varepsilon \|\omega_g\|_{1,1} \le (1 + \varepsilon) \|g\|_{\mathcal{G}_1}.$$

From Theorems 1.2 and 1.3 we deduce the following:

Corollary 1.5 *Assume that X_1 is strongly non-lattice. Then there exists a constant c depending only on the law of X_1 such that for any $g \in \mathcal{G}_0$, $y > 0$ and $n \ge 1$ it holds*

$$Q_n g(y) \equiv \mathbb{E}\left(g(y + S_n); \tau_y > n\right) \le c \|g\|_{\mathcal{G}_0} \frac{1+y}{n}.$$

Moreover, for any $g \in \mathcal{G}_1$, $y > 0$ and $n \ge 1$.

$$Q_n g(y) \equiv \mathbb{E}\left(g(y + S_n); \tau_y > n\right) \le c \|g\|_{\mathcal{G}_1} \frac{1}{n}$$

and

$$Q_n g(y) \equiv \mathbb{E}\left(g(y + S_n); \tau_y > n\right) \le c \|g\|_{\mathcal{G}_1} \frac{1+y}{n^{3/2}}.$$

We end this section by recalling some notations used in this paper: $\mathbb{R}_+ = [0, \infty)$ is the nonnegative part of the real line $\mathbb{R}$, $\mathbb{R}_+^* = (0, \infty)$ is the set of positive numbers. Denote by $\phi(t) = \frac{1}{\sqrt{2\pi}} e^{-t^2/2}$, $t \in \mathbb{R}$ the standard normal density. The normal density of zero mean and variance σ^2 is denoted by $\phi_{\sigma^2}(t) := \phi(t/\sigma)/\sigma$. By $c, c_0, c_1, \dots$ we denote absolute constants and $c_{\alpha,\beta,\dots}, c'_{\alpha,\beta,\dots}, c''_{\alpha,\beta,\dots}, \dots$ denote constants depending only on the indices $\alpha, \beta, \dots$. All these constants are not always the same when used in different formulas. Occasionally, the constants will be specifically mentioned in the text.

2 Duality Lemma for Random Walks

The next key properties are crucial in the proof of the duality lemma below.

We associate with the condition that the random walk $(y + S_k)_{k \ge 1}$ stays positive the function

$$J(y, x_1, \dots, x_n) := 1_{\mathbb{R}_+^*}(y) \, 1_{\mathbb{R}_+^*}(y + x_1) \, 1_{\mathbb{R}_+^*}(y + x_1 + x_2) \dots 1_{\mathbb{R}_+^*}(y + x_1 + \dots + x_n),$$

which is defined for any real $x_1, \dots, x_n$ and y. We readily verify the following property:
Antisymmetry: For any real $x_1, \dots, x_n$, starting point $y \in \mathbb{R}_+^*$ and terminal point $z \in \mathbb{R}_+^*$ satisfying $z = x_n + \dots + x_1 + y$, it holds

$$J(y, x_1, \dots, x_n) = J(z, -x_n, \dots, -x_1). \tag{2.1}$$

Proof Note that

$$J(y, x_1, ..., x_n) = 1\,(y \geq M_n\,(x_1, ..., x_n))$$
$$= 1\,(z \geq x_1 + ... + x_n + M_n\,(x_1, ..., x_n)),$$

where

$$M_n\,(x_1, ..., x_n) := \max\,\{0, -x_1, -x_1 - x_2, ..., -x_1 - ... - x_n\} \geq 0.$$

Since

$$x_1 + ... + x_n + M_n\,(x_1, ..., x_n)$$
$$= x_1 + ... + x_n + \max\,\{0, -x_1, -x_1 - x_2, ..., -x_1 - ... - x_n\}$$
$$= \max\,\{x_1 + ... + x_n, x_2 + ... + x_n, ..., x_n, 0\}$$
$$= M_n\,(-x_n, -x_{n-1}, ..., -x_1),$$

we have

$$J(y, x_1, ..., x_n) = 1\,(z \geq M_n\,(-x_n, -x_{n-1}, ..., -x_1))$$
$$= J(z, -x_n, ..., -x_1).$$

$\square$

This (elementary) property turns out to be one of the key points in proving the duality lemma below. The second key point is the elementary fact that the Lebesgue measure is shift-invariant on $\mathbb{R}$

Shift-Invariance: For any nonnegative bounded measurable function f on $\mathbb{R}$ with compact support and any $a \in \mathbb{R}$ it holds

$$\int_{\mathbb{R}} f(y)\,dy = \int_{\mathbb{R}} f(z - a)\,dz. \tag{2.2}$$

Introduce the following transition kernels from $\mathbb{R}_+^*$ to $\mathbb{R}_+^*$:

$$Q_n\,(y, dz) = \mathbb{P}\,(y + S_n \in dz, \tau_y > n)$$
$$= \mathbb{P}\,(y + S_n \in dz, y + S_1 \geq 0, ..., y + S_{n-1} \geq 0) \tag{2.3}$$

and

$$Q_n^*\,(z, dy) = \mathbb{P}\,(z + S_n^* \in dy, \tau_z^* > n)$$
$$= \mathbb{P}\,(z + S_n^* \in dy, z + S_1^* \geq 0, ..., z + S_{n-1}^* \geq 0). \tag{2.4}$$

Define the transition operators

$$\mathbf{Q}_n g\,(\cdot) = \int_{\mathbb{R}_+^*} g\,(x)\,Q_n\,(\cdot, dx) \tag{2.5}$$

and

$$\mathbf{Q}_n^* g\,(\cdot) = \int_{\mathbb{R}_+^*} g\,(x)\, Q_n^*\,(\cdot, dx), \tag{2.6}$$

for any bounded measurable function g on $\mathbb{R}$.

The actions of $\mathbf{Q}_n$ and $\mathbf{Q}_n^*$ on a positive bounded measurable function g in terms of the joint law of $X_1, \dots, X_n$ can be computed as follows:

$$\mathbf{Q}_n g\,(y) = \int_{\mathbb{R}^n} F_{X_1,\dots,X_n}\,(dx_1, \dots, dx_n)\, g\,(y + x_1 + \dots + x_n)\, J\,(y, x_1, \dots, x_n) \tag{2.7}$$

and, in the same way,

$$\mathbf{Q}_n^* g\,(z) = \int_{\mathbb{R}^n} F_{X_1^*,\dots,X_n^*}\,(dx_1^*, \dots, dx_n^*)\, g\,(z + x_1^* + \dots + x_n^*)\, J\,(z, x_1^*, \dots, x_n^*)$$

$$= \int_{\mathbb{R}^n} F_{X_1,\dots,X_n}\,(dx_1, \dots, dx_n)\, g\,(z - x_n - \dots - x_1)\, J\,(z, -x_n, \dots, -x_1). \tag{2.8}$$

The following lemma establishes a duality relation between $\mathbf{Q}_n^*$ and $\mathbf{Q}_n$.

Lemma 2.1 (Duality) *Let g and h be two nonnegative bounded measurable functions with support in $\mathbb{R}_+^*$. Assume that one of the functions f or g has a compact support. Then*

$$\int_{\mathbb{R}_+^*} h\,(y)\, \mathbf{Q}_n g\,(y)\, dy = \int_{\mathbb{R}_+^*} g\,(z)\, \mathbf{Q}_n^* h\,(z)\, dz.$$

Proof Note that the function gh has a compact support. Using (2.7) and Fubini's theorem, we have

$$\int_{\mathbb{R}_+^*} h\,(y)\, \mathbf{Q}_n g\,(y)\, dy = \int_{\mathbb{R}^n} I\,(x_1, \dots, x_n)\, F_{X_1,\dots,X_n}\,(dx_1, \dots, dx_n), \tag{2.9}$$

where we denoted for brevity

$$I\,(x_1, \dots, x_n) = \int_{\mathbb{R}_+^*} h\,(y)\, g\,(y + x_1 + \dots + x_n)\, J\,(y, x_1, \dots, x_n)\, dy.$$

In the same way, using (2.8), we have

$$\int_{\mathbb{R}_+^*} g\,(z)\, \mathbf{Q}_n^* h\,(z)\, dz = \int_{\mathbb{R}^n} I^*\,(x_1, \dots, x_n)\, F_{X_1,\dots,X_n}\,(dx_1, \dots, dx_n),$$

with

$$I^*\,(x_1, \dots, x_n) = \int_{\mathbb{R}_+^*} g\,(z)\, h\,(z - x_n - \dots - x_1)\, J\,(z, -x_n, \dots, -x_1)\, dy.$$

To finish the proof of the lemma we show that, for any real $x_1, \ldots, x_n$,

$$I(x_1, \ldots, x_n) = I^*(x_1, \ldots, x_n). \tag{2.10}$$

For this we extend the functions h and g to the whole $\mathbb{R}$ by setting $h(y) = 0$ and $g(y) = 0$ for $y \notin \mathbb{R}_+^*$. Since $J(x_n, \ldots, x_1, y) = 1 (y > M_n(x_1, \ldots, x_n)) = 0$ for $y \leq 0$ we get

$$I(x_1, \ldots, x_n) = \int_{\mathbb{R}} h(y) g(x_n + \ldots + x_1 + y) J(y, x_1, \ldots, x_n) \, dy.$$

Using the shift-invariance property (2.2) of the Lebesgue integral on $\mathbb{R}$ it follows that

$$I(x_1, \ldots, x_n) = \int_{\mathbb{R}} h(z - x_n - \ldots - x_1) g(z) J(z - x_n - \ldots - x_1, x_1, \ldots, x_n) \, dz.$$

Since by antisymmetry property, we have

$$J(z - x_1 - \ldots - x_n, x_1, \ldots, x_n) = J(z, -x_n, \ldots, -x_1),$$

we conclude that (2.10) is true and so

$$\int_{\mathbb{R}_+^*} h(y) \mathbf{Q}_n g(y) \, dy = \int_{\mathbb{R}_+^*} g(z) \mathbf{Q}_n^* h(z) \, dz. \tag{2.11}$$

□

The duality stated in Lemma 2.1 can be rewritten in the following equivalent way. For any two functions g and h satisfying the conditions of Lemma 2.1 it holds

$$\int_{\mathbb{R}_+^*} h(y) \int_{\mathbb{R}_+^*} g(z) \mathbb{P}_n \left(y + S_n \in dz; \tau_y > n \right) dy$$
$$= \int_{\mathbb{R}_+^*} g(z) \int_{\mathbb{R}_+^*} h(y) \mathbb{P}_n \left(z + S_n^* \in dy; \tau_z^* > n \right) dz. \tag{2.12}$$

It is easy to see that the condition that one of the functions g or h has compact support in the previous lemma can be replaced by the condition that, one of the function g or h is integrable. The usefulness of Lemma 2.1 is explained by the following:

Corollary 2.2 *For any nonnegative bounded measurable function g on $\mathbb{R}_+^*$ it holds*

$$\int_{\mathbb{R}_+^*} \mathbb{E}_n \left(g(y + S_n); \tau_y > n \right) dy = \int_{\mathbb{R}_+^*} g(z) \mathbb{P}_n \left(\tau_z^* > n \right) dz.$$

Proof Let $h = 1_{[0,a]}$ with $a > 0$. By duality Lemma 2.1,

$$\int_{\mathbb{R}_+} 1_{[0,a]}(y) \mathbb{E}_n \left(g(y + S_n); \tau_y > n \right) dy = \int_{\mathbb{R}_+^*} 1_{[0,a]}(y) \, \mathbf{Q}_n g(y) \, dy$$

$$= \int_{\mathbb{R}_+^*} g(z) \, \mathbf{Q}_n^* 1_{[0,a]}(z) \, dz \leq \int_{\mathbb{R}_+^*} g(z) \, \mathbb{P}_n \left(\tau_z^* > n \right) dz.$$

Taking the limit as $a \to \infty$, by the Lebesgue monotone convergence theorem, we get

$$\int_{\mathbb{R}_+^*} \mathbb{E}_n \left(g(y + S_n); \tau_y > n \right) dy \leq \int_{\mathbb{R}_+} g(z) \, \mathbb{P}_n \left(\tau_z^* > n \right) dz.$$

In the same way, we obtain the opposite bound, which finishes the proof of the corollary. □

This corollary will be used in Lemma 4.2 to prove that $h(\cdot) = \mathbb{E}_n \left(g(\cdot + S_n) \right)$; $\tau_y > n \right)$ is integrable with respect to the Lebesgue measure.

3 A Non-asymptotic Version of the Local Limit Theorem

Local limit theorems have attracted much attention since the seminal papers by Gnedenko [10], Stone [15] and Shepp [14]. In this section, we give a version the local limit theorem for functions h with a non-integrable Fourier transform. The peculiarity of our result is that it is non-asymptotic, i.e., holds for any $n \geq 1$. We also give explicit dependence of the constants on the properties of the function h, which to the best of our knowledge is not given in the previous papers. The explicit dependence of the constants turns out to be crucial in proving the main results of the present paper. We conclude this section by showing how a Stone's type local limit theorem can be obtained from our result.

3.1 Smoothing and Some Related Bounds

In the sequel, we use a random variable with a compact support and with integrable Fourier transform. Define the triangular density $\kappa(\cdot)$ by $\kappa(x) = 1 - |x|$, for $|x| \leq 1$ and $\kappa(x) = 0$ otherwise (which is the density of a sum of two independent uniform random variables on $[-1/2, 1/2]$). Note that the support of the function $\kappa(\cdot)$ is the interval $[-1, 1]$ and its Fourier transform $\widehat{\kappa}(t) = \frac{1}{2\pi} \left(\frac{\sin(2t)}{2t} \right)^2$ is integrable:

$$\|\widehat{\kappa}\|_1 = \int_{-\infty}^{\infty} \widehat{\kappa}(t)\, dt = \frac{1}{2\pi} \int_{-\infty}^{\infty} \left(\frac{\sin(2t)}{2t}\right)^2 dt < \infty.$$

Let η be an extra random variable with density κ independent of $X_1, ..., X_n$. Let $y > 0$ and $\varepsilon \in (0, 1/2)$. Set $\eta_\varepsilon = \varepsilon\eta$. The density of η_ε is $\kappa_\varepsilon(x) = \kappa(x/\varepsilon)/\varepsilon$. Moreover, its characteristic function $\widehat{\kappa}_\varepsilon(t) = \mathbb{E}e^{it\varepsilon\eta} = \widehat{\kappa}(\varepsilon t)$ is integrable

$$\|\widehat{\kappa}_\varepsilon\|_1 = \int_{-\infty}^{\infty} |\widehat{\kappa}(\varepsilon t)|\, dt = \frac{1}{\varepsilon} \int_{-\infty}^{\infty} |\widehat{\kappa}(t)|\, dt = \frac{1}{\varepsilon}\|\widehat{\kappa}\|_1.$$

Let $g : \mathbb{R} \to \mathbb{R}_+$ be a bounded measurable function. Along with the definition (1.6), for any $x \in \mathbb{R}$, set

$$g_\varepsilon(x) := \sup_{u \in [x-\varepsilon, x+\varepsilon]} g(u) \quad \text{and} \quad g_{-\varepsilon}(x) = \inf_{u \in [x-\varepsilon, x+\varepsilon]} g(u). \tag{3.1}$$

Note that

$$g_{\pm\varepsilon} * \kappa_\varepsilon(x) = \mathbb{E}g_{\pm\varepsilon}(x - \eta_\varepsilon) = \int_{-\infty}^{\infty} g_{\pm\varepsilon}(x - u)\kappa_\varepsilon(u)\, du. \tag{3.2}$$

Lemma 3.1 *For any $x \in \mathbb{R}$,*

$$g_{-\varepsilon}(x) \leq g(x) \leq g_\varepsilon(x) \tag{3.3}$$

and

$$g_{-2\varepsilon}(x) \leq g_{-\varepsilon} * \kappa_\varepsilon(x) \leq g(x) \leq g_\varepsilon * \kappa_\varepsilon(x) \leq g_{2\varepsilon}(x). \tag{3.4}$$

Proof By (3.1), for any $x \in \mathbb{R}$ and $u \in [-\varepsilon, \varepsilon]$ it holds $g_\varepsilon(x - u) \geq g(x)$ and $g_{-\varepsilon}(x - u) \leq g(x)$. In particular, with $u = 0$ we have $g_\varepsilon(x) \geq g(x)$ and $g_{-\varepsilon}(x) \leq g(x)$. Since the support of the random variable η_ε is $[-\varepsilon, \varepsilon]$, we have $g(x) \leq g_\varepsilon(x - \eta_\varepsilon)$ and $g(x) \geq g_{-\varepsilon}(x - \eta_\varepsilon)$ for any $x \in \mathbb{R}$. From this, taking the expectation, we get

$$g(x) \leq \mathbb{E}g_\varepsilon(x - \eta_\varepsilon) = g_\varepsilon * \kappa_\varepsilon(x), \quad x \in \mathbb{R}$$

and

$$g(x) \geq \mathbb{E}g_{-\varepsilon}(x - \eta_\varepsilon) = g_{-\varepsilon} * \kappa_\varepsilon(x), \quad x \in \mathbb{R}.$$

On the other hand, since $g_\varepsilon(x - u) \leq g_{2\varepsilon}(x)$ for any $x \in \mathbb{R}_+^*$ and $|u| \leq \varepsilon$, it holds

$$g_\varepsilon * \kappa_\varepsilon(x) = \int_{-\infty}^{\infty} g_\varepsilon(x - u)\kappa_\varepsilon(u)\, du \leq g_{2\varepsilon}(x) \int_{-\infty}^{\infty} \kappa_\varepsilon(u)\, du = g_{2\varepsilon}(x), \quad x \in \mathbb{R}.$$

In the same way we obtain

$$g_{-\varepsilon} * \kappa_\varepsilon(x) = \int_{-\infty}^{\infty} g_{-\varepsilon}(x - u)\kappa_\varepsilon(u)\,du \geq g_{-2\varepsilon}(x) \int_{-\infty}^{\infty} \kappa_\varepsilon(u)\,du = g_{-2\varepsilon}(x), \quad x \in \mathbb{R}.$$

□

In the sequel, denote by $\widehat{g}$ the Fourier transform of g whenever the latter is integrable.

Lemma 3.2 *Assume that $g_{2\varepsilon}$ is integrable. For any $x \in \mathbb{R}$,*

$$\left\| \widehat{g_\varepsilon * \kappa_\varepsilon} \right\|_\infty \leq \|g_{2\varepsilon}\|_1, \qquad \left\| \widehat{g_{-\varepsilon} * \kappa_\varepsilon} \right\|_\infty \leq \|g\|_1 \tag{3.5}$$

and

$$\left\| \widehat{g_\varepsilon * \kappa_\varepsilon} \right\|_1 \leq \|g_\varepsilon\|_1 \frac{\|\widehat{\kappa}\|_1}{\varepsilon}, \qquad \left\| \widehat{g_{-\varepsilon} * \kappa_\varepsilon} \right\|_1 \leq \|g\|_1 \frac{\|\widehat{\kappa}\|_1}{\varepsilon}. \tag{3.6}$$

Proof Using Lemma 3.1, we have

$$\left\| \widehat{g_\varepsilon * \kappa_\varepsilon} \right\|_\infty \leq \|g_\varepsilon * \kappa_\varepsilon\|_1 = \int_{-\infty}^{\infty} g_\varepsilon * \kappa_\varepsilon dx \leq \int_{-\infty}^{\infty} g_{2\varepsilon}(x)\,dx = \|g_{2\varepsilon}\|_1$$

and

$$\left\| \widehat{g_{-\varepsilon} * \kappa_\varepsilon} \right\|_\infty \leq \|g_{-\varepsilon} * \kappa_\varepsilon\|_1 \leq \|g\|_1.$$

Since $\widehat{g_\varepsilon * \kappa_\varepsilon} = \widehat{g}_\varepsilon \widehat{\kappa}_\varepsilon$, we have

$$\left\| \widehat{g_\varepsilon * \kappa_\varepsilon} \right\|_1 = \|\widehat{g}_\varepsilon \widehat{\kappa}_\varepsilon\|_1 \leq \|\widehat{g}_\varepsilon\|_\infty \|\widehat{\kappa}_\varepsilon\|_1 \leq \|g_\varepsilon\|_1 \frac{\|\widehat{\kappa}\|_1}{\varepsilon}$$

and

$$\left\| \widehat{g_{-\varepsilon} * \kappa_\varepsilon} \right\|_1 = \|\widehat{g}_{-\varepsilon} \widehat{\kappa}_\varepsilon\|_1 \leq \|\widehat{g}_{-\varepsilon}\|_\infty \|\widehat{\kappa}_\varepsilon\|_1 \leq \|g_{-\varepsilon}\|_1 \|\widehat{\kappa}_\varepsilon\|_1 \leq \|g\|_1 \frac{\|\widehat{\kappa}\|_1}{\varepsilon}.$$

□

3.2 A Non-asymptotic Local Limit Theorem for Functions with Integrable Fourier Transform

Let $X_1, X_2, \ldots$ be i.i.d. random variables of means 0 and unit variances: $\mathbb{E}X_1 = 0$ and $\mathbb{E}X_1^2 = 1$. Let $F(x) = \mathbb{P}(X_1 \leq x)$, $x \in \mathbb{R}$ be the distribution function of X_1.

Let $\mathcal{H}$ be the set of bounded nonnegative functions h with support in $\mathbb{R}$ and bounded integrable Fourier transform $\widehat{h}$. We apply the convention $0/0 = 0$ whenever the indeterminacy $0/0$ occurs.

Theorem 3.3 *Suppose that X_1 is strongly non-lattice. Then there is a decreasing sequence of positive numbers $(r_n)_{n\geq 1}$ depending only on the law of X_1, such that $\lim_{n\to\infty} r_n = 0$ and for any $n \geq 1$,*

$$\sup_{h\in\mathcal{H}} \sup_{y\in\mathbb{R}} \frac{\left| \sqrt{n}\mathbb{E}h\,(y+S_n) - \int_{\mathbb{R}} h\,(x)\,\phi\left(\frac{x-y}{\sqrt{n}}\right) dx \right|}{\|\widehat{h}\|_1 + \|\widehat{h}\|_\infty} \leq r_n.$$

Proof Let $h \in \mathcal{H}$. Without loss of generality we assume that $\sigma = 1$. By inversion formula we have

$$h\,(x) = \frac{1}{2\pi} \int_{\mathbb{R}} e^{\mathbf{i}xt}\widehat{h}\,(t)\,dt, \quad x \in \mathbb{R}_+^*.$$

Denote $P_n\,(dx) = \mathbb{P}\,(S_n \in dx)$. Let $\widehat{P}_n\,(t) = \int_{\mathbb{R}_+} e^{\mathbf{i}tx} P_n\,(dx)$ be its Fourier transform. By Fubini's theorem, for any $y \in \mathbb{R}$,

$$\mathbb{E}h\,(y+S_n) = \int_{\mathbb{R}} h\,(y+x)\,P_n\,(dx)$$
$$= \int_{\mathbb{R}} \frac{1}{2\pi} \int_{\mathbb{R}} e^{\mathbf{i}(y+x)t}\widehat{h}\,(t)\,dt\,P_n\,(dx)$$
$$= \frac{1}{2\pi} \int_{\mathbb{R}} e^{\mathbf{i}yt}\widehat{h}\,(t)\,\widehat{P}_n\,(t)\,dt.$$

Changing the variable $t = \frac{u}{\sqrt{n}}$, we obtain

$$\sqrt{n}\mathbb{E}h\,(y+S_n) = \frac{1}{2\pi} \int_{\mathbb{R}} e^{\mathbf{i}\frac{yu}{\sqrt{n}}}\widehat{h}\left(\frac{u}{\sqrt{n}}\right)\widehat{P}_n\left(\frac{u}{\sqrt{n}}\right) du$$
$$= \frac{1}{2\pi} \int_{\mathbb{R}} e^{\mathbf{i}\frac{yu}{\sqrt{n}}}\widehat{h}\left(\frac{u}{\sqrt{n}}\right)\widehat{\phi}\,(u)\,du + I, \qquad (3.7)$$

where

$$I = \frac{1}{2\pi} \int_{\mathbb{R}} e^{\mathbf{i}\frac{yu}{\sqrt{n}}}\widehat{h}\left(\frac{u}{\sqrt{n}}\right)\left(\widehat{P}_n\left(\frac{u}{\sqrt{n}}\right) - \widehat{\phi}\,(u)\right) du.$$

Let $\varepsilon > 0$. Decompose the integral I into three parts: $I = I_1 + I_2 + I_3$, where

$$I_1 = \frac{1}{2\pi} \int_{|u|\leq\varepsilon\sqrt{n}} e^{\mathbf{i}\frac{yu}{\sqrt{n}}}\widehat{h}\left(\frac{u}{\sqrt{n}}\right)\left(\widehat{P}_n\left(\frac{u}{\sqrt{n}}\right) - \widehat{\phi}\,(u)\right) du,$$
$$I_2 = -\frac{1}{2\pi} \int_{|u|>\varepsilon\sqrt{n}} e^{\mathbf{i}\frac{yu}{\sqrt{n}}}\widehat{h}\left(\frac{u}{\sqrt{n}}\right)\widehat{\phi}\,(u)\,du,$$
$$I_3 = \frac{1}{2\pi} \int_{|u|>\varepsilon\sqrt{n}} e^{\mathbf{i}\frac{yu}{\sqrt{n}}}\widehat{h}\left(\frac{u}{\sqrt{n}}\right)\widehat{P}_n\left(\frac{u}{\sqrt{n}}\right) du.$$

First we control I_1. We shall prove that, for $|u| \leq \varepsilon \sqrt{n}$,

$$\left| \widehat{P}_n \left(\frac{u}{\sqrt{n}} \right) - \widehat{\phi}(u) \right| \leq u^2 r_F \left(\frac{u}{\sqrt{n}} \right) \exp \left(-\frac{u^2}{2} + u^2 r_F \left(\frac{u}{\sqrt{n}} \right) \right), \qquad (3.8)$$

where $r_F(v)$ is a real function satisfying $r_F(t) \to 0$ as $t \to 0$. Denote $\psi_F(t) = \log \widehat{F}(t)$, where $\widehat{F}(t) = \mathbb{E} \exp(it X_1)$. Since $\mathbb{E} X_1 = 0$ and $\mathbb{E} X_1^2 = 1$, by Taylor's expansion, there exists $\varepsilon > 0$ and a complex function $R_F(\cdot)$ such that $|R_F(t)| \to 0$ as $t \to 0$ and $\psi_F(t) = -\frac{t^2}{2} + t^2 R_F(t)$, for $|t| \leq \varepsilon$. Taking into account that $\widehat{P}_n(t) = \left(\widehat{F}(t) \right)^n$, for any u satisfying $|u| \leq \varepsilon$, we have

$$\log \widehat{P}_n \left(\frac{u}{\sqrt{n}} \right) = n \psi_F \left(\frac{u}{\sqrt{n}} \right) = -\frac{u^2}{2} + u^2 R_F \left(\frac{u}{\sqrt{n}} \right).$$

Since $e^x = 1 + \eta x e^x$, for some $|\eta| \leq 2$ and $|x|$ sufficiently small, this implies that, for any $|u| \leq \varepsilon \sqrt{n}$,

$$\widehat{P}_n \left(\frac{u}{\sqrt{n}} \right) = \exp \left(-\frac{u^2}{2} + u^2 R_F \left(\frac{u}{\sqrt{n}} \right) \right)$$

$$= \exp \left(-\frac{u^2}{2} \right) \left(1 + \theta u^2 R_F \left(\frac{u}{\sqrt{n}} \right) \exp \left(u^2 R_F \left(\frac{u}{\sqrt{n}} \right) \right) \right),$$

where $|\theta| \leq 2$, which proves (3.8) with $r_F(t) = |R_F(t)|$.

Using (3.8) we get

$$|I_1| \leq \frac{1}{2\pi} \int_{|u| \leq \varepsilon \sqrt{n}} \left| \widehat{h} \left(\frac{u}{\sqrt{n}} \right) \right| \left| \widehat{P}_n \left(\frac{u}{\sqrt{n}} \right) - \widehat{\phi}(u) \right| du$$

$$\leq c \int_{|u| \leq \varepsilon \sqrt{n}} u^2 r_F \left(\frac{u}{\sqrt{n}} \right) \exp \left(-\frac{u^2}{2} + u^2 r_F \left(\frac{u}{\sqrt{n}} \right) \right) \left| \widehat{h} \left(\frac{u}{\sqrt{n}} \right) \right| du. \quad (3.9)$$

Since $r_F(t) \to 0$ as $t \to 0$ one can choose a positive ε depending only on the law of X_1 so small that $\sup_{|t| \leq \varepsilon} r_F(t) \leq 1/8$, which implies $-\frac{u^2}{2} + u^2 r_F \left(\frac{u}{\sqrt{n}} \right) \geq -3u^2/8$. Therefore

$$|I_1| \leq c \int_{|u| \leq \varepsilon \sqrt{n}} u^2 r_F \left(\frac{u}{\sqrt{n}} \right) \exp \left(-3u^2/8 \right) \left| \widehat{h} \left(\frac{u}{\sqrt{n}} \right) \right| du$$

$$\leq c \int_{|u| \leq \varepsilon \sqrt{n}} r_F \left(\frac{u}{\sqrt{n}} \right) \exp \left(-u^2/4 \right) \left| \widehat{h} \left(\frac{u}{\sqrt{n}} \right) \right| du,$$

where we use the bound $u^2 \exp \left(-u^2/8 \right) \leq c$, $u \in \mathbb{R}$. Since the sequence $r_n' = \sup_{v \in [0, \varepsilon n^{-1/4}]} r_F(v)$ decreases as $n \to \infty$ and $r_n' \leq c_F'$ for some positive constant c_F' depending only on the law of X_1, we have

$$|I_1| \leq c \int_{|u| \leq \varepsilon n^{1/4}} r_F \left(\frac{u}{\sqrt{n}}\right) \exp\left(-u^2/4\right) \left|\widehat{h}\left(\frac{u}{\sqrt{n}}\right)\right| du$$

$$+ c \int_{\varepsilon n^{1/4} \leq |u| \leq \varepsilon \sqrt{n}} r_F \left(\frac{u}{\sqrt{n}}\right) \exp\left(-u^2/4\right) \left|\widehat{h}\left(\frac{u}{\sqrt{n}}\right)\right| du$$

$$\leq c r_n' \int_{\mathbb{R}} \exp\left(-u^2/4\right) \left|\widehat{h}\left(\frac{u}{\sqrt{n}}\right)\right| du$$

$$+ c_F' e^{-\varepsilon^2 \sqrt{n}/4} \int_{\mathbb{R}} \left|\widehat{h}\left(\frac{u}{\sqrt{n}}\right)\right| du.$$

Since $\widehat{\phi}_\sigma(t) = e^{-t^2 \sigma^2/2}$ is the Fourier transform of $\phi_{\sigma^2}(u) = \frac{1}{\sqrt{2\pi}\sigma} e^{-\frac{t^2}{2\sigma^2}}$, we obtain

$$|I_1| \leq c r_n' \int_{\mathbb{R}} \left|\widehat{h}(u) \sqrt{n} e^{-nu^2/4}\right| du + c_F' \sqrt{n} e^{-\varepsilon^2 \sqrt{n}/4} \int_{\mathbb{R}} \left|\widehat{h}(u)\right| du.$$

$$= c r_n' \left\|\widehat{h}\sqrt{n}\widehat{\phi}_{n/2}\right\|_1 + c_F' \sqrt{n} e^{-\varepsilon^2 \sqrt{n}/4} \left\|\widehat{h}\right\|_1. \tag{3.10}$$

Control of I_2. Obviously

$$|I_2| \leq \frac{1}{2\pi} \int_{|u| > \varepsilon \sqrt{n}} \left|\widehat{h}\left(\frac{u}{\sqrt{n}}\right)\right| \widehat{\phi}(u) du$$

$$\leq \frac{1}{2\pi} e^{-\varepsilon^2 n/2} \int_{\mathbb{R}} \left|\widehat{h}\left(\frac{u}{\sqrt{n}}\right)\right| du$$

$$= \frac{\sqrt{n}}{2\pi} e^{-\varepsilon^2 n/2} \left\|\widehat{h}\right\|_1. \tag{3.11}$$

Control of I_3. Since X_1 is strongly non-lattice there exists a positive constant $q_{F,\varepsilon} < 1$ depending on the distribution function F and on ε such that $\left|\widehat{P}_n(t)\right| \leq q_{F,\varepsilon}^n$, for any $|t| > \varepsilon$. Using this we get

$$|I_3| \leq \frac{1}{2\pi} \int_{|u| > \varepsilon \sqrt{n}} \left|\widehat{h}\left(\frac{u}{\sqrt{n}}\right)\right| q_{F,\varepsilon}^n du$$

$$\leq \frac{1}{2\pi} e^{-c_{F,\varepsilon}'' n} \int_{\mathbb{R}} \left|\widehat{h}\left(\frac{u}{\sqrt{n}}\right)\right| du$$

$$= \frac{\sqrt{n}}{2\pi} e^{-c_{F,\varepsilon}'' n} \left\|\widehat{h}\right\|_1, \tag{3.12}$$

for some positive constant $c_{F,\varepsilon}''$. Collecting the bounds (3.10), (3.11) and (3.12), we obtain

$$|I| \leq c r_n' \left\|\widehat{h}\sqrt{n}\widehat{\phi}_{n/2}\right\|_1 + \frac{e^{-c_F''' n}}{c_F'''} \left\|\widehat{h}\right\|_1, \tag{3.13}$$

for some constant $c_F''' > 0$ depending on the law of X_1 and ε. Changing the variable $u = t\sqrt{n}$, from (3.7) and (3.13) it follows that

$$\left| \sqrt{n}\mathbb{E}h\left(y + S_n\right) - \frac{1}{2\pi} \int_{-\infty}^{\infty} e^{-ity} \widehat{h}\left(t\right) \sqrt{n}\widehat{\phi}\left(t\sqrt{n}\right) dt \right| \le cr_n' \left\| \widehat{h}\sqrt{n}\,\widehat{\phi}_{n/2} \right\|_1 + \frac{e^{-c_F''' n}}{c_F'''} \left\| \widehat{h} \right\|_1 .$$
(3.14)

Note that $\sqrt{n}\widehat{\phi}\left(t\sqrt{n}\right)$ is the Fourier transform of $\phi\left(\frac{u}{\sqrt{n}}\right)$:

$$\sqrt{n}\widehat{\phi}\left(t\sqrt{n}\right) = \sqrt{n} \int_{-\infty}^{\infty} e^{-itx\sqrt{n}} \phi\left(x\right) dx = \int_{-\infty}^{\infty} e^{-itu} \phi\left(\frac{u}{\sqrt{n}}\right) du.$$

Using the inversion formula we get

$$\frac{1}{2\pi} \int_{-\infty}^{\infty} e^{-ity} \widehat{h}\left(t\right) \sqrt{n}\widehat{\phi}\left(t\sqrt{n}\right) dt = \frac{1}{2\pi} \int_{-\infty}^{\infty} \phi\left(\frac{u}{\sqrt{n}}\right) \int_{-\infty}^{\infty} e^{-it(y+u)} \widehat{h}\left(t\right) dt\, du$$

$$= \frac{1}{2\pi} \int_{-\infty}^{\infty} h\left(y + u\right) \phi\left(\frac{u}{\sqrt{n}}\right) du. \qquad (3.15)$$

From (3.14) and (3.15) we obtain

$$\left| \sqrt{n}\mathbb{E}h\left(y + S_n\right) - \int_{\mathbb{R}} h\left(y + x\right) \phi\left(\frac{x}{\sqrt{n}}\right) dx \right| \le cr_n' \left\| \widehat{h}\sqrt{n}\,\widehat{\phi}_{n/2} \right\|_1 + \frac{e^{-c_F''' n}}{c_F'''} \left\| \widehat{h} \right\|_1 .$$

Since ε depend only on the law of X_1, to finish the proof of Theorem 3.3 it is enough to note that

$$\left\| \widehat{h}\sqrt{n}\,\widehat{\phi}_{n/2} \right\|_1 = \int_{\mathbb{R}} \left| \widehat{h}\left(\frac{u}{\sqrt{n}}\right) e^{-u^2/4} \right| du \le c \left\| \widehat{h} \right\|_\infty .$$

$\square$

3.3 Non-asymptotic Local Theorem for Functions with Non-integrable Fourier Transform

In this section, we give an extension of Theorem 3.3 for functions with non-integrable Fourier transforms. Our result is non-asymptotic, i.e., holds for any $n \ge 1$. Recall that for any positive bounded measurable function h on $\mathbb{R}$ and $\varepsilon > 0$ the extension h_ε is defined by (3.1).

Theorem 3.4 *Assume that X_1 is strongly non-lattice. Then there exist a constant c and a decreasing sequence of positive numbers $(r_n)_{n\ge1}$, $\lim_{n\to\infty} r_n = 0$, both depending only on the law of X_1, such that for any positive bounded measurable function h on $\mathbb{R}$ and $n \ge 1$,*

$$\sup_{y \in \mathbb{R}} \left(\sqrt{n} \mathbb{E} h \left(y + S_n \right) - \int_{\mathbb{R}} h_{r_n} \left(x \right) \phi \left(\frac{x - y}{\sigma \sqrt{n}} \right) dx \right) \le c r_n \left\| h_{r_n} \right\|_1$$

and

$$\sup_{y \in \mathbb{R}} \left(\int_{\mathbb{R}} h_{-r_n} \left(x \right) \phi \left(\frac{x - y}{\sigma \sqrt{n}} \right) dx - \sqrt{n} \mathbb{E} h \left(y + S_n \right) \right) \le c r_n \left\| h_{r_n} \right\|_1 .$$

Proof Without loss of generality we consider that $\sigma = 1$. Let $\varepsilon \in (0, 1/2)$ and $h_\varepsilon^* = h_\varepsilon * \kappa_\varepsilon$. Using the bound (3.4) of Lemma 3.1,

$$\sqrt{n} \mathbb{E} h \left(y + S_n \right) \le \sqrt{n} \mathbb{E} h_\varepsilon^* \left(y + S_n \right) .$$

By Theorem 3.3 there exist a constant c and a sequence $(r_n)_{n \ge 1}$, $r_n \to 0$ as $n \to \infty$, depending only on the law of X_1 such that

$$\sup_{y \in \mathbb{R}} \left| \sqrt{n} \mathbb{E} h_\varepsilon^* \left(y + S_n \right) - \int_{\mathbb{R}} h_\varepsilon^* \left(x \right) \phi \left(\frac{x - y}{\sqrt{n}} \right) dx \right| \le c r_n \left(\left\| \widehat{h}_\varepsilon^* \right\|_\infty + \left\| \widehat{h}_\varepsilon^* \right\|_1 \right),$$

(3.16)

where $\widehat{h}_\varepsilon^*$ is the Fourier transform of h_ε^*. By Lemma 3.2,

$$\left\| \widehat{h}_\varepsilon^* \right\|_\infty \le \left\| h_{2\varepsilon} \right\|_1 , \qquad \left\| \widehat{h}_\varepsilon^* \right\|_1 \le \left\| h_\varepsilon \right\|_1 \frac{\left\| \widehat{\kappa} \right\|_1}{\varepsilon} = \frac{c}{\varepsilon} \left\| h_\varepsilon \right\|_1 .$$

Moreover, again by (3.4) of Lemma 3.1 $h_\varepsilon^* \left(x \right) \le h_{2\varepsilon} \left(x \right)$, so that

$$\sqrt{n} \mathbb{E} h \left(y + S_n \right) \le \int_{\mathbb{R}} h_{2\varepsilon} \left(x \right) \phi \left(\frac{x - y}{\sqrt{n}} \right) dx + c r_n \left\| h_{2\varepsilon} \right\|_1 + c r_n \varepsilon^{-1} \left\| h_\varepsilon \right\|_1 .$$

Since $\left\| h_\varepsilon \right\|_1 \le \left\| h_{2\varepsilon} \right\|_1$, choosing $\varepsilon = r_n' := \sqrt{r_n}$ we obtain, for $n \ge 1$,

$$\sqrt{n} \mathbb{E} h \left(y + S_n \right) \le \int_{\mathbb{R}} h_{2r_n'} \left(x \right) \phi \left(\frac{x - y}{\sqrt{n}} \right) dx + c' r_n' \left\| h_{2r_n'} \right\|_1 ,$$

for some constant $c' > 0$ depending only on the law of X_1.

The lower bound is proved in the same way, thus finishing the proof. $\square$

3.4 Stone's Type Local Limit Theorem

We shall derive from Theorem 3.4 the following version of the local limit theorem due to Stone [15] under the condition that X_1 is strongly non-lattice. Let $X_1, X_2, ...$ be i.i.d. random variables of means 0 and unit variances: $\mathbb{E} X_1 = 0$ and $\mathbb{E} X_1^2 = 1$.

Theorem 3.5 *Assume that X_1 is strongly non-lattice. Then, there exist a constant c and a decreasing sequence $(r_n)_{n\geq 1}$, $\lim_{n\to\infty} r_n = 0$, both depending only on the law of X_1, such that for any $n \geq 1$,*

$$\sup_{\Delta \geq r_n} \sup_{x \in \mathbb{R}} \left| \frac{1}{\Delta} \sqrt{n} \mathbb{P}\left(S_n \in [x, x+\Delta]\right) - \phi\left(x/\sqrt{n}\right) \right| \leq c r_n.$$

Proof Let $\Delta > 0$. Consider the indicator function $h = 1_{[0,\Delta]}$. Then $h_{r_n} = 1_{[-r_n, \Delta+r_n]}$. By Theorem 3.4 there exists a sequence $(r_n)_{n\geq 1}$, $\lim_{n\to\infty} r_n = 0$, depending only on the law of X_1 such that, uniformly in $y \in \mathbb{R}$,

$$\sqrt{n}\mathbb{E}h\left(-y + S_n\right) \leq \int_{\mathbb{R}} h_{r_n}(x) \phi\left(\frac{x+y}{\sqrt{n}}\right) dx + \left\|h_{r_n}\right\|_1 r_n.$$

Since $\left\|h_{r_n}\right\|_1 = \Delta + 2r_n$ and

$$\int_{\mathbb{R}} h_{r_n}(x) \phi\left(\frac{x+y}{\sqrt{n}}\right) dx \leq \int_{-r_n}^{\Delta + r_n} \phi\left(\frac{x+y}{\sqrt{n}}\right) dx \leq (\Delta + 2r_n)\phi(y/\sqrt{n}),$$

we obtain

$$\sqrt{n}\mathbb{P}\left(S_n \in [y, y+\Delta]\right) \leq (\Delta + 2r_n)\phi(y/\sqrt{n}) + (\Delta + 2r_n)r_n.$$

This implies

$$\sqrt{n}\mathbb{P}\left(S_n \in [y, y+\Delta]\right) - \Delta\phi(y/\sqrt{n}) \leq 2r_n + (\Delta + 2r_n)r_n.$$

Choosing $r'_n = r_n^{1/2}$, for any $\Delta > r'_n$ one gets

$$\sqrt{n}\mathbb{P}\left(S_n \in [y, y+\Delta]\right) - \Delta\phi(y/\sqrt{n}) \leq \Delta(2r'_n + (1 + 2r'_n)r_n) \leq c\Delta r'_n.$$

A lower bound is proved in the same way, which ends the proof.   □

4 Proof of the Main Results

Recall the following notations which will be used all over this section: for any $n \geq 1$ and $y \in \mathbb{R}_+^*$,

$$Q_n(y, dz) := \mathbb{P}\left(y + S_n \in dz, \tau_y > n\right)$$

and, for any bounded measurable function $g : \mathbb{R}_+^* \to \mathbb{R}_+$,

$$Q_n g(y) := \int_{\mathbb{R}_+} g(z) Q_n(y, dz) = \mathbb{E}\left(g(y + S_n); \tau_n > n\right), \quad y \in \mathbb{R}_+^*.$$

4.1 Boundedness and Integrability of $\mathbf{Q}_n g$

Let $g : \mathbb{R}_+^* \to \mathbb{R}_+$ be a bounded measurable function. It is easy to see that the function $\mathbf{Q}_n g$ is bounded

$$\|\mathbf{Q}_n g\|_\infty \le \int_{\mathbb{R}_+} g(z) Q_n(y, dz) \le \|g\|_\infty \int_{\mathbb{R}_+} Q_n(y, dz) \le \|g\|_\infty. \tag{4.1}$$

Moreover, using Theorem 1.1 we obtain, for any $y > 0$,

$$\mathbf{Q}_n g(y) = \int_{\mathbb{R}_+} g(x) \mathbb{P}(y + S_n \in dx; \tau_y > n) \le \|g\|_\infty \mathbb{P}(\tau_y > n) \le c\|g\|_\infty \frac{1+y}{\sqrt{n}} \tag{4.2}$$

and a similar inequality for $\mathbf{Q}_n^* g(\cdot)$ holds true.

Recall that $g_\varepsilon(u) = \sup_{|v-u|\le\varepsilon} g(v)$, where $\varepsilon > 0$. The following lemma shows that when g_ε is integrable, the functions $\sqrt{n}\mathbf{Q}_n g(\cdot)$ are bounded in L^∞ uniformly in $n \ge 1$.

Lemma 4.1 *There exists a sequence of numbers $(r_n)_{n\ge1}$ depending only on the law of X_1 and satisfying $r_m \to 0$ as $n \to \infty$ such that*

$$\sqrt{n}\,\|\mathbf{Q}_n g\|_\infty \le \|g_{r_n}\|_1 \left(\frac{1}{\sqrt{2\pi}} + r_n\right).$$

Proof We have

$$\sqrt{n}\mathbf{Q}_n g(u) = \sqrt{n}\int_{\mathbb{R}_+^*} g(z)\mathbb{P}(u + S_n \in dz; \tau_u > n)$$
$$\le \sqrt{n}\int_{\mathbb{R}_+^*} g(z)\mathbb{P}(u + S_n \in dz). \tag{4.3}$$

Using Theorem 3.4, it follows that there is a sequence of numbers $(r_n)_{n\ge1}$, depending only on the law of X_1, such that $\lim_{n\to\infty} r_n = 0$ and uniformly in $u > 0$

$$\sqrt{n}\int_{\mathbb{R}} g(z)\mathbb{P}(u + S_n \in dz) \le V_n(u) + \|g_{r_n}\|_1 r_n, \tag{4.4}$$

where

$$V_n(u) = \int_{-\infty}^{+\infty} g_{r_n}(z)\frac{1}{\sqrt{2\pi}}e^{-\frac{(z-u)^2}{2n}}dz \le \frac{1}{\sqrt{2\pi}}\|g_{r_n}\|_1. \tag{4.5}$$

From (4.3), (4.4) and (4.5) the claim follows. □

The next lemma shows that the L_1 norm of the function $\mathbf{Q}_n g$ is of order $n^{-1/2}$. This turns out to be one of the key points in the sequel. The proof is based upon the duality Lemma 2.1 and Theorem 1.1. Recall that the weighted L_1 norm $\|g\|_{1,p}$ used below is defined by (1.7).

Lemma 4.2 *There is an absolute constant c such that, for any bounded and measurable function $g : \mathbb{R}_+^* \to \mathbb{R}_+$, it holds*

$$\sup_{n\geq 1} \sqrt{n}\, \|Q_n g\|_1 := \sup_{n\geq 1} \sqrt{n} \int_{\mathbb{R}_+} Q_n g\,(y)\, dy \leq c\, \|g\|_{1,1}\,.$$

Proof Let $a > 0$ and $n \geq 1$. By duality Lemma 2.1,

$$\int_{\mathbb{R}_+} 1_{[0,a]}\,(y)\, Q_n g\,(y)\, dy = \int_{\mathbb{R}_+} 1_{[0,a]}\,(y) \left(\int_{\mathbb{R}_+} g\,(z)\, Q_n\,(y, dz) \right) dy$$

$$= \int_{\mathbb{R}_+} g\,(z) \left(\int_{\mathbb{R}_+} 1_{[0,a]}\,(y)\, Q_n^*\,(z, dy) \right) dz$$

$$\leq \int_{\mathbb{R}_+} g\,(z) \left(\int_{\mathbb{R}_+} Q_n^*\,(z, dy) \right) dz.$$

By Theorem 1.1, there exists a constant c such that, for any $z \geq 0$,

$$\int_{\mathbb{R}_+} Q_n^*\,(z, dy) = \int_{\mathbb{R}_+} \mathbb{P}\left(z + S_n^* \in dy; \tau_z^* > n\right) = \mathbb{P}\left(\tau_z^* > n\right) \leq c\, \frac{1+z}{\sqrt{n}}.$$

Therefore,

$$\int_{\mathbb{R}_+} 1_{[0,a]}\,(y)\, Q_n g\,(y)\, dy \leq \frac{c}{\sqrt{n}} \int_{\mathbb{R}_+} g\,(z)\,(1+z)\, dz.$$

Taking the limit as $a \to \infty$, by monotone convergence theorem, we obtain

$$\int_{\mathbb{R}_+} Q_n g\,(y)\, dy \leq \frac{c}{\sqrt{n}} \int_{\mathbb{R}_+} g\,(z)\,(1+z)\, dz. \tag{4.6}$$

□

Let $\varepsilon \in (0, 1/2)$. For any bounded measurable function $g : \mathbb{R}_+^* \to \mathbb{R}_+$, introduce the upper right ε-bound of g by setting

$$\bar{g}_\varepsilon\,(s) = \sup_{u \in [s-\varepsilon, s] \cap \mathbb{R}_+^*} g\,(u) \quad \text{for } s \in \mathbb{R}, \tag{4.7}$$

where $\sup \emptyset = 0$. With this definition $\bar{g}_\varepsilon(s) = 0$ for $s \leq 0$. Note also that, in this case, $\bar{g}_\varepsilon\,(s) \leq g_\varepsilon\,(s)$, for all $s \in \mathbb{R}$, where g_ε is defined by (1.6).

Recall the triangular density $\kappa\,(x) = 1 - |x|$, for $|x| \leq 1$ and $\kappa\,(x) = 0$ otherwise. Let η be a random variable with density κ independent of $X_1, ..., X_n$. Let

$\varepsilon \in (0, 1/2)$ and $\eta_\varepsilon = \varepsilon\eta$. Setting $\zeta_\varepsilon = \frac{1}{2}(\eta_\varepsilon + \varepsilon) \geq 0$, for any $s > 0$, we obtain a new smoothing variable whose support is the interval $[0, \varepsilon]$. Denote by $k_\varepsilon^+(\cdot)$ the density of ζ_ε.

Lemma 4.3 *For any bounded measurable function* $g : \mathbb{R}_+^* \to \mathbb{R}_+$, $s > 0$ *and* $n \geq 1$,

$$\mathbf{Q}_n g(s) := \mathbb{E}(g(s + S_n); \tau_s > n) \leq \mathbb{E}\mathbf{Q}_n \bar{g}_\varepsilon(s + \zeta_\varepsilon) = (\mathbf{Q}_n \bar{g}_\varepsilon) * k_\varepsilon^+(s).$$

Proof Note that $\zeta_\varepsilon \in (0, \varepsilon)$ and that by the definition of $\bar{g}_\varepsilon$, for any $s > 0$,

$$\bar{g}_\varepsilon(s + \zeta_\varepsilon) = \sup_{u \in [s+\zeta_\varepsilon-\varepsilon, s+\zeta_\varepsilon] \cap \mathbb{R}_+^*} g(u) \geq g(s), \tag{4.8}$$

where the for the last inequality we use the fact that the interval $[s + \zeta_\varepsilon - \varepsilon, s + \zeta_\varepsilon] \cap \mathbb{R}_+^*$ contains s. Using (4.8) with $s + S_n$ instead of s and the fact that ζ_ε is independent of the sequence $(X_i)_{i \geq 1}$ we have, for any $s > 0$,

$$\begin{aligned}
\mathbf{Q}_n g(s) &= \mathbb{E}(g(s + S_n); \tau_s > n)\\
&= \mathbb{E}(g(s + S_n); s + S_1 > 0, ..., s + S_n > 0)\\
&\leq \mathbb{E}(\bar{g}_\varepsilon(s + S_n + \zeta_\varepsilon); s + S_1 + \zeta_\varepsilon > 0, ..., s + S_n + \zeta_\varepsilon > 0)\\
&= \mathbb{E}(\bar{g}_\varepsilon(s + S_n + \zeta_\varepsilon); \tau_{s+\zeta_\varepsilon} > n)\\
&= \mathbb{E}\mathbf{Q}_n \bar{g}_\varepsilon(s + \zeta_\varepsilon). \qquad \square
\end{aligned}$$

4.2 Proof of Theorem 1.2

First we prove the inequality (1.8).

Assume that n is large enough and that $k = [n/2]$ and $m = n - k$. By the Markov property, for any $y > 0$.

$$\mathbf{Q}_n g(y) = \int_{\mathbb{R}_+^*} Q_k(y, ds) \int_{\mathbb{R}_+^*} Q_m(s, dz) g(z). \tag{4.9}$$

Since $Q_m(s, dz) = \mathbb{P}(s + S_m \in dz; \tau_s > m) \leq \mathbb{P}(s + S_m \in dz)$,

$$\begin{aligned}
\mathbf{Q}_n g(y) &\leq \int_{\mathbb{R}_+^*} Q_k(y, ds) \int_{\mathbb{R}_+^*} g(z) \mathbb{P}(s + S_m \in dz)\\
&= \int_{\mathbb{R}_+^*} Q_k(y, ds) \int_{\mathbb{R}} g(z) \mathbb{P}(s + S_m \in dz). \tag{4.10}
\end{aligned}$$

By Theorem 3.4, there exists a constant c and a decreasing sequence $(r_m)_{m \geq 1}$, $r_m \to 0$ as $m \to \infty$, depending only on the law of X_1 such that, for any $m \geq 1$,

$$\sup_{s \in \mathbb{R}} \left(\sqrt{m} \int_{\mathbb{R}} g(z) \mathbb{P}(s + S_m \in dz) - \int_{\mathbb{R}} g_{r_n}(z) \phi \left(\frac{z - s}{\sqrt{m}} \right) dz \right) \le cr_n \left\| g_{r_n} \right\|_1$$

form which we have

$$\sqrt{m} \sup_{s \in \mathbb{R}} \int_{\mathbb{R}} g(z) \mathbb{P}(s + S_m \in dz) \le cr_n \left\| g_{r_n} \right\|_1. \tag{4.11}$$

Substituting (4.11) into (4.10) we obtain

$$\sqrt{m} \mathbf{Q}_n g(y) \le cr_n \left\| g_{r_n} \right\|_1 \int_{\mathbb{R}_+^*} Q_n(y, ds). \tag{4.12}$$

By Theorem 1.1, for any $y \ge 0$,

$$\int_{\mathbb{R}_+^*} Q_k(y, ds) = \int_{\mathbb{R}_+^*} \mathbb{P}(y + S_k \in ds; \tau_y > k) = \mathbb{P}(\tau_y > k) \le c \frac{1 + y}{\sqrt{k}}. \tag{4.13}$$

Substituting (4.13) into (4.12) the result follows.

Now we prove the bound (1.9). In the proof of this assertion we use the duality implicitly, through Lemma 4.2 whose proof is based on the duality.

As before, let $k = [n/2]$ and $m = n - k$. By the Markov property (4.9), we have, for any $y > 0$,

$$\mathbf{Q}_n g(y) = \int_{\mathbb{R}_+^*} \mathbf{Q}_m g(s) Q_k(y, ds).$$

Since $Q_k(y, ds) = \mathbb{P}(y + S_k \in ds; \tau_y > k) \le \mathbb{P}(y + S_k \in ds)$, we get

$$\mathbf{Q}_n g(y) \le \int_{\mathbb{R}} h_m(s) \mathbb{P}(y + S_k \in ds), \tag{4.14}$$

where $h_m(s) = \mathbf{Q}_m g(s)$ for $s > 0$ and $h_m(s) = 0$ otherwise. We are going to apply the local limit Theorem 3.3 with $h = h_m$. However, the function h_m may have non-integrable Fourier transform. To overcome this difficulty, we shall substitute it by a function with bounded integrable Fourier transform.

For any $\varepsilon \in (0, 1/2)$ define $\overline{g}_\varepsilon$ by (4.7) and set for brevity

$$\overline{h}_{m,\varepsilon}(s) := \mathbf{Q}_m \overline{g}_\varepsilon(s), \quad s > 0.$$

We extend g_ε and $\overline{h}_{m,\varepsilon}$ to the whole real line by setting $g_\varepsilon = 0$ and $\overline{h}_{m,\varepsilon}(s) = 0$ for $s \le 0$. Then, for any $s \in \mathbb{R}$,

$$\overline{h}_{m,\varepsilon}^*(s) := \mathbb{E} \overline{h}_{m,\varepsilon}(s + \zeta_\varepsilon) \ge 0. \tag{4.15}$$

By Lemma 4.3, for any $s > 0$,

$$\mathbf{Q}_m g(s) = \mathbb{E}\left(g(s + S_m); \tau_s > m\right)$$
$$\leq \mathbb{E}\mathbf{Q}_m \overline{g}_\varepsilon (s + \zeta_\varepsilon) = \mathbb{E}\overline{h}_{m,\varepsilon}(s + \zeta_\varepsilon) =: \overline{h}^*_{m,\varepsilon}(s).$$

This and the previous inequality imply, for any $s \in \mathbb{R}$,

$$h_m(s) \leq \mathbb{E}\mathbf{Q}_n \overline{g}_\varepsilon (s + \zeta_\varepsilon) =: \overline{h}^*_{m,\varepsilon}(s). \tag{4.16}$$

From (4.16) and (4.14) we obtain,

$$\mathbf{Q}_n g(y) \leq \int_{\mathbb{R}} \overline{h}^*_{m,\varepsilon}(s) \, \mathbb{P}(y + S_k \in ds). \tag{4.17}$$

Denote by $\widehat{h}^*_{m,\varepsilon}$ the Fourier transform of $\overline{h}^*_{m,\varepsilon}$, which, as we shall see below, is bounded and integrable. By Theorem 3.3, there is a decreasing sequence of real numbers $(r_n)_{n\geq 1}$ depending only on the law of X_1, such that $\lim_{n\to\infty} r_n = 0$ and for any $n \geq 1$ uniformly in $y > 0$,

$$\sqrt{k} \int_{\mathbb{R}} \overline{h}^*_{m,\varepsilon}(s) \, \mathbb{P}(y + S_k \in ds)$$
$$\leq \frac{1}{\sqrt{2\pi}} \int_{\mathbb{R}} \overline{h}^*_{m,\varepsilon}(s) \exp\left(-\frac{(s-y)^2}{2k}\right) ds + \left(\left\|\widehat{h}^*_{m,\varepsilon}\right\|_\infty + \left\|\widehat{h}^*_{m,\varepsilon}\right\|_1\right) r_k$$
$$\leq \frac{1}{\sqrt{2\pi}} \left\|\overline{h}^*_{m,\varepsilon}\right\|_1 + \left(\left\|\widehat{h}^*_{m,\varepsilon}\right\|_\infty + \left\|\widehat{h}^*_{m,\varepsilon}\right\|_1\right) r_k. \tag{4.18}$$

Note that, for $s > 0$, we have $\overline{h}_{m,\varepsilon}(s) = \mathbb{E}\left(\overline{g}_\varepsilon(s + S_m); \tau_s > m\right)$, while for $s \leq 0$, we have $\overline{h}_{m,\varepsilon}(s) := 0 \leq \mathbb{E}\left(\overline{g}_\varepsilon(s + S_m); \tau_s > m\right)$, which proves that, for any $s \in \mathbb{R}$,

$$\overline{h}_{m,\varepsilon}(s) \leq \mathbb{E}\left(\overline{g}_\varepsilon(s + S_m); \tau_s > m\right).$$

Therefore, conditioning with respect to ζ_s, for any $s \in \mathbb{R}$, we get

$$\overline{h}^*_{m,\varepsilon}(s) = \mathbb{E}\left(\mathbb{E}\overline{h}_{m,\varepsilon}(s + \zeta_\varepsilon) \big| \zeta_s\right)$$
$$\leq \mathbb{E}\left(\mathbb{E}\left(\overline{g}_\varepsilon(s + \zeta_\varepsilon + S_m); \tau_{s+\zeta_\varepsilon} > m\right) \big| \zeta_s\right)$$
$$= \mathbb{E}\left(\mathbb{E}\left(\overline{g}_\varepsilon(s + \zeta_\varepsilon + S_m); s + S_1 + \zeta_\varepsilon > 0, ..., s + S_m + \zeta_\varepsilon > 0\right) \big| \zeta_s\right)$$
$$\leq \mathbb{E}\left(\overline{g}_{2\varepsilon}(s + \varepsilon + S_m); s + S_1 + \varepsilon > 0, ..., s + S_m + \varepsilon > 0\right)$$
$$= \mathbf{Q}_m \overline{g}_{2\varepsilon}(s + \varepsilon).$$

Using Lemma 4.2,

$$\left\|\widehat{h}^*_{m,\varepsilon}\right\|_\infty \leq \left\|\overline{h}^*_{m,\varepsilon}\right\|_1 = \int_0^\infty \overline{h}^*_{m,\varepsilon}(s) \, ds \leq \int_0^\infty \mathbf{Q}_m \overline{g}_{2\varepsilon}(s + \varepsilon) \, ds$$

$$\leq \int_0^\infty \mathbf{Q}_m \overline{g}_{2\varepsilon} \, (s) \, ds = \left\| \mathbf{Q}_m \overline{g}_{2\varepsilon} \right\|_1 \leq \frac{c}{\sqrt{m}} \left\| \overline{g}_{2\varepsilon} \right\|_{1,1} \leq \frac{c}{\sqrt{m}} \left\| g_{2\varepsilon} \right\|_{1,1},$$

(4.19)

which proves that $\widehat{h}^*_{m,\varepsilon}$ is bounded. Since by (4.15), $\overline{h}^*_{m,\varepsilon}$ is a convolution, we have, for any $s \in \mathbb{R}$,

$$\widehat{h}^*_{m,\varepsilon} \, (s) = \widehat{h}_{m,\varepsilon} \, (s) \, \mathbb{E} e^{-is\zeta_\varepsilon} = e^{-is\frac{\varepsilon}{2}} \widehat{h}_{m,\varepsilon} \, (s) \, \widehat{\kappa}_\varepsilon \, (s/2),$$

where $\widehat{h}_{m,\varepsilon}$ is the Fourier transform of $\overline{h}_{m,\varepsilon}$. Then, using Lemma 4.2, as in (4.19), this proves that $\widehat{h}^*_{m,\varepsilon}$ is integrable

$$\begin{aligned}
\left\| \widehat{h}^*_{m,\varepsilon} \right\|_1 &= \int_{\mathbb{R}} \left| \widehat{h}_{m,\varepsilon} \, (t) \, \widehat{\kappa}_\varepsilon \, (t/2) \right| dt \leq \left\| \widehat{h}_{m,\varepsilon} \right\|_\infty \int_{\mathbb{R}} \left| \widehat{\kappa}_\varepsilon \, (t/2) \right| dt \\
&= \frac{2}{\varepsilon} \left\| \widehat{h}_{m,\varepsilon} \right\|_\infty \int_{\mathbb{R}} \left| \widehat{\kappa} \, (t) \right| dt \leq \frac{c}{\varepsilon} \left\| \overline{h}_{m,\varepsilon} \right\|_1 = \frac{c}{\varepsilon} \left\| \mathbf{Q}_m \overline{g}_\varepsilon \right\|_1 \\
&\leq \frac{c}{\varepsilon \sqrt{m}} \left\| \overline{g}_\varepsilon \right\|_{1,1} \leq \frac{c}{\varepsilon \sqrt{m}} \left\| g_{2\varepsilon} \right\|_{1,1}.
\end{aligned}$$

(4.20)

Implementing (4.18) into (4.17) and using the bounds (4.19), (4.20), we obtain,

$$\begin{aligned}
\sqrt{k} \mathbf{Q}_n g \, (y) &\leq \sqrt{k} \int_{\mathbb{R}_+} h^*_{m,\varepsilon} \, (s) \, \mathbb{P} \, (y + S_k \in ds) \\
&\leq \frac{1}{\sqrt{2\pi}} \left\| h^*_{m,\varepsilon} \right\|_1 + \left(\left\| \widehat{h}^*_{m,\varepsilon} \right\|_\infty + \left\| \widehat{h}^*_{m,\varepsilon} \right\|_1 \right) r_k \\
&\leq \frac{c}{\sqrt{m}} \left\| g_{2\varepsilon} \right\|_{1,1} \left(1 + \left(1 + \frac{1}{\varepsilon} \right) r_k \right).
\end{aligned}$$

Choosing $\varepsilon = \sqrt{r_k}$ proves inequality (1.9).

4.3 Proof of Theorem 1.3

In the proof of this statement the duality is used implicitly through Theorem 1.2. Assume that $k = [n/2]$ and $m = n - k$. By the Markov property

$$\begin{aligned}
\mathbf{Q}_n g \, (y) &= \int_{\mathbb{R}_+} g \, (z) \, Q_n \, (y, dz) \\
&= \int_{\mathbb{R}_+} Q_k \, (y, ds) \int_{\mathbb{R}_+} g \, (z) \, Q_m \, (s, dz).
\end{aligned}$$

(4.21)

By Theorem 1.2, there exists a sequence $(r_n)_{n \geq 1}$, $r_n \to 0$ as $n \to \infty$, depending only on the law of X_1, such that

$$\int_{\mathbb{R}_+} g(z) Q_m(s, dz) \leq \frac{c(1 + r_n)}{m} \|g_{r_n}\|_{1,1} \leq \frac{c}{m} \|g_{r_n}\|_{1,1}. \qquad (4.22)$$

From (4.21) and (4.22),

$$\mathbf{Q}_n g(y) \leq \int_{\mathbb{R}_+} Q_k(y, ds) \frac{c}{m} \|g_{r_n}\|_{1,1}. \qquad (4.23)$$

By Theorem 1.1, there exists a constant c such that, for any $y \geq 0$,

$$\int_{\mathbb{R}_+} Q_k(y, ds) = \int_{\mathbb{R}_+} \mathbb{P}(y + S_k \in ds; \tau_y > k) \leq \mathbb{P}(\tau_y > k) \leq c \frac{1 + y}{\sqrt{k}}. \qquad (4.24)$$

From this and (4.23),

$$\mathbf{Q}_n g(y) \leq c \frac{1 + y}{m\sqrt{k}} \|g_{r_n}\|_{1,1} \leq c \frac{1 + y}{n^{3/2}} \|g_{r_n}\|_{1,1},$$

which proves the theorem.

Remark 4.4 Inspecting the proof of Theorem 1.3 one could think to improve the rate $n^{3/2}$ using instead of the bound (4.24) the more precise bounds (1.8) and (1.9). To do so the inequalities (1.8) and (1.9) should be applied with g being the unity function: $g(x) = e(x) = 1$. However, since the unity function e is not in $\mathbb{L}^1$, we have $\|g_{r_n}\|_1 = \|e_{r_n}\|_1 = \infty$. Recall that our bounds (1.8) and (1.9) can be applied only for functions g with $\|g_{r_n}\|_{1,1} < +\infty$. In the particular case considered here we have $\|e_{r_n}\|_{1,1} = \|e_{r_n}\|_1 = +\infty$ which makes such an improvement impossible.

References

1. Bertoin, J., Doney, R.A.: On conditioning a random walk to stay nonnegative. Ann. Probab. **22**(4), 2152–2167 (1994)
2. Borovkov, A.A.: On the asymptotic behavior of the distributions of first-passage times. I. Math. Notes **75**(1), 23–37 (2004)
3. Borovkov, A.A.: On the asymptotic behavior of distributions of first-passage times. II. Math. Notes **75**(3), 322–330 (2004)
4. Borovkov, A.A.: On the rate of convergence in the invariance principle. Probab. Theory Appl. **18**(2), 217–234 (1973)
5. Caravenna, F.: A local limit theorem for random walks conditioned to stay positive. Probab. Theory Relat. Fields. **133**(4), 508–530 (2005)
6. Denisov, D., Wachtel, V.: Conditional limit theorems for ordered random walks. Electron. J. Probab. **15**, 292–322 (2010)
7. Denisov, D., Wachtel, V.: Random walks in cones. Ann. Probab. **43**(3), 992–1044 (2015)

8. Doney, R.A.: Conditional limit theorems for asymptotically stable random walks. Z. Wahrscheinlichkeitsth. **70**, 351–360 (1985)
9. Eichelsbacher, P., König, W.: Ordered random walks. Electron. J. Probab. **13**(46), 1307–1336 (2008)
10. Gnedenko, B.V.: On a local limit theorem of the theory of probability. Uspekhi Mat. Nauk **3**(3), 187–194 (1948)
11. Grama, I., Lauvergnat, R., Le Page, E.: Limit theorems for affine Markov walks conditioned to stay positive. To appear in Ann. I.H.P. (2016). arXiv:1601.02991
12. Iglehart, D.L.: Functional central limit theorems for random walks conditioned to stay positive. Ann. Probab. **2**(4), 608–619 (1974)
13. Spitzer, F.: Principles of Random Walk, Second edn. Springer, Berlin (1976)
14. Shepp, L.A.: A local limit theorem. Ann. Math. Statist. **35**(1), 419–423 (1964)
15. Stone, L.A.: A local limit theorem for nonlattice multi-dimensional distribution functions Ann. Math. Statist. **36**(2), 546–551 (1964)
16. Vatutin, V.A., Wachtel, V.: Local probabilities for random walks conditioned to stay positive. Probab. Theory Relat. Fields **143**(1–2), 177–217 (2009)

Part IV
Approximation of Stochastic Processes

Regression-Based Variance Reduction Approach for Strong Approximation Schemes

Denis Belomestny, Stefan Häfner and Mikhail Urusov

Abstract In this paper, we present a novel approach towards variance reduction for discretised diffusion processes. The proposed approach involves specially constructed control variates and allows for a significant reduction in the variance for the terminal functionals. In this way, the complexity order of the standard Monte Carlo algorithm (ε^{-3}) can be reduced down to $\varepsilon^{-2}\sqrt{|\log(\varepsilon)|}$ in case of the Euler scheme with ε being the precision to be achieved. These theoretical results are illustrated by several numerical examples.

Keywords Monte Carlo methods · Regression methods · Control variates Stochastic differential equations · Strong schemes

1 Introduction

Let $T > 0$ be a fixed time horizon. Consider a d-dimensional diffusion process $(X_t)_{t \in [0,T]}$ defined on a filtered probability space $(\Omega, \mathscr{F}, (\mathscr{F}_t)_{t \in [0,T]}, \mathbb{P})$ by the Itô stochastic differential equation

$$dX_t = \mu(X_t)\,dt + \sigma(X_t)\,dW_t, \quad X_0 = x_0 \in \mathbb{R}^d, \tag{1}$$

The study has been funded by the Russian Academic Excellence Project '5–100'.

D. Belomestny (✉) · M. Urusov
Duisburg-Essen University, Essen, Germany
e-mail: denis.belomestny@uni-due.de

D. Belomestny
National Research University Higher School of Economics, Moscow, Russia

S. Häfner
PricewaterhouseCoopers GmbH, Frankfurt, Germany
e-mail: stefan.haefner@de.pwc.com

M. Urusov
e-mail: mikhail.urusov@uni-due.de

© Springer International Publishing AG 2017
V. Panov (ed.), *Modern Problems of Stochastic Analysis and Statistics*,
Springer Proceedings in Mathematics & Statistics 208,
DOI 10.1007/978-3-319-65313-6_7

131

for Lipschitz continuous functions $\mu\colon \mathbb{R}^d \to \mathbb{R}^d$ and $\sigma\colon \mathbb{R}^d \to \mathbb{R}^{d \times m}$, where $(W_t)_{t \in [0,T]}$ is a standard m-dimensional $(\mathscr{F}_t)$-Brownian motion. Suppose we want to find a continuous function

$$u = u(t, x)\colon [0, T] \times \mathbb{R}^d \to \mathbb{R},$$

which has a continuous first derivative with respect to t and continuous first and second derivatives with respect to the components of x on $[0, T) \times \mathbb{R}^d$, such that it solves the partial differential equation

$$\frac{\partial u}{\partial t} + \mathscr{L}u = 0 \quad \text{on } [0, T) \times \mathbb{R}^d, \tag{2}$$

$$u(T, x) = f(x) \quad \text{for } x \in \mathbb{R}^d, \tag{3}$$

where f is a given Borel function on $\mathbb{R}^d$. Here, $\mathscr{L}$ is the differential operator associated with the Eq. (1):

$$(\mathscr{L}u)(t, x) := \sum_{k=1}^{d} \mu_k(x) \frac{\partial u}{\partial x_k}(t, x) + \frac{1}{2} \sum_{k,l=1}^{d} (\sigma \sigma^\top)_{kl}(x) \frac{\partial^2 u}{\partial x_k \partial x_l}(t, x),$$

where $\sigma^\top$ denotes the transpose of σ. Under appropriate conditions on μ, σ and f, there is a solution of the Cauchy problem (2)–(3), which is unique in the class of solutions satisfying certain growth conditions, and it has the following Feynman-Kac stochastic representation

$$u(t, x) = \mathbb{E}[f(X_T^{t,x})] \tag{4}$$

(see Sect. 5.7 in [5]), where $X^{t,x}$ denotes the solution started at time t in point x. Moreover, it holds

$$\mathbb{E}[f(X_T^{0,x}) | X_t^{0,x}] = u(t, X_t^{0,x}), \quad \text{a.s.}$$

for $t \in [0, T]$ and

$$f(X_T^{0,x}) = \mathbb{E}[f(X_T^{0,x})] + M_T^*, \quad \text{a.s.} \tag{5}$$

with

$$M_T^* := \int_0^T \nabla_x u(t, X_t^{0,x}) \, \sigma(X_t^{0,x}) \, dW_t \equiv \int_0^T \sum_{k=1}^{d} \frac{\partial u}{\partial x_k}(t, X_t^{0,x}) \sum_{i=1}^{m} \sigma_{ki}(X_t^{0,x}) \, dW_t^i. \tag{6}$$

The standard Monte Carlo (SMC) approach for computing $u(0, x)$ at a fixed point $x \in \mathbb{R}^d$ basically consists of three steps. First, an approximation $\overline{X}_T$ for $X_T^{0,x}$ is constructed via a time discretisation in Eq. (1) (we refer to [6] for a nice overview of various discretisation schemes). In this paper, we focus on the Euler–Maruyama approximation to the exact solution (the Euler scheme). Next, N_0 independent copies of the approximation $\overline{X}_T$ are generated, and, finally, a Monte Carlo estimate V_{N_0} is defined as the average of the values of f at simulated points:

$$V_{N_0} := \frac{1}{N_0} \sum_{n=1}^{N_0} f\left(\overline{X}_T^{(n)}\right). \tag{7}$$

In the computation of $u(0, x) = \mathbb{E}[f(X_T^{0,x})]$ by the SMC approach, there are two types of error inherent: the discretisation error $\mathbb{E}[f(X_T^{0,x})] - \mathbb{E}[f(\overline{X}_T)]$ and the Monte Carlo (statistical) error, which results from the substitution of $\mathbb{E}[f(\overline{X}_T)]$ with the sample average V_{N_0}. The aim of variance reduction methods is to reduce the statistical error. For example, in the so-called control variate variance reduction approach, one looks for a random variable ξ with $\mathbb{E}\xi = 0$, which can be simulated, such that the variance of the difference $f(\overline{X}_T) - \xi$ is minimised, that is,

$$\text{Var}[f(\overline{X}_T) - \xi] \to \min \text{ under } \mathbb{E}\xi = 0.$$

The use of control variates for solving (1) via Monte Carlo path simulation approach was initiated by Newton [10] and further developed in Milstein and Tretyakov [8]. In fact, the construction of the appropriate control variates in the above two papers essentially relies on identities (5) and (6) implying that the zero-mean random variable M_T^* can be viewed as an optimal control variate, since

$$\text{Var}[f(X_T^{0,x}) - M_T^*] = \text{Var}[\mathbb{E}f(X_T^{0,x})] = 0.$$

Let us note that it would be desirable to have a control variate reducing the variance of $f(\overline{X}_T)$ rather than the one of $f(X_T^{0,x})$ because we simulate from the distribution of $f(\overline{X}_T)$ and not from the one of $f(X_T^{0,x})$. Moreover, the control variate M_T^* cannot be directly computed, since the function $u(t, x)$ is unknown. This is why Milstein and Tretyakov [8] proposed to use regression for getting a preliminary approximation for $u(t, x)$ in a first step.

The contribution of our work is as follows. We propose an approach for the construction of control variates that reduce the variance of $f(\overline{X}_T)$, i.e. we perform variance reduction not for the exact but rather for the discretised process. A nice by-product is that our control variates can be computed in a rather simple way, and less assumptions are required in our case, than one would require to construct control variates based on the exact solution. Moreover, we present bounds for the regression error involved in the construction of our control variates and perform the complexity analysis (these are not present in [8]), which is also helpful for designing numerical experiments. We are able to achieve a sufficient convergence order of the resulting variance, which in turn leads to a significant complexity reduction as compared to the SMC algorithm. Other examples of algorithms with this property include the analogous regression-based variance reduction approach for weak approximation schemes of [2], the multilevel Monte Carlo (MLMC) algorithm of [3] and the quadrature-based algorithm of [9].

Summing up, we propose a new regression-type approach for the construction of control variates in case of the Euler scheme. It takes advantage of the smoothness in μ, σ and f (which is needed for nice convergence properties of regression methods) in order to significantly reduce the variance of the random variable $f(\overline{X}_T)$.

This work is organised as follows. In Sect. 2, we describe the construction of control variates for strong approximation schemes. Section 3 describes the use of regression algorithms for the construction of control variates and analyses their convergence. A complexity analysis of the variance reduced Monte Carlo algorithm is conducted in Sect. 4. Section 5 is devoted to a simulation study. Finally, all proofs are collected in Sect. 6.

Notational convention. Throughout, elements of $\mathbb{R}^d$ (resp. $\mathbb{R}^{1 \times d}$) are understood as column vectors (resp. row vectors). Generally, most vectors in what follows are column vectors. However, gradients of functions and some vectors defined via them are row vectors. Finally, we record our standing assumption that we do not repeat explicitly in the sequel.

Standing assumption. The coefficients μ and σ in (1) are globally Lipschitz functions.

2   Control Variates for Strong Approximation Schemes

To begin with, we introduce some notations, which will be frequently used in the sequel. Throughout this paper, $\mathbb{N}_0 := \mathbb{N} \cup \{0\}$ denotes the set of nonnegative integers, $J \in \mathbb{N}$ denotes the time discretisation parameter, we set $\Delta := T/J$ and consider discretisation schemes defined on the grid $\{t_j = j\Delta : j = 0, \ldots, J\}$. We set $\Delta_j W := W_{j\Delta} - W_{(j-1)\Delta}$, and by W^i we denote the ith component of the vector W. Further, for $k \in \mathbb{N}_0$, $H_k \colon \mathbb{R} \to \mathbb{R}$ stands for the (normalised) kth Hermite polynomial, i.e.

$$H_k(x) := \frac{(-1)^k}{\sqrt{k!}} e^{\frac{x^2}{2}} \frac{d^k}{dx^k} e^{-\frac{x^2}{2}}, \quad x \in \mathbb{R}.$$

Notice that $H_0 \equiv 1$, $H_1(x) = x$, $H_2(x) = \frac{1}{\sqrt{2}}(x^2 - 1)$.

2.1   Series Representation

Let us consider a scheme, where d-dimensional approximations $X_{\Delta, j\Delta}, j = 0, \ldots, J$, satisfy $X_{\Delta, 0} = x_0$ and

$$X_{\Delta,j\Delta} = \Phi_\Delta \left(X_{\Delta,(j-1)\Delta}, \Delta_j W \right), \tag{8}$$

where $\Delta_j W := W_{j\Delta} - W_{(j-1)\Delta}$, for some Borel measurable functions $\Phi_\Delta : \mathbb{R}^{d\times m} \to \mathbb{R}^d$ (clearly, the Euler scheme is a special case of this setting).

Theorem 1 *Let* $f : \mathbb{R}^d \to \mathbb{R}$ *be a Borel measurable function such that it holds* $\mathbb{E}|f(X_{\Delta,T})|^2 < \infty$. *Then, we have the representation (cf. Theorem 2.1 in [2])*

$$f(X_{\Delta,T}) = \mathbb{E}[f(X_{\Delta,T})] + \sum_{j=1}^{J} \sum_{k\in\mathbb{N}_0^m\setminus\{0_m\}} a_{j,k}(X_{\Delta,(j-1)\Delta}) \prod_{r=1}^{m} H_{k_r} \left(\frac{\Delta_j W^r}{\sqrt{\Delta}} \right), \tag{9}$$

where $k = (k_1, \ldots, k_m)$ *and* $0_m := (0, \ldots, 0) \in \mathbb{R}^m$ *(in the second summation), and the coefficients* $a_{j,k} : \mathbb{R}^d \to \mathbb{R}$ *are given by the formula*

$$a_{j,k}(x) = \mathbb{E}\left[f(X_{\Delta,T}) \prod_{r=1}^{m} H_{k_r} \left(\frac{\Delta_j W^r}{\sqrt{\Delta}} \right) \,\middle|\, X_{\Delta,(j-1)\Delta} = x \right], \tag{10}$$

for all $j \in \{1, \ldots, J\}$ *and* $k \in \mathbb{N}_0^m \setminus \{0_m\}$.

Remark 1 Representation (9) shows that we have a perfect control variate, namely

$$M_{\Delta,T} := \sum_{j=1}^{J} \sum_{k\in\mathbb{N}_0^m\setminus\{0_m\}} a_{j,k}(X_{\Delta,(j-1)\Delta}) \prod_{r=1}^{m} H_{k_r} \left(\frac{\Delta_j W^r}{\sqrt{\Delta}} \right), \tag{11}$$

for the functional $f(X_{\Delta,T})$, i.e. $\mathrm{Var}[f(X_{\Delta,T}) - M_{\Delta,T}] = 0$.

The control variate $M_{\Delta,T}$ is not implementable because of the infinite summation in (11) and because the coefficients $a_{j,k}$ are unknown. In the later sections, we estimate the unknown coefficients in this and other (related) representations via regression and present bounds for the estimation error.

Now we introduce the following 'truncated' control variate

$$M_{\Delta,T}^{ser,1} := \sum_{j=1}^{J} \sum_{i=1}^{m} a_{j,e_i}(X_{\Delta,(j-1)\Delta}) \frac{\Delta_j W^i}{\sqrt{\Delta}}, \tag{12}$$

where e_i denotes the ith unit vector in $\mathbb{R}^m$. The superscript 'ser' comes from 'series'. In the next subsection, performing a quite different argumentation, we derive another control variate, which will turn out to be theoretically equivalent to $M_{\Delta,T}^{ser,1}$.

2.2 Integral Representation

Integral representation for the exact solution. We first motivate what we call 'integral representation for the discretisation', which will be presented below in this subsection, in that we recall in more detail the main idea of constructing control variates in Milstein and Tretyakov [8]. As was already mentioned in the introduction, the control variate in [8] is an approximation of M_T^* of (6), where the function u is given in (4) and is therefore unknown, which raises the question about a possible practical implementation of (6).

To this end, let us define the 'derivative processes' $\delta^i X_{s,x}^k(t) := \frac{\partial X_{s,x}^k(t)}{\partial x_i}$ for $i, k \in \{1, \ldots, d\}$, where $X_{s,x}^k(t)$ means the kth component of the solution of (1) started at time s in x evaluated at time $t \geq s$, and simply write $\delta^i X_t^k$ rather than $\delta^i X_{0,x_0}^k(t)$ below. Further, we define the matrix $\delta X_t := \begin{pmatrix} \delta^1 X_t^1 & \cdots & \delta^d X_t^1 \\ \vdots & \ddots & \vdots \\ \delta^1 X_t^d & \cdots & \delta^d X_t^d \end{pmatrix} \in \mathbb{R}^{d \times d}$ as well as

the vectors $\delta^i X_t := \left(\delta^i X_t^1 \cdots \delta^i X_t^d \right)^\top \in \mathbb{R}^d$. Assuming $\mu, \sigma \in C^1$, we notice that $\delta^i X_t$ satisfies the following SDE

$$d\delta^i X_t = \sum_{k=1}^d \delta^i X_t^k \left[\frac{\partial \mu(X_t)}{\partial x_k} dt + \frac{\partial \sigma(X_t)}{\partial x_k} dW_t \right], \quad \delta^i X_0^k = \begin{cases} 1, i = k \\ 0, i \neq k \end{cases}. \quad (13)$$

Milstein and Tretyakov [8] exploit (13) to prove that, provided $f, \mu, \sigma \in C^1$, the integral in (6) can be expressed by means of δX_t as follows

$$M_T^* := \int_0^T \nabla_x u(t, X_t) \sigma(X_t) dW_t = \int_0^T \mathbb{E}\left[\nabla f(X_T) \delta X_T \mid X_t \right] \delta X_t^{-1} \sigma(X_t) dW_t,$$

$$(14)$$

where $\nabla_x u(t, x) \in \mathbb{R}^{1 \times d}$ denotes the gradient of u w.r.t. x. The second integral here can be used for a practical construction of an approximation of M_T^* because the conditional expectation can be approximated via regression.

The preceding description lacks assumptions under which the procedure works (the mentioned ones are not enough). We refer to [8] for more detail.

Integral representation for the discretisation. As was mentioned in the introduction, we are going to reduce not the variance in $f(X_T)$ but rather the one in $f(X_{\Delta,T})$, that is, we aim at constructing control variates directly for the discretised process. The fine details of the construction must of course depend on the discretisation scheme. For the rest of the paper, we focus on the Euler scheme, that is, we have

$$\Phi_\Delta(x, y) = x + \mu(x)\Delta + \sigma(x)y. \tag{15}$$

We define the 'discretised derivative process' $\delta^i X^k_{t_j,x}(\Delta, t_l) := \frac{\partial X^k_{t_j,x}(\Delta,t_l)}{\partial x_i}$, for $l \geq j$ and $i, k \in \{1, \ldots, d\}$, where $X^k_{t_j,x}(\Delta, t_l)$ means the kth component of the (Euler) discretisation for (1) started at time t_j in x and evaluated at time t_l ($\geq t_j$), and use $\delta^i X^k_{\Delta,t_l}$ as an abbreviation of $\delta^i X^k_{0,x_0}(\Delta, t_l)$. Assuming $\mu, \sigma \in C^1$, we get that the process $(\delta^i X_{\Delta,j\Delta})_{j=1,\ldots,J}$ has the dynamics

$$\delta^i X_{\Delta,j\Delta} = \delta^i X_{\Delta,(j-1)\Delta} + \sum_{k=1}^d \delta^i X^k_{\Delta,(j-1)\Delta} \left[\frac{\partial \mu(X_{\Delta,(j-1)\Delta})}{\partial x_k} \Delta + \frac{\partial \sigma(X_{\Delta,(j-1)\Delta})}{\partial x_k} \Delta_j W \right], \tag{16}$$

(cf. (13)), where $\delta X_{\Delta,0} = I_d$, and in what follows I_d denotes the identity matrix of size d.

Given a Borel function $f : \mathbb{R}^d \to \mathbb{R}$ satisfying $\mathbb{E}\left|f(X_{\Delta,T})\right| < \infty$, it can be verified by a direct calculation that, for $t \in [t_{j-1}, t_j)$,

$$\mathbb{E}[f(X_{\Delta,T})|\mathscr{F}_t] = u_\Delta(t, X_{\Delta,t_{j-1}}, W_t - W_{t_{j-1}}), \tag{17}$$

where the function $u_\Delta : [0, T] \times \mathbb{R}^{d+m} \to \mathbb{R}$ is constructed via the backward recursion as follows

$$u_\Delta(t, x, y) = \mathbb{E}[u_\Delta(t_j, \Phi_\Delta(x, y + z_j\sqrt{t_j - t}), 0)], \quad t \in [t_{j-1}, t_j), \tag{18}$$
$$u_\Delta(T, x, 0) = f(x), \tag{19}$$

where $t_j := \frac{jT}{J}$, $j \in \{0, \ldots, J\}$, and $z_1, \ldots, z_J \overset{\text{i.i.d.}}{\sim} \mathscr{N}(0_m, I_m)$.

We now introduce the following assumptions: for any $j \in \{1, \ldots, J\}$ and $x \in \mathbb{R}^d$, it holds

(Ass1) $f(X_{t_{j-1},x}(\Delta, T)) \in L^1$,
(Ass2)$_n$ $|\Delta_j W|^n \, \mathbb{E}[f(X_{t_{j-1},x}(\Delta, T))|\mathscr{F}_{t_j}] \in L^1$.

(Ass1) is just a minimal assumption that allows to have (17) with the function u_Δ constructed via (18)–(19). (Ass2)$_n$ is a technical assumption, which depends on n, allowing to replace integration and differentiation in several cases of interest (see below). In most places, we need the variant (Ass2)$_1$, i.e. with $n = 1$, but at a couple of instances, we will need stronger variants (Ass2)$_n$ with $n \geq 1$. That is why we have the parameter n in the formulation of that assumption.

An attractive feature of such an approach via the discretised process (in contrast to the one via the exact solution) is that, under (Ass1) and (Ass2)$_1$, due to the smoothness of the Gaussian density, the function u_Δ is continuously differentiable in y regardless of whether f is smooth, and, moreover, u_Δ is continuously differentiable in x, provided f, μ, σ are continuously differentiable. More precisely, we obtain the above statements because, for $t \in [t_{j-1}, t_j)$, we can write (for simplicity, in the one-dimensional case)

$$u_\Delta(t, x, y) = \int_{\mathbb{R}} u_\Delta\left(t_j, \Phi_\Delta(x, w), 0\right) \frac{1}{\sqrt{2\pi(t_j - t)}} e^{-\frac{(w-y)^2}{2(t_j - t)}} dw,$$

and differentiation under the integral applies due to $(Ass2)_1$ together with the dominated convergence theorem (notice that the expression $\mathbb{E}[f(X_{t_{j-1},x}(\Delta, T))|\mathscr{F}_{t_j}]$ in $(Ass2)_n$ is nothing else than $u_\Delta(t_j, \Phi_\Delta(x, \Delta_j W), 0)$).

Theorem 2 *Suppose (Ass1) and $(Ass2)_1$.*

(i) It holds

$$f(X_{\Delta,T}) = \mathbb{E}[f(X_{\Delta,T})] + \sum_{j=1}^{J} \int_{t_{j-1}}^{t_j} \nabla_y u_\Delta(t, X_{\Delta,t_{j-1}}, W_t - W_{t_{j-1}}) \, dW_t,$$

where $\nabla_y u_\Delta(t, x, y) \in \mathbb{R}^{1 \times m}$ denotes the gradient of u_Δ w.r.t. y.

(ii) Assume additionally that $f, \mu, \sigma \in C^1$. Then, we also have the alternative representation

$$f(X_{\Delta,T}) = \mathbb{E}[f(X_{\Delta,T})] + \sum_{j=1}^{J} \int_{t_{j-1}}^{t_j} \mathbb{E}\left[\nabla f(X_{\Delta,T})\delta X_{\Delta,T}\delta X_{\Delta,t_j}^{-1} \mid \mathscr{F}_t\right] \sigma(X_{\Delta,t_{j-1}}) \, dW_t.$$

Let us define the function $g_j \colon \mathbb{R}^d \to \mathbb{R}^{1 \times d}$, $j \in \{1, \dots, J\}$, through

$$g_j(x) = \left(g_{j,1}(x), \dots, g_{j,d}(x)\right) := \mathbb{E}\left[\nabla f(X_{\Delta,T})\delta X_{\Delta,T}\delta X_{\Delta,t_j}^{-1} \mid X_{\Delta,t_{j-1}} = x\right]. \tag{20}$$

Note that it holds (see the proof of Theorem 2)

$$g_j(x) = \mathbb{E}\left[\nabla_x u_\Delta(t_j, X_{\Delta,t_j}, 0) \mid X_{\Delta,t_{j-1}} = x\right], \tag{21}$$

$$\nabla_y u_\Delta(t_{j-1}, x, 0) = g_j(x)\sigma(x), \tag{22}$$

where $\nabla_x u_\Delta(t, x, y)$ denotes the gradient of u_Δ w.r.t. x, and we conditioned on $X_{\Delta,t_{j-1}}$ instead of $\mathscr{F}_{t_{j-1}}$ because $(X_{\Delta,t_j})_{j=0,\dots,J}$ is a Markov chain (one can do that for grid points only). Theorem 2 inspires to introduce the control variate

$$M_{\Delta,T}^{int,1} := \sum_{j=1}^{J} \sum_{i=1}^{m} \frac{\partial u_\Delta(t_{j-1}, X_{\Delta,t_{j-1}}, 0)}{\partial y_i} \Delta_j W^i$$

$$= \sum_{j=1}^{J} \sum_{k=1}^{d} g_{j,k}(X_{\Delta,t_{j-1}}) \sum_{i=1}^{m} \sigma_{ki}(X_{\Delta,t_{j-1}}) \Delta_j W^i. \tag{23}$$

It will turn out that $M_{\Delta,T}^{int,1} = M_{\Delta,T}^{ser,1}$. To this end, we derive a connection between the series and integral representations.

Theorem 3 *Under (Ass1) and (Ass2)$_n$ for all $n \in \mathbb{N}$, provided that it holds*

$$\left| D^\alpha \left(\frac{\partial}{\partial y_r} u_\Delta(t, x, y) \right) \right| := \left| \frac{\partial^K \left(\frac{\partial}{\partial y_r} u_\Delta(t, x, y) \right)}{\partial t^{\alpha_1} \partial y_1^{\alpha_2} \cdots \partial y_m^{\alpha_{m+1}}} \right| \leq C^K \tag{24}$$

for all $K \in \mathbb{N}$, $r \in \{1, \ldots, m\}$, $|\alpha| = K$, $t \in [t_{j-1}, t_j)$, $x \in \mathbb{R}^d$, $y \in \mathbb{R}^m$, with some constant $C > 0$, we have for the Euler scheme

$$f(X_{\Delta,T}) = \mathbb{E}[f(X_{\Delta,T})] + \sum_{j=1}^{J} \sum_{l=1}^{\infty} \Delta^{l/2} \sum_{\substack{k \in \mathbb{N}_0^m \\ \sum_{r=1}^m k_r = l}} \frac{\partial^l u_\Delta(t_{j-1}, X_{\Delta,t_{j-1}}, 0)}{\partial y_1^{k_1} \cdots \partial y_m^{k_m}} \prod_{r=1}^{m} \frac{H_{k_r} \left(\frac{\Delta_j W^r}{\sqrt{\Delta}} \right)}{\sqrt{k_r!}}$$

$$\tag{25}$$

whenever $0 < \Delta < \frac{1}{C^2}$. (The series converge in L^2.) Consequently, we obtain for $l = \sum_{r=1}^m k_r \in \mathbb{N}$

$$\frac{\Delta^{l/2}}{\sqrt{k_1!} \cdots \sqrt{k_m!}} \cdot \frac{\partial^l u_\Delta(t_{j-1}, X_{\Delta,t_{j-1}}, 0)}{\partial y_1^{k_1} \cdots \partial y_m^{k_m}} = a_{j,k}(X_{\Delta,t_{j-1}}). \tag{26}$$

Remark 2 In the one-dimensional case ($d = m = 1$), a representation of a similar type as (25) appears in [1] in a somewhat different form. Our form is aimed at constructing control variates via regression methods.

In particular, we see from Theorem 3 that $M_{\Delta,T}^{int,1} = M_{\Delta,T}^{ser,1}$ provided that (24) holds. However, we can prove the equality of the aforementioned control variates without assuming (24):

Theorem 4 *Under (Ass1) and (Ass2)$_1$, we have for $i \in \{1, \ldots, m\}$*

$$a_{j,e_i}(x) = \sqrt{\Delta} \frac{\partial}{\partial y_i} u_\Delta(t_{j-1}, x, 0),$$

and consequently,

$$M_{\Delta,T}^{int,1} = M_{\Delta,T}^{ser,1}.$$

It is interesting to remark that, although we assumed $f(X_{\Delta,T}) \in L^2$ when speaking about the series representation, the coefficients a_{j,e_i} are well-defined already under (Ass1) and (Ass2)$_1$.

We can now investigate the order of the truncation error, which arises when we replace the control variate $M_{\Delta,T}$ of (11) with the control variate $M_{\Delta,T}^{ser,1}$ of (12).

Theorem 5 *Suppose (Ass1) and (Ass2)₃. Provided that the function $u_\Delta(t, x, y)$ has bounded partial derivatives in y of orders 2 and 3, it holds*

$$\text{Var}\left[f(X_{\Delta,T}) - M_{\Delta,T}^{int,1}\right] = \text{Var}\left[f(X_{\Delta,T}) - M_{\Delta,T}^{ser,1}\right] \lesssim \Delta. \tag{27}$$

Remark 3 (i) Below we will present sufficient conditions in terms of the functions f, μ, σ that ensure the assumption on u_Δ in Theorem 5 (see Theorem 6 in Sect. 3).

(ii) The control variate $M_{\Delta,T}^{int,1}$ differs from the one suggested in [8] only in an index concerning the inverted matrix, i.e. we have $\delta X_{\Delta,t_j}^{-1}$ inside of $g_j(X_{\Delta,t_{j-1}})$ rather than the $\mathcal{F}_{t_{j-1}}$-measurable random variable $\delta X_{\Delta,t_{j-1}}^{-1}$ which arises in case of the exact solution $f(X_T)$ from a simple discretisation of the stochastic integral in (14).

Regarding the weak convergence order of the Euler scheme, we have the following result (cf. Theorem 2.1 in [7]).

Proposition 1 *Assume that μ and σ in (1) are Lipschitz continuous with components $\mu_k, \sigma_{ki}: \mathbb{R}^d \to \mathbb{R}, k = 1, \ldots, d, i = 1, \ldots, m$, being 4 times continuously differentiable with their partial derivatives of orders up to 4 having polynomial growth. Let $f: \mathbb{R}^d \to \mathbb{R}$ be 4 times continuously differentiable with partial derivatives of orders up to 4 having polynomial growth. Then, for the Euler scheme (15), we have*

$$\left|\mathbb{E}f(X_T) - \mathbb{E}f(X_{\Delta,T})\right| \le c\Delta, \tag{28}$$

where the constant c does not depend on Δ.

We remark that the assumption that, for sufficiently large $n \in \mathbb{N}$, the expectations $\mathbb{E}|X_{\Delta,j\Delta}|^{2n}$ are uniformly bounded in J and $j = 0, \ldots, J$ (cf. Theorem 2.1 in [7]) is automatically satisfied for the Euler scheme because μ and σ, being globally Lipschitz, have at most linear growth.

3 Regression Analysis

In the previous sections, we have given several representations for the control variates. Now we discuss how to compute the coefficients in these representations via regression. For the sake of clarity, we will focus on the control variate given by (23), that is, we will estimate the functions $g_{j,k}$ in (20) via linear regression. Let us start with a general description of the global Monte Carlo regression algorithm.

3.1 Global Monte Carlo Regression Algorithm

Fix a q-dimensional vector of real-valued functions $\psi = (\psi^1, \ldots, \psi^q)$ on $\mathbb{R}^d$. Simulate a set of N 'training paths' of the Markov chains $X_{\Delta,j\Delta}$ and $\delta X_{\Delta,j\Delta}, j = 0, \ldots, J$.

We should choose $N > q$. In what follows these N training paths are denoted by D_N^{tr}:

$$D_N^{tr} := \left\{ (X_{\Delta,j\Delta}^{tr,(n)}, \delta X_{\Delta,j\Delta}^{tr,(n)})_{j=0,\dots,J} : n = 1, \dots, N \right\}.$$

Let $\alpha_{j,k} = (\alpha_{j,k}^1, \dots, \alpha_{j,k}^q)$, where $j \in \{1, \dots, J\}$, $k \in \{1, \dots, d\}$, be a solution of the following least squares optimisation problem:

$$\operatorname{argmin}_{\alpha \in \mathbb{R}^q} \sum_{n=1}^{N} \left[\zeta_{j,k}^{tr,(n)} - \alpha^1 \psi^1 (X_{\Delta,(j-1)\Delta}^{tr,(n)}) - \dots - \alpha^q \psi^q (X_{\Delta,(j-1)\Delta}^{tr,(n)}) \right]^2$$

with

$$\zeta_j^{tr,(n)} = \left(\zeta_{j,1}^{tr,(n)}, \dots, \zeta_{j,d}^{tr,(n)} \right) := \nabla f (X_{\Delta,T}^{tr,(n)}) \delta X_{\Delta,T}^{tr,(n)} \left(\delta X_{\Delta,j\Delta}^{tr,(n)} \right)^{-1}.$$

Define an estimate for the coefficient function $g_{j,k}$ via

$$\hat{g}_{j,k}(z) := \alpha_{j,k}^1 \psi^1(z) + \dots + \alpha_{j,k}^q \psi^q(z), \quad z \in \mathbb{R}^d.$$

The cost of computing $\alpha_{j,k}$ is of order $O(Nq^2)$, since each $\alpha_{j,k}$ is of the form $\alpha_{j,k} = B^{-1} b$ with

$$B_{l,o} := \frac{1}{N} \sum_{n=1}^{N} \psi^l (X_{\Delta,(j-1)\Delta}^{tr,(n)}) \psi^o (X_{\Delta,(j-1)\Delta}^{tr,(n)}) \tag{29}$$

and

$$b_l := \frac{1}{N} \sum_{n=1}^{N} \psi^l (X_{\Delta,(j-1)\Delta}^{tr,(n)}) \zeta_{j,k}^{tr,(n)},$$

$l, o \in \{1, \dots, q\}$. The cost of approximating the family of the coefficient functions $g_{j,k}$, $j \in \{1, \dots, J\}$, $k \in \{1, \dots, d\}$, is of order $O(JdNq^2)$.

3.2 Piecewise Polynomial Regression

There are different ways to choose the basis functions $\psi = (\psi^1, \dots, \psi^q)$. In this section, we describe piecewise polynomial partitioning estimates and present L^2-upper bounds for the estimation error.

From now on, we fix some $p \in \mathbb{N}_0$, which will denote the maximal degree of polynomials involved in our basis functions. The piecewise polynomial partitioning estimate of $g_{j,k}$ works as follows: consider some $R > 0$ and an equidistant partition of $[-R, R]^d$ in Q^d cubes $K_1, \ldots, K_{Q^d}$. Further, consider the basis functions $\psi^{l,1}, \ldots, \psi^{l,q}$ with $l \in \{1, \ldots, Q^d\}$ and $q = \binom{p+d}{d}$ such that $\psi^{l,1}(x), \ldots, \psi^{l,q}(x)$ are polynomials with degree less than or equal to p for $x \in K_l$ and $\psi^{l,1}(x) = \cdots = \psi^{l,q}(x) = 0$ for $x \notin K_l$. Then we obtain the least squares regression estimate $\hat{g}_{j,k}(x)$ for $x \in \mathbb{R}^d$ as described in Sect. 3.1, based on $Q^d q = O(Q^d p^d)$ basis functions. In particular, we have $\hat{g}_{j,k}(x) = 0$ for any $x \notin [-R, R]^d$. We note that the cost of computing $\hat{g}_{j,k}$ for all j, k is of order $O(JdNQ^d p^{2d})$ rather than $O(JdNQ^{2d} p^{2d})$ due to a block diagonal matrix structure of B in (29). An equivalent approach, which leads to the same estimator $\hat{g}_{j,k}(x)$, is to perform separate regressions for each cube $K_1, \ldots, K_{Q^d}$. Here, the number of basis functions at each regression is of order $O(p^d)$ so that the overall cost is of order $O(JdNQ^d p^{2d})$, too. For $x = (x_1, \ldots, x_d) \in \mathbb{R}^d$ and $h \in [1, \infty)$, we will use the notations

$$|x|_h := \left(\sum_{k=1}^{d} |x_k|^h \right)^{1/h}, \quad |x|_\infty := \max_{k=1,\ldots,d} |x_k|.$$

For $s \in \mathbb{N}_0, C > 0$ and $h \in [1, \infty]$, we say that a function $F : \mathbb{R}^d \to \mathbb{R}$ is $(s + 1, C)$-smooth w.r.t. the norm $|\cdot|_h$ whenever, for all $\alpha = (\alpha_1, \ldots, \alpha_d) \in \mathbb{N}_0^d$ with $\sum_{k=1}^{d} \alpha_k = s$, we have

$$|D^\alpha F(x) - D^\alpha F(y)| \le C|x - y|_h, \quad x, y \in \mathbb{R}^d,$$

i.e. the function $D^\alpha F$ is globally Lipschitz with the Lipschitz constant C with respect to the norm $|\cdot|_h$ on $\mathbb{R}^d$ (cf. Definition 3.3 in [4]). In what follows, we use the notation $\mathbb{P}_{\Delta, j-1}$ for the distribution of $X_{\Delta,(j-1)\Delta}$. In particular, we will work with the corresponding L^2-norm:

$$\|F\|_{L^2(\mathbb{P}_{\Delta, j-1})}^2 := \int_{\mathbb{R}^d} F^2(x) \, \mathbb{P}_{\Delta, j-1}(dx) = \mathbb{E}\left[F^2\left(X_{\Delta,(j-1)\Delta} \right) \right].$$

We now define $\zeta_{j,k}$ as the kth component of the vector $\zeta_j = (\zeta_{j,1}, \ldots, \zeta_{j,d}) := \nabla f(X_{\Delta,\tau}) \delta X_{\Delta,\tau} \delta X_{\Delta,j\Delta}^{-1}$ and remark that $g_{j,k}(x) = \mathbb{E}[\zeta_{j,k}|X_{\Delta,(j-1)\Delta} = x]$. In what follows, we consider the following assumptions: there exist $h \in [1, \infty]$ and positive constants $\Sigma, A, C_h, \nu, B_\nu$ such that, for all $J \in \mathbb{N}, j \in \{1, \ldots, J\}$ and $k \in \{1, \ldots, d\}$, it holds

(A1) $\sup_{x \in \mathbb{R}^d} \mathrm{Var}[\zeta_{j,k}|X_{\Delta,(j-1)\Delta} = x] \le \Sigma < \infty$,
(A2) $\sup_{x \in \mathbb{R}^d} |g_{j,k}(x)| \le A < \infty$,
(A3) $g_{j,k}$ is $(p + 1, C_h)$-smooth w.r.t. the norm $|\cdot|_h$,
(A4) $\mathbb{P}(|X_{\Delta,(j-1)\Delta}|_\infty > R) \le B_\nu R^{-\nu}$ for all $R > 0$.

Remark 4 Let us notice that it is only a matter of convenience which h to choose in (A3) because all norms $|\cdot|_h$ are equivalent. Furthermore, since μ and σ are assumed to be globally Lipschitz, hence have linear growth, then, given any $v > 0$, (A4) is satisfied with a sufficiently large $B_v > 0$. In other words, (A4) is needed only to introduce the constant B_v, which appears in the formulations below.

In the next theorem we, in particular, present sufficient conditions in terms of the functions μ, σ and f that imply the preceding assumptions.

Theorem 6 *(i) Under (Ass1) and (Ass2)$_1$, let all functions f, μ_k, σ_{ki}, $k \in \{1, \ldots, d\}$, $i \in \{1, \ldots, m\}$, be continuously differentiable with bounded partial derivatives. Then (A1) and (A2) hold with appropriate constants Σ and A.*

(ii) If, moreover, (Ass1) and (Ass2)$_3$ are satisfied, all functions σ_{ki} are bounded and all functions f, μ_k, σ_{ki} are 3 times continuously differentiable with bounded partial derivatives up to order 3, then the function $u_\Delta(t, x, y)$ has bounded partial derivatives in y up to order 3. In particular, (27) holds true.

Remark 5 As a generalisation of Theorem 6, it is natural to expect that (A3) is satisfied with a sufficiently large constant $C_h > 0$ if, under (Ass1) and (Ass2)$_{p+2}$, all functions f, μ_k, σ_{ki} are $p + 2$ times continuously differentiable with bounded partial derivatives up to order $p + 2$.

Let $\hat{g}_{j,k}$ be the piecewise polynomial partitioning estimate of $g_{j,k}$. By $\tilde{g}_{j,k}$ we denote the truncated estimate, which is defined as

$$\tilde{g}_{j,k}(x) := T_A \hat{g}_{j,k}(x) := \begin{cases} \hat{g}_{j,k}(x) & \text{if } |\hat{g}_{j,k}(x)| \leq A, \\ A \operatorname{sgn} \hat{g}_{j,k}(x) & \text{otherwise,} \end{cases}$$

where A is the bound from (A2).

Lemma 1 *Under (A1)–(A4), we have*

$$\mathbb{E}\|\tilde{g}_{j,k} - g_{j,k}\|^2_{L^2(\mathbb{P}_{\Delta,j-1})} \leq \tilde{c} \left(\Sigma + A^2(\log N + 1)\right) \frac{\binom{p+d}{d} Q^d}{N} \tag{30}$$

$$+ \frac{8 C_h^2}{(p+1)!^2 d^{2-2/h}} \left(\frac{Rd}{Q}\right)^{2p+2} + 8A^2 B_v R^{-v},$$

where $\tilde{c}$ is a universal constant.

It is worth noting that the expectation in the left-hand side of (30) accounts for the averaging over the randomness in D_N^{tr}. To explain this in more detail, let $(X_{\Delta,j\Delta})_{j=0,\ldots,J}$ be a 'testing path' which is independent of the training paths D_N^{tr}. Then it holds

$$\|\tilde{g}_{j,k} - g_{j,k}\|^2_{L^2(\mathbb{P}_{\Delta,j-1})} \equiv \|\tilde{g}_{j,k}(\cdot, D_N^{tr}) - g_{j,k}(\cdot)\|^2_{L^2(\mathbb{P}_{\Delta,j-1})}$$

$$= \mathbb{E}\left[\left(\tilde{g}_{j,k}(X_{\Delta,(j-1)\Delta}, D_N^{tr}) - g_{j,k}(X_{\Delta,(j-1)\Delta})\right)^2 \mid D_N^{tr}\right],$$

hence,

$$\mathbb{E}\|\tilde{g}_{j,k} - g_{j,k}\|^2_{L^2(\mathbb{P}_{\Delta,j-1})} = \mathbb{E}\left[\left(\tilde{g}_{j,k}(X_{\Delta,(j-1)\Delta}, D_N^{tr}) - g_{j,k}(X_{\Delta,(j-1)\Delta})\right)^2\right], \quad (31)$$

which provides an alternative form for the expression in the left-hand side of (30).

Let us now estimate the variance of the random variable $f(X_{\Delta,T}) - \tilde{M}_{\Delta,T}^{int,1}$, where

$$\tilde{M}_{\Delta,T}^{int,1} := \sum_{j=1}^{J}\sum_{k=1}^{d}\tilde{g}_{j,k}(X_{\Delta,(j-1)\Delta}, D_N^{tr})\sum_{i=1}^{m}\sigma_{ki}(X_{\Delta,(j-1)\Delta})\Delta_j W^i. \quad (32)$$

Theorem 7 *Let us assume* $\sup_{x\in\mathbb{R}^d}|\sigma_{ki}(x)| \leq \sigma_{\max} < \infty$ *for all* $k \in \{1,\dots,d\}$ *and* $i \in \{1,\dots,m\}$. *Then we have under (A1)–(A4)*

$$\mathrm{Var}[f(X_{\Delta,T}) - \tilde{M}_{\Delta,T}^{int,1}] \lesssim \frac{1}{J} + d^2 T m \sigma_{\max}^2 \left\{ \tilde{c}\left(\Sigma + A^2(\log N + 1)\right)\frac{\binom{p+d}{d}Q^d}{N} \right.$$

$$\left. + \frac{8\,C_h^2}{(p+1)!^2 d^{2-2/h}}\left(\frac{Rd}{Q}\right)^{2p+2} + 8A^2 B_\nu R^{-\nu}\right\}. \quad (33)$$

We finally stress that $\tilde{M}_{\Delta,T}^{int,1}$ is a valid control variate in that it does not introduce bias, i.e. $\mathbb{E}[\tilde{M}_{\Delta,T}^{int,1}|D_N^{tr}] = 0$, which follows from the martingale transform structure in (32).

3.3 Summary of the Algorithm

The algorithm of the 'integral approach' consists of two phases: training phase and testing phase. In the training phase, we simulate N independent training paths D_N^{tr} and construct regression estimates $\tilde{g}_{j,k}(\cdot, D_N^{tr})$ for the coefficients $g_{j,k}(\cdot), k \in \{1,\dots,d\}$. In the testing phase, independently from D_N^{tr} we simulate N_0 independent testing paths $(X_{\Delta,j\Delta}^{(n)})_{j=0,\dots,J}, n = 1,\dots,N_0$, and build the Monte Carlo estimator for $\mathbb{E}f(X_T)$ as

$$\frac{1}{N_0}\sum_{n=1}^{N_0}\left(f(X_{\Delta,T}^{(n)}) - \tilde{M}_{\Delta,T}^{int,1,(n)}\right). \quad (34)$$

The expectation of this estimator equals $\mathbb{E}f(X_{\Delta,T})$, and the upper bound for the variance is $\frac{1}{N_0}$ times the expression in (33).

4 Complexity Analysis

The results presented in previous sections provide us with 'building blocks' to perform the complexity analysis.

Standing assumption for Complexity Analysis consists in

$$(Ass1), (Ass2)_1, (27) \text{ and } (28).$$

Combining Theorems 5, 6 and Proposition 1, we recall that this standing assumption is satisfied whenever we have (Ass1), (Ass2)$_3$, σ is bounded, $f, \mu, \sigma \in C^4$, the partial derivatives of f, μ and σ up to order 3 are bounded and of order 4 have polynomial growth. However, we prefer to formulate the standing assumption for complexity analysis as above because one might imagine other sufficient conditions for it.

4.1 Integral Approach

Below we present a complexity analysis which explains how we can approach the complexity order $\varepsilon^{-2}\sqrt{|\log(\varepsilon)|}$ with ε being the precision to be achieved.

For the integral approach, we perform d regressions in the training phase and d evaluations of $\tilde{g}_{j,k}$ in the testing phase (using the regression coefficients from the training phase) at each time step. Therefore, the overall cost is of order

$$J Q^d d c_{p,d} \max \{c_{p,d} N, N_0\}, \tag{35}$$

where $c_{p,d} := \binom{p+d}{p}$. Under (A1)–(A4) and boundedness of σ (cf. Theorem 7), we have the following constraints

$$\max \left\{ \frac{1}{J^2}, \frac{1}{J N_0}, \frac{Q^d d^2 m c_{p,d} \log(N)}{N N_0}, \frac{d^2 m}{(p+1)!^2 N_0} \left(\frac{Rd}{Q} \right)^{2(p+1)}, \frac{d^2 m B_v}{N_0 R^v} \right\} \lesssim \varepsilon^2, \tag{36}$$

to ensure a *mean squared error* (MSE) of order ε^2. Note that the first term in (36) comes from the squared bias of the estimator (due to (28) and $\mathbb{E}[\tilde{M}^{int,1}_{\Delta,T}] = 0$) and the remaining four ones come from the variance of the estimator (see (33) and (34)).

Theorem 8 *Under (A1)–(A4) and boundedness of σ, we obtain the following solution for the integral approach:*

$$J \asymp \varepsilon^{-1}, \quad Q \asymp \left[\frac{B_\nu^{4(p+1)} d^{2\nu+4(p+1)(\nu+1)} m^{\nu+2(p+1)}}{\varepsilon^{2\nu+4(p+1)} c_{p,d}^{2\nu+4(p+1)}(p+1)!^{4\nu}}\right]^{\frac{1}{d\nu+2(p+1)(d+2\nu)}}, \tag{37}$$

$$N \asymp \left[\frac{B_\nu^{2d(p+1)} d^{2d\nu+2(p+1)(d\nu+2d+2\nu)} m^{d\nu+2(p+1)(d+\nu)}}{\varepsilon^{2d\nu+4(p+1)(d+\nu)} c_{p,d}^{d\nu+2d(p+1)}(p+1)!^{2d\nu}}\right]^{\frac{1}{d\nu+2(p+1)(d+2\nu)}}$$

$$\cdot \sqrt{\log\left(\varepsilon^{-\frac{2d\nu+4(p+1)(d+\nu)}{d\nu+2(p+1)(d+2\nu)}}\right)}, \tag{38}$$

$$N_0 \asymp N c_{p,d}$$

$$\asymp \left[\frac{B_\nu^{2d(p+1)} c_{p,d}^{4\nu(p+1)} d^{2d\nu+2(p+1)(d\nu+2d+2\nu)} m^{d\nu+2(p+1)(d+\nu)}}{\varepsilon^{2d\nu+4(p+1)(d+\nu)}(p+1)!^{2d\nu}}\right]^{\frac{1}{d\nu+2(p+1)(d+2\nu)}}$$

$$\cdot \sqrt{\log\left(\varepsilon^{-\frac{2d\nu+4(p+1)(d+\nu)}{d\nu+2(p+1)(d+2\nu)}}\right)}, \tag{39}$$

$$R \asymp \left[\frac{B_\nu^{d+4(p+1)}(p+1)!^{2d} m^{2(p+1)}}{\varepsilon^{4(p+1)} c_{p,d}^{4(p+1)} d^{2(p+1)(d-2)}}\right]^{\frac{1}{d\nu+2(p+1)(d+2\nu)}}, \tag{40}$$

provided that $2(p+1) > d$ *and* $\nu > \frac{2d(p+1)}{2(p+1)-d}$.[1] *Thus, we have for the complexity*

$$\mathscr{C}_{int} \asymp J Q^d d c_{p,d}^2 N \asymp J Q^d d c_{p,d} N_0$$

$$\asymp \left[\frac{B_\nu^{6d(p+1)} c_{p,d}^{2(p+1)(4\nu-d)-d\nu} d^{5d\nu+2(p+1)(3d\nu+5d+4\nu)} m^{3d\nu+6(p+1)(d+\nu)}}{\varepsilon^{5d\nu+2(p+1)(5d+4\nu)}(p+1)!^{6d\nu}}\right]^{\frac{1}{d\nu+2(p+1)(d+2\nu)}}$$

$$\cdot \sqrt{\log\left(\varepsilon^{-\frac{2d\nu+4(p+1)(d+\nu)}{d\nu+2(p+1)(d+2\nu)}}\right)}. \tag{41}$$

Remark 6 (i) For the sake of comparison with the SMC and MLMC approaches, we recall at this point that their complexities are

$$\mathscr{C}_{SMC} \asymp \varepsilon^{-3} \quad \text{and} \quad \mathscr{C}_{MLMC} \asymp \varepsilon^{-2}$$

at best.[2] Complexity estimate (41) shows that one can approach the complexity order $\varepsilon^{-2}\sqrt{|\log(\varepsilon)|}$, when $p, \nu \to \infty$, i.e. if the coefficients $g_{j,k}$ are smooth enough and the solution X of SDE (1) lives in a compact set.

---

[1] Performing the full complexity analysis via Lagrange multipliers one can see that these parameter values are *not* optimal if $2(p+1) \le d$ or $\nu \le \frac{2d(p+1)}{2(p+1)-d}$ (a Lagrange multiplier corresponding to a '≤ 0' constraint is negative, cf. proof of Theorem 8). Therefore, the recommendation is to choose the power p for our basis functions according to $p > \frac{d-2}{2}$. The opposite choice is allowed as well (the method converges), but theoretical complexity of the method would be then worse than that of the SMC, namely, ε^{-3}.

[2] For the Euler scheme, there is an additional logarithmic factor in the complexity of the MLMC algorithm (see [3]).

(ii) Note that we would have obtained the same complexity even when the variance in (27) were of order Δ^K with $K > 1$. This is due to the fact that the second constraint in (36) is the only inactive one and this would still hold if the condition were $\frac{1}{J^K N_0} \lesssim \varepsilon^2$. Hence, it is not useful to derive a control variate with a higher variance order for the Euler scheme.

4.2 Series Approach

Below we present a complexity analysis for the series representation, defined in Sect. 2.1. Again we focus on the Euler scheme (15). Then we compare the resulting complexity with the one in (41).

Similarly to Sect. 3.2, we define $\zeta_{j,i}$ as the ith component of the vector $\zeta_j = (\zeta_{j,1}, \ldots, \zeta_{j,m})^\top := f(X_{\Delta,T}) \frac{\Delta_j W}{\sqrt{\Delta}}$ and remark that $a_{j,e_i}(x) = \mathbb{E}[\zeta_{j,i} | X_{\Delta,(j-1)\Delta} = x]$ (compare with (10)). We will work under the following assumptions: there exist $h \in [1, \infty]$ and positive constants Σ, A, C_h such that, for all $J \in \mathbb{N}$, $j \in \{1, \ldots, J\}$ and $i \in \{1, \ldots, m\}$, it holds:

(B1) $\sup_{x \in \mathbb{R}^d} \mathrm{Var}[\zeta_{j,i} | X_{\Delta,(j-1)\Delta} = x] \leq \Sigma < \infty$,
(B2) $\sup_{x \in \mathbb{R}^d} |a_{j,e_i}(x)| \leq A\sqrt{\Delta} < \infty$,
(B3) a_{j,e_i} is $(p + 1, C_h)$-smooth w.r.t. the norm $|\cdot|_h$.

Note the difference between (B2) and (A2) of Sect. 3.2, while (B1) has the same form as (A1). This is due to (26), hence the additional factor $\sqrt{\Delta}$ in (B2).

In what follows the N training paths are denoted by

$$D_N^{tr} := \left\{ (X_{\Delta, j\Delta}^{tr,(n)})_{j=0,\ldots,J} : n = 1, \ldots, N \right\},$$

that is, we do not need to simulate paths for the derivative processes $\delta X_{\Delta, j\Delta}$. Let $\hat{a}_{j,e_i}$ be the piecewise polynomial partitioning estimate of a_{j,e_i} described in Sect. 3.2. By $\tilde{a}_{j,e_i}$ we denote the truncated estimate, which is defined as follows:

$$\tilde{a}_{j,e_i}(x) := T_{A\sqrt{\Delta}} \hat{a}_{j,e_i}(x) := \begin{cases} \hat{a}_{j,e_i}(x) & \text{if } |\hat{a}_{j,e_i}(x)| \leq A\sqrt{\Delta}, \\ A\sqrt{\Delta} \, \mathrm{sgn}\, \hat{a}_{j,e_i}(x) & \text{otherwise.} \end{cases}$$

Lemma 2 *Under (B1)–(B3) and (A4), we have*

$$\mathbb{E}\|\tilde{a}_{j,e_i} - a_{j,e_i}\|_{L^2(\mathbb{P}_{\Delta,j-1})}^2 \leq \tilde{c} \left(\Sigma + A^2 \Delta (\log N + 1)\right) \frac{c_{p,d} Q^d}{N} \tag{42}$$

$$+ \frac{8 C_h^2}{(p+1)!^2 d^{2-\frac{2}{h}}} \left(\frac{R}{Q}\right)^{2p+2} + 8A^2 \Delta B_\nu R^{-\nu},$$

where $\tilde{c}$ is a universal constant.

Let us now estimate the variance of the random variable $f(X_{\Delta,T}) - \tilde{M}_{\Delta,T}^{ser,1}$, where

$$\tilde{M}_{\Delta,T}^{ser,1} := \sum_{j=1}^{J} \sum_{i=1}^{m} \tilde{a}_{j,e_i}(X_{\Delta,(j-1)\Delta}, D_N^{tr}) \frac{\Delta_j W^i}{\sqrt{\Delta}}. \tag{43}$$

Theorem 9 *Under (B1)–(B3) and (A4), we have*

$$\mathrm{Var}[f(X_{\Delta,T}) - \tilde{M}_{\Delta,T}^{ser,1}] \lesssim \frac{1}{J} + Jm \left\{ \tilde{c} \left(\Sigma + A^2 \Delta (\log N + 1) \right) \frac{c_{p,d} Q^d}{N} \right.$$

$$\left. + \frac{8 C_h^2}{(p+1)!^2 d^{2-\frac{2}{h}}} \left(\frac{R}{Q} \right)^{2p+2} + 8 A^2 \Delta B_\nu R^{-\nu} \right\}. \tag{44}$$

Let us study the complexity of the following 'series approach': In the training phase, we simulate N independent training paths D_N^{tr} and construct regression estimates $\tilde{a}_{j,e_i}(\cdot, D_N^{tr})$ for the coefficients $a_{j,e_i}(\cdot)$, $i \in \{1, \ldots, m\}$. In the testing phase, independently from D_N^{tr}, we simulate N_0 independent testing paths $(X_{\Delta,j\Delta}^{(n)})_{j=0,\ldots,J}$, $n = 1, \ldots, N_0$, and build the Monte Carlo estimator for $\mathbb{E} f(X_T)$ as

$$\frac{1}{N_0} \sum_{n=1}^{N_0} \left(f(X_{\Delta,T}^{(n)}) - \tilde{M}_{\Delta,T}^{ser,1,(n)} \right). \tag{45}$$

Therefore, the overall cost is of order

$$J Q^d m c_{p,d} \max \left\{ c_{p,d} N, N_0 \right\}. \tag{46}$$

The expectation of the estimator in (45) equals $\mathbb{E} f(X_{\Delta,T})$, and the upper bound for the variance is $\frac{1}{N_0}$ times the expression in (44). Hence, we have the following constraints

$$\max \left\{ \frac{1}{J^2}, \frac{1}{JN_0}, \frac{J Q^d m c_{p,d}}{N N_0}, \frac{Jm}{(p+1)!^2 N_0} \left(\frac{Rd}{Q} \right)^{2(p+1)}, \frac{m B_\nu}{N_0 R^\nu} \right\} \lesssim \varepsilon^2, \tag{47}$$

to ensure a MSE of order ε^2 (due to $\mathbb{E}[M_{\Delta,T}^{ser,1}] = 0$ as well as (44) and (45)). Note that there is no longer a log term in (47). This is due to the factor Δ in (44) such that Σ is of a higher order, compared to $\Delta(\log N + 1)$.

Theorem 10 *Under (B1)–(B3) and (A4), we obtain the following solution for the series approach:*

$$J \asymp \varepsilon^{-1}, \quad Q \asymp \left[\frac{B_\nu^{4(p+1)} d^{4\nu(p+1)} m^{\nu+2(p+1)}}{\varepsilon^{3\nu+2(p+1)} c_{p,d}^{2\nu+4(p+1)} (p+1)!^{4\nu}} \right]^{\frac{1}{d\nu+2(p+1)(d+2\nu)}}, \tag{48}$$

$$N \asymp \left[\frac{B_\nu^{2d(p+1)} d^{2d\nu(p+1)} m^{d\nu+2(p+1)(d+\nu)}}{\varepsilon^{3d\nu+2(p+1)(2d+3\nu)} c_{p,d}^{d\nu+2d(p+1)} (p+1)!^{2d\nu}} \right]^{\frac{1}{d\nu+2(p+1)(d+2\nu)}}, \tag{49}$$

$$N_0 \asymp N c_{p,d} \asymp \left[\frac{B_\nu^{2d(p+1)} c_{p,d}^{4\nu(p+1)} d^{2d\nu(p+1)} m^{d\nu+2(p+1)(d+\nu)}}{\varepsilon^{3d\nu+2(p+1)(2d+3\nu)} (p+1)!^{2d\nu}} \right]^{\frac{1}{d\nu+2(p+1)(d+2\nu)}}, \tag{50}$$

$$R \asymp \left[\frac{B_\nu^{d+4(p+1)} (p+1)!^{2d} m^{2(p+1)}}{\varepsilon^{2(p+1)-d} c_{p,d}^{4(p+1)} d^{2d(p+1)}} \right]^{\frac{1}{d\nu+2(p+1)(d+2\nu)}}, \tag{51}$$

provided that $2(p+1) > d$ *and* $\nu > \frac{2(p+1)}{2(p+1)-d}$.[3] *Thus, we have for the complexity*

$$\mathscr{C}_{ser} \asymp J Q^d m c_{p,d}^2 N \asymp J Q^d m c_{p,d} N_0$$

$$\asymp \left[\frac{B_\nu^{6d(p+1)} c_{p,d}^{2(p+1)(4\nu-d)-d\nu} d^{6d\nu(p+1)} m^{3d\nu+6(p+1)(d+\nu)}}{\varepsilon^{7d\nu+2(p+1)(4d+5\nu)} (p+1)!^{6d\nu}} \right]^{\frac{1}{d\nu+2(p+1)(d+2\nu)}}. \tag{52}$$

Remark 7 (i) Complexity estimate (52) shows that one cannot go beyond the complexity order $\varepsilon^{-2.5}$ in this case, no matter how large p, ν are. This is mainly due to the factor J within the third constraint in (47) which does not arise in (36).

(ii) Similarly to Sect. 4.1, we would have obtained the same complexity even when we used a control variate with a higher variance order Δ^K for some $K > 1$.

(iii) When comparing (52) with (41), one clearly sees that (41) always achieves a better complexity for $\nu > \frac{2(p+1)}{2(p+1)-d}$ (in terms of ε).

(iv) Furthermore, also from the pure computational point of view, it is preferable to consider the integral approach rather than the series approach, even though the control variates $M_{\Delta,T}^{ser,1}$ and $M_{\Delta,T}^{int,1}$ are theoretically equivalent (recall Theorem 4). This is mainly due to the factor $\Delta_j W^i$ in a_{j,e_i} (see (10)), which is independent of $X_{\Delta,(j-1)\Delta}$ and has zero expectation and thus may lead to poor regression results (cf. 'RCV approach' in [2]). Regarding the integral approach, such a destabilising factor is not present in $g_{j,k}$ (see (20)).

5 Numerical Results

In this section, we consider the Euler scheme and compare the numerical performance of the SMC, MLMC, series and integral approaches. For simplicity, we implemented

---

[3]Compare with footnote 1 on p. 16.

a global regression (i.e. the one without truncation and partitioning). Regarding the choice of basis functions, we use in both series and integral approaches the same polynomials $\psi(x) = \prod_{k=1}^{d} x_k^{l_k}$, where $l_1, \ldots, l_d \in \{0, 1, \ldots, p\}$ and $\sum_{k=1}^{d} l_k \leq p$. In addition to the polynomials, we consider the function f as a basis function. Hence, we have overall $\binom{p+d}{d} + 1$ basis functions in each regression. As for the MLMC approach, we use the same simulation results as in [2].

The following results are based on program codes written and vectorised in MATLAB and running on a Linux 64-bit operating system.

5.1 One-Dimensional Example

Here $d = m = 1$. We consider the following SDE (cf. [2])

$$dX_t = -\frac{1}{2} \tanh(X_t) \operatorname{sech}^2(X_t)\, dt + \operatorname{sech}(X_t)\, dW_t, \quad X_0 = 0, \tag{53}$$

for $t \in [0, 1]$, where $\operatorname{sech}(x) := \frac{1}{\cosh(x)}$. This SDE has an exact solution $X_t = \operatorname{arsinh}(W_t)$. Furthermore, we consider the functional $f(x) = \operatorname{sech}(x) + 15 \arctan(x)$, that is, we have

$$\mathbb{E}[f(X_1)] = \mathbb{E}[\operatorname{sech}(\operatorname{arsinh}(W_1))] = \mathbb{E}\left[\frac{1}{\sqrt{1 + W_1^2}}\right] \approx 0.789640. \tag{54}$$

We choose $p = 3$ (that is, 5 basis functions) and, for each $\varepsilon = 2^{-i}, i \in \{2, 3, 4, 5, 6\}$, we set the parameters J, N and N_0 as follows (compare with the formulas in Sect. 4 for $\nu \to \infty$, $\lim_{\nu \to \infty} B_\nu = 1$ and ignore the log terms for the integral approach):

$$J = \lceil \varepsilon^{-1} \rceil, \quad N = 256 \cdot \begin{cases} \lceil 0.6342 \cdot \varepsilon^{-1.0588} \rceil & \text{integral approach,} \\ \lceil 0.6342 \cdot \varepsilon^{-1.5882} \rceil & \text{series approach,} \end{cases}$$

$$N_0 = 256 \cdot \begin{cases} \lceil 2.5367 \cdot \varepsilon^{-1.0588} \rceil & \text{integral approach,} \\ \lceil 2.5367 \cdot \varepsilon^{-1.5882} \rceil & \text{series approach.} \end{cases}$$

Regarding the SMC approach, the number of paths is set $N_0 = 256 \cdot \varepsilon^{-2}$. The factor 256 is here for stability purposes. As for the MLMC approach, we set the initial number of paths in the first level ($l = 0$) equal to 10^3 as well as the 'discretisation parameter' $M = 4$, which leads to time steps of the length $\frac{1}{4^l}$ at level l (the notation here is as in [3]). Next, we compute the numerical RMSE (the exact value is known, see (54)) by means of 100 independent repetitions of the algorithm. As can be seen from left-hand side in Fig. 1, the estimated numerical complexity is about RMSE$^{-1.82}$ for the integral approach, RMSE$^{-2.43}$ for the series approach, RMSE$^{-1.99}$ for the MLMC approach and RMSE$^{-3.02}$ for the SMC approach, which we get by regressing the log time (logarithmic computing time of the whole algorithm in seconds) versus log RMSE. Thus, the complexity reduction works best with the integral approach.

5.2 Five-Dimensional Example

Here $d = m = 5$. We consider the SDE (cf. [2])

$$dX_t^i = -\sin\left(X_t^i\right)\cos^3\left(X_t^i\right)dt + \cos^2\left(X_t^i\right)dW_t^i, \quad X_0^i = 0, \quad i \in \{1, 2, 3, 4\},$$

$$dX_t^5 = \sum_{i=1}^{4}\left[-\frac{1}{2}\sin\left(X_t^i\right)\cos^2\left(X_t^i\right)dt + \cos\left(X_t^i\right)dW_t^i\right] + dW_t^5, \quad X_0^5 = 0. \quad (55)$$

The solution of (55) is given by

$$X_t^i = \arctan\left(W_t^i\right), \quad i \in \{1, 2, 3, 4\},$$

$$X_t^5 = \sum_{i=1}^{4}\operatorname{arsinh}\left(W_t^i\right) + W_t^5.$$

for $t \in [0, 1]$. Further, we consider the functional

$$f(x) = \cos\left(\sum_{i=1}^{5} x_i\right) - 20\sum_{i=1}^{4}\sin\left(x_i\right),$$

that is, we have

$$\mathbb{E}\left[f\left(X_1\right)\right] = \left(\mathbb{E}\left[\cos\left(\arctan\left(W_1^1\right) + \operatorname{arsinh}\left(W_1^1\right)\right)\right]\right)^4 \mathbb{E}\left[\cos\left(W_1^5\right)\right] \approx 0.002069.$$

We again choose $p = 3$ (this now results in 57 basis functions), consider the same values of ε as above (and, in addition, consider the values $\varepsilon = 2^{-7}$ and $\varepsilon = 2^{-8}$ for the SMC approach to obtain similar computing times as for the series and integral approaches). Moreover, we set (compare with the formulas in Sect. 4 for $v \to \infty$, $\lim_{v \to \infty} B_v = 1$ and ignore the log terms for the integral approach):

$$J = \lceil \varepsilon^{-1} \rceil, \quad N = \begin{cases} \lceil 35.9733 \cdot \varepsilon^{-1.2381} \rceil & \text{integral approach,} \\ 4 \cdot \lceil 4.9044 \cdot \varepsilon^{-1.8571} \rceil & \text{series approach,} \end{cases}$$

$$N_0 = \begin{cases} \lceil 2014.5030 \cdot \varepsilon^{-1.2381} \rceil & \text{integral approach,} \\ 4 \cdot \lceil 274.6480 \cdot \varepsilon^{-1.8571} \rceil & \text{series approach.} \end{cases}$$

The number of paths for the SMC approach is again set $N_0 = 256 \cdot \varepsilon^{-2}$. Regarding the MLMC approach, we again choose $M = 4$, but the initial number of paths in the first level is increased to 10^4. As in the one-dimensional case, we compute the

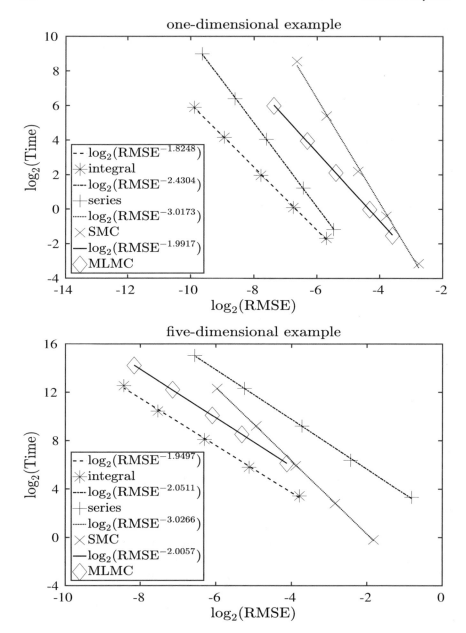

Fig. 1 Numerical complexities of the integral, series, SMC and MLMC approaches in the one- and five-dimensional cases

numerical RMSE by means of 100 independent repetitions of the algorithm. Our empirical findings are illustrated on the right-hand side in Fig. 1. We observe the numerical complexity RMSE$^{-1.95}$ for the integral approach, RMSE$^{-2.05}$ for the series approach, RMSE$^{-2.01}$ for the MLMC approach and RMSE$^{-3.03}$ for the SMC approach. Even though here the complexity order of the series approach is better than that of the SMC approach and close to that of MLMC approach, the series approach is practically outperformed by the other approaches (see Fig. 1; the multiplicative constant influencing the computing time is obviously very big). However, the integral approach remains numerically the best one also in this five-dimensional example.

6 Proofs

Proof of Theorem 1

Cf. the proof of Theorem 2.1 in [2].

Proof of Theorem 2

First of all, we derive

$$
\lim_{t \nearrow t_j} u_\Delta(t, X_{\Delta,t_{j-1}}, W_t - W_{t_{j-1}}) \tag{56}
$$

$$
= \lim_{t \nearrow t_j} \mathbb{E}\left[u_\Delta(t_j, \Phi_\Delta(x, y + z_j\sqrt{t_j - t}), 0)\right]\Big|_{x=X_{\Delta,(j-1)\Delta},\, y=W_t-W_{t_{j-1}}}
$$

$$
= u_\Delta(t_j, \Phi_\Delta(X_{\Delta,(j-1)\Delta}, \Delta_j W), 0) = u_\Delta(t_j, X_{\Delta,t_j}, 0).
$$

By means of Itô's lemma and the fact that u_Δ satisfies the heat equation

$$
\frac{\partial u_\Delta}{\partial t} + \frac{1}{2} \sum_{i=1}^{m} \frac{\partial^2 u_\Delta}{\partial y_i^2} = 0 \tag{57}
$$

due to its relation to the normal distribution, we then obtain

$$
f(X_{\Delta,T}) - \mathbb{E}[f(X_{\Delta,T})] \tag{58}
$$

$$
= u_\Delta(T, X_{\Delta,T}, 0) - u_\Delta(0, x_0, 0)
$$

$$
= \sum_{j=1}^{J} \left(u_\Delta(t_j, X_{\Delta,t_j}, 0) - u_\Delta(t_{j-1}, X_{\Delta,t_{j-1}}, 0)\right)
$$

$$
= \sum_{j=1}^{J} \lim_{t \nearrow t_j} \left(u_\Delta(t, X_{\Delta,t_{j-1}}, W_t - W_{t_{j-1}}) - u_\Delta(t_{j-1}, X_{\Delta,t_{j-1}}, 0)\right)
$$

$$= \sum_{j=1}^{J} \sum_{i=1}^{m} \lim_{t \nearrow t_j} \int_{t_{j-1}}^{t} \frac{\partial u_\Delta}{\partial y_i}(s, X_{\Delta, t_{j-1}}, W_s - W_{t_{j-1}}) \, dW_s^i$$

$$= \sum_{j=1}^{J} \int_{t_{j-1}}^{t_j} \nabla_y u_\Delta(s, X_{\Delta, t_{j-1}}, W_s - W_{t_{j-1}}) \, dW_s.$$

Next, let us derive a relation between $\nabla_y u_\Delta$ and $\nabla_x u_\Delta$. We have for $t \in [t_{j-1}, t_j)$

$$\nabla_y u_\Delta(t, x, y) = \nabla_y \mathbb{E}[u_\Delta(t_j, \Phi_\Delta(x, y + z_j \sqrt{t_j - t}), 0)]$$
$$= \nabla_x \mathbb{E}[u_\Delta(t_j, \Phi_\Delta(x, y + z_j \sqrt{t_j - t}), 0)] \sigma(x).$$

Thus, the term $\nabla_y u_\Delta(s, X_{\Delta, t_{j-1}}, W_s - W_{t_{j-1}})$ in (58) takes the form

$$\nabla_y u_\Delta(s, X_{\Delta, t_{j-1}}, W_s - W_{t_{j-1}}) = \mathbb{E}[\nabla_x u_\Delta(t_j, X_{\Delta, t_j}, 0) \mid \mathscr{F}_s] \sigma(X_{\Delta, t_{j-1}}). \quad (59)$$

Note that it holds

$$u_\Delta(t_j, x, 0) = \mathbb{E}[f(X_{t_j, x}(\Delta, T))],$$

where we recall that $X_{t_j, x}(\Delta, t_l)$, for $l \geq j$, denotes the Euler discretisation starting at time t_j in x (analogous to $X_{s,x}(t)$ for the exact solution). Hence, we have for $\nabla_x u_\Delta$

$$\nabla_x u_\Delta(t_j, x, 0) = \mathbb{E}[\nabla f(X_{t_j, x}(\Delta, T)) \delta X_{t_j, x}(\Delta, T)]$$

or, in another form,

$$\nabla_x u_\Delta(t_j, X_{\Delta, t_j}, 0) = \mathbb{E}\left[\nabla f(X_{t_j, X_{\Delta, t_j}}(\Delta, T)) \delta X_{t_j, X_{\Delta, t_j}}(\Delta, T) \mid \mathscr{F}_{t_j}\right],$$

where $\delta^i X_{t_j, x}^k(\Delta, t_l) := \frac{\partial X_{t_j, x}^k(\Delta, t_l)}{\partial x_i}$ with $l \geq j$ and $i, k \in \{1, \ldots, d\}$. We also notice at this point that $X_{\Delta, t_l} = X_{0, x_0}(\Delta, t_l)$ and $\delta X_{\Delta, t_l} = \delta X_{0, x_0}(\Delta, t_l)$.

Let us define $\sigma_k(x) := (\sigma_{k,1}(x), \ldots, \sigma_{k,m}(x))^\top$ for $k \in \{1, \ldots, d\}$. Further, we denote with $\mathscr{J}_\mu \in \mathbb{R}^{d \times d}$, $\mathscr{J}_{\sigma_k} \in \mathbb{R}^{m \times d}$ the Jacobi matrices of the functions μ, σ_k. Regarding the discretisation $\delta X_{\Delta, j\Delta}$ of δX_t we can use, alternatively to (16), the matrix form

$$\delta X_{\Delta, j\Delta} = A_j \delta X_{\Delta, (j-1)\Delta} = A_j A_{j-1} \cdots A_1, \quad (60)$$

where

$$A_k := I_d + \mathscr{J}_\mu(X_{\Delta,(k-1)\Delta})\Delta + \begin{pmatrix} \Delta_k W^\top \mathscr{J}_{\sigma_1}(X_{\Delta,(k-1)\Delta}) \\ \vdots \\ \Delta_k W^\top \mathscr{J}_{\sigma_d}(X_{\Delta,(k-1)\Delta}) \end{pmatrix}.$$

This gives us

$$X_{t_j, X_{\Delta,t_j}}(\Delta, t_l) = \Phi_\Delta(\cdots(\Phi_\Delta(X_{\Delta,t_j}, \Delta_{j+1}W), \cdots, \Delta_l W)$$

$$= \Phi_\Delta(\cdots(\Phi_\Delta(X_{\Delta,0}, \Delta_1 W), \cdots, \Delta_l W) = X_{\Delta,t_l},$$

$$\delta X_{t_j, X_{\Delta,t_j}}(\Delta, t_l) = A_l A_{l-1}\cdots A_{j+1} = A_l A_{l-1}\cdots A_1 \left(A_j A_{j-1}\cdots A_1\right)^{-1}$$

$$= \delta X_{\Delta,t_l} \delta X_{\Delta,t_j}^{-1},$$

where Φ_Δ is defined through (15). Finally, we obtain for $s \in [t_{j-1}, t_j)$

$$\nabla_y u_\Delta(s, X_{\Delta,t_{j-1}}, W_s - W_{t_{j-1}}) = \mathbb{E}\left[\mathbb{E}\left[\nabla f(X_{\Delta,T})\delta X_{\Delta,T}\delta X_{\Delta,t_j}^{-1} \mid \mathscr{F}_{t_j}\right] \mid \mathscr{F}_s\right]\sigma(X_{\Delta,t_{j-1}})$$

$$= \mathbb{E}\left[\nabla f(X_{\Delta,T})\delta X_{\Delta,T}\delta X_{\Delta,t_j}^{-1} \mid \mathscr{F}_s\right]\sigma(X_{\Delta,t_{j-1}}).$$

Proof of Theorem 3

Below we simply write $u_{\Delta,t_{j-1}}$ rather than $u_\Delta(t_{j-1}, X_{\Delta,t_{j-1}}, 0)$. Let us consider the Taylor expansion for $\frac{\partial}{\partial y_r}u_\Delta(t, X_{\Delta,t_{j-1}}, W_t - W_{t_{j-1}})$ of order $K \in \mathbb{N}_0$ around $(t_{j-1}, X_{\Delta,t_{j-1}}, 0)$, with $r \in \{1, \ldots, m\}$, that is, for $t \in [t_{j-1}, t_j)$, we set

$$T_{j,r}^K(t) := \sum_{|\alpha| \leq K} \frac{D^\alpha\left(\frac{\partial}{\partial y_r}u_{\Delta,t_{j-1}}\right)}{\alpha_1!\cdots\alpha_{m+1}!}(t - t_{j-1})^{\alpha_1}(W_t^1 - W_{t_{j-1}}^1)^{\alpha_2}\cdots(W_t^m - W_{t_{j-1}}^m)^{\alpha_{m+1}},$$

(61)

where $\alpha \in \mathbb{N}_0^{m+1}$ and $D^\alpha\left(\frac{\partial}{\partial y_r}u_{\Delta,t_{j-1}}\right) = \frac{\partial^{|\alpha|}\left(\frac{\partial}{\partial y_m}u_{\Delta,t_{j-1}}\right)}{\partial t^{\alpha_1}\partial y_1^{\alpha_2}\cdots\partial y_m^{\alpha_{m+1}}}$. Via Taylor's theorem we obtain

$$\frac{\partial}{\partial y_r}u_\Delta(t, X_{\Delta,t_{j-1}}, W_t - W_{t_{j-1}}) - T_{j,r}^K(t)$$

$$= \sum_{|\alpha|=K+1} \left[\frac{(K+1)!}{\alpha_1!\cdots\alpha_{m+1}!}\int_0^1 (1-z)^K D^\alpha\left(\frac{\partial}{\partial y_r}u_\Delta(t_{j-1} + z(t-t_{j-1}), X_{\Delta,t_{j-1}}, z(W_t - W_{t_{j-1}}))\right) dz\right.$$

$$\left. \cdot(t - t_{j-1})^{\alpha_1}(W_t^1 - W_{t_{j-1}}^1)^{\alpha_2}\cdots(W_t^m - W_{t_{j-1}}^m)^{\alpha_{m+1}}\right].$$

Provided that (24) holds, we get

$$\text{Var}\left[\sum_{j=1}^{J}\sum_{r=1}^{m}\int_{t_{j-1}}^{t_j}\left(\frac{\partial}{\partial y_r}u_\Delta(t, X_{\Delta, t_{j-1}}, W_t - W_{t_{j-1}}) - T_{j,r}^K(t)\right)dW_t^r\right]$$

$$=\sum_{j=1}^{J}\sum_{r=1}^{m}\int_{t_{j-1}}^{t_j}\mathbb{E}\left[\left(\frac{\partial}{\partial y_r}u_\Delta(t, X_{\Delta, t_{j-1}}, W_t - W_{t_{j-1}}) - T_{j,r}^K(t)\right)^2\right]dt$$

$$\lesssim C^{2(K+1)}\sum_{j=1}^{J}\sum_{|\alpha|=K+1}\int_{t_{j-1}}^{t_j}\mathbb{E}\left[(t-t_{j-1})^{2\alpha_1}(W_t^1 - W_{t_{j-1}}^1)^{2\alpha_2}\cdots(W_t^m - W_{t_{j-1}}^m)^{2\alpha_{m+1}}\right]dt$$

$$\lesssim(C^2\Delta)^{K+1}\xrightarrow{K\to\infty}0,$$

and thus $T_{j,r}^K$ converges for $K \to \infty$ in $L^2(\Omega \times [0,T])$ to $\frac{\partial u_\Delta}{\partial y_r}(t, X_{\Delta, t_{j-1}}, W_t - W_{t_{j-1}})$. Moreover, due to (57), the limit of $T_{j,r}^K$ simplifies to (cf. (61))

$$\frac{\partial u_{\Delta, t_{j-1}}}{\partial y_r} + \sum_{i=1}^{m}\frac{\partial^2 u_{\Delta, t_{j-1}}}{\partial y_r \partial y_i}(W_t^i - W_{t_{j-1}}^i)$$

$$+\frac{1}{2}\sum_{i=1}^{m}\frac{\partial^3 u_{\Delta, t_{j-1}}}{\partial y_r \partial y_i^2}((W_t^i - W_{t_{j-1}}^i)^2 - (t - t_{j-1}))$$

$$+\sum_{\substack{i_1, i_2=1 \\ i_1 < i_2}}^{m}\frac{\partial^3 u_{\Delta, t_{j-1}}}{\partial y_r \partial y_{i_1} \partial y_{i_2}}(W_t^{i_1} - W_{t_{j-1}}^{i_1})(W_t^{i_2} - W_{t_{j-1}}^{i_2})$$

$$+\left[\frac{1}{6}\sum_{i=1}^{m}\frac{\partial^4 u_{\Delta, t_{j-1}}}{\partial y_r \partial y_i^3}((W_t^i - W_{t_{j-1}}^i)^3 - 3(W_t^i - W_{t_{j-1}}^i)(t - t_{j-1}))\right.$$

$$+\frac{1}{2}\sum_{\substack{i_1, i_2=1 \\ i_1 < i_2}}^{m}\frac{\partial^4 u_{\Delta, t_{j-1}}}{\partial y_r \partial y_{i_1}^2 \partial y_{i_2}}((W_t^{i_1} - W_{t_{j-1}}^{i_1})^2 - (t - t_{j-1}))(W_t^{i_2} - W_{t_{j-1}}^{i_2})$$

$$\left.+\sum_{\substack{i_1, i_2, i_3=1 \\ i_1 < i_2 < i_3}}^{m}\frac{\partial^4 u_{\Delta, t_{j-1}}}{\partial y_r \partial y_{i_1} \partial y_{i_2} \partial y_{i_3}}(W_t^{i_1} - W_{t_{j-1}}^{i_1})(W_t^{i_2} - W_{t_{j-1}}^{i_2})(W_t^{i_3} - W_{t_{j-1}}^{i_3})\right]$$

$$+\dots$$

$$=\sum_{l=1}^{\infty}(t-t_{j-1})^{\frac{l-1}{2}}\sum_{\substack{k\in\mathbb{N}_0^m \\ \sum_{i=1}^{m}k_i=l-1}}{}'\frac{\partial^l u_{\Delta, t_{j-1}}}{\partial y_r \partial y_1^{k_1}\cdots\partial y_m^{k_m}}\prod_{i=1}^{m}\frac{H_{k_i}\left(\frac{W_t^i - W_{t_{j-1}}^i}{\sqrt{t - t_{j-1}}}\right)}{\sqrt{k_i!}}.$$

To compute the stochastic integral

$$\int_{t_{j-1}}^{t_j} \nabla_y u_\Delta(t, X_{\Delta,t_{j-1}}, W_t - W_{t_{j-1}}) \, dW_t$$

$$= \sum_{l=1}^{\infty} \sum_{r=1}^{m} \int_{t_{j-1}}^{t_j} (t-t_{j-1})^{\frac{l-1}{2}} \sum_{\substack{k\in\mathbb{N}_0^m \\ \sum_{i=1}^m k_i = l-1}} \frac{\partial^l u_{\Delta,t_{j-1}}}{\partial y_r \partial y_1^{k_1} \cdots \partial y_m^{k_m}} \prod_{i=1}^{m} \frac{H_{k_i}\left(\frac{W_t^i - W_{t_{j-1}}^i}{\sqrt{t-t_{j-1}}}\right)}{\sqrt{k_i!}} \, dW_t^r,$$

we apply Itô's lemma w.r.t. the functions $F_k(t, y_1, \ldots, y_m) := t^{l/2} \prod_{i=1}^{m} \frac{H_{k_i}\left(\frac{y_i}{\sqrt{t}}\right)}{\sqrt{k_i!}}$, where $\sum_{i=1}^{m} k_i = l$. Thus, we obtain

$$dF_k(t-t_{j-1}, W_t^1 - W_{t_{j-1}}^1, \ldots, W_t^m - W_{t_{j-1}}^m) \qquad (62)$$

$$= (t-t_{j-1})^{\frac{l-1}{2}} \sum_{r=1}^{m} \frac{H_{k_r-1}\left(\frac{W_t^r - W_{t_{j-1}}^r}{\sqrt{t-t_{j-1}}}\right)}{\sqrt{(k_r-1)!}} \prod_{\substack{i=1 \\ i\neq r}}^{m} \frac{H_{k_i}\left(\frac{W_t^i - W_{t_{j-1}}^i}{\sqrt{t-t_{j-1}}}\right)}{\sqrt{k_i!}} \, dW_t^r.$$

This gives us finally

$$\int_{t_{j-1}}^{t_j} \nabla_y u_\Delta(t, X_{\Delta,t_{j-1}}, W_t - W_{t_{j-1}}) \, dW_t$$

$$= \sum_{l=1}^{\infty} \Delta^{l/2} \sum_{\substack{k\in\mathbb{N}_0^m \\ \sum_{i=1}^m k_i = l}} \frac{\partial^l u_\Delta(t_{j-1}, X_{\Delta,t_{j-1}}, 0)}{\partial y_1^{k_1} \cdots \partial y_m^{k_m}} \prod_{i=1}^{m} \frac{H_{k_i}\left(\frac{\Delta_j W^i}{\sqrt{\Delta}}\right)}{\sqrt{k_i!}}.$$

Proof of Theorem 4

We define the (random) function $G_{l,j}(x)$ for $J \geq l \geq j \geq 0$, $x \in \mathbb{R}^d$, as follows

$$G_{l,j}(x) = \Phi_{\Delta,l} \circ \Phi_{\Delta,l-1} \circ \ldots \circ \Phi_{\Delta,j+1}(x), \quad l > j, \qquad (63)$$
$$G_{l,j}(x) = x, \quad l = j,$$

where $\Phi_{\Delta,l}(x) := \Phi_\Delta(x, \Delta_l W)$ for $l = 1, \ldots, J$. Note that it holds

$$u_\Delta(t_j, x, 0) = \mathbb{E}\left[f(G_{J,j}(x))\right]. \qquad (64)$$

Similar to G, we define the function $\tilde{G}_j(x, z)$, $0 \leq j < J$, $x \in \mathbb{R}^d$, $z := (z_1, \ldots, z_{J-j}) \in \mathbb{R}^{m\times(J-j)}$, $z_l := (z_l^1, \ldots, z_l^m)^\top \in \mathbb{R}^m$ for $l = 1, \ldots, J - j$, as follows

$$\tilde{G}_j(x, z) := \tilde{\Phi}_{\Delta,z_{J-j}} \circ \ldots \circ \tilde{\Phi}_{\Delta,z_1}(x),$$

where $\tilde{\Phi}_{\Delta,z_l}(x) := \Phi_\Delta\left(x, z_l\sqrt{\Delta}\right)$. Note that G and $\tilde{G}$ are in the following relation

$$G_{J,j}(x) = \tilde{G}_j\left(x, \frac{1}{\sqrt{\Delta}}\left(\Delta_{j+1}W, \Delta_{j+2}W, \dots, \Delta_J W\right)\right), \quad j < J. \quad (65)$$

Let us represent $\sqrt{\Delta}\frac{\partial}{\partial y_i}u_\Delta(t_{j-1}, x, 0)$, where $j \in \{1, \dots, J\}$ and $i \in \{1, \dots, m\}$, as a $(J - j + 1)m$-dimensional integral, that is (cf. (65))

$$\sqrt{\Delta}\frac{\partial}{\partial y_i}u_\Delta(t_{j-1}, x, 0) = \sqrt{\Delta}\frac{\partial}{\partial y_i}\mathbb{E}\left[f\left(G_{J,j}\left(\Phi_\Delta\left(x, \Delta_j W + y\right)\right)\right)\right]\Big|_{y=0_m}$$

$$= \int_{\mathbb{R}^{(J-j+1)m}} \sqrt{\Delta}\frac{\partial}{\partial y_i}\left[f\left(\tilde{G}_{j-1}\left(x, \left(z_1 + \frac{y}{\sqrt{\Delta}}, z_2, \dots, z_{J-j+1}\right)\right)\right)\right]\varphi_{(J-j+1)m}(z)\,dz\Big|_{y=0_m},$$

where $\varphi_{(J-j+1)m}$ denotes the $(J - j + 1)m$-dimensional standard normal density function. Since it holds

$$\sqrt{\Delta}\frac{\partial}{\partial y_i}\left[f\left(\tilde{G}_{j-1}\left(x, \left(z_1 + \frac{y}{\sqrt{\Delta}}, z_2, \dots, z_{J-j+1}\right)\right)\right)\right]$$

$$= \frac{\partial}{\partial z_1^i}\left[f\left(\tilde{G}_{j-1}\left(x, \left(z_1 + \frac{y}{\sqrt{\Delta}}, z_2, \dots, z_{J-j+1}\right)\right)\right)\right],$$

we obtain via integration by parts

$$\sqrt{\Delta}\frac{\partial}{\partial y_i}u_\Delta(t_{j-1}, x, 0)$$

$$= \int_{\mathbb{R}^{(J-j+1)m}} \frac{\partial}{\partial z_1^i}\left[f\left(\tilde{G}_{j-1}(x, z)\right)\right]\varphi_{(J-j+1)m}(z)\,dz$$

$$= -\int_{\mathbb{R}^{(J-j+1)m}} f\left(\tilde{G}_{j-1}(x, z)\right)\frac{\partial}{\partial z_1^i}\varphi_{(J-j+1)m}(z)\,dz$$

$$= \int_{\mathbb{R}^{(J-j+1)m}} f\left(\tilde{G}_{j-1}(x, z)\right)z_1^i\varphi_{(J-j+1)m}(z)\,dz$$

$$= \mathbb{E}\left[f(G_{J,j-1}(x))\frac{\Delta_j W^i}{\sqrt{\Delta}}\right] = \mathbb{E}\left[f(X_{\Delta,T})\frac{\Delta_j W^i}{\sqrt{\Delta}}\,\Big|\,X_{\Delta,(j-1)\Delta} = x\right] = a_{j,e_i}(x).$$

We finally remark that we have only the integral term in the integration by parts above because the function $z_1 \mapsto f(\tilde{G}_{j-1}(x, z))\varphi_{(J-j+1)m}(z)$ is integrable over $\mathbb{R}$ w.r.t. the Lebesgue measure.

Proof of Theorem 5

Via Taylor's theorem we get

$$\frac{\partial u_\Delta(t, X_{\Delta,t_{j-1}}, W_t - W_{t_{j-1}})}{\partial y_i}$$

$$= \frac{\partial u_\Delta(t_{j-1}, X_{\Delta,t_{j-1}}, 0)}{\partial y_i} + (t - t_{j-1}) \int_0^1 \frac{\partial^2 u_\Delta(t_{j-1} + z(t - t_{j-1}), X_{\Delta,t_{j-1}}, z(W_t - W_{t_{j-1}}))}{\partial y_i \partial t} \, dz$$

$$+ \sum_{r=1}^m (W_t^r - W_{t_{j-1}}^r) \int_0^1 \frac{\partial^2 u_\Delta(t_{j-1} + z(t - t_{j-1}), X_{\Delta,t_{j-1}}, z(W_t - W_{t_{j-1}}))}{\partial y_i \partial y_r} \, dz. \qquad (66)$$

Due to (57), (66) simplifies to

$$\frac{\partial u_\Delta(t, X_{\Delta,t_{j-1}}, W_t - W_{t_{j-1}})}{\partial y_i} = \frac{\partial u_\Delta(t_{j-1}, X_{\Delta,t_{j-1}}, 0)}{\partial y_i}$$

$$- \frac{1}{2}(t - t_{j-1}) \int_0^1 \sum_{r=1}^m \frac{\partial^3 u_\Delta(t_{j-1} + z(t - t_{j-1}), X_{\Delta,t_{j-1}}, z(W_t - W_{t_{j-1}}))}{\partial y_i \partial y_r^2} \, dz$$

$$+ \sum_{r=1}^m (W_t^r - W_{t_{j-1}}^r) \int_0^1 \frac{\partial^2 u_\Delta(t_{j-1} + z(t - t_{j-1}), X_{\Delta,t_{j-1}}, z(W_t - W_{t_{j-1}}))}{\partial y_i \partial y_r} \, dz.$$

Provided that the second and third derivatives of u_Δ w.r.t. y are bounded, we have

$$\mathrm{Var}\left[\int_{t_{j-1}}^{t_j} \frac{\partial u_\Delta(t, X_{\Delta,t_{j-1}}, W_t - W_{t_{j-1}})}{\partial y_i} \, dW_t^i - \frac{\partial u_\Delta(t_{j-1}, X_{\Delta,t_{j-1}}, 0)}{\partial y_i} \Delta_j W^i \right]$$

$$= \int_{t_{j-1}}^{t_j} \mathbb{E}\left[\left(\int_0^1 \sum_{r=1}^m \left((W_t^r - W_{t_{j-1}}^r) \frac{\partial^2 u_\Delta(t_{j-1} + z(t - t_{j-1}), X_{\Delta,t_{j-1}}, z(W_t - W_{t_{j-1}}))}{\partial y_i \partial y_r} \right. \right. \right.$$

$$\left. \left. \left. - \frac{1}{2}(t - t_{j-1}) \frac{\partial^3 u_\Delta(t_{j-1} + z(t - t_{j-1}), X_{\Delta,t_{j-1}}, z(W_t - W_{t_{j-1}}))}{\partial y_i \partial y_r^2} \right) dz \right)^2 \right] dt$$

$$\lesssim \sum_{r=1}^m \int_{t_{j-1}}^{t_j} \mathbb{E}\left[(W_t^r - W_{t_{j-1}}^r)^2 + (t - t_{j-1})^2 \right] dt \lesssim \Delta^2.$$

Thus, we finally obtain

$$\mathrm{Var}\left[f(X_{\Delta,T}) - M_{\Delta,T}^{int,1} \right] \lesssim \Delta.$$

Proof of Theorem 6

We start the calculations, which will lead to the proof of part (ii). At some point, we will get the proof of part (i) as a by-product.

In this proof, we will use the shorthand notation $\xi_k := \Delta_k W, k \in \{1, \ldots, J\}$. For $j \in \{0, \ldots, J-1\}$, we have

$$u_\Delta(t_j, x, y) = \mathbb{E}\left[f\left(\Phi_{\Delta,J} \circ \Phi_{\Delta,J-1} \circ \ldots \circ \Phi_{\Delta,j+2} \circ \Phi_\Delta(x, y + \xi_{j+1}))\right)\right],$$

where $\Phi_{\Delta,k}(x) := \Phi_\Delta(x, \xi_k)$. Denote, for $k > j$,

$$G_{k,j}(x, y) := \Phi_{\Delta,k} \circ \Phi_{\Delta,k-1} \circ \ldots \circ \Phi_{\Delta,j+2} \circ \Phi_\Delta(x, y + \xi_{j+1}).$$

Assume that for any $n \in \mathbb{N}, l \in \{1, \ldots, d\}, \alpha \in \mathbb{N}_0^d$,

$$\left|\mathbb{E}\left[\left(D^\alpha \Phi_{\Delta,k+1}^l(G_{k,j}(x, y))\right)^n \middle| \mathscr{F}_k\right]\right| \leq \begin{cases} (1 + A_{n,l}\Delta), & \beta = \alpha_l = 1 \\ B_{n,l,\alpha}\Delta, & (\beta > 1) \vee (\alpha_l \neq 1) \end{cases} \tag{67}$$

with probability one for $\beta = |\alpha| \in \mathbb{N}$ and some constants $A_{n,l} > 0, B_{n,l,\alpha} > 0$. We recall the notation $D^\alpha f(x) = \frac{\partial^{|\alpha|} f(x)}{\partial x_1^{\alpha_1} \cdots \partial x_d^{\alpha_d}}$, which was used here. Clearly, for the Euler scheme (15), condition (67) is satisfied if all the derivatives of order β for $\mu_k, \sigma_{ki}, k \in \{1, \ldots, d\}, i \in \{1, \ldots, m\}$, are bounded. Moreover, suppose that for any $n_1, n_2 \in \mathbb{N}, l \in \{1, \ldots, d\}, \alpha_1, \alpha_2 \in \mathbb{N}_0^d$, with $\beta_1 = |\alpha_1| > 0, \beta_2 = |\alpha_2| > 0, (\beta_1 > 1) \vee (\beta_2 > 1) \vee ((\alpha_1)_l \neq 1) \vee ((\alpha_2)_l \neq 1)$,

$$\left|\mathbb{E}\left[\left(D^{\alpha_1} \Phi_{\Delta,k+1}^l(G_{k,j}(x, y))\right)^{n_1} \left(D^{\alpha_2} \Phi_{\Delta,k+1}^l(G_{k,j}(x, y))\right)^{n_2} \middle| \mathscr{F}_k\right]\right| \leq C_{n_1,n_2,l,\alpha_1,\alpha_2}\Delta \tag{68}$$

for some constant $C_{n_1,n_2,l,\alpha_1,\alpha_2} > 0$. Again, for the Euler scheme (15), condition (68) is satisfied if all the derivatives of orders β_1 and β_2 for μ_k, σ_{ki} are bounded.

We have for some $i \in \{1, \ldots, m\}$ and $l \in \{1, \ldots, d\}$

$$\frac{\partial}{\partial y_i} G_{k+1,j}^l(x, y) = \sum_{s=1}^d \frac{\partial}{\partial x_s} \Phi_{\Delta,k+1}^l(G_{k,j}(x, y)) \frac{\partial}{\partial y_i} G_{k,j}^s(x, y)$$

and $\frac{\partial}{\partial y_i} G_{j+1,j}^s(x, y) = \frac{\partial}{\partial y_i} \Phi_\Delta^s(x, y + \xi_{j+1})$. Hence

$$\mathbb{E}\left[\left(\frac{\partial}{\partial y_i} G_{k+1,j}^l(x, y)\right)^2\right]$$

$$\leq \mathbb{E}\left[\left(\frac{\partial}{\partial x_l} \Phi_{\Delta,k+1}^l(G_{k,j}(x, y)) \frac{\partial}{\partial y_i} G_{k,j}^l(x, y)\right)^2\right.$$

$$\left. + \sum_{s \neq l} \left\{2\frac{\partial}{\partial x_l} \Phi_{\Delta,k+1}^l(G_{k,j}(x, y)) \frac{\partial}{\partial x_s} \Phi_{\Delta,k+1}^l(G_{k,j}(x, y)) \frac{\partial}{\partial y_i} G_{k,j}^l(x, y) \frac{\partial}{\partial y_i} G_{k,j}^s(x, y)\right.\right.$$

$$+(d-1)\left(\frac{\partial}{\partial x_s}\Phi^l_{\Delta,k+1}(G_{k,j}(x,y))\frac{\partial}{\partial y_i}G^s_{k,j}(x,y)\right)^2\right\}\right]$$

Denote

$$\rho^{i,s}_{k+1,n}=\mathbb{E}\left[\left(\frac{\partial}{\partial y_i}G^s_{k+1,j}(x,y)\right)^n\right],\tag{69}$$

then, due to $2ab\le a^2+b^2$, we get for $k=j+1,\ldots,J-1$,

$$\rho^{i,l}_{k+1,2}\le(1+A_{2,l}\Delta)\rho^{i,l}_{k,2}+\sum_{s\neq l}\left\{C_{1,1,l,e_l,e_s}\Delta(\rho^{i,l}_{k,2}+\rho^{i,s}_{k,2})+(d-1)B_{2,l,e_s}\Delta\rho^{i,s}_{k,2}\right\}.$$

Further, denote

$$\rho^i_{k+1,n}=\sum_{l=1}^{d}\rho^{i,l}_{k+1,n},$$

then we get for $k=j+1,\ldots,J-1$,

$$\rho^i_{k+1,2}\le(1+A_2\Delta)\rho^i_{k,2}+2(d-1)C_{1,1}\Delta\rho^i_{k,2}+(d-1)^2B_2\Delta\rho^i_{k,2}.$$

where $A_2:=\max\limits_{l=1,\ldots,d}A_{2,l}$, $B_2:=\max\limits_{l,s=1,\ldots,d}B_{2,l,e_s}$ and $C_{1,1}:=\max\limits_{l,s=1,\ldots,d}C_{1,1,l,e_l,e_s}$. This gives us

$$\rho^i_{k+1,2}\le(1+\kappa_1\Delta)\rho^i_{k,2},\quad k=j+1,\ldots,J-1$$

for some constant $\kappa_1>0$, leading to

$$\rho^i_{k,2}\le(1+\kappa_1\Delta)^{k-j-1}\rho^i_{j+1,2},\ k=j+1,\ldots,J-1,$$

where

$$\rho^i_{j+1,2}=\sum_{s=1}^{d}\mathbb{E}\left[\left(\frac{\partial}{\partial y_i}\Phi^s_\Delta(x,y+\xi_{j+1})\right)^2\right]=\sum_{s=1}^{d}\sigma^2_{si}(x).$$

Thus, we obtain the boundedness of

$$\frac{\partial}{\partial y_i}u_\Delta(t_j,x,y)=\sum_{s=1}^{d}\mathbb{E}\left[\frac{\partial}{\partial x_s}f(G_{J,j}(x,y))\frac{\partial}{\partial y_i}G^s_{J,j}(x,y)\right],$$

provided that σ_{ki} and all the derivatives of order 1 of f, μ_k, σ_{ki} are bounded.

Similar calculations show that the boundedness of σ_{ki} is not necessary to assume in order to get that $\frac{\partial}{\partial x_i}u_\Delta(t_j,x,y)$ and consequently $g_{j,l}(x)$ for $l\in\{1,\ldots,d\}$ are bounded (recall (21)). This yields (A2) under the assumptions in part (i) of Theorem 6 (that is, the boundedness of σ_{ki} is not needed).

Furthermore, we have, due to $(\sum_{k=1}^{d} a_k)^n \leq d^{n-1} \sum_{k=1}^{d} a_k^n$,

$$\mathbb{E}\left[\left(\frac{\partial}{\partial y_i} G_{k+1,j}^l(x,y)\right)^4\right]$$

$$\leq \mathbb{E}\left[\left(\frac{\partial}{\partial x_l}\Phi_{\Delta,k+1}^l(G_{k,j}(x,y))\frac{\partial}{\partial y_i}G_{k,j}^l(x,y)\right)^4\right.$$

$$+\sum_{s\neq l}\left\{4\left(\frac{\partial}{\partial x_l}\Phi_{\Delta,k+1}^l(G_{k,j}(x,y))\frac{\partial}{\partial y_i}G_{k,j}^l(x,y)\right)^3\right.$$

$$\frac{\partial}{\partial x_s}\Phi_{\Delta,k+1}^l(G_{k,j}(x,y))\frac{\partial}{\partial y_i}G_{k,j}^s(x,y)$$

$$+6(d-1)\left(\frac{\partial}{\partial x_l}\Phi_{\Delta,k+1}^l(G_{k,j}(x,y))\frac{\partial}{\partial y_i}G_{k,j}^l(x,y)\right.$$

$$\left.\frac{\partial}{\partial x_s}\Phi_{\Delta,k+1}^l(G_{k,j}(x,y))\frac{\partial}{\partial y_i}G_{k,j}^s(x,y)\right)^2$$

$$+4(d-1)^2\frac{\partial}{\partial x_l}\Phi_{\Delta,k+1}^l(G_{k,j}(x,y))\frac{\partial}{\partial y_i}G_{k,j}^l(x,y)$$

$$\left(\frac{\partial}{\partial x_s}\Phi_{\Delta,k+1}^l(G_{k,j}(x,y))\frac{\partial}{\partial y_i}G_{k,j}^s(x,y)\right)^3$$

$$\left.\left.+(d-1)^3\left(\frac{\partial}{\partial x_s}\Phi_{\Delta,k+1}^l(G_{k,j}(x,y))\frac{\partial}{\partial y_i}G_{k,j}^s(x,y)\right)^4\right\}\right]$$

and thus, due to $4a^3b \leq 3a^4 + b^4$ and $2a^2b^2 \leq a^4 + b^4$,

$$\rho_{k+1,4}^{i,l} \leq (1 + A_{4,l}\Delta)\rho_{k,4}^{i,l}$$

$$+\sum_{s\neq l}\left\{C_{3,1,l,e_l,e_s}\Delta(3\rho_{k,4}^{i,l} + \rho_{k,4}^{i,s}) + 3(d-1)C_{2,2,l,e_l,e_s}\Delta(\rho_{k,4}^{i,l} + \rho_{k,4}^{i,s})\right.$$

$$\left.+(d-1)^2 C_{1,3,l,e_l,e_s}\Delta(\rho_{k,4}^{i,l} + 3\rho_{k,4}^{i,s}) + (d-1)^3 B_{4,l,e_s}\Delta\rho_{k,4}^{i,s}\right\}$$

This gives us

$$\rho_{k+1,4}^i \leq (1 + A_4\Delta)\rho_{k,4}^i + 4(d-1)C_{3,1}\Delta\rho_{k,4}^i + 6(d-1)^2 C_{2,2}\Delta\rho_{k,4}^i$$

$$+4(d-1)^3 C_{1,3}\Delta\rho_{k,4}^i + (d-1)^4 B_4\Delta\rho_{k,4}^i,$$

where $A_4 := \max\limits_{l=1,\ldots,d} A_{4,l}$, $B_4 := \max\limits_{l,s=1,\ldots,d} B_{4,l,e_s}$, $C_{3,1} := \max\limits_{l,s=1,\ldots,d} C_{3,1,l,e_l,e_s}$, $C_{2,2} := \max\limits_{l,s=1,\ldots,d} C_{2,2,l,e_l,e_s}$ and $C_{1,3} := \max\limits_{l,s=1,\ldots,d} C_{1,3,l,e_l,e_s}$. Hence, we obtain

$$\rho_{k+1,4}^i \leq (1 + \kappa_2 \Delta)\rho_{k,4}^i, \quad k = j+1, \ldots, J-1$$

for some constant $\kappa_2 > 0$, leading to

$$\rho_{k,4}^i \leq (1 + \kappa_2 \Delta)^{k-j-1}\rho_{j+1,4}^i, \ k = j+1, \ldots, J-1,$$

where

$$\rho_{j+1,4}^i = \sum_{s=1}^{d} \mathbb{E}\left[\left(\frac{\partial}{\partial y_i}\Phi_\Delta^s(x, y + \xi_{j+1})\right)^4\right] = \sum_{s=1}^{d} \sigma_{si}^4(x).$$

Thus, we obtain boundedness of $\rho_{k,4}^i$ uniformly in x, y, j, $k \in \{j+1, \ldots, J\}$ and J, for all $i \in \{1, \ldots, m\}$, provided σ_{ki} and all derivatives of order 1 of f, μ_k, σ_{ki} are bounded.

Now we set[4] $\widetilde{G}_{J,j}(x) := G_{J,j}(x, 0)$ and observe that similar calculations involving derivatives w.r.t. x_k show that the quantities

$$\mathbb{E}\left[\left(\frac{\partial}{\partial x_k}\widetilde{G}_{J,j}^s(x)\right)^4\right]$$

(cf. with (69)) are all bounded uniformly in x, J and $j \in \{0, \ldots, J-1\}$, provided all derivatives of order 1 of f, μ_k, σ_{ki} are bounded (that is, boundedness of σ_{ki} is not needed at this point). Using the identity $\widetilde{G}_{J,j}(X_{\Delta,t_j}) = X_{\Delta,T}$ one can check that

$$\mathcal{J}_{\widetilde{G}_{J,j}}(X_{\Delta,t_j}) = \delta X_{\Delta,T}\delta X_{\Delta,t_j}^{-1}, \tag{70}$$

where $\mathcal{J}_{\widetilde{G}_{J,j}}$ denotes the Jacobi matrix of the function $\widetilde{G}_{J,j}$. Recalling the definition $\zeta_j = (\zeta_{j,1}, \ldots, \zeta_{j,d}) := \nabla f(X_{\Delta,T})\delta X_{\Delta,T}\delta X_{\Delta,t_j}^{-1}$ of the vector ζ_j, we get from (70) that

$$\zeta_{j,k} = \sum_{s=1}^{d} \frac{\partial}{\partial x_s}f(\widetilde{G}_{J,j}(X_{\Delta,t_j}))\frac{\partial}{\partial x_k}\widetilde{G}_{J,j}^s(X_{\Delta,t_j}).$$

Then we obtain for $k \in \{1, \ldots, d\}$ and $j \in \{1, \ldots, J\}$

$$\begin{aligned}
&\text{Var}\left[\zeta_{j,k} \mid X_{\Delta,t_{j-1}} = x\right] \\
&\leq \mathbb{E}\left[\zeta_{j,k}^2 \mid X_{\Delta,t_{j-1}} = x\right] \\
&= \mathbb{E}\left[\left(\sum_{s=1}^{d} \frac{\partial}{\partial x_s}f(\widetilde{G}_{J,j}(X_{\Delta,t_j}))\frac{\partial}{\partial x_k}\widetilde{G}_{J,j}^s(X_{\Delta,t_j})\right)^2 \mid X_{\Delta,t_{j-1}} = x\right] \\
&\leq d\sum_{s=1}^{d} \mathbb{E}\left[\left(\frac{\partial}{\partial x_s}f(\widetilde{G}_{J,j-1}(x))\frac{\partial}{\partial x_k}\widetilde{G}_{J,j}^s(\Phi_{\Delta,j}(x))\right)^2\right]
\end{aligned}$$

---

[4]Notice that thus defined $\widetilde{G}_{J,j}$ is the same as $G_{J,j}$ of (63) (in the proof of Theorem 4).

$$\leq d \sum_{s=1}^{d} \sqrt{\mathbb{E}\left[\left(\frac{\partial}{\partial x_s} f(\widetilde{G}_{J,j-1}(x))\right)^4\right] \mathbb{E}\left[\left(\frac{\partial}{\partial x_k} \widetilde{G}_{J,j}^s(\Phi_{\Delta_j}(x))\right)^4\right]}.$$

Due to the discussion above, the latter expression is bounded in x, provided all derivatives of order 1 of f, μ_k, σ_{ki} are bounded. That is, we get (A1), and the proof of part (i) is completed.

Proceeding with part (ii), we have

$$\mathbb{E}\left[\left(\frac{\partial}{\partial y_i} G_{k+1,j}^l(x,y)\right)^6\right]$$

$$\leq \mathbb{E}\left[\left(\frac{\partial}{\partial x_l} \Phi_{\Delta,k+1}^l(G_{k,j}(x,y)) \frac{\partial}{\partial y_i} G_{k,j}^l(x,y)\right)^6\right.$$

$$+ \sum_{s\neq l}\left\{6\left(\frac{\partial}{\partial x_l} \Phi_{\Delta,k+1}^l(G_{k,j}(x,y)) \frac{\partial}{\partial y_i} G_{k,j}^l(x,y)\right)^5\right.$$

$$\frac{\partial}{\partial x_s} \Phi_{\Delta,k+1}^l(G_{k,j}(x,y)) \frac{\partial}{\partial y_i} G_{k,j}^s(x,y)$$

$$+ 15(d-1)\left(\frac{\partial}{\partial x_l} \Phi_{\Delta,k+1}^l(G_{k,j}(x,y)) \frac{\partial}{\partial y_i} G_{k,j}^l(x,y)\right)^4$$

$$\left(\frac{\partial}{\partial x_s} \Phi_{\Delta,k+1}^l(G_{k,j}(x,y)) \frac{\partial}{\partial y_i} G_{k,j}^s(x,y)\right)^2$$

$$+ 20(d-1)^2\left(\frac{\partial}{\partial x_l} \Phi_{\Delta,k+1}^l(G_{k,j}(x,y)) \frac{\partial}{\partial y_i} G_{k,j}^l(x,y)\right.$$

$$\left.\frac{\partial}{\partial x_s} \Phi_{\Delta,k+1}^l(G_{k,j}(x,y)) \frac{\partial}{\partial y_i} G_{k,j}^s(x,y)\right)^3$$

$$+ 15(d-1)^3\left(\frac{\partial}{\partial x_l} \Phi_{\Delta,k+1}^l(G_{k,j}(x,y)) \frac{\partial}{\partial y_i} G_{k,j}^l(x,y)\right)^2$$

$$\left(\frac{\partial}{\partial x_s} \Phi_{\Delta,k+1}^l(G_{k,j}(x,y)) \frac{\partial}{\partial y_i} G_{k,j}^s(x,y)\right)^4$$

$$+ 6(d-1)^4 \frac{\partial}{\partial x_l} \Phi_{\Delta,k+1}^l(G_{k,j}(x,y)) \frac{\partial}{\partial y_i} G_{k,j}^l(x,y)$$

$$\left(\frac{\partial}{\partial x_s} \Phi_{\Delta,k+1}^l(G_{k,j}(x,y)) \frac{\partial}{\partial y_i} G_{k,j}^s(x,y)\right)^5$$

$$+(d-1)^5 \left(\frac{\partial}{\partial x_s}\Phi^l_{\Delta,k+1}(G_{k,j}(x,y))\frac{\partial}{\partial y_i}G^s_{k,j}(x,y)\right)^6\Bigg]\Bigg]$$

and thus, due to $6a^5 b \le 5a^6 + b^6$, $3a^4 b^2 \le 2a^6 + b^6$ and $2a^3 b^3 \le a^6 + b^6$,

$$\rho^{i,l}_{k+1,6} \le (1 + A_{6,l}\Delta)\rho^{i,l}_{k,6}$$
$$+ \sum_{s \neq l} \Big\{ C_{5,1,l,e_l,e_s}\Delta(5\rho^{i,l}_{k,6} + \rho^{i,s}_{k,6}) + 5(d-1)C_{4,2,l,e_l,e_s}\Delta(2\rho^{i,l}_{k,6} + \rho^{i,s}_{k,6})$$
$$+ 10(d-1)^2 C_{3,3,l,e_l,e_s}\Delta(\rho^{i,l}_{k,6} + \rho^{i,s}_{k,6}) + 5(d-1)^3 C_{2,4,l,e_l,e_s}\Delta(\rho^{i,l}_{k,6} + 2\rho^{i,s}_{k,6})$$
$$+ (d-1)^4 C_{1,5,l,e_l,e_s}\Delta(\rho^{i,l}_{k,6} + 5\rho^{i,s}_{k,6}) + (d-1)^5 B_{6,l,e_s}\Delta\rho^{i,s}_{k,6} \Big\}.$$

This gives us

$$\rho^i_{k+1,6} \le (1 + A_6\Delta)\rho^i_{k,6} + 6(d-1)C_{5,1}\Delta\rho^i_{k,6} + 15(d-1)^2 C_{4,2}\Delta\rho^i_{k,6}$$
$$+ 20(d-1)^3 C_{3,3}\Delta\rho^i_{k,6}$$
$$+ 15(d-1)^4 C_{2,4}\Delta\rho^i_{k,6} + 6(d-1)^5 C_{1,5}\Delta\rho^i_{k,6} + (d-1)^6 B_6\Delta\rho^i_{k,6},$$

where $A_6 := \max_{l=1,\dots,d} A_{6,l}$, $B_6 := \max_{l,s=1,\dots,d} B_{6,l,e_s}$, $C_{5,1} := \max_{l,s=1,\dots,d} C_{5,1,l,e_l,e_s}$, $C_{4,2} := \max_{l,s=1,\dots,d} C_{4,2,l,e_l,e_s}$, $C_{3,3} := \max_{l,s=1,\dots,d} C_{3,3,l,e_l,e_s}$, $C_{2,4} := \max_{l,s=1,\dots,d} C_{2,4,l,e_l,e_s}$ and $C_{1,5} := \max_{l,s=1,\dots,d} C_{1,5,l,e_l,e_s}$. Hence, we obtain

$$\rho^i_{k+1,6} \le (1 + \kappa_3\Delta)\rho^i_{k,6}, \quad k = j+1,\dots,J-1$$

for some constant $\kappa_3 > 0$, leading to

$$\rho^i_{k,6} \le (1 + \kappa_3\Delta)^{k-j-1}\rho^i_{j+1,6}, \quad k = j+1,\dots,J-1,$$

where

$$\rho^i_{j+1,6} = \sum_{s=1}^{d} \mathbb{E}\left[\left(\frac{\partial}{\partial y_i}\Phi^s_\Delta(x,y+\xi_{j+1})\right)^6\right] = \sum_{s=1}^{d}\sigma^6_{si}(x).$$

Moreover, we have

$$\mathbb{E}\left[\left(\frac{\partial}{\partial y_i}G^l_{k+1,j}(x,y)\right)^8\right]$$
$$\le \mathbb{E}\left[\left(\frac{\partial}{\partial x_l}\Phi^l_{\Delta,k+1}(G_{k,j}(x,y))\frac{\partial}{\partial y_i}G^l_{k,j}(x,y)\right)^8\right.$$

$$+ \sum_{s \neq l} \Bigg\{ 8 \left(\frac{\partial}{\partial x_l} \Phi^l_{\Delta, k+1}(G_{k,j}(x, y)) \frac{\partial}{\partial y_i} G^l_{k,j}(x, y) \right)^7$$

$$\frac{\partial}{\partial x_s} \Phi^l_{\Delta, k+1}(G_{k,j}(x, y)) \frac{\partial}{\partial y_i} G^s_{k,j}(x, y)$$

$$+ 28(d-1) \left(\frac{\partial}{\partial x_l} \Phi^l_{\Delta, k+1}(G_{k,j}(x, y)) \frac{\partial}{\partial y_i} G^l_{k,j}(x, y) \right)^6$$

$$\left(\frac{\partial}{\partial x_s} \Phi^l_{\Delta, k+1}(G_{k,j}(x, y)) \frac{\partial}{\partial y_i} G^s_{k,j}(x, y) \right)^2$$

$$+ 56(d-1)^2 \left(\frac{\partial}{\partial x_l} \Phi^l_{\Delta, k+1}(G_{k,j}(x, y)) \frac{\partial}{\partial y_i} G^l_{k,j}(x, y) \right)^5$$

$$\left(\frac{\partial}{\partial x_s} \Phi^l_{\Delta, k+1}(G_{k,j}(x, y)) \frac{\partial}{\partial y_i} G^s_{k,j}(x, y) \right)^3$$

$$+ 70(d-1)^3 \left(\frac{\partial}{\partial x_l} \Phi^l_{\Delta, k+1}(G_{k,j}(x, y)) \frac{\partial}{\partial y_i} G^l_{k,j}(x, y) \right.$$

$$\left. \frac{\partial}{\partial x_s} \Phi^l_{\Delta, k+1}(G_{k,j}(x, y)) \frac{\partial}{\partial y_i} G^s_{k,j}(x, y) \right)^4$$

$$+ 56(d-1)^4 \left(\frac{\partial}{\partial x_l} \Phi^l_{\Delta, k+1}(G_{k,j}(x, y)) \frac{\partial}{\partial y_i} G^l_{k,j}(x, y) \right)^3$$

$$\left(\frac{\partial}{\partial x_s} \Phi^l_{\Delta, k+1}(G_{k,j}(x, y)) \frac{\partial}{\partial y_i} G^s_{k,j}(x, y) \right)^5$$

$$+ 28(d-1)^5 \left(\frac{\partial}{\partial x_l} \Phi^l_{\Delta, k+1}(G_{k,j}(x, y)) \frac{\partial}{\partial y_i} G^l_{k,j}(x, y) \right)^2$$

$$\left(\frac{\partial}{\partial x_s} \Phi^l_{\Delta, k+1}(G_{k,j}(x, y)) \frac{\partial}{\partial y_i} G^s_{k,j}(x, y) \right)^6$$

$$+ 8(d-1)^6 \frac{\partial}{\partial x_l} \Phi^l_{\Delta, k+1}(G_{k,j}(x, y)) \frac{\partial}{\partial y_i} G^l_{k,j}(x, y)$$

$$\left(\frac{\partial}{\partial x_s} \Phi^l_{\Delta, k+1}(G_{k,j}(x, y)) \frac{\partial}{\partial y_i} G^s_{k,j}(x, y) \right)^7$$

$$+ (d-1)^7 \left(\frac{\partial}{\partial x_s} \Phi^l_{\Delta, k+1}(G_{k,j}(x, y)) \frac{\partial}{\partial y_i} G^s_{k,j}(x, y) \right)^8 \Bigg\} \Bigg]$$

and thus, due to $8a^7b \leq 7a^8 + b^8$, $4a^6b^2 \leq 3a^8 + b^8$, $8a^5b^3 \leq 5a^8 + 3b^8$ and $2a^4b^4 \leq a^8 + b^8$,

$$
\rho_{k+1,8}^{i,l} \leq (1 + A_{8,l}\Delta)\rho_{k,8}^{i,l}
$$

$$
+ \sum_{s \neq l} \Big\{ C_{7,1,l,e_l,e_s}\Delta(7\rho_{k,8}^{i,l} + \rho_{k,8}^{i,s}) + 7(d-1)C_{6,2,l,e_l,e_s}\Delta(3\rho_{k,8}^{i,l} + \rho_{k,8}^{i,s})
$$

$$
+ 7(d-1)^2 C_{5,3,l,e_l,e_s}\Delta(5\rho_{k,8}^{i,l} + 3\rho_{k,8}^{i,s}) + 35(d-1)^3 C_{4,4,l,e_l,e_s}\Delta(\rho_{k,8}^{i,l} + \rho_{k,8}^{i,s})
$$

$$
+ 7(d-1)^4 C_{3,5,l,e_l,e_s}\Delta(3\rho_{k,8}^{i,l} + 5\rho_{k,8}^{i,s}) + 7(d-1)^5 C_{2,6,l,e_l,e_s}\Delta(\rho_{k,8}^{i,l} + 3\rho_{k,8}^{i,s})
$$

$$
+ (d-1)^6 C_{1,7,l,e_l,e_s}\Delta(\rho_{k,8}^{i,l} + 7\rho_{k,8}^{i,s}) + (d-1)^7 B_{8,l,e_s}\Delta\rho_{k,8}^{i,s} \Big\}.
$$

This gives us

$$
\rho_{k+1,8}^{i} \leq (1 + A_8\Delta)\rho_{k,8}^{i} + 8(d-1)C_{7,1}\Delta\rho_{k,8}^{i} + 28(d-1)^2 C_{6,2}\Delta\rho_{k,8}^{i} + 56(d-1)^3 C_{5,3}\Delta\rho_{k,8}^{i}
$$

$$
+ 70(d-1)^4 C_{4,4}\Delta\rho_{k,8}^{i} + 56(d-1)^5 C_{3,5}\Delta\rho_{k,8}^{i} + 28(d-1)^6 C_{2,6}\Delta\rho_{k,8}^{i}
$$

$$
+ 8(d-1)^7 C_{1,7}\Delta\rho_{k,8}^{i} + (d-1)^8 B_8\Delta\rho_{k,8}^{i},
$$

where $A_8 := \max_{l=1,\dots,d} A_{8,l}$, $B_8 := \max_{l,s=1,\dots,d} B_{8,l,e_s}$, $C_{7,1} := \max_{l,s=1,\dots,d} C_{7,1,l,e_l,e_s}$, $C_{6,2} := \max_{l,s=1,\dots,d} C_{6,2,l,e_l,e_s}$, $C_{5,3} := \max_{l,s=1,\dots,d} C_{5,3,l,e_l,e_s}$, $C_{4,4} := \max_{l,s=1,\dots,d} C_{4,4,l,e_l,e_s}$, $C_{3,5} := \max_{l,s=1,\dots,d} C_{3,5,l,e_l,e_s}$, $C_{2,6} := \max_{l,s=1,\dots,d} C_{2,6,l,e_l,e_s}$ and $C_{1,7} := \max_{l,s=1,\dots,d} C_{1,7,l,e_l,e_s}$. Hence, we obtain

$$
\rho_{k+1,8}^{i} \leq (1 + \kappa_4\Delta)\rho_{k,8}^{i}, \quad k = j+1, \dots, J-1
$$

for some constant $\kappa_4 > 0$, leading to

$$
\rho_{k,8}^{i} \leq (1 + \kappa_4\Delta)^{k-j-1}\rho_{j+1,8}^{i}, \quad k = j+1, \dots, J-1,
$$

where

$$
\rho_{j+1,8}^{i} = \sum_{s=1}^{d} \mathbb{E}\left[\left(\frac{\partial}{\partial y_i}\Phi_\Delta^s(x, y + \xi_{j+1}) \right)^8 \right] = \sum_{s=1}^{d} \sigma_{si}^8(x).
$$

Next, we have for some $i, o \in \{1, \dots, m\}$ and $l \in \{1, \dots, d\}$

$$
\frac{\partial^2}{\partial y_i \partial y_o} G_{k+1,j}^l(x, y) = \sum_{s=1}^{d} \frac{\partial}{\partial x_s}\Phi_{\Delta,k+1}^l(G_{k,j}(x, y)) \frac{\partial^2}{\partial y_i \partial y_o} G_{k,j}^s(x, y)
$$

$$
+ \sum_{s,u=1}^{d} \frac{\partial^2}{\partial x_s \partial x_u}\Phi_{\Delta,k+1}^l(G_{k,j}(x, y)) \frac{\partial}{\partial y_i} G_{k,j}^s(x, y) \frac{\partial}{\partial y_o} G_{k,j}^u(x, y)
$$

and $\dfrac{\partial^2}{\partial y_i \partial y_o} G_{j+1,j}^s(x, y) = \dfrac{\partial^2}{\partial y_i \partial y_o}\Phi_\Delta^s(x, y + \xi_{j+1})$. Hence

$$\mathbb{E}\left[\left(\frac{\partial^2}{\partial y_i \partial y_o} G^l_{k+1,j}(x,y)\right)^2\right]$$

$$\leq \mathbb{E}\left[\left(\frac{\partial}{\partial x_l}\Phi^l_{\Delta,k+1}(G_{k,j}(x,y))\frac{\partial^2}{\partial y_i \partial y_o}G^l_{k,j}(x,y)\right)^2\right.$$

$$+\sum_{s\neq l}\left\{2\frac{\partial}{\partial x_l}\Phi^l_{\Delta,k+1}(G_{k,j}(x,y))\frac{\partial}{\partial x_s}\Phi^l_{\Delta,k+1}(G_{k,j}(x,y))\frac{\partial^2}{\partial y_i \partial y_o}G^l_{k,j}(x,y)\right.$$

$$\left.\frac{\partial^2}{\partial y_i \partial y_o}G^s_{k,j}(x,y)+(d-1)\left(\frac{\partial}{\partial x_s}\Phi^l_{\Delta,k+1}(G_{k,j}(x,y))\frac{\partial^2}{\partial y_i \partial y_o}G^s_{k,j}(x,y)\right)^2\right\}$$

$$+2\sum_{s,u,v=1}^d \frac{\partial}{\partial x_v}\Phi^l_{\Delta,k+1}(G_{k,j}(x,y))\frac{\partial^2}{\partial x_s \partial x_u}\Phi^l_{\Delta,k+1}(G_{k,j}(x,y))$$

$$\frac{\partial^2}{\partial y_i \partial y_o}G^v_{k,j}(x,y)\frac{\partial}{\partial y_i}G^s_{k,j}(x,y)\frac{\partial}{\partial y_o}G^u_{k,j}(x,y)$$

$$\left.+d^2\sum_{s,u=1}^d\left(\frac{\partial^2}{\partial x_s \partial x_u}\Phi^l_{\Delta,k+1}(G_{k,j}(x,y))\frac{\partial}{\partial y_i}G^s_{k,j}(x,y)\frac{\partial}{\partial y_o}G^u_{k,j}(x,y)\right)^2\right]$$

Denote

$$\psi^{i,o,s}_{k+1,n}=\mathbb{E}\left[\left(\frac{\partial^2}{\partial y_i \partial y_o}G^s_{k+1,j}(x,y)\right)^n\right]$$

and $e_{s,u}:=e_s+e_u$, then we get, due to

$$2\mathbb{E}\left[XYZ\right]\leq 2\sqrt{\mathbb{E}\left[X^2\right]}\sqrt[4]{\mathbb{E}\left[Y^4\right]}\sqrt[4]{\mathbb{E}\left[Z^4\right]}\leq \mathbb{E}\left[X^2\right]+\sqrt{\mathbb{E}\left[Y^4\right]}\sqrt{\mathbb{E}\left[Z^4\right]}\leq \mathbb{E}\left[X^2\right]$$

$$+\frac{1}{2}(\mathbb{E}[Y^4]+\mathbb{E}[Z^4]),$$

for $k=j+1,\ldots,J-1$,

$$\psi^{i,o,l}_{k+1,2}\leq (1+A_{2,l}\Delta)\psi^{i,o,l}_{k,2}+\sum_{s\neq l}\left\{C_{1,1,l,e_l,e_s}\Delta(\psi^{i,o,l}_{k,2}+\psi^{i,o,s}_{k,2})+(d-1)B_{2,l,e_s}\Delta\psi^{i,o,s}_{k,2}\right\}$$

$$+\sum_{s,u,v=1}^d C_{1,1,l,e_v,e_{s,u}}\Delta\left(\psi^{i,o,v}_{k,2}+\frac{1}{2}\left(\rho^{i,s}_{k,4}+\rho^{o,u}_{k,4}\right)\right)$$

$$+d^2\sum_{s,u=1}^d B_{2,l,e_{s,u}}\Delta\frac{1}{2}\left(\rho^{i,s}_{k,4}+\rho^{o,u}_{k,4}\right).$$

Further, denote

$$\psi^{i,o}_{k+1,n}=\sum_{l=1}^d \psi^{i,o,l}_{k+1,n},$$

then we get for $k=j+1,\ldots,J-1$,

$$\psi_{k+1,2}^{i,o} \leq (1 + A_2\Delta)\psi_{k,2}^{i,o} + 2(d-1)C_{1,1}\Delta\psi_{k,2}^{i,o} + (d-1)^2 B_2\Delta\psi_{k,2}^{i,o}$$

$$+ d^3\tilde{C}_{1,1}\Delta\left(\psi_{k,2}^{i,o} + \frac{1}{2}\left(\rho_{k,4}^i + \rho_{k,4}^o\right)\right) + d^4\tilde{B}_2\Delta\frac{1}{2}\left(\rho_{k,4}^i + \rho_{k,4}^o\right).$$

where $\tilde{C}_{1,1} := \max\limits_{l,s,u,v=1,\ldots,d} C_{1,1,l,e_v,e_{s,u}}$ and $\tilde{B}_2 := \max\limits_{l,s,u=1,\ldots,d} B_{2,l,e_{s,u}}$. This gives us

$$\psi_{k+1,2}^{i,o} \leq (1 + \kappa_5\Delta)\psi_{k,2}^{i,o} + \kappa_6, \quad k = j+1, \ldots, J-1$$

for some constants $\kappa_5, \kappa_6 > 0$, leading to

$$\psi_{k,2}^{i,o} \leq (1 + \kappa_5\Delta)^{k-j-1}\psi_{j+1,2}^{i,o} + \kappa_7 = \kappa_7, \, k = j+1, \ldots, J-1,$$

where $\kappa_7 > 0$ and

$$\psi_{j+1,2}^{i,o} = \sum_{s=1}^{d}\mathbb{E}\left[\left(\frac{\partial^2}{\partial y_i\partial y_o}\Phi_\Delta^s(x, y + \xi_{j+1})\right)^2\right] = 0.$$

Thus, we obtain the boundedness of

$$\frac{\partial^2}{\partial y_i\partial y_o}u_\Delta(t_j, x, y) = \mathbb{E}\left[\sum_{s=1}^{d}\frac{\partial}{\partial x_s}f(G_{J,j}(x, y))\frac{\partial^2}{\partial y_i\partial y_o}G_{J,j}^s(x, y)\right.$$

$$\left. + \sum_{s,u=1}^{d}\frac{\partial^2}{\partial x_s\partial x_u}f(G_{J,j}(x, y))\frac{\partial}{\partial y_i}G_{J,j}^s(x, y)\frac{\partial}{\partial y_o}G_{J,j}^u(x, y)\right],$$

provided that σ_{ki} and all the derivatives of order 1 and 2 for f, μ_k, σ_{ki} are bounded. Moreover, we have

$$\mathbb{E}\left[\left(\frac{\partial^2}{\partial y_i\partial y_o}G_{k+1,j}^l(x, y)\right)^4\right]$$

$$\leq \mathbb{E}\left[\left(\frac{\partial}{\partial x_l}\Phi_{\Delta,k+1}^l(G_{k,j}(x, y))\frac{\partial^2}{\partial y_i\partial y_o}G_{k,j}^l(x, y)\right)^4\right.$$

$$+ \sum_{s\neq l}\left\{4\left(\frac{\partial}{\partial x_l}\Phi_{\Delta,k+1}^l(G_{k,j}(x, y))\frac{\partial^2}{\partial y_i\partial y_o}G_{k,j}^l(x, y)\right)^3\right.$$

$$\frac{\partial}{\partial x_s}\Phi_{\Delta,k+1}^l(G_{k,j}(x, y))\frac{\partial^2}{\partial y_i\partial y_o}G_{k,j}^s(x, y)$$

$$+ 6(d-1)\left(\frac{\partial}{\partial x_l}\Phi_{\Delta,k+1}^l(G_{k,j}(x, y))\frac{\partial^2}{\partial y_i\partial y_o}G_{k,j}^l(x, y)\right.$$

$$\frac{\partial}{\partial x_s}\Phi^l_{\Delta,k+1}(G_{k,j}(x,y))\frac{\partial^2}{\partial y_i\partial y_o}G^s_{k,j}(x,y)\Bigg)^2$$

$$+4(d-1)^2\frac{\partial}{\partial x_l}\Phi^l_{\Delta,k+1}(G_{k,j}(x,y))\frac{\partial^2}{\partial y_i\partial y_o}G^l_{k,j}(x,y)$$

$$\left(\frac{\partial}{\partial x_s}\Phi^l_{\Delta,k+1}(G_{k,j}(x,y))\frac{\partial^2}{\partial y_i\partial y_o}G^s_{k,j}(x,y)\right)^3$$

$$+(d-1)^3\left(\frac{\partial}{\partial x_s}\Phi^l_{\Delta,k+1}(G_{k,j}(x,y))\frac{\partial^2}{\partial y_i\partial y_o}G^s_{k,j}(x,y)\right)^4\Bigg\}$$

$$+\sum_{s,u,v=1}^{d}\Bigg\{4d^2\left(\frac{\partial}{\partial x_v}\Phi^l_{\Delta,k+1}(G_{k,j}(x,y))\frac{\partial^2}{\partial y_i\partial y_o}G^v_{k,j}(x,y)\right)^3$$

$$\frac{\partial^2}{\partial x_s\partial x_u}\Phi^l_{\Delta,k+1}(G_{k,j}(x,y))\cdot\frac{\partial}{\partial y_i}G^s_{k,j}(x,y)\frac{\partial}{\partial y_o}G^u_{k,j}(x,y)$$

$$+6d^3\left(\frac{\partial}{\partial x_v}\Phi^l_{\Delta,k+1}(G_{k,j}(x,y))\frac{\partial^2}{\partial y_i\partial y_o}G^v_{k,j}(x,y)\right.$$

$$\left.\frac{\partial^2}{\partial x_s\partial x_u}\Phi^l_{\Delta,k+1}(G_{k,j}(x,y))\right)^2$$

$$\cdot\left(\frac{\partial}{\partial y_i}G^s_{k,j}(x,y)\frac{\partial}{\partial y_o}G^u_{k,j}(x,y)\right)^2$$

$$+4d^4\frac{\partial}{\partial x_v}\Phi^l_{\Delta,k+1}(G_{k,j}(x,y))\frac{\partial^2}{\partial y_i\partial y_o}G^v_{k,j}(x,y)$$

$$\cdot\left(\frac{\partial^2}{\partial x_s\partial x_u}\Phi^l_{\Delta,k+1}(G_{k,j}(x,y))\frac{\partial}{\partial y_i}G^s_{k,j}(x,y)\frac{\partial}{\partial y_o}G^u_{k,j}(x,y)\right)^3\Bigg\}$$

$$+d^6\sum_{s,u}^{d}\left(\frac{\partial^2}{\partial x_s\partial x_u}\Phi^l_{\Delta,k+1}(G_{k,j}(x,y))\frac{\partial}{\partial y_i}G^s_{k,j}(x,y)\frac{\partial}{\partial y_o}G^u_{k,j}(x,y)\right)^4\Bigg]$$

and thus, due to $4a^3bc \leq 3a^4 + \frac{1}{2}\left(b^8+c^8\right)$, $2a^2b^2c^2 \leq a^4 + \frac{1}{2}\left(b^8+c^8\right)$ and $4ab^3c^3 \leq a^4 + \frac{3}{2}\left(b^8+c^8\right)$,

$$\psi_{k+1,4}^{i,o,l} \le (1 + A_{4,l}\Delta)\psi_{k,4}^{i,o,l}$$

$$+ \sum_{s\neq l} \left\{ C_{3,1,l,e_l,e_s}\Delta(3\psi_{k,4}^{i,o,l} + \psi_{k,4}^{i,o,s}) + 3(d-1)C_{2,2,l,e_l,e_s}\Delta(\psi_{k,4}^{i,o,l} + \psi_{k,4}^{i,o,s}) \right.$$

$$\left. +(d-1)^2 C_{1,3,l,e_l,e_s}\Delta(\psi_{k,4}^{i,o,l} + 3\psi_{k,4}^{i,o,s}) + (d-1)^3 B_{4,l,e_s}\Delta\psi_{k,4}^{i,o,s} \right\}$$

$$+ \sum_{s,u,v=1}^{d} \left\{ d^2 C_{3,1,l,e_v,e_{s,u}}\Delta\left(3\psi_{k,4}^{i,o,v} + \frac{1}{2}\left(\rho_{k,8}^{i,s} + \rho_{k,8}^{o,u}\right)\right) \right.$$

$$+ 3d^3 C_{2,2,l,e_v,e_{s,u}}\Delta\left(\psi_{k,4}^{i,o,v} + \frac{1}{2}\left(\rho_{k,8}^{i,s} + \rho_{k,8}^{o,u}\right)\right)$$

$$\left. + d^4 C_{1,3,l,e_v,e_{s,u}}\Delta\left(\psi_{k,4}^{i,o,v} + \frac{3}{2}\left(\rho_{k,8}^{i,s} + \rho_{k,8}^{o,u}\right)\right)\right\}$$

$$+ d^6 \sum_{s,u=1}^{d} B_{4,l,e_{s,u}}\Delta\frac{1}{2}\left(\rho_{k,8}^{i,s} + \rho_{k,8}^{o,u}\right).$$

This gives us

$$\psi_{k+1,4}^{i,o} \le (1 + A_4\Delta)\psi_{k,4}^{i,o} + 4(d-1)C_{3,1}\Delta\psi_{k,4}^{i,o} + 6(d-1)^2 C_{2,2}\Delta\psi_{k,4}^{i,o}$$

$$+ 4(d-1)^3 C_{1,3}\Delta\rho_{k,4}^{i} + (d-1)^4 B_4\Delta\psi_{k,4}^{i,o} + d^5\tilde{C}_{3,1}\Delta\left(3\psi_{k,4}^{i,o} + \frac{1}{2}\left(\rho_{k,8}^{i} + \rho_{k,8}^{o}\right)\right)$$

$$+ 3d^6\tilde{C}_{2,2}\Delta\left(\psi_{k,4}^{i,o} + \frac{1}{2}\left(\rho_{k,8}^{i} + \rho_{k,8}^{o}\right)\right) + d^7\tilde{C}_{1,3}\Delta\left(\psi_{k,4}^{i,o} + \frac{3}{2}\left(\rho_{k,8}^{i} + \rho_{k,8}^{o}\right)\right)$$

$$+ d^8\tilde{B}_4\Delta\frac{1}{2}\left(\rho_{k,8}^{i} + \rho_{k,8}^{o}\right),$$

where $\tilde{C}_{3,1} := \max\limits_{l,s,u,v=1,\ldots,d} C_{3,1,l,e_v,e_{s,u}}$, $\tilde{C}_{2,2} := \max\limits_{l,s,u,v=1,\ldots,d} C_{2,2,l,e_v,e_{s,u}}$, $\tilde{C}_{1,3} :=$ $\max\limits_{l,s,u,v=1,\ldots,d} C_{1,3,l,e_v,e_{s,u}}$ and $\tilde{B}_4 := \max\limits_{l,s,u=1,\ldots,d} B_{4,l,e_{s,u}}$. Hence, we obtain

$$\psi_{k+1,4}^{i,o} \le (1 + \kappa_8\Delta)\psi_{k,4}^{i,o} + \kappa_9, \quad k = j+1,\ldots,J-1$$

for some constants $\kappa_8, \kappa_9 > 0$, leading to

$$\psi_{k,4}^{i,o} \le (1 + \kappa_8\Delta)^{k-j-1}\psi_{j+1,4}^{i,o} + \kappa_{10} = \kappa_{10}, \, k = j+1,\ldots,J-1,$$

where $\kappa_{10} > 0$ and

$$\psi_{j+1,4}^{i,o} = \sum_{s=1}^{d}\mathbb{E}\left[\left(\frac{\partial^2}{\partial y_i\partial y_o}\Phi_\Delta^s(x, y + \xi_{j+1})\right)^4\right] = 0.$$

Next, we have for some $i, o, r \in \{1,\ldots,m\}$ and $l \in \{1,\ldots,d\}$

$$\frac{\partial^3}{\partial y_i \partial y_o \partial y_r} G^l_{k+1,j}(x,y)$$

$$= \sum_{s=1}^{d} \frac{\partial}{\partial x_s} \Phi^l_{\Delta,k+1}(G_{k,j}(x,y)) \frac{\partial^3}{\partial y_i \partial y_o \partial y_r} G^s_{k,j}(x,y)$$

$$+ \sum_{s,u=1}^{d} \frac{\partial^2}{\partial x_s \partial x_u} \Phi^l_{\Delta,k+1}(G_{k,j}(x,y)) \left(\frac{\partial^2}{\partial y_i \partial y_o} G^s_{k,j}(x,y) \frac{\partial}{\partial y_r} G^u_{k,j}(x,y) \right.$$

$$+ \frac{\partial^2}{\partial y_i \partial y_r} G^s_{k,j}(x,y) \frac{\partial}{\partial y_o} G^u_{k,j}(x,y)$$

$$+ \left. \frac{\partial}{\partial y_i} G^s_{k,j}(x,y) \frac{\partial^2}{\partial y_o \partial y_r} G^u_{k,j}(x,y) \right)$$

$$+ \sum_{s,u,v=1}^{d} \frac{\partial^3}{\partial x_s \partial x_u \partial x_v} \Phi^l_{\Delta,k+1}(G_{k,j}(x,y)) \frac{\partial}{\partial y_i} G^s_{k,j}(x,y) \frac{\partial}{\partial y_o} G^u_{k,j}(x,y) \frac{\partial}{\partial y_r} G^v_{k,j}(x,y)$$

and $\frac{\partial^3}{\partial y_i \partial y_o \partial y_r} G^s_{j+1,j}(x,y) = \frac{\partial^3}{\partial y_i \partial y_o \partial y_r} \Phi^s_{\Delta}(x, y + \xi_{j+1})$. Hence

$$\mathbb{E}\left[\left(\frac{\partial^3}{\partial y_i \partial y_o \partial y_r} G^l_{k+1,j}(x,y) \right)^2 \right]$$

$$\leq \mathbb{E}\left[\left(\frac{\partial}{\partial x_l} \Phi^l_{\Delta,k+1}(G_{k,j}(x,y)) \frac{\partial^3}{\partial y_i \partial y_o \partial y_r} G^l_{k,j}(x,y) \right)^2 \right.$$

$$+ \sum_{s \neq l} \left\{ 2 \frac{\partial}{\partial x_l} \Phi^l_{\Delta,k+1}(G_{k,j}(x,y)) \frac{\partial}{\partial x_s} \Phi^l_{\Delta,k+1}(G_{k,j}(x,y)) \right.$$

$$\frac{\partial^3}{\partial y_i \partial y_o \partial y_r} G^l_{k,j}(x,y) \frac{\partial^3}{\partial y_i \partial y_o \partial y_r} G^s_{k,j}(x,y)$$

$$+ \left. \left. (d-1) \left(\frac{\partial}{\partial x_s} \Phi^l_{\Delta,k+1}(G_{k,j}(x,y)) \frac{\partial^3}{\partial y_i \partial y_o \partial y_r} G^s_{k,j}(x,y) \right)^2 \right\} \right.$$

$$+ 2 \sum_{s,u,v=1}^{d} \frac{\partial^2}{\partial x_s \partial x_u} \Phi^l_{\Delta,k+1}(G_{k,j}(x,y)) \frac{\partial}{\partial x_v} \Phi^l_{\Delta,k+1}(G_{k,j}(x,y)) \frac{\partial^3}{\partial y_i \partial y_o \partial y_r} G^v_{k,j}(x,y)$$

$$\cdot \left(\frac{\partial^2}{\partial y_i \partial y_o} G^s_{k,j}(x,y) \frac{\partial}{\partial y_r} G^u_{k,j}(x,y) + \frac{\partial^2}{\partial y_i \partial y_r} G^s_{k,j}(x,y) \frac{\partial}{\partial y_o} G^u_{k,j}(x,y) \right.$$

$$+ \left. \frac{\partial}{\partial y_i} G^s_{k,j}(x,y) \frac{\partial^2}{\partial y_o \partial y_r} G^u_{k,j}(x,y) \right)$$

$$+ 2 \sum_{s,u,v,w=1}^{d} \frac{\partial^3}{\partial x_s \partial x_u \partial x_v} \Phi^l_{\Delta,k+1}(G_{k,j}(x,y))$$

$$\frac{\partial}{\partial x_w} \Phi^l_{\Delta,k+1}(G_{k,j}(x,y)) \frac{\partial^3}{\partial y_i \partial y_o \partial y_r} G^w_{k,j}(x,y)$$

$$\cdot \frac{\partial}{\partial y_i} G_{k,j}^s(x, y) \frac{\partial}{\partial y_o} G_{k,j}^u(x, y) \frac{\partial}{\partial y_r} G_{k,j}^v(x, y)$$

$$+ 6d^2 \sum_{s,u=1}^{d} \left(\frac{\partial^2}{\partial x_s \partial x_u} \Phi_{\Delta,k+1}^l(G_{k,j}(x, y)) \right)^2 \left(\left(\frac{\partial^2}{\partial y_i \partial y_o} G_{k,j}^s(x, y) \frac{\partial}{\partial y_r} G_{k,j}^u(x, y) \right)^2 \right.$$

$$+ \left(\frac{\partial^2}{\partial y_i \partial y_r} G_{k,j}^s(x, y) \frac{\partial}{\partial y_o} G_{k,j}^u(x, y) \right)^2$$

$$\left. + \left(\frac{\partial}{\partial y_i} G_{k,j}^s(x, y) \frac{\partial^2}{\partial y_o \partial y_r} G_{k,j}^u(x, y) \right)^2 \right)$$

$$+ 2d^3 \sum_{s,u,v=1}^{d} \left(\frac{\partial^3}{\partial x_s \partial x_u \partial x_v} \Phi_{\Delta,k+1}^l(G_{k,j}(x, y)) \frac{\partial}{\partial y_i} G_{k,j}^s(x, y) \frac{\partial}{\partial y_o} G_{k,j}^u(x, y) \right.$$

$$\left. \left. \frac{\partial}{\partial y_r} G_{k,j}^v(x, y) \right)^2 \right]$$

Denote

$$\zeta_{k+1}^{i,o,r,s} = \mathbb{E} \left[\left(\frac{\partial^3}{\partial y_i \partial y_o \partial y_r} G_{k+1,j}^s(x, y) \right)^2 \right]$$

and $e_{s,u,v} := e_s + e_u + e_v$, then we get, due to $3a^2 b^2 c^2 \le a^6 + b^6 + c^6$ and

$$2\mathbb{E}[XYZU] \le 2\sqrt{\mathbb{E}[X^2]} \sqrt[6]{\mathbb{E}[Y^6]} \sqrt[6]{\mathbb{E}[Z^6]} \sqrt[6]{\mathbb{E}[U^6]}$$

$$\le \mathbb{E}[X^2] + \sqrt[3]{\mathbb{E}[Y^6]} \sqrt[3]{\mathbb{E}[Z^6]} \sqrt[3]{\mathbb{E}[U^6]}$$

$$\le \mathbb{E}[X^2] + \frac{1}{3} \left(\mathbb{E}[Y^6] + \mathbb{E}[Z^6] + \mathbb{E}[U^6] \right),$$

for $k = j + 1, \dots, J - 1$,

$$\zeta_{k+1}^{i,o,r,l} \le (1 + A_{2,l}\Delta)\zeta_k^{i,o,r,l} + \sum_{s \neq l} \left\{ C_{1,1,l,e_l,e_s} \Delta(\zeta_k^{i,o,r,l} + \zeta_k^{i,o,r,s}) + (d-1)B_{2,l,e_s} \Delta \zeta_k^{i,o,r,s} \right\}$$

$$+ \sum_{s,u,v=1}^{d} C_{1,1,l,e_v,e_{s,u}} \Delta \left(\zeta_{k,2}^{i,o,r,v} + \frac{1}{2} \left(\rho_{k,4}^{i,s} + \rho_{k,4}^{o,u} + \rho_{k,4}^{r,u} + \psi_{k,4}^{i,o,s} + \psi_{k,4}^{i,r,s} + \psi_{k,4}^{o,r,u} \right) \right)$$

$$+ \sum_{s,u,v,w=1}^{d} C_{1,1,l,e_w,e_{s,u,v}} \Delta \left(\zeta_{k,2}^{i,o,r,w} + \frac{1}{3} \left(\rho_{k,6}^{i,s} + \rho_{k,6}^{o,u} + \rho_{k,6}^{r,v} \right) \right)$$

$$+ 3d^2 \sum_{s,u=1}^{d} B_{2,l,e_{s,u}} \Delta \left(\rho_{k,4}^{i,s} + \rho_{k,4}^{o,u} + \rho_{4,k}^{r,u} + \psi_{k,4}^{i,o,s} + \psi_{k,4}^{i,r,s} + \psi_{k,4}^{o,r,u} \right)$$

$$+ d^3 \sum_{s,u,v=1}^{d} B_{2,l,e_{s,u,v}} \Delta \frac{1}{3} \left(\rho_{k,6}^{i,s} + \rho_{k,6}^{o,u} + \rho_{k,6}^{r,w} \right).$$

Further, denote

$$\zeta_{k+1}^{i,o,r} = \sum_{l=1}^{d} \zeta_{k+1}^{i,o,r,l},$$

then we get for $k = j + 1, \ldots, J - 1$,

$$\zeta_{k+1,2}^{i,o,r} \le (1 + A_2\Delta)\zeta_{k,2}^{i,o,r} + 2(d-1)C_{1,1}\Delta\zeta_{k,2}^{i,o,r} + (d-1)^2 B_2\Delta\zeta_{k,2}^{i,o,r}$$

$$+ d^3\tilde{C}_{1,1}\Delta \left(\zeta_{k,2}^{i,o,r} + \frac{1}{2}\left(\rho_{k,4}^i + \rho_{k,4}^o + \rho_{k,4}^r + \psi_{k,4}^{i,o} + \psi_{k,4}^{i,r} + \psi_{k,4}^{o,r} \right) \right)$$

$$+ d^4\tilde{C}_{1,1}\Delta \left(\zeta_{k,2}^{i,o,r} + \frac{1}{3}\left(\rho_{k,6}^i + \rho_{k,6}^o + \rho_{k,6}^r \right) \right)$$

$$+ 3d^4\tilde{B}_2\Delta \left(\rho_{k,4}^i + \rho_{k,4}^o + \rho_{k,4}^r + \psi_{k,4}^{i,o} + \psi_{k,4}^{i,r} + \psi_{k,4}^{o,r} \right)$$

$$+ d^6\tilde{B}_2\Delta\frac{1}{3}\left(\rho_{k,6}^i + \rho_{k,6}^o + \rho_{k,6}^r \right).$$

where $\tilde{C}_{1,1} := \max\limits_{l,s,u,v,w=1,\ldots,d} C_{1,1,l,e_w,e_{s,u,v}}$ and $\tilde{B}_2 := \max\limits_{l,s,u,v=1,\ldots,d} B_{2,l,e_{s,u,v}}$. This gives us

$$\zeta_{k+1,2}^{i,o,r} \le (1 + \kappa_{11}\Delta)\zeta_{k,2}^{i,o,r} + \kappa_{12}, \quad k = j+1, \ldots, J-1$$

for some constants $\kappa_{11}, \kappa_{12} > 0$, leading to

$$\zeta_{k,2}^{i,o,r} \le (1 + \kappa_{11}\Delta)^{k-j-1}\zeta_{j+1,2}^{i,o,r} + \kappa_{13} = \kappa_{13}, \, k = j+1, \ldots, J-1,$$

where $\kappa_{13} > 0$ and

$$\zeta_{j+1,2}^{i,o,r} = \sum_{s=1}^{d} \mathbb{E}\left[\left(\frac{\partial^3}{\partial y_i \partial y_o \partial y_r}\Phi_\Delta^s(x, y + \xi_{j+1}) \right)^2 \right] = 0.$$

Thus, we obtain the boundednesss of

$$\frac{\partial^3}{\partial y_i \partial y_o \partial y_r}u_\Delta(t_j, x, y)$$

$$= \mathbb{E}\left[\sum_{s=1}^{d} \frac{\partial}{\partial x_s}f(G_{J,j}(x, y))\frac{\partial^3}{\partial y_i \partial y_o \partial y_r}G_{J,j}^s(x, y) \right.$$

$$+ \sum_{s,u=1}^{d} \frac{\partial^2}{\partial x_s \partial x_u}f(G_{J,j}(x, y))\left(\frac{\partial^2}{\partial y_i \partial y_o}G_{J,j}^s(x, y)\frac{\partial}{\partial y_r}G_{J,j}^u(x, y) \right.$$

$$+ \frac{\partial^2}{\partial y_i \partial y_r}G_{J,j}^s(x, y)\frac{\partial}{\partial y_o}G_{J,j}^u(x, y)$$

$$\left. \left. + \frac{\partial}{\partial y_i}G_{J,j}^s(x, y)\frac{\partial^2}{\partial y_o \partial y_r}G_{J,j}^u(x, y) \right) \right.$$

$$+ \sum_{s,u,v=1}^{d} \frac{\partial^3}{\partial x_s \partial x_u \partial x_v} f(G_{J,j}(x,y)) \frac{\partial}{\partial y_i} G_{J,j}^s(x,y) \frac{\partial}{\partial y_o} G_{J,j}^u(x,y) \frac{\partial}{\partial y_r} G_{J,j}^v(x,y) \Bigg],$$

provided that σ_{ki} and all the derivatives of order 1, 2 and 3 for f, μ_k, σ_{ki} are bounded.

Proof of Lemma 1

Cf. Theorem 5.2 in [2].

Proof of Theorem 7

We have, by the martingale property of $(\tilde{M}_{\Delta,j\Delta}^{int,1})_{j=0,...,J}$, where $\tilde{M}_{\Delta,j\Delta}^{int,1}$ is given by (32) with J being replaced by j, and by the orthogonality of the system $\Delta_j W^i$,

$$\mathrm{Var}[f(X_{\Delta,T}) - \tilde{M}_{\Delta,T}^{int,1}] = \mathrm{Var}[f(X_{\Delta,T}) - M_{\Delta,T}^{int,1}] + \mathrm{Var}[M_{\Delta,T}^{int,1} - \tilde{M}_{\Delta,T}^{int,1}]$$

$$\lesssim \frac{1}{J} + \Delta \sum_{j=1}^{J} \sum_{i=1}^{m} \mathbb{E}\| \sum_{k=1}^{d} (\tilde{g}_{j,k} - g_{j,k})\sigma_{ki}\|_{L^2(\mathbb{P}_{\Delta,j-1})}^2$$

$$\leq \frac{1}{J} + d\Delta \sum_{j=1}^{J} \sum_{i=1}^{m} \sum_{k=1}^{d} \mathbb{E}\|(\tilde{g}_{j,k} - g_{j,k})\sigma_{ki}\|_{L^2(\mathbb{P}_{\Delta,j-1})}^2$$

$$\leq \frac{1}{J} + d^2 Tm\sigma_{max}^2 \Bigg\{ \tilde{c} \left(\Sigma + A^2(\log N + 1)\right) \frac{\binom{p+d}{d} Q^d}{N}$$

$$+ \frac{8 C_h^2}{(p+1)!^2 d^{2-2/h}} \left(\frac{Rd}{Q}\right)^{2p+2} + 8A^2 B_v R^{-v} \Bigg\}.$$

Proof of Theorem 8

Let us, for simplicity, first ignore the $\log(N)$-term in (36) and only consider the terms w.r.t. the variables J, N, N_0, Q, R which shall be optimised, since the constants $d, m, c_{p,d}, (p+1)!, B_v$ do not affect the terms on ε. Further, we consider the log cost and log constraints rather than (35) and (36). Let us subdivide the optimisation problem into two cases:

1. $N \lesssim N_0$. This gives us the Lagrange function

$$\begin{aligned}
L_{\lambda_1,...,\lambda_6}&(J, N, N_0, Q, R) \qquad\qquad\qquad\qquad\qquad\qquad (71)\\
&:= \log(J) + \log(N_0) + d\log(Q) + \lambda_1(-2\log(J) - 2\log(\varepsilon))\\
&\quad + \lambda_2(-\log(J) - \log(N_0) - 2\log(\varepsilon))\\
&\quad + \lambda_3(d\log(Q) - \log(N) - \log(N_0) - 2\log(\varepsilon))\\
&\quad + \lambda_4(2(p+1)(\log(R) - \log(Q)) - \log(N_0) - 2\log(\varepsilon))\\
&\quad + \lambda_5(-v\log(R) - \log(N_0) - 2\log(\varepsilon)) + \lambda_6(\log(N) - \log(N_0)),
\end{aligned}$$

where $\lambda_1, \ldots, \lambda_6 \geq 0$. Thus, considering of the conditions $\frac{\partial L}{\partial J} = \frac{\partial L}{\partial N} = \frac{\partial L}{\partial N_0} = \frac{\partial L}{\partial Q} = \frac{\partial L}{\partial R} \stackrel{!}{=} 0$ gives us the following relations

$$\lambda_1 = \frac{1 - \lambda_2}{2},$$

$$\lambda_3 = \frac{2(p+1)(\nu(1-\lambda_2) - d) - d\nu}{d\nu + 2(p+1)(d+2\nu)} = \lambda_6,$$

$$\lambda_4 = \frac{d\nu(3 - \lambda_2)}{d\nu + 2(p+1)(d+2\nu)},$$

$$\lambda_5 = \frac{2d(p+1)(3 - \lambda_2)}{d\nu + 2(p+1)(d+2\nu)}.$$

The case $\lambda_1, \ldots, \lambda_6 > 0$ is not feasible, since all constraints in (71) cannot be active, that is they cannot become zero simultaneously because of six (linearly independent) equalities on five unknowns. Hence, we derive the solutions under $\lambda_i = 0$ for different i and observe which one is actually optimal.

a. $\lambda_1 = 0 \Rightarrow \lambda_3 = \lambda_6 = -\frac{d(2(p+1)+\nu)}{d\nu+2(p+1)(d+2\nu)} < 0$. Due to negative λ_3, λ_6, this case is not optimal.

b. $\lambda_2 = 0 \Rightarrow \lambda_1, \lambda_4, \lambda_5 > 0$, $\lambda_3 = \lambda_6 = \frac{2(p+1)(\nu-d)-d\nu}{d\nu+2(p+1)(d+2\nu)}$. Again, we make a case distinction:

   i. $\lambda_3 = \lambda_6 = 0 \Rightarrow \nu = \frac{2d(p+1)}{2(p+1)-d}$ for $2(p+1) > d$. This gives us, due to $\lambda_1, \lambda_4, \lambda_5 > 0$,

$$J \asymp \varepsilon^{-1},$$

$$Q \asymp \left[\frac{1}{N_0\varepsilon^2}\right]^{\frac{1}{d}},$$

$$JQ^d N_0 \asymp \varepsilon^{-3}.$$

This solution is no improvement compared to the SMC approach.

   ii. $\lambda_3 = \lambda_6 > 0 \Rightarrow \nu > \frac{2d(p+1)}{2(p+1)-d}$ for $2(p+1) > d$. In this case, all constraints apart from the second one in (71), corresponding to λ_2, are active. Then we obtain

$$J \asymp \varepsilon^{-1},$$

$$Q \asymp \varepsilon^{-\frac{2\nu+4(p+1)}{d\nu+2(p+1)(d+2\nu)}},$$

$$N_0 \asymp \varepsilon^{-\frac{2d\nu+4(p+1)(d+\nu)}{d\nu+2(p+1)(d+2\nu)}},$$

$$JQ^d N_0 \asymp \varepsilon^{-\frac{5d\nu+2(p+1)(5d+4\nu)}{d\nu+2(p+1)(d+2\nu)}},$$

which is a better solution than the previous one. Moreover, the remaining constraint $\frac{1}{JN_0} \lesssim \varepsilon^2$ is also satisfied under this solution.

c. $\lambda_3 = \lambda_6 = 0 \Rightarrow \lambda_1, \lambda_4, \lambda_5 > 0, \lambda_2 = \frac{2(p+1)(v-d)-dv}{2(p+1)v}$. The case $\lambda_2 = 0$ is the same as the last but one and thus gives us $JQ^d N_0 \asymp \varepsilon^{-3}$. The case $\lambda_2 > 0$ leads to four active constraints in (71), namely the ones corresponding to $\lambda_1, \lambda_2, \lambda_4, \lambda_5$, such that

$$J \asymp \varepsilon^{-1},$$

$$Q \asymp \varepsilon^{-\frac{v+2(p+1)}{2v(p+1)}},$$

$$N_0 \asymp \varepsilon^{-1},$$

$$JQ^d N_0 \asymp \varepsilon^{-\frac{dv+2(p+1)(d+2v)}{2v(p+1)}}.$$

This solution seems to be nice at the first moment. However, it does not satisfy both constraints corresponding to λ_3, λ_6. On the one hand, we have for the third constraint $N \gtrsim \varepsilon^{-1-\frac{dv+2d(p+1)}{2v(p+1)}}$. On the other hand, we have for the sixth constraint $N \lesssim \varepsilon^{-1}$. Hence, this is not an admissible solution.

d. $\lambda_4 = 0 \Rightarrow \lambda_1 = -1$. Since λ_1 is negative, this case is not optimal.

e. $\lambda_5 = 0 \Rightarrow \lambda_1 = -1$. As for the previous one, this case is not optimal.

2. $N \gtrsim N_0$. This gives us the Lagrange function

$$\begin{aligned}
\tilde{L}_{\lambda_1,\ldots,\lambda_6}&(J, N, N_0, Q, R) \\
:=& \log(J) + \log(N) + d \log(Q) + \lambda_1(-2\log(J) - 2\log(\varepsilon)) \\
&+ \lambda_2(-\log(J) - \log(N_0) - 2\log(\varepsilon)) \\
&+ \lambda_3(d\log(Q) - \log(N) - \log(N_0) - 2\log(\varepsilon)) \\
&+ \lambda_4(2(p+1)(\log(R) - \log(Q)) - \log(N_0) - 2\log(\varepsilon)) \\
&+ \lambda_5(-v\log(R) - \log(N_0) - 2\log(\varepsilon)) + \lambda_6(\log(N_0) - \log(N)).
\end{aligned}$$

Analogously to the procedure above we get the same optimal solution, that is

$$J \asymp \varepsilon^{-1},$$

$$Q \asymp \varepsilon^{-\frac{2v+4(p+1)}{dv+2(p+1)(d+2v)}},$$

$$N \asymp \varepsilon^{-\frac{2dv+4(p+1)(d+v)}{dv+2(p+1)(d+2v)}},$$

$$JQ^d N \asymp \varepsilon^{-\frac{5dv+2(p+1)(5d+4v)}{dv+2(p+1)(d+2v)}}.$$

Now we consider also the remaining terms $c_{p,d}$, $(p+1)!$, B_v and obtain (37)–(41) via equalising all constraints in (36) apart from the second one. Finally, we add the log term concerning ε in the parameters N, N_0 to ensure that all constraints are really satisfied.

Proof of Lemma 2

Cf. Theorem 5.2 in [2].

Proof of Theorem 9

We have, by the martingale property of $(\tilde{M}^{ser,1}_{\Delta,j\Delta})_{j=0,\dots,J}$, where $\tilde{M}^{ser,1}_{\Delta,j\Delta}$ is given by (43) with J being replaced by j, and by the orthonormality of the system $\frac{\Delta_j W}{\sqrt{\Delta}}$,

$$
\mathrm{Var}[f(X_{\Delta,T}) - \tilde{M}^{ser,1}_{\Delta,T}] = \mathrm{Var}[f(X_{\Delta,T}) - M^{ser,1}_{\Delta,T}] + \mathrm{Var}[M^{ser,1}_{\Delta,T} - \tilde{M}^{ser,1}_{\Delta,T}]
$$

$$
\lesssim \frac{1}{J} + \sum_{j=1}^{J}\sum_{i=1}^{m} \mathbb{E}\|\tilde{a}_{j,e_i} - a_{j,e_i}\|^2_{L^2(\mathbb{P}_{\Delta,j-1})}
$$

$$
\leq \frac{1}{J} + Jm\left\{ \tilde{c}\left(\Sigma + A^2 \Delta (\log N + 1)\right) \frac{c_{p,d}\, Q^d}{N} \right.
$$

$$
\left. + \frac{8\, C_h^2}{(p+1)!^2}\left(\frac{R}{Q}\right)^{2p+2} + 8A^2 \Delta B_\nu R^{-\nu}\right\}.
$$

Proof of Theorem 10

The proof is similar to the one of Theorem 8.

Acknowledgements Stefan Häfner thanks the Faculty of Mathematics of the University of Duisburg-Essen, where this work was carried out.

References

1. Akahori, J., Amaba, T., Okuma, K.: A discrete-time Clark-Ocone formula and its application to an error analysis (2013). arXiv:1307.0673v2
2. Belomestny, D., Häfner, S., Nagapetyan, T., Urusov, M.: Variance reduction for discretised diffusions via regression (2016). arXiv:1510.03141v3
3. Giles, M.B.: Multilevel Monte Carlo path simulation. Op. Res. **56**(3), 607–617 (2008)
4. Györfi, L., Kohler, M., Krzyżak, A., Walk, H.: A distribution-free theory of nonparametric regression. Springer Series in Statistics. Springer, New York (2002)
5. Karatzas, I., Shreve, S.: Brownian Motion and Stochastic Calculus, vol. 113. Springer Science & Business Media, Berlin (2012)
6. Kloeden, P., Platen, E.: Numerical Solution of Stochastic Differential Equations, vol. 23. Springer, Berlin (1992)
7. Milstein, G.N., Tretyakov, M.V.: Stochastic numerics for mathematical physics. Scientific Computation. Springer, Berlin (2004)
8. Milstein, G.N., Tretyakov, M.V.: Practical variance reduction via regression for simulating diffusions. SIAM J. Numer. Anal. **47**(2), 887–910 (2009)
9. Müller-Gronbach, T., Ritter, K., Yaroslavtseva, L.: On the complexity of computing quadrature formulas for marginal distributions of SDEs. J. Complex. **31**(1), 110–145 (2015)
10. Newton, N.J.: Variance reduction for simulated diffusions. SIAM J. Appl. Math. **54**(6), 1780–1805 (1994)

Quadratic Approximation
for Log-Likelihood Ratio Processes

Alexander Gushchin and Esko Valkeila

Abstract We consider a sequence of general filtered statistical models with a finite-dimensional parameter. It is tacitly assumed that a proper rescaling of the parameter space is already done (so we deal with a local parameter) and also time rescaling is done if necessary. Our first and main purpose is to give sufficient conditions for the existence of certain uniform in time linear–quadratic approximations of log-likelihood ratio processes. Second, we prove general theorems establishing LAN, LAMN and LAQ properties for these models based on these linear–quadratic approximations. Our third purpose is to prove three theorems related to the necessity of the conditions in our main result. These theorems assert that these conditions are necessarily satisfied if (1) an approximation of a much more general form exists and a (necessary) condition of asymptotic negligibility of jumps of likelihood ratio processes holds, or (2) we have LAN property at every moment of time and the limiting models are continuous in time, or (3) we have LAN property, Hellinger processes are asymptotically degenerate at the terminal times, and the condition of asymptotic negligibility of jumps holds.

Keywords Contiguity · Filtered statistical experiment · Hellinger process
Likelihood ratio process · Limit theorems · Local asymptotic mixed normality
Local asymptotic normality · Local asymptotic quadraticity

Esko Valkeila—Deceased

A. Gushchin (✉)
Steklov Mathematical Institute, Gubkina 8, 119991 Moscow, Russia
e-mail: gushchin@mi.ras.ru

A. Gushchin
Laboratory of Stochastic Analysis and its Applications, National Research University
Higher School of Economics, Myasnitskaya 20, 101000 Moscow, Russia

E. Valkeila
Aalto University, P.O. Box 11100,
00076 Aalto, Finland

© Springer International Publishing AG 2017
V. Panov (ed.), *Modern Problems of Stochastic Analysis and Statistics*,
Springer Proceedings in Mathematics & Statistics 208,
DOI 10.1007/978-3-319-65313-6_8

1 Introduction

Local quadratic approximations to the logarithms of likelihood ratios play a significant role in the classical asymptotic statistics. Many results in the asymptotic decision theory are proved under the property of local asymptotic normality (LAN) introduced by Le Cam [22]. The LAN property means that the log-likelihoods admit a specific quadratic approximation in local neighbourhoods of a fixed parameter value. Sometimes, the LAN property is not valid but nevertheless the log-likelihoods admit local quadratic approximations. The local asymptotic quadraticity (LAQ) property formalizes this more general situation. An intermediate case between LAN and LAQ is local asymptotic mixed normality (LAMN) which is statistically a more rich property than LAQ. We refer to Le Cam and Yang [27, Chap. 6] and to Höpfner [10] for the definition of LAN, LAMN and LAQ, and for statistical assertions resulting from these properties. The unexplained terminology and notation are explained later on.

We work with general filtered statistical models, see e.g. Shiryaev and Spokoiny [35]. We make no assumptions on the filtrations such as quasi-left continuity, and so our results also cover the discrete-time filtrations. In this framework, we give sufficient conditions for certain linear–quadratic approximations of log-likelihood processes. Moreover, we study the connection of this approximation to LAN, LAMN and LAQ properties.[1]

In the case of discrete-time filtrations, Fabian and Hannan [1] used such an approach to study LAN and LAMN properties of the log-likelihoods. More precisely, they performed approximations by constructing appropriate martingales, see [1, Theorem 3.9], and then the LAN or LAMN property follows from the properties of approximating martingales, see e.g. [1, Theorem 3.14].

We use a similar scheme. Let

$$(\Omega^n, \mathscr{F}^n, \mathbb{F}^n = (\mathscr{F}^n_t)_{t \in \mathbb{R}_+}, (\mathsf{P}^{n,\vartheta})_{\vartheta \in \Theta})$$

be a sequence of filtered statistical models, where Θ is an open subset of $\mathbb{R}^k$. Let also an $\mathbb{F}^n$-stopping time T_n be given for every n, which may be interpreted as the duration of observations in the nth experiment. One of our purposes is to find sufficient conditions for LAN, LAMN or LAQ properties of the experiments $\mathbb{E}^n = (\Omega^n, \mathscr{F}^n_{T_n}, (\mathsf{P}^{n,\vartheta}_{T_n})_{\vartheta \in \Theta})$ at some fixed point $\vartheta_0 \in \Theta$.

Let $Z^{n,\vartheta}$ be the generalized density process of $\mathsf{P}^{n,\vartheta_0 + \varphi_n \vartheta}$ with respect to $\mathsf{P}^n := \mathsf{P}^{n,\vartheta_0}$, where $\{\varphi_n\}$ is a normalizing sequence of $k \times k$ matrices. We tacitly assume that the sequence $\{\varphi_n\}$ is chosen in a 'correct' way; however, the only formal restriction on the sequence $\{\varphi_n\}$ is that the sequence (P^n_0) is contiguous with respect to $(\mathsf{P}^{n,\vartheta_0 + \varphi_n \vartheta_n}_0)$ for every bounded sequence $\{\vartheta_n\}$ in $\mathbb{R}^k$. Denote by $\mathscr{W} = \mathscr{W}(\{T_n\})$ the set of all sequences $\{w^n\}$ with the following properties: $w^n = (w^{n,1}, \dots, w^{n,k})$, $w^n_0 = 0$, is a

---

[1]To be more precise, approximations and limits are assumed to be uniform on all compact parameter subsets. The corresponding properties are often called ULAN (uniform LAN), ULAMN, etc. However, we omit the letter 'U' in the notation.

locally square-integrable martingale on $(\Omega^n, \mathscr{F}^n, \mathbb{F}^n, \mathsf{P}^n)$ with values in $\mathbb{R}^k$ for each n, the quadratic characteristic $\langle w^n, w^n \rangle_{T_n}$ is bounded in P^n-probability, i.e.

$$
\text{the sequence} \quad \left(\sum_{i=1}^{k} \langle w^{n,i}, w^{n,i} \rangle_{T_n} \middle| \mathsf{P}^n \right) \quad \text{is } \mathbb{R}\text{-tight,}
$$

and the Lindeberg-type condition on jumps of w^n holds, i.e.

$$
\|x\|^2 \mathbf{1}_{\{\|x\| > \varepsilon\}} \star v_{T_n}^{w^n} \xrightarrow{\mathsf{P}^n} 0, \quad n \to \infty, \quad \text{for all } \varepsilon > 0.
$$

Our first and main objective is to find conditions that imply the existence of a sequence $\{w^n\} \in \mathscr{W}$ such that the following uniform in time quadratic approximation

$$
\sup_{s \leq T_n} \left| \log Z_s^{n, \vartheta_n} - \log Z_0^{n, \vartheta_n} - \left(\vartheta_n^\top w_s^n - \frac{1}{2} \vartheta_n^\top \langle w^n, w^n \rangle_s \vartheta_n \right) \right| \xrightarrow{\mathsf{P}^n} 0, \quad n \to \infty, \quad (1)
$$

holds for each bounded sequence $\{\vartheta_n\}$ in $\mathbb{R}^k$.

The existence of the quadratic approximation (1) with $\{w^n\} \in \mathscr{W}$ has a number of immediate benefits:

• Due to the boundedness assumption on $\langle w^n, w^n \rangle_{T_n}$, we obtain the contiguity

$$
(\mathsf{P}_{T_n}^n) \lhd (\mathsf{P}_{T_n}^{n, \vartheta_0 + \varphi_n \vartheta_n})
$$

for every bounded sequence ϑ_n, which is necessary for the LAQ property.
• Limit theorems for the likelihoods will follow now from limit theorems for locally square-integrable martingales. Because the approximation is uniform in time, this carries over to functional limit theorems as well.
• To obtain LAN, LAMN or LAQ property for $\mathbb{E}^n$, it is sufficient to study properties of w_n only.
• We need no additional efforts to obtain LAN, LAMN or LAQ property for the experiments $(\Omega^n, \mathscr{F}_{S_n}^n, (\mathsf{P}_{S_n}^{n, \vartheta})_{\vartheta \in \Theta})$ at ϑ_0 with stopping times $S_n \leq T_n$.

Our second objective is to prove LAN, LAMN and LAQ properties, also in functional form, from the quadratic approximation.

Finally, our third objective is to study the relationships between our results and assumptions. We prove several theorems illustrating the necessity of conditions under which the approximation (1) and other results are obtained. In particular, our assumptions are necessary and sufficient for the LAN property (with a given sequence $\{\varphi_n\}$) in the case of i.i.d. observations. Let us mention here that if a quadratic approximation (1) with $\{w^n\} \in \mathscr{W}$ exists, then

$$
\sup_{s \leq T_n} |\Delta \log Z_s^{n, \vartheta_n}| \xrightarrow{\mathsf{P}^n} 0, \quad n \to \infty,
$$

for every bounded sequence ϑ_n. This condition outlines the range of applicability of our method.

We formulate our main approximation result under two different equivalent groups of conditions. The first group is characterized in terms of intrinsic properties of the models, and in this case we construct explicitly an approximating sequence $\{w^n\} \in \mathcal{W}$ satisfying (1). The second group says what are sufficient conditions in predictable terms for the approximation (1) if we already have a candidate for a sequence $\{w^n\} \in \mathcal{W}$. The second approach is similar to earlier works by Luschgy [31–33] but he proved his results under additional assumptions on the structure of the likelihood processes and the filtrations. This second approach might be convenient in applications if our models are locally differentiable at ϑ_0, see Jacod [15] for the precise definition. In this case, the normalized score process $w^n = \varphi_n v_n$, where v_n is the score process at ϑ_0, is a P^n-locally square-integrable martingale, and this may be a natural choice. However, we would like to emphasize that local differentiability properties of the models are in no way required for the existence of the approximation (1).

Since the normalizing sequence $\{\varphi_n\}$ is assumed to be fixed, we use the notation $\mathsf{P}^{n,\vartheta}$ instead of $\mathsf{P}^{n,\vartheta_0+\varphi_n\vartheta}$ in the rest of the paper except Sect. 5. We do not discuss here how to choose $\{\varphi_n\}$; however, understanding what is required may be useful for finding an appropriate normalizing sequence. Let us note that the paper is mainly aimed to find conditions for the existence of the approximation (1). However, this approximation is meaningless from the statistical point of view if the matrices $\langle w^n, w^n \rangle_{T_n}$ are asymptotically singular (noninvertible) with positive probability. As an example, we mention the model considered by Gushchin and Küchler [4], where the log-likelihoods are already quadratic and hence the approximation (1) holds trivially. Correspondingly, the invertibility of the corresponding matrix plays a decisive role in determining normalizing matrices $\{\varphi_n\}$. It turns out that there are 11 different cases (depending on ϑ_0) for a correct choice of $\{\varphi_n\}$. This choice is far from being trivial in most cases, especially in Case M3. Another instructive model is considered by Höpfner and Jacod [11], where nonlinear transformations of the parameter space are needed to ensure the invertibility of the matrix in the quadratic term of limiting log-likelihood.

Let us also mention that some of our results tacitly assume that (deterministic linear) time changes in filtered statistical models are already done. There are also models where nonlinear time changes may be useful, see examples in Höpfner [10, Chap. 8].

As explained above, in the discrete-time case our main results generalize those of Fabian and Hannan [1], where the references to earlier works can be found; see also Greenwood and Shiryaev [2, Sect. 8], Le Cam [25, Chap. 9, Sect. 5], and Hallin et al. [7]. For continuous-time filtrations, we have already mentioned the results by Luschgy [31–33], where more information on earlier works can be found; for related results see also Linkov [28].

This paper can be considered as the second part of our paper [6] where corresponding results were proved for binary experiments and where the reader can find more detailed discussions on the relationship between different assumptions. Our proofs rely heavily on the results in [6]. In the both papers the use of Hellinger processes plays an essential rôle. We refer to [6] for literature on Hellinger processes in limit theorems for binary experiments. In parametric models, limit theorems for likelihoods using Hellinger processes were proved in Vostrikova [38, 39] and Jacod [14].

In Sect. 5, we apply the theory developed in the previous sections to i.i.d. models and obtain 'minimal' conditions for the LAN property. Perhaps it would have been natural to obtain similar results also in a number of other sufficiently simple models including autoregressive models, cf. e.g. Shiryaev and Spokoiny [35], Markov step processes, cf. Höpfner [8, 9], one-dimensional ergodic diffusions, cf. e.g. Kutoyants [21].

For standard notation and results concerning general theory of processes, stochastic integration and semimartingales we refer to Jacod and Shiryaev [16]. We shall deal with different filtered spaces $(\Omega, \mathscr{F}, \mathbb{F} = (\mathscr{F}_t)_{t \in \mathbb{R}_+})$; the filtration $\mathbb{F}$ is always right-continuous, but no completeness assumption is made, cf. [16]. If P is a probability measure on $(\Omega, \mathscr{F})$ and T is a stopping time relative to $\mathbb{F}$, then P_T is the restriction of P onto $\mathscr{F}_T$. An increasing process is always assumed to be right-continuous. If X is a semimartingale, then X^c is its continuous martingale part and $[X, X]$ is its quadratic variation; the angle brackets $\langle M, M \rangle$ stand for the quadratic characteristic of a locally square-integrable martingale M. The notation $H \cdot X_t = \int_0^t H_s \, dX_s$ and $W \star \mu_t = \int_0^t \int_{\mathbb{R}^d} W(s, x) \, \mu(ds, dx)$ is used for the (ordinary or stochastic) integral processes, where X is a semimartingale and $\mu = \mu(\omega, ds, dx)$ is a random measure on $\mathbb{R}_+ \times \mathbb{R}^d$.

We shall consider also stochastic processes defined only on predictable stochastic intervals of the form $\Gamma = \bigcup_k [\![0, T_k]\!]$, where (T_k) is an increasing sequence of stopping times. We refer to Jacod [12, Chap. 5] for more details on such processes. If X is defined on Γ, then the process $\mathrm{Var}(X)$ is defined also on Γ in the following way: if $(\omega, t) \in \Gamma$ then $\mathrm{Var}(X)_t(\omega)$ is the total variation of $X_{\cdot}(\omega)$ on $[0, t]$.

Let E be a Polish space and $\mathscr{E}$ its Borel σ-field. $\mathscr{P}(E)$ is the space of all probability measures on $(E, \mathscr{E})$ endowed with the weak topology. The distribution of a random element X with values in E under a probability measure P, i.e. the image $\mathsf{P} \circ X^{-1} \in \mathscr{P}(E)$ of P under X, is denoted by $\mathscr{L}(X \mid \mathsf{P})$. The space $\mathbb{D}(E)$ of all càdlàg functions $\alpha : \mathbb{R}_+ \to E$ equipped with the Skorokhod topology is also a Polish space. The Borel σ-field in $\mathbb{D}(E)$ is denoted by $\mathscr{D}(E)$. The corresponding notation $\mathbb{C}(E)$ and $\mathscr{C}(E)$ is used for the space of all continuous functions from $\mathbb{R}_+$ to E equipped with the local uniform topology and its Borel σ-field. If $E = \mathbb{R}$, we shall sometimes write $\mathbb{D}$ and $\mathbb{C}$ instead of $\mathbb{D}(\mathbb{R})$ and $\mathbb{C}(\mathbb{R})$, respectively.

The weak convergence of distributions in $\mathscr{P}(\mathbb{R}^d)$ is denoted by $\Rightarrow$, while the symbol $\xrightarrow{d}$ is used for the weak convergence of distributions in $\mathscr{P}(\mathbb{D}(E))$. To avoid ambiguities, we shall add that the convergence is in $\mathbb{D}(E)$ if $E \neq \mathbb{R}$. On the other hand, the symbol $\xrightarrow{d_f(S)}$ is used for the finite-dimensional convergence along a set S, i.e. $\mathscr{L}(X^n \mid \mathsf{P}^n) \xrightarrow{d_f(S)} \mathscr{L}(X \mid \mathsf{P})$, $n \to \infty$, means that $\mathscr{L}(X^n_{t_1}, \ldots, X^n_{t_p} \mid \mathsf{P}^n) \Rightarrow \mathscr{L}(X_{t_1}, \ldots, X_{t_p} \mid \mathsf{P})$, $n \to \infty$, for any $p = 1, 2, \ldots$ and $t_1, \ldots, t_p \in S$.

We say that a sequence $(X^n \mid \mathsf{P}^n)$ is $\mathbb{D}$-tight if X^n are P^n-a.s. càdlàg processes with values in $\mathbb{R}$ and the laws $\mathscr{L}(X^n \mid \mathsf{P}^n)$ are tight in $\mathbb{D}$; if, moreover, all cluster points of the sequence $\mathcal{L}(X^n \mid \mathsf{P}^n)$ are laws of continuous processes, we say that the sequence $(X^n \mid \mathsf{P}^n)$ is $\mathbb{C}$-tight.

If ξ_n are random variables with values in $[-\infty, +\infty]$ on probability spaces $(\Omega^n, \mathscr{F}^n,$
$\mathsf{P}^n)$, we write

$$\xi_n \xrightarrow{\mathsf{P}^n} 0 \quad \text{if} \quad \lim_{n \to \infty} \mathsf{P}^n(|\xi_n| > \varepsilon) = 0 \quad \text{for every } \varepsilon > 0,$$

and we say that the sequence

$$(\xi_n \mid \mathsf{P}^n) \quad \text{is } \mathbb{R}\text{-tight} \quad \text{if} \quad \lim_{N \uparrow \infty} \limsup_{n \to \infty} \mathsf{P}^n(|\xi_n| > N) = 0.$$

We shall also use this notation even if ξ_n are not well defined everywhere on Ω^n; it is sufficient to assume that ξ_n are defined on subsets $B_n \in \mathscr{F}$ and $\lim_{n \to \infty} \mathsf{P}^n(B_n) = 1$.

If P^n and P'^n are probability measures on measurable spaces $(\Omega^n, \mathscr{F}^n)$, $n = 1, 2, \ldots$, then $(\mathsf{P}^n) \lhd (\mathsf{P}'^n)$ means that the sequence (P^n) is contiguous to the sequence (P'^n).

For probability measures P and P' on the same measurable space the squared Hellinger distance is defined as

$$\rho^2(\mathsf{P}, \mathsf{P}') = \frac{1}{2} \int \left[\left(\frac{d\mathsf{P}}{d\mathsf{Q}} \right)^{1/2} - \left(\frac{d\mathsf{P}'}{d\mathsf{Q}} \right)^{1/2} \right]^2 d\mathsf{Q},$$

where $\mathsf{Q} = \frac{1}{2}(\mathsf{P} + \mathsf{P}')$ (or any other measure dominating P and P').

$\mathbb{M}_+^k$ stands for the set of all symmetric positive semidefinite $k \times k$ matrices, and $\mathscr{S}$ is the set of all bounded sequences in $\mathbb{R}^k$.

2   Quadratic Approximation

In Sect. 2.1, we introduce the objects that are needed to formulate our main result in Sect. 2.2.

2.1   Basic Ingredients

Let $(\Omega^n, \mathscr{F}^n, \mathbb{F}^n = (\mathscr{F}_t^n)_{t \in \mathbb{R}_+}, (\mathsf{P}^{n,\vartheta})_{\vartheta \in \Theta})$ be a sequence of filtered statistical experiments, where $\Theta = \mathbb{R}^k$. Denote $\mathsf{P}^n := \mathsf{P}^{n,0}$. For processes defined on Ω^n stochastic integrals, angle and square brackets, compensators (of increasing processes and random measures) are taken with respect to P^n.

For $\vartheta \in \Theta$ let $Z^{n,\vartheta}$ be the (generalized) density process of $\mathsf{P}^{n,\vartheta}$ with respect to P^n, i.e. a right-continuous (and admitting left-hand limits P^n- and $\mathsf{P}^{n,\vartheta}$-a.s.) adapted process $(Z_t^{n,\vartheta})_{t\in\mathbb{R}_+}$ with values in $[0,\infty]$ such that for any $\mathbb{F}^n$-stopping time T_n

$$\mathsf{P}^{n,\vartheta}(B) = \int_B Z_{T_n}^{n,\vartheta}\, d\mathsf{P}^n + \mathsf{P}^{n,\vartheta}(B \cap \{Z_{T_n}^{n,\vartheta} = \infty\}), \quad B \in \mathscr{F}_{T_n}^n.$$

Of course, $\mathsf{P}^n(Z_{T_n}^{n,\vartheta} < \infty) = 1$ and $Z_{T_n}^{n,\vartheta}$ coincides P^n-a.s. with the Radon–Nikodým derivative of the part of the measure $\mathsf{P}_{T_n}^{n,\vartheta}$ which is absolutely continuous with respect to $\mathsf{P}_{T_n}^n$. Moreover, $Z^{n,\vartheta}$ is a P^n-supermartingale and

$$\mathsf{P}^n(\sup_t Z_t^{n,\vartheta} \geq a) \leq a^{-1} \quad \text{for any } a > 0 \text{ and } \vartheta \in \Theta. \tag{2}$$

Let $T_k^{n,\vartheta} := \inf\{t\colon Z_t^{n,\vartheta} < 1/k\}$ and $\Gamma^{n,\vartheta} := \bigcup_{k=1}^\infty [\![0, T_k^{n,\vartheta}]\!]$, then $\Gamma^{n,\vartheta} = [\![0]\!] \cup \{Z_-^{n,\vartheta} > 0\}$ P^n- and $\mathsf{P}^{n,\vartheta}$-a.s. Put also $T^{n,\vartheta} := T_n^{n,\vartheta}$. Note that the contiguity

$$(\mathsf{P}_{T_n}^n) \lhd (\mathsf{P}_{T_n}^{n,\vartheta_n}), \quad \{\vartheta_n\} \in \mathscr{S},$$

where T_n is an $\mathbb{F}^n$-stopping time for each n, is equivalent to the property

$$\lim_{\varepsilon \downarrow 0} \limsup_{n\to\infty} \mathsf{P}^n(\inf_{s\leq T_n} Z_s^{n,\vartheta_n} < \varepsilon) = 0, \tag{3}$$

see [16, Lemma V.1.19], which implies

$$\lim_{n\to\infty} \mathsf{P}^n(T^{n,\vartheta_n} < T_n) = 0; \tag{4}$$

in particular,

$$\lim_{n\to\infty} \mathsf{P}^n\{\omega\colon (\omega, t) \in \Gamma^{n,\vartheta_n} \text{for all } t \leq T_n(\omega)\} = 1. \tag{5}$$

Put $Y^{n,\vartheta} := \sqrt{Z^{n,\vartheta}}$. The process $Y^{n,\vartheta}$ is a P^n-supermartingale. In what follows, $h^{n,\vartheta}$ and $\iota^{n,\vartheta}$ are *arbitrary* versions of the Hellinger processes $h(\frac{1}{2}; \mathsf{P}^n, \mathsf{P}^{n,\vartheta})$ and $h(0; \mathsf{P}^n, \mathsf{P}^{n,\vartheta})$ of orders $1/2$ and 0, respectively, for P^n and $\mathsf{P}^{n,\vartheta}$. In other words, $h^{n,\vartheta}$ and $\iota^{n,\vartheta}$ are predictable increasing processes with values in $[0,\infty]$ such that $h_0^n = \iota_0^n = 0$,

$$Y^{n,\vartheta} + Y_-^{n,\vartheta} \cdot h^{n,\vartheta} \quad \text{is a } \mathsf{P}^n\text{-martingale.} \tag{6}$$

$$Z^{n,\vartheta} + Z_-^{n,\vartheta} \cdot \iota^{n,\vartheta} \quad \text{is a } \mathsf{P}^n\text{-local martingale.} \tag{7}$$

The processes $h^{n,\vartheta}$ and $\iota^{n,\vartheta}$ are P^n-a.s. unique and finite on $\Gamma^{n,\vartheta}$. If $\mathsf{P}^{n,\vartheta} \overset{\text{loc}}{\ll} \mathsf{P}^n$ then one can take $\iota^{n,\vartheta} = 0$. We refer to Jacod and Shiryaev [16, Chap. IV] for the definition and properties of Hellinger processes and to Gushchin and Valkeila [6] for the above description of $h^{n,\vartheta}$ and $\iota^{n,\vartheta}$.

Define now processes $y^{n,\vartheta}$ and $m^{n,\vartheta}$ on the predictable interval $\Gamma^{n,\vartheta}$ by

$$y^{n,\vartheta} := (1/Y_-^{n,\vartheta}) \cdot Y^{n,\vartheta} \quad \text{and} \quad m^{n,\vartheta} := y^{n,\vartheta} + h^{n,\vartheta}. \tag{8}$$

The process $m^{n,\vartheta}$ is a P^n-locally square-integrable martingale on $\varGamma^{n,\vartheta}$, see Lemma 4.1 in [6]. Define also a stopped process $\widetilde{m}^{n,\vartheta} := (m^{n,\vartheta})^{T^{n,\vartheta}}$, which is a P^n-square-integrable martingale on the whole time interval up to ∞ due to [6, Lemma 4.1] and the definition of $T^{n,\vartheta}$.

If $\vartheta, \eta \in \Theta$, let $h^{n,\vartheta,\eta}$ be an *arbitrary* version of the Hellinger process $h(\frac{1}{2}; \mathsf{P}^{n,\vartheta}, \mathsf{P}^{n,\eta})$ of order $1/2$ for $\mathsf{P}^{n,\vartheta}$ and $\mathsf{P}^{n,\eta}$. It is convenient for us to introduce also a related process $\overline{h}^{n,\vartheta,\eta}$, which is calculated from $Z^{n,\vartheta}$ and $Z^{n,\eta}$ with respect to P^n. Namely, let $\overline{Y}^{n,\vartheta,\eta} := \sqrt{Z^{n,\vartheta} Z^{n,\eta}}$ and define $\overline{h}^{n,\vartheta,\eta}$ as any predictable increasing process with values in $[0, \infty]$ such that $\overline{h}_0^{n,\vartheta,\eta} = 0$ and

$$\overline{Y}^{n,\vartheta,\eta} + \overline{Y}_-^{n,\vartheta,\eta} \cdot \overline{h}^{n,\vartheta,\eta} \quad \text{is a } \mathsf{P}^n\text{-local martingale.} \tag{9}$$

Since $\overline{Y}^{n,\vartheta,\eta}$ is a nonnegative P^n-supermartingale, the existence of $\overline{h}^{n,\vartheta,\eta}$ and its P^n-uniqueness on $\varGamma^{n,\vartheta} \cap \varGamma^{n,\eta}$ follow from standard arguments as in the case of Hellinger processes. If $\mathsf{P}^{n,\vartheta} \overset{\mathrm{loc}}{\ll} \mathsf{P}^n$ and $\mathsf{P}^{n,\eta} \overset{\mathrm{loc}}{\ll} \mathsf{P}^n$, then any version of $h^{n,\vartheta,\eta}$ can be taken as $\overline{h}^{n,\vartheta,\eta}$ and vice versa. It follows from (6) and (9) that one can take $h^{n,\vartheta}$ as $\overline{h}^{n,\vartheta,0}$ and vice versa. Similarly, one can take $\iota^{n,\vartheta}$ as $\overline{h}^{n,\vartheta,\vartheta}$ and vice versa, cf. (7) and (9).

We prefer to use the processes $\overline{h}^{n,\vartheta,\eta}$ in all our results. However, they can be everywhere replaced by $h^{n,\vartheta,\eta}$ as it follows from the proofs and from the next proposition.

Proposition 1 *Let* $(\mathsf{P}_{T_n}^n) \lhd (\mathsf{P}_{T_n}^{n,\vartheta_n})$ *and* $\iota_{T_n}^{n,\vartheta_n} \overset{\mathsf{P}^n}{\longrightarrow} 0$, $n \to \infty$, *for each* $\{\vartheta_n\} \in \mathscr{S}$. *Then*

$$\mathrm{Var}\,(\overline{h}^{n,\vartheta_n,\eta_n} - h^{n,\vartheta_n,\eta_n})_{T_n} \overset{\mathsf{P}^n}{\longrightarrow} 0$$

for all $\{\vartheta_n\}, \{\eta_n\} \in \mathscr{S}$.

The proof of Proposition 1 follows from Lemma 2 and (5).

2.2 Quadratic Approximation

In what follows a sequence $\{T_n\}$ is fixed, where T_n is a stopping time relative to $\mathbb{F}^n$ for every n.

Let us denote by $\mathscr{W}$ the set of all sequences $\{w^n\}$ satisfying the following properties: $w^n = (w^{n,1}, \ldots, w^{n,k})$, $w_0^n = 0$, is a locally square-integrable martingale on $(\Omega^n, \mathscr{F}^n, \mathbb{F}^n, \mathsf{P}^n)$ with values in $\mathbb{R}^k$ for each n,

$$\text{the sequence } \left(\sum_{i=1}^k \langle w^{n,i}, w^{n,i} \rangle_{T_n} \middle| \mathsf{P}^n \right) \text{ is } \mathbb{R}\text{-tight,} \tag{10}$$

and

$$\|x\|^2 \mathbf{1}_{\{\|x\|>\varepsilon\}} \star v_{T_n}^{w^n} \xrightarrow{\mathsf{P}^n} 0, \quad n \to \infty, \quad \text{for all } \varepsilon > 0. \tag{11}$$

Introduce the following assumptions:

(O) For every $\{\vartheta_n\} \in \mathscr{S}$,

$$(\mathsf{P}_0^n) \lhd (\mathsf{P}_0^{n,\vartheta_n})$$

and

$$\iota_{T_n}^{n,\vartheta_n} \xrightarrow{\mathsf{P}^n} 0, \quad n \to \infty. \tag{12}$$

(H) There is a sequence $\{H^n\}$ of random matrices on $(\Omega^n, \mathscr{F}_{T_n}^n)$ with values in $\mathbb{M}_+^k$ such that the sequence $(\operatorname{tr} H^n | \mathsf{P}^n)$ is $\mathbb{R}$-tight and, for all $\{\vartheta_n\}$ and $\{\eta_n\}$ in $\mathscr{S}$,

$$\overline{h}_{T_n}^{n,\vartheta_n,\eta_n} - (\vartheta_n - \eta_n)^\top H^n (\vartheta_n - \eta_n) \xrightarrow{\mathsf{P}^n} 0, \quad n \to \infty. \tag{13}$$

(L) For every $\{\vartheta_n\} \in \mathscr{S}$,

$$x^2 \mathbf{1}_{\{|x|>\varepsilon\}} \star v_{T_n}^{m^{n,\vartheta_n}} \xrightarrow{\mathsf{P}^n} 0, \quad n \to \infty, \quad \text{for all } \varepsilon > 0. \tag{14}$$

(W) There is a sequence $\{w^n\} \in \mathscr{W}$ such that, for each $\{\vartheta_n\} \in \mathscr{S}$,

$$\left\langle m^{n,\vartheta_n} - \frac{1}{2}\vartheta_n^\top w^n, m^{n,\vartheta_n} - \frac{1}{2}\vartheta_n^\top w^n \right\rangle_{T_n} \xrightarrow{\mathsf{P}^n} 0, \quad n \to \infty. \tag{15}$$

Note that conditions (O) and (H) are overlapping: (12) is a special case of (13) with $\eta_n = \vartheta_n$. However, it is not the case if we replace $\overline{h}^{n,\vartheta_n,\eta_n}$ by h^{n,ϑ_n,η_n} in (H).

Theorem 1 (a) *Let conditions* (O), (H), *and* (L) *be satisfied. Then*

$$(\mathsf{P}_{T_n}^n) \lhd (\mathsf{P}_{T_n}^{n,\vartheta_n}) \quad \text{for each } \{\vartheta_n\} \in \mathscr{S} \tag{16}$$

and condition (W) *holds true. Moreover, with* $\{w^n\}$ *from* (W) *we have*

$$\operatorname{Var}\left(\overline{h}^{n,\vartheta_n,\eta_n} - \frac{1}{8}(\vartheta_n - \eta_n)^\top \langle w^n, w^n \rangle (\vartheta_n - \eta_n)\right)_{T_n} \xrightarrow{\mathsf{P}^n} 0, \quad n \to \infty, \tag{17}$$

for all sequences $\{\vartheta_n\}, \{\eta_n\} \in \mathscr{S}$.

(b) *Assume that conditions* (O) *and* (W) *are satisfied. Then we have* (16), (H) *with* $H^n = \frac{1}{8}\langle w^n, w^n \rangle_{T_n}$, *and* (L).

(c) *Assume that conditions* (O) *and* (W) *are satisfied. Then*

$$\sup_{s \le T_n} \left| \log Z_s^{n,\vartheta_n} - \log Z_0^{n,\vartheta_n} - \left(\vartheta_n^\top w_s^n - \frac{1}{2}\vartheta_n^\top \langle w^n, w^n \rangle_s \vartheta_n \right) \right| \xrightarrow{\mathsf{P}^n} 0, \quad n \to \infty, \tag{18}$$

for each $\{\vartheta_n\} \in \mathscr{S}$, *with* $\{w^n\}$ *from* (W).

Remark 1 The contiguity (16) implies

$$\lim_{n \to \infty} \mathsf{P}^n \left(\inf_{s \le T_n} Z_s^{n, \vartheta_n} = 0 \right) = 0,$$

cf. (5). Hence the process $\log Z_s^{n, \vartheta_n} - \log Z_0^{n, \vartheta_n}$, $s \le T_n$, in (18) is well defined and takes finite values on a set, whose P^n-probability tends to 1 as $n \to \infty$.

Remark 2 The processes in conditions (O), (L) and (W) are P^n-a.s. uniquely defined only on the set Γ^{n, ϑ_n}, and the process $\overline{h}^{n, \vartheta_n, \eta_n}$ in (H) is P^n-a.s. unique on the set $\Gamma^{n, \vartheta_n} \cap \Gamma^{n, \eta_n}$. Theorem 1 says that in order to obtain its statement, in particular, the contiguity (16), it is sufficient to check its assumptions for some versions of these processes. On the other hand, as soon as the contiguity (16) is established, these conditions do not depend on the choice of corresponding versions, see (5).

Remark 3 In Theorem 1 and all subsequent theorems, one can replace the measure $\nu^{m^{n, \vartheta_n}}$ by the measure $\nu^{y^{n, \vartheta_n}}$ in the Lindeberg-type condition (14). This follows from the proofs and from Proposition 2.6 in [6]. For connections between condition (14) and some other conditions see [6].

Remark 4 Let $(\mathsf{P}_0^{n, \vartheta_n}) \lhd (\mathsf{P}_0^n)$. We cannot assert under the assumptions of Theorem 1 that $(\mathsf{P}_{T_n}^{n, \vartheta_n}) \lhd (\mathsf{P}_{T_n}^n)$. A simple modification of our Example 6.1 in [6] yields a counterexample.

It is clear that if (W) is satisfied with some $\{w^n\}$ and we have another sequence $\{w'^n\}$, each $w'^n = (w'^{n, 1}, \ldots, w'^{n, k})$, $w_0'^n = 0$, being a locally square-integrable martingale on $(\Omega^n, \mathscr{F}^n, \mathbb{F}^n, \mathsf{P}^n)$, such that

$$\sum_{i=1}^{k} \langle w^{n, i} - w'^{n, i}, w^{n, i} - w'^{n, i} \rangle_{T_n} \xrightarrow{\mathsf{P}^n} 0, \quad n \to \infty, \tag{19}$$

then $\{w'^n\} \in \mathscr{W}$ and (15) holds with w'^n instead of w^n. But (19) is a special case of (15). This simple observation shows that the following choice of $\{w^n\}$ is always possible in (W) if this condition is satisfied with some $\{w^n\}$ and $(\mathsf{P}_{T_n}^n) \lhd (\mathsf{P}_{T_n}^{n, \vartheta_n})$, $\{\vartheta_n\} \in \mathscr{S}$. Namely, $w^n = (w^{n, 1}, \ldots, w^{n, k})$ can be defined as follows:

$$w^{n, i} = 2\widetilde{m}^{n, e_i}, \quad i = 1, \ldots, k, \tag{20}$$

where the processes $\widetilde{m}^{n, \vartheta}$ are defined after (8) and $e_1, \ldots, e_k$ are coordinate unit vectors. Moreover, this sequence has an additional property that each w^n is a P^n-square-integrable martingale.

The next proposition gives an equivalent form of condition (H). The statement is simple and of little interest by itself, and we leave its proof to the reader. The reason for which we present it here, is that it is connected with a much more difficult problem of characterizing filtered statistical models admitting approximations of the form (44) with (43) but without assumption (42). For a nonfiltered version of this problem, see [5, Theorem 4.1].

Proposition 2 *Assume that conditions* (O) *and* (L) *are satisfied. Then condition* (H) *holds if and only if*

$$\text{the sequence } (h_{T_n}^{n,\vartheta_n}|\mathbf{P}^n) \text{ is } \mathbb{R}\text{-tight}$$

and

$$\alpha \overline{h}_{T_n}^{n,\vartheta_n,\alpha\vartheta_n+(1-\alpha)\eta_n} + (1-\alpha)\overline{h}_{T_n}^{n,\eta_n,\alpha\vartheta_n+(1-\alpha)\eta_n} - \alpha(1-\alpha)\overline{h}_{T_n}^{n,\vartheta_n,\eta_n} \xrightarrow{\mathbf{P}^n} 0$$

for all $\alpha \in (0,1)$ and all $\{\vartheta_n\}, \{\eta_n\} \in \mathscr{S}$.

3   Limit Theorems

We consider the same setting as in Sect. 2. We are given a sequence $(\Omega^n, \mathscr{F}^n, \mathbb{F}^n = (\mathscr{F}_t^n)_{t\in\mathbb{R}_+}, (\mathbf{P}^{n,\vartheta})_{\vartheta\in\Theta})$ of filtered statistical experiments, where $\Theta = \mathbb{R}^k$, and, for every n, an $\mathbb{F}^n$-stopping time T_n. $\mathbb{E}_{T_n}^n$ stands for the (nonfiltered) statistical experiment $(\Omega^n, \mathscr{F}_{T_n}^n, (\mathbf{P}_{T_n}^{n,\vartheta})_{\vartheta\in\Theta})$.

3.1   Preliminaries

In this subsection, we recall the definitions of the properties that we want to obtain additionally to the conclusion of Theorem 1. As it was explained in introduction, it is tacitly assumed that a proper rescaling of the parameter space is already done, so ϑ is a local parameter. This is why we omit the letter 'L' in the abbreviations. The first definition is of preparatory character. It includes properties that we already know how to prove. Statistically meaningful concepts appear in the next definitions.

Definition 1 The sequence $\{\mathbb{E}_{T_n}^n\}$ is said to admit a quadratic approximation for the log-likelihood ratios if

$$(\mathbf{P}_{T_n}^n) \lhd (\mathbf{P}_{T_n}^{n,\vartheta}) \quad \text{for every } \vartheta \in \Theta \tag{21}$$

and there are $\mathscr{F}_{T_n}$-measurable random vectors V_n with values in $\mathbb{R}^k$ and random matrices K_n with values in $\mathbb{M}_+^k$ such that, for each $\{\vartheta_n\} \in \mathscr{S}$,

$$\log Z_{T_n}^{n,\vartheta_n} - \left(\vartheta_n^\top V_n - \frac{1}{2}\vartheta_n^\top K_n \vartheta_n \right) \xrightarrow{\mathbf{P}^n} 0, \quad n \to \infty. \tag{22}$$

Remark 5 The contiguity (21) is equivalent to the property that the sequence of distributions $\mathscr{L}(\log Z_{T_n}^{n,\vartheta} | \mathsf{P}^n)$ is $\mathbb{R}$-tight, and then it follows easily from (22) that the sequence $\mathscr{L}(V_n, K_n | \mathsf{P}^n)$ is $\mathbb{R}^{k+k^2}$-tight. Conversely, if we have (22) and the sequence $\mathscr{L}(V_n, K_n | \mathsf{P}^n)$ is tight, then

$$(\mathsf{P}_{T_n}^n) \lhd (\mathsf{P}_{T_n}^{n,\vartheta_n}) \quad \text{for each } \{\vartheta_n\} \in \mathscr{S}.$$

Definition 2 The sequence $\{\mathbb{E}_{T_n}^n\}$ is said to be asymptotically quadratic (AQ) if it satisfies Definition 1,

$$(\mathsf{P}_{T_n}^{n,\vartheta}) \lhd (\mathsf{P}_{T_n}^n) \quad \text{for every } \vartheta \in \Theta, \tag{23}$$

and for any cluster point $\mathscr{L}(K)$ of $\mathscr{L}(K_n | \mathsf{P}^n)$ the matrix K is almost surely invertible.

Remark 6 If we have (21) and (22), then, by Le Cam's first lemma, the contiguity (23) is equivalent to

$$\mathsf{E} \exp\left(\vartheta^\top V - \frac{1}{2}\vartheta^\top K\vartheta\right) = 1 \tag{24}$$

for any cluster point $\mathscr{L}(V, K)$ of $\mathscr{L}(V_n, K_n | \mathsf{P}^n)$. Therefore, if the sequence $\{\mathbb{E}_{T_n}^n\}$ is AQ, then

$$(\mathsf{P}_{T_n}^n) \lhd \rhd (\mathsf{P}_{T_n}^{n,\vartheta_n}) \quad \text{for each } \{\vartheta_n\} \in \mathscr{S}.$$

Definition 3 The sequence $\{\mathbb{E}_{T_n}^n\}$ is said to be asymptotically mixed normal (AMN) if it satisfies Definition 1 and for any cluster point $\mathscr{L}(V, K)$ of the sequence $\mathscr{L}(V_n, K_n | \mathsf{P}^n)$, the matrix K is almost surely invertible and, conditionally on K, the vector V is normal with zero mean and the covariance matrix K.

Remark 7 AMN implies AQ. Indeed, if the sequence $\{\mathbb{E}_{T_n}^n\}$ is AMN, then (24) is automatically satisfied, and we have (23) due to the previous remark.

Definition 4 The sequence $\{\mathbb{E}_{T_n}^n\}$ is said to be asymptotically normal (AN) if it satisfies Definition 1 and for any cluster point $\mathscr{L}(V, K)$ of the sequence $\mathscr{L}(V_n, K_n | \mathsf{P}^n)$, the matrix K is deterministic and invertible, and the vector V is normal with zero mean and the covariance matrix K.

It is clear that AN is a special case of AMN and, hence, of AQ. In what follows, it is convenient for us to have a relaxed form of AN. Namely, let us say, that the sequence $\{\mathbb{E}_{T_n}^n\}$ is asymptotically normal* (AN*) if it satisfies all the requirements of Definition 4 except that K is invertible.

Our definition of AQ, AMN, and AN are in accordance with the definitions of LAQ, LAMN, and LAN in Le Cam and Yang [27, pp. 120–121]. It is more usual, especially in the case of asymptotic normality, to require convergence in law of distributions $\mathscr{L}(V_n, K_n | \mathsf{P}^n)$. Under the assumptions of Theorems 2–6 below such convergence does take place.

3.2 Asymptotic Normality

In this subsection, we state two results concerning asymptotic normality. Instead of
(O), we assume the following stronger hypothesis:

(O*) For every $\{\vartheta_n\} \in \mathscr{S}$, we have (12) and $Z_0^{n,\vartheta_n} \xrightarrow{\mathsf{P}^n} 1$.

This is not harmless because conditions (14) or (11) do not allow us to change time
$t \rightsquigarrow t + 1$ and to put $\mathscr{F}_t^n$ = trivial σ-field for $t < 1$. However, it is possible to work
under condition (O) in Theorems 2 and 3 if one assumes additionally that $\Omega^n \equiv \Omega$
and the densities $Z_0^{n,\vartheta}$ are $\bigcap_n \mathscr{F}_0^n$-measurable. In such a case, one obtains (with no
changes in the proofs) that the convergence in (26) and (30) is $\bigcap_n \mathscr{F}_0^n$-mixing, see
Liptser and Shiryayev [29, Theorems 5.5.4 and 7.1.4] and also Jacod and Shiryaev
[16, Chap. VIII, Sect. 5]. Therefore, the variables $\log Z_0^{n,\vartheta_n}$ and the processes w^n in
(18) are asymptotically independent under P^n. We leave details to the reader.

Theorem 2 *Let conditions (O*) and (L) be satisfied and (H) hold with $H^n \equiv H$,
where $H = (H^{ij})_{i,j=1,\dots,k}$ is a deterministic matrix. Then*

$$(\mathsf{P}_{T_n}^n) \lhd \rhd (\mathsf{P}_{T_n}^{n,\vartheta_n}) \quad \text{for each } \{\vartheta_n\} \in \mathscr{S} \tag{25}$$

and there is a sequence $\{w^n\} \in \mathscr{W}(\{T_n\})$ such that

$$\mathscr{L}(w_{T_n}^n | \mathsf{P}^n) \Rightarrow \mathscr{N}(0, 8H) \tag{26}$$

and

$$\langle w^{n,i}, w^{n,j} \rangle_{T_n} \xrightarrow{\mathsf{P}^n} 8H^{ij}, \quad i,j = 1,\dots,k, \tag{27}$$

as $n \to \infty$, and

$$\sup_{s \le T_n} \left| \log Z_s^{n,\vartheta_n} - \left(\vartheta_n^\top w_s^n - \frac{1}{2} \vartheta_n^\top \langle w^n, w^n \rangle_s \vartheta_n^\top \right) \right| \xrightarrow{\mathsf{P}^n} 0, \quad n \to \infty, \tag{28}$$

for each $\{\vartheta_n\} \in \mathscr{S}$. The sequence $\mathbb{E}_{T_n}^n$ is asymptotically normal if H is nonsingular.

Assume that $t \rightsquigarrow H_t$, $H_t = (H_t^{ij})$ is a continuous increasing function with values
in $\mathbb{M}_+^k$, $H_0 = 0$, M is a continuous Gaussian martingale with values in $\mathbb{R}^k$ with
$M_0 = 0$ and $\langle M^i, M^j \rangle_t = 8H_t^{ij}$, $i,j = 1,\dots,k$, $t \in [0, T]$, on some stochastic basis
$(\Omega, \mathscr{F}, \mathbb{F}, \mathbb{P})$.

Theorem 3 *Let $T \in \mathbb{R}_+$ and $T_n \equiv T$. Assume that (O*), (H) and (L) are satisfied
and*

$$h_t^{n,\vartheta} \xrightarrow{\mathsf{P}^n} \vartheta^\top H_t \vartheta, \quad n \to \infty, \quad \text{for all } t \in S \text{ and } \vartheta \in \Theta, \tag{29}$$

*where S is a dense subset of $[0, T]$ containing 0 and T. Then (25) holds and there is
a sequence $\{w^n\} \in \mathscr{W}(\{T_n\})$ such that*

$$\mathcal{L}(w^n|\mathsf{P}^n) \xrightarrow{d} \mathcal{L}(M|\mathsf{P}), \quad n \to \infty, \quad in \ \mathbb{D}([0, T], \mathbb{R}^k), \tag{30}$$

$$\sup_{s \leq T} \left| \langle w^{n,i}, w^{n,j} \rangle_s - 8H_s^{ij} \right| \xrightarrow{\mathsf{P}^n} 0, \quad n \to \infty, \quad i, j = 1, \ldots, k, \tag{31}$$

and (28) holds for each $\{\vartheta_n\} \in \mathcal{S}$. The sequence $\mathbb{E}_t^n$, $t \in (0, T]$, is asymptotically normal if H_t is nonsingular.

A converse (in a sense) statement is given in Theorem 8.

As a simple exercise, we leave to the reader the question what has to be added to conditions (O^*) and (W) to obtain the same conclusions as in Theorems 2 and 3.

3.3 Asymptotic Mixed Normality

In contrast to wide applicability of the results in the previous subsection, Theorems 4 and 5 below are restricted to particular (L)AMN situations, where the Hellinger process for the limit model can be defined on the space of the original experiments and there is the convergence in probability of the Hellinger processes. There are broad classes of examples where (L)AMN occurs, but the Helinger processes converge only in law.

We impose the following assumptions.

First, the *nesting* condition is satisfied: $\Omega^n = \Omega$, $\mathcal{F}^n = \mathcal{F}$, and $\mathsf{P}^n = \mathsf{P}$ for every n, and there is a sequence of numbers (s_n), decreasing to 0, such that $\mathcal{F}_{s_n}^n \subseteq \mathcal{F}_{s_{n+1}}^{n+1}$ for all n and $\mathcal{G} := \bigvee_n \mathcal{F}_\infty^n = \bigvee_n \mathcal{F}_{s_n}^n$.

Second, there is given a continuous increasing process $C = (C_t)_{t \in \mathbb{R}_+}$ with values in $\mathbb{M}_+^k$ such that $C_0 = 0$ and C_t are $\mathcal{G}$-measurable for all t. Let $\mathbb{C} = \mathbb{C}(\mathbb{R}^k)$ be the space of continuous functions $\alpha = (\alpha(t))$ on $\mathbb{R}_+$ with values in $\mathbb{M}_+^k$ and $\mathcal{C}$ the Borel σ-field on $\mathbb{C}$. Let X be the canonical process on $\mathbb{C}$, i.e. $X_t(\alpha) = \alpha(t)$. For every $\vartheta \in \Theta$, there is a Markov kernel $\mathsf{Q}^\vartheta(\omega, d\alpha)$ from $(\Omega, \mathcal{G})$ into $(\mathbb{C}, \mathcal{C})$ such that for each $\omega \in \Omega$ $X_0 = 0$ $\mathsf{Q}^\vartheta(\omega, d\alpha)$-a.s. and $X_t - \vartheta^\top C_t(\omega)$ is a continuous Gaussian martingale under $\mathsf{Q}^\vartheta(\omega, d\alpha)$ with the quadratic characteristic $C_t(\omega)$. Put $\mathsf{P}^\vartheta(d\omega, d\alpha) = \mathsf{P}(d\omega)\mathsf{Q}^\vartheta(\omega, d\alpha)$, $\mathsf{P} = \mathsf{P}^0$. Consider the filtered model $(\Omega \times \mathbb{C}, \mathcal{G} \otimes \mathcal{C}, \mathbf{F}, (\mathsf{P}^\vartheta)_{\vartheta \in \Theta})$, where $\mathbf{F} = (\mathcal{F}_t)$ is the smallest filtration of $\Omega \times \mathbb{C}$ to which X (naturally extended to $\Omega \times \mathbb{C}$) is adapted and such that $\mathcal{G} \subseteq \mathcal{F}_0$. It is clear that $\mathsf{P}^\vartheta \overset{loc}{\sim} \mathsf{P}$ and the density process $Z^\vartheta = (Z_t^\vartheta(\omega, \alpha))$ is given by

$$Z_t^\vartheta(\omega, \alpha) = \exp(\vartheta^\top X_t(\omega) - \frac{1}{2}\vartheta^\top C_t(\alpha)\vartheta).$$

We use the notion of $\mathcal{G}$-stable convergence in the same sense as in [6].

Theorem 4 *Assume that the above assumptions are satisfied. Let $T \in \mathbb{R}_+$ and $T_n \equiv T$. Assume that conditions (O*) and (L) are satisfied and (H) holds with $H^n \equiv \frac{1}{8}C_T$. Moreover, assume that $h_{s_n}^{n,\vartheta} \xrightarrow{\mathsf{P}} 0$, $n \to \infty$, for each $\vartheta \in \Theta$. Then*

$$(\mathsf{P}_{T_n}^n) \vartriangleleft \vartriangleright (\mathsf{P}_{T_n}^{n,\vartheta_n}) \quad \text{for each } \{\vartheta_n\} \in \mathscr{S} \tag{32}$$

and there is a sequence $\{w^n\} \in \mathscr{W}$ such that

$$\mathscr{L}(w_{T_n}^n, \langle w^n, w^n \rangle_{T_n} | \mathsf{P}) \Rightarrow \mathscr{L}(X_T, C_T | \mathsf{P})), \quad n \to \infty, \quad (\mathscr{G}\text{-stably}) \tag{33}$$

and

$$\sup_{s \le T_n} \left| \log Z_s^{n,\vartheta_n} - \left(\vartheta_n^\top w_s^n - \frac{1}{2} \vartheta_n^\top \langle w^n, w^n \rangle_s \vartheta_n^\top \right) \right| \xrightarrow{\mathsf{P}^n} 0, \quad n \to \infty, \tag{34}$$

for each $\{\vartheta_n\} \in \mathscr{S}$. The sequence $\mathbb{E}_{T_n}^n$ is asymptotically mixed normal if C_T is P-a.s. nonsingular.

Theorem 5 *Assume that the above assumptions are satisfied. Let $T \in \mathbb{R}_+$ and $T_n \equiv T$. Assume that (O*), (H), and (L) are satisfied and*

$$h_t^{n,\vartheta} \xrightarrow{\mathsf{P}} \frac{1}{8} \vartheta^\top C_t \vartheta, \quad n \to \infty, \quad \text{for all } t \in S \text{ and } \vartheta \in \Theta,$$

where S is a dense subset of $[0, T]$ containing 0 and T. Then (32) holds and there is a sequence $\{w^n\} \in \mathscr{W}(\{T_n\})$ such that

$$\mathscr{L}(w^n, \langle w^n, w^n \rangle | \mathsf{P}) \xrightarrow{d} \mathscr{L}(X, C | \mathsf{P}), \quad n \to \infty, \quad (\mathscr{G}\text{-stably})$$

in $\mathbb{D}([0, T], \mathbb{R}^{k+k^2})$, and (34) holds for each $\{\vartheta_n\} \in \mathscr{S}$. The sequence $\mathbb{E}_t^n$, $t \in (0, T]$, is asymptotically mixed normal if C_t is P-a.s. nonsingular.

3.4 Asymptotic Quadraticity

In this subsection, we consider a general sequence $(\Omega^n, \mathscr{F}^n, \mathbb{F}^n = (\mathscr{F}_t^n)_{t \in \mathbb{R}_+}$, $(\mathsf{P}^{n,\vartheta})_{\vartheta \in \Theta})$ of filtered statistical experiments, where $\Theta = \mathbb{R}^k$, as in Sect. 2. We are interested in the case where the limiting density process is of the form $\mathscr{E}(\vartheta^\top M)$, M being a continuous local martingale (not necessarily Gaussian or conditionally Gaussian). General limit theorems for likelihood processes, corresponding to such a limit, e.g. Theorems X.1.59 and X.1.65 in Jacod and Shiryaev [16] and Theorem 3.9

in Gushchin and Valkeila [6], have certain drawbacks. First, the majoration conditions X.1.57 (c) in [16] and M (c) in [6] are quite restrictive. Second, in many models
the process M happens to be of the form $\int K\,dB$, where B is a Brownian motion and
K is adapted with respect to the filtration $\mathbb{F}^B$ generated by B. Thus, it is inconvenient
to represent the quadratic characteristic of M as a functional of M or of the density
process as is needed in the above-mentioned theorems.

In Theorem 6 below, we have tried to avoid these drawbacks. Though a majoration
condition is still imposed, it refers to another process which is a Gaussian martingale
in many applications, and then the condition is trivially satisfied. However, this
theorem is oriented towards rather specific models in the broad range of (L)AQ
situations.

Introduce the following assumptions:

(B) (a) $(\Omega, \mathscr{F}, \mathbb{F}) = (\mathbb{D}(\mathbb{R}^q), \mathscr{D}(\mathbb{R}^q), \mathscr{D}(\mathbb{R}^q))$ is the Skorokhod space with the
Borel σ-field $\mathscr{D}(\mathbb{R}^q)$ and the filtration $\mathscr{D}(\mathbb{R}^q)$ generated by the canonical process
denoted by B.
(b) $C = (C^{ij})_{i,j \leq q}$ is an adapted continuous increasing process with values in
$\mathbb{M}_+^q$, defined on $(\Omega, \mathscr{F}, \mathbb{F})$, $C_0 = 0$.
(c) There is a continuous and deterministic increasing function $t \rightsquigarrow F_t$ with
$F_0 = 0$, such that $F - \sum_{i=1}^{q} C^{ii}(\alpha)$ is nondecreasing for all $\alpha \in \Omega$.
(d) $\alpha \rightsquigarrow C_t(\alpha)$ is Skorokhod-continuous for all $t \in \mathbb{R}_+$.
(e) There is a unique probability measure P on $(\Omega, \mathscr{F})$ under which B is a
continuous local martingale with $B_0 = 0$ and $\langle B, B \rangle = C$.
(G) (a) There are adapted càdlàg processes $G^n = (G^{n,ij})_{i \leq k,\, j \leq q}$ and $G =$
$(G^{ij})_{i \leq k,\, j \leq q}$ with values in $\mathbb{R}^{k \times q}$, defined on $(\Omega, \mathscr{F}, \mathbb{F})$.
(b) If $\alpha_n \to \alpha \in \mathbb{C}(\mathbb{R}^q)$ in the Skorokhod topology on $\mathbb{D}(\mathbb{R}^q)$ (i.e. locally uniformly), then $G^n(\alpha_n) \to G(\alpha)$ in the Skorokhod topology on $\mathbb{D}(\mathbb{R}^{k \times q})$.

It follows from (B) (c) that there is a predictable process $c = (c^{ij})_{i,j \leq q}$ with values
in $\mathbb{M}_+^q$, defined on $(\Omega, \mathscr{F}, \mathbb{F})$, such that $C_t^{ij} = c^{ij} \cdot F_t, i, j \leq q$, and $\operatorname{tr} c_t \leq 1$ for all
$t \in \mathbb{R}_+$ P-a.s.

In what follows, we use the notation $G^n \circ B^n$, which is understood as the
composition of the mappings $B^n \colon \Omega^n \to \Omega$ and $G^n \colon \Omega \to \mathbb{D}(\mathbb{R}^{k \times q})$. Note that
$G \circ B = G$. For a $(k \times q)$-dimensional adapted càdlàg process $K = (K^{ij})_{i \leq k,\, j \leq q}$
and a q-dimensional locally square-integrable martingale $M = (M^j)_{j \leq q}$, the process
$Y := K_- \cdot M$ is understood as a k-dimensional locally square-integrable martingale
$Y = (Y^i)_{i \leq k}$ such that $Y^i = \sum_{j=1}^{q} K_-^{ij} \cdot M^j$.

Theorem 6 (i) *Let* (O*), (B), *and* (G) *be satisfied,* $T \in \mathbb{R}_+$ *and* $T_n \equiv T$. *Assume that
there is a sequence* $\{B^n\}$ *such that the following holds:* $B^n = (B^{n,j})_{j \leq q}$, $B_0^n = 0$, *is
a locally square-integrable martingale on* $(\Omega^n, \mathscr{F}^n, \mathbb{F}^n, \mathsf{P}^n)$ *with values in* $\mathbb{R}^q$ *for
each* n,

$$\langle B^n, B^n \rangle_t - C_t \circ B^n \xrightarrow{\mathsf{P}^n} 0, \quad n \to \infty, \quad \text{for all } t \in S, \tag{35}$$

where S is a dense subset of $[0, T]$ *containing* 0 *and* T,

$$\|x\|^2 \mathbf{1}_{\{\|x\|>\varepsilon\}} \star v_T^{B^n} \xrightarrow{\mathsf{P}^n} 0, \quad n \to \infty, \quad \text{for all } \varepsilon > 0, \tag{36}$$

and

$$\left\langle m^{n,\vartheta_n} - \frac{1}{2}\vartheta_n^\top w^n, m^{n,\vartheta_n} - \frac{1}{2}\vartheta_n^\top w^n \right\rangle_T \xrightarrow{\mathsf{P}^n} 0, \quad n \to \infty, \tag{37}$$

for each $\{\vartheta_n\} \in \mathcal{S}$, *where* $w^n := K_-^n \cdot B^n$, $K^n := G^n \circ B^n$. *Then* $\{w^n\} \in \mathcal{W}$ *and* (W) *is satisfied,*

$$(\mathsf{P}_T^n) \lhd (\mathsf{P}_T^{n,\vartheta_n}) \quad \text{for each } \{\vartheta_n\} \in \mathcal{S}, \tag{38}$$

$$\mathscr{L}(w^n, \langle w^n, w^n \rangle | \mathsf{P}^n) \xrightarrow{d} \mathscr{L}(G_- \cdot B, (G_-cG_-^\top) \cdot F | \mathsf{P}), \quad n \to \infty, \quad \text{in } \mathbb{D}([0, T], \mathbb{R}^{k+k^2}), \tag{39}$$

and

$$\sup_{s \le T} \left| \log Z_s^{n,\vartheta_n} - \left(\vartheta_n^\top w_s^n - \frac{1}{2}\vartheta_n^\top \langle w^n, w^n \rangle_s \vartheta_n^\top \right) \right| \xrightarrow{\mathsf{P}^n} 0, \quad n \to \infty,$$

for each $\{\vartheta_n\} \in \mathcal{S}$.

(ii) *Assume additionally that*

$$\mathsf{E} \exp \left((\vartheta^\top G_-) \cdot B_T - \frac{1}{2}(\vartheta^\top G_-cG_-^\top \vartheta) \cdot F_T \right) = 1 \tag{40}$$

for any $\vartheta \in \mathbb{R}^k$. *Then*

$$(\mathsf{P}_T^n) \lhd \rhd (\mathsf{P}_T^{n,\vartheta_n}) \quad \text{for each } \{\vartheta_n\} \in \mathcal{S},$$

Assumption (40) *is automatically satisfied if* G *is a Gaussian process on* $(\Omega, \mathcal{F}, \mathsf{P})$.

(iii) *Assume additionally to* (i) *and* (ii) *that* $(G_-cG_-^\top) \cdot F_t$, $t \in (0, T]$, *is* P-*a.s. nonsingular. Then the sequence* $\mathbb{E}_t^n$ *is asymptotically quadratic.*

Remark 8 A sufficient condition for the process G to be Gaussian on $(\Omega, \mathcal{F}, \mathsf{P})$, see (ii), is that C is a deterministic function (so B is a Gaussian martingale) and $G^{ij}(\alpha)_t = \sum_{l=1}^q \int_0^t \alpha^l(s) \zeta_l(ds)$ for all $t \in \mathbb{R}$, $\alpha \in \mathbb{C}(\mathbb{R}^q)$, $i \le k$, $j \le q$, where ζ_l is a finite signed measure on $[0, t]$, depending in general also on t, i, and j.

4 Necessity of Conditions

In this section, we state three theorems demonstrating the necessity of conditions in the theorems in Sects. 2 and 3. The first theorem says, in particular, that if one assumes the mutual contiguity (41), then the conditions of Theorem 1 are satisfied if and only if there exists an approximation (44) with (43) and condition (42) of asymptotic negligibility of jumps of likelihood ratio processes holds true. Recall that the conditions of Theorem 1 imply (42), see Propositions 2.6 and 2.8 in [6].

Theorem 7 *Let*

$$(\mathsf{P}_{T_n}^{n,\vartheta_n}) \vartriangleleft \vartriangleright (\mathsf{P}_{T_n}^{n}) \tag{41}$$

and

$$\sup_{s \leq T_n} |\Delta Z_s^{n,\vartheta_n}| \xrightarrow{\mathsf{P}^n} 0, \quad n \to \infty, \tag{42}$$

for each $\{\vartheta_n\} \in \mathscr{S}$. Assume also that there exist càdlàg processes X^n with values in $\mathbb{R}^k$ and predictable processes $B^{n,\vartheta}$ with finite variation such that for every $\{\vartheta_n\} \in \mathscr{S}$

$$\text{the sequence} \quad \left(\text{Var}\,(B^{n,\vartheta})_{T_n}\big|\mathsf{P}^n\right) \quad \text{is } \mathbb{R}\text{-tight}, \tag{43}$$

and

$$\sup_{s \leq T_n} \left|\log Z_s^{n,\vartheta_n} - \log Z_0^{n,\vartheta_n} - \left(\vartheta_n^\top X_s^n - B_s^{n,\vartheta_n}\right)\right| \xrightarrow{\mathsf{P}^n} 0, \quad n \to \infty. \tag{44}$$

Then assumptions (O), (H), (L), and (W) of Sect. 2.2 are satisfied. In particular, by Theorem 1 there is a sequence $\{w^n\} \in \mathscr{W}(\{T_n\})$ of P^n-locally square-integrable martingales such that one can replace X^n by w^n and B^{n,ϑ_n} by $\vartheta_n^\top \langle w^n, w^n \rangle \vartheta_n$ in (44).

The next theorem says that if at every time t (here it is assumed that $T_n \equiv T$ and deterministic), our models are asymptotically normal* and the limiting models are continuous in t (this condition replaces (42)), then all assumptions of Theorem 1 are satisfied. It is assumed that there is given a continuous increasing function $K_t = (K_t^{ij})$, $t \in [0, T]$, with values in $\mathbb{M}_+^k$. Denote by N a continuous Gaussian martingale with values in $\mathbb{R}^k$ on some stochastic basis $(\Omega, \mathscr{F}, \mathbb{F}, \mathsf{P})$ with $\mathscr{L}(N_0|\mathsf{P}) = \mathscr{N}(0, K_0)$ and $\langle N^i, N^j \rangle_t = K_t^{ij} - K_0^{ij}$, $i, j = 1, \ldots, k$, $t \in [0, T]$.

Theorem 8 *Let $T \in \mathbb{R}_+$ and $T_n \equiv T$. Assume that, for every $t \in S$, where S is a dense subset of $[0, T]$ containing 0 and T, the sequence $\mathbb{E}_t^n$ of experiments is asymptotically normal* with random vectors $V_n = V_t^n$ and random matrices $K_n = K_t^n$, and $K_t^n \xrightarrow{\mathsf{P}^n} K_t$, $n \to \infty$. Then conditions (O), (H), (L) and (W) of Sect. 2.2 are satisfied,*

$$\mathscr{L}(w^n|\mathsf{P}^n) \xrightarrow{d} \mathscr{L}(N - N_0|\mathsf{P}), \quad n \to \infty, \quad \text{in } \mathbb{D}([0, T], \mathbb{R}^k), \tag{45}$$

$$\sup_{s \leq T} \left|\langle w^{n,i}, w^{n,j} \rangle_s - (K_s^{ij} - K_0^{ij})\right| \xrightarrow{\mathsf{P}^n} 0, \quad n \to \infty, \quad i, j = 1, \ldots, k, \tag{46}$$

V_0^n and $(w^n)_{t \in [0,T]}$ are asymptotically independent under P^n and

$$\sup_{s \leq T} \left|\log Z_s^{n,\vartheta_n} - \left(\vartheta_n^\top (V_0^n + w_s^n) - \frac{1}{2}\vartheta_n^\top \left(K_0^n + \langle w^n, w^n \rangle_s\right)\vartheta_n\right)\right| \xrightarrow{\mathsf{P}^n} 0, \quad n \to \infty, \tag{47}$$

for each $\{\vartheta_n\} \in \mathscr{S}$.

This theorem should be also compared with Theorem 5.3 in Strasser [37].

In the last theorem, in contrast to the previous one, we assume asymptotic normality* only at terminal times and impose condition (42) again. Moreover, we introduce the following additional assumption:

(D) For every $\{\vartheta_n\}$ and $\{\eta_n\}$ in $\mathscr{S}$ the sequence $h_{T_n}^{n,\vartheta_n,\eta_n}$ is asymptotically degenerate, i.e. every subsequence contains a further subsequence tending to a nonrandom limit in P^{n,η_n}-probability.

Of course, (D) is satisfied if all the processes $h^{n,\vartheta,\eta}$ admit deterministic versions and T_n are deterministic, in particular, if our experiments correspond to independent observations on a nonrandom time interval. For a detailed discussion of the property of all the Hellinger processes to be deterministic, we refer to Jacod [13].

Theorem 9 *Assume that the sequence* $\{\mathbb{E}_{T_n}^n\}$ *is asymptotically normal**, $Z_0^{n,\vartheta_n} \xrightarrow{\mathsf{P}^n} 1$ *for every* $\{\vartheta_n\} \in \mathscr{S}$, *and conditions* (42) *and* (D) *hold. Then assumptions* (O), (H), (L), *and* (W) *of Sect. 2.2 are satisfied and we have the uniform in s approximation* (18) *with* $\{w^n\} \in \mathscr{W}(\{T_n\})$.

Remark 9 In the case $k = 1$, we are able to prove the same statement replacing assumption (D) by a weaker one, namely, that $h_{T_n}^{n,\vartheta_n}$ are asymptotically degenerate for each $\{\vartheta_n\} \in \mathscr{S}$. The proof is much more laborious and is not given here.

5 Independent Observations

In this section, we consider a special case where our experiments have a product structure. We show that the quadratic approximation (1) is necessary for the LAN property under a standard additional assumption, see (54) below. This assumption is not needed if the factors in every experiment are copies of each other (but may be different in different experiments). Thus, in such a case the quadratic approximation (1) always takes place if the LAN occurs.

We assume throughout this section that an open subset Θ of $\mathbb{R}^k$ is given. Let $\left(X_i^n, \mathscr{X}_i^n, (\mathsf{Q}_i^{n,\vartheta})_{\vartheta \in \Theta}\right)$ be statistical models, $i = 1, 2, \ldots, k_n$, $n = 1, 2, \ldots, k_n \to \infty$ as $n \to \infty$. For simplicity of notation, we shall assume that $k_n = n$. Put

$$\Omega^n = \prod_{i=1}^n X_i^n, \quad \mathscr{F}^n = \bigotimes_{i=1}^n \mathscr{X}_i^n, \quad \mathsf{P}^{n,\vartheta} = \prod_{i=1}^n \mathsf{Q}_i^{n,\vartheta},$$

and introduce the filtrations $\mathbb{F}^n = (\mathscr{F}_t^n)_{t \in \mathbb{R}_+}$ and the stopping times T_n by

$$\mathscr{F}_t^n = \mathscr{G}_{[nt] \wedge n}^n, \quad T_n = 1,$$

where $\mathscr{G}^n_m$ is the sub-σ-field of $\mathscr{F}^n$ generated by the projections of Ω^n onto $X^n_1, \ldots, X^n_m$.

Fix $\vartheta_0 \in \Theta$ and take a sequence $\{\varphi_n\}$ of nonsingular $k \times k$ matrices such that $\varphi_n \to 0$ as $n \to \infty$. Put

$$\mathsf{P}^n = \mathsf{P}^{n,\vartheta_0}, \quad \mathsf{Q}^n_i = \mathsf{Q}^{n,\vartheta_0}_i;$$

E^n stands for the expectation with respect to P^n.

Let $\alpha^{n,\vartheta}_i$ be the density of the absolutely continuous part of $\mathsf{Q}^{n,\vartheta_0+\varphi_n\vartheta}_i$ with respect to Q^n_i. The generalized density process $Z^{n,\vartheta}$ of $\mathsf{P}^{n,\vartheta_0+\varphi_n\vartheta}$ with respect to P^n satisfies

$$Z^{n,\vartheta}_t = \prod_{i=1}^{[nt]\wedge n} \alpha^{n,\vartheta}_i \quad \mathsf{P}^n\text{-a.s.}$$

Now, we can construct different processes from $Z^{n,\vartheta}$ as it was done in Sect. 2.1. Namely, let

$$h^{n,\vartheta}_t = \sum_{i=1}^{[nt]\wedge n} \mathsf{E}^n\left(1 - \sqrt{\alpha^{n,\vartheta}_i}\right) = \sum_{i=1}^{[nt]\wedge n} \rho^2\left(\mathsf{Q}^n_i, \mathsf{Q}^{n,\vartheta_0+\varphi_n\vartheta}_i\right), \tag{48}$$

$$\iota^{n,\vartheta}_t = \sum_{i=1}^{[nt]\wedge n} \left(1 - \mathsf{E}^n\alpha^{n,\vartheta}_i\right), \tag{49}$$

$$\overline{h}^{n,\vartheta,\eta}_t = \sum_{i=1}^{[nt]\wedge n} \mathsf{E}^n\left(1 - \sqrt{\alpha^{n,\vartheta}_i \alpha^{n,\eta}_i}\right). \tag{50}$$

$$h^{n,\vartheta,\eta}_t = \sum_{i=1}^{[nt]\wedge n} \rho^2\left(\mathsf{Q}^{n,\vartheta_0+\varphi_n\vartheta}_i, \mathsf{Q}^{n,\vartheta_0+\varphi_n\eta}_i\right), \tag{51}$$

$$y^{n,\vartheta}_t = \sum_{i=1}^{[nt]\wedge n} \left(\sqrt{\alpha^{n,\vartheta}_i} - 1\right), \tag{52}$$

$$m^{n,\vartheta}_t = \sum_{i=1}^{[nt]\wedge n} \left(\sqrt{\alpha^{n,\vartheta}_i} - \mathsf{E}^n\sqrt{\alpha^{n,\vartheta}_i}\right). \tag{53}$$

It is easy to see that the processes in (48), (49), and (50) do satisfy (6), (7), and (9), respectively, and, similarly, the process $h^{n,\vartheta,\eta}$ in (51) is a version of the Hellinger process of order $1/2$ for $\mathsf{P}^{n,\vartheta_0+\varphi_n\vartheta}$ and $\mathsf{P}^{n,\vartheta_0+\varphi_n\eta}$, and that the processes in (52) and (53) coincide with the corresponding processes in (8) on the stochastic intervals where the latter ones were defined. According to Remark 2, we can use the versions introduced in (48)–(53) in all subsequent considerations. Similarly, we can use the above version of m^{n,e_i} instead of $\widetilde{m}^{n,e_i}$ in (20), which makes w^n to be a sum of square-integrable zero mean independent random vectors (with respect to P^n). Note also that here it seems to be more convenient to check the Lindeberg-type condition (14) with $\nu^{y^{n,\vartheta_n}}$ instead of $\nu^{m^{n,\vartheta_n}}$, see Remark 3. Then (14) takes the form of the standard Lindeberg condition:

$$\sum_{i=1}^{n} \mathsf{E}^n \left(\sqrt{\alpha_i^{n,\vartheta_n}} - 1 \right)^2 \mathbf{1}_{\left\{ \left| \sqrt{\alpha_i^{n,\vartheta_n}} - 1 \right| > \varepsilon \right\}} \to 0, \quad n \to \infty, \quad \text{for all } \varepsilon > 0$$

for each $\{\vartheta_n\} \in \mathscr{S}$.

Now assume that (O), (H) and (L) hold. Since the processes $\overline{h}^{n,\vartheta,\eta}$ are deterministic, we may assume that the matrices H^n in (H) are deterministic. Hence, if one assumes additionally that $\liminf_{n\to\infty} \det H^n > 0$, then it follows from Theorem 2 that the sequence $\left(\Omega^n, \mathscr{F}^n, (\mathsf{P}^{n,\vartheta_0+\varphi_n\vartheta})_{\vartheta \in \mathbb{R}^k} \right)$ is asymptotically normal, which amounts to say that the sequence $\left(\Omega^n, \mathscr{F}^n, (\mathsf{P}^{n,\vartheta})_{\vartheta \in \Theta} \right)$ is locally asymptotically normal at ϑ_0.

Let us now assume that the sequence $\left(\Omega^n, \mathscr{F}^n, (\mathsf{P}^{n,\vartheta_0+\varphi_n\vartheta})_{\vartheta \in \mathbb{R}^k} \right)$ is asymptotically normal. We assert that if

$$\lim_{n\to\infty} \sup_{i \le n} \rho^2 (\mathsf{Q}_i^{n,\vartheta_0}, \mathsf{Q}_i^{n,\vartheta_0+\varphi_n\vartheta_n}) = 0 \tag{54}$$

for any $\{\vartheta_n\} \in \mathscr{S}$, then (O), (H) and (L) hold, and hence we have the quadratic approximation (1) with $w^n = (w^{n,1}, \ldots, w^{n,k})$ defined by

$$w_t^{n,m} = 2 \sum_{i=1}^{[nt] \wedge n} \left(\sqrt{\alpha_i^{n,e_m}} - \mathsf{E}^n \sqrt{\alpha_i^{n,e_m}} \right),$$

as explained above.

To prove this statement, it is enough to show according Theorem 9 that condition (42) is satisfied. Take a sequence $\{\vartheta_n\} \in \mathscr{S}$ and let (V_n, K_n) be the sequence from the definition of AN. Similarly to the proof of Theorem 9 it is enough to check (42) under the assumption that $\vartheta_n \to \vartheta$ and K_n tends (in P^n-probability) to a (deterministic) matrix K. Then the distributions $\mathscr{L}(\log Z_1^{n,\vartheta_n} \mid \mathsf{P}^n)$ weakly converge to the normal distribution with mean $-\frac{1}{2}\vartheta^\top K \vartheta$ and variance $\vartheta^\top K \vartheta$. In particular,

$$\mathsf{P}^n(Z_1^{n,\vartheta_n} = 0) = 1 - \prod_{i=1}^{n} \left(1 - \mathsf{P}^n(\alpha_i^{n,\vartheta_n} = 0) \right) \to 0,$$

which implies

$$\sum_{i=1}^{n} \mathsf{P}^n(\alpha_i^{n,\vartheta_n} = 0) \to 0, \quad n \to \infty. \tag{55}$$

Put $\eta_{n,i} = (\log \alpha_i^{n,\vartheta_n})\mathbf{1}_{\{\alpha_i^{n,\vartheta_n} > 0\}}$. Then $\eta_{n,i}$, $i = 1, \ldots, n$, are independent and $(\eta_{n,i})_{i \leq n, \, n=1,2,\ldots}$ is an infinitesimal (or a null) array of random variables in the sense that

$$\lim_{n \to \infty} \sup_i \mathsf{P}^n(|\eta_{n,i}| > \varepsilon) = 0 \quad \text{for every } \varepsilon > 0,$$

the last property is due to (54) because of

$$\rho^2(\mathsf{Q}_i^{n,\vartheta_0}, \mathsf{Q}_i^{n,\vartheta_0+\varphi_n\vartheta_n}) = \mathsf{E}^n\left(1 - \sqrt{\alpha_i^{n,\vartheta_n}}\right) \geq \frac{1}{2}\mathsf{E}^n\left(1 - \sqrt{\alpha_i^{n,\vartheta_n}}\right)^2.$$

On the other hand, in view of (55),

$$\mathscr{L}\left(\sum_{i=1}^n \eta_{n,i} \,\bigg|\, \mathsf{P}^n\right) \Rightarrow \mathscr{N}(-\tfrac{1}{2}\vartheta^\top K\vartheta, \vartheta^\top K\vartheta).$$

It is well known that the weak convergence for infinitesimal arrays to a Gaussian law implies

$$\lim_{n \to \infty} \sum_{i=1}^n \mathsf{P}^n(|\eta_{n,i}| > \varepsilon) = 0 \quad \text{for every } \varepsilon > 0,$$

see e.g. Kallenberg [20, Theorem 5.15]. Combining this relation with (55), we get

$$\mathsf{P}^n(\sup_i |\alpha_i^{n,\vartheta_n} - 1| > \varepsilon) \leq \sum_{i=1}^n \mathsf{P}^n(|\alpha_i^{n,\vartheta_n} - 1| > \varepsilon) \to 0 \quad \text{for every } \varepsilon > 0.$$

The claim follows now from (2).

Remark 10 The above statements concerning necessary and sufficient conditions for AN are similar to Proposition 6 in Le Cam [23], see also Theorem 1 in Le Cam [25, Chap. 16, Sect. 3, p. 472].

Remark 11 Let J_n be nonempty subsets of $\{1, \ldots, n\}$, $\widetilde{\mathscr{F}}^n$ generated by the projections of Ω^n onto X_j^n, $j \in J_n$, $\widetilde{\mathsf{P}}^{n,\vartheta} = \mathsf{P}^{n,\vartheta}|_{\widetilde{\mathscr{F}}^n}$. If the sequence $\mathbb{E}^n = \left(\Omega^n, \mathscr{F}^n, (\mathsf{P}^{n,\vartheta_0+\varphi_n\vartheta})_{\vartheta \in \mathbb{R}^k}\right)$ is AN and (54) holds, then the sequence $\widetilde{\mathbb{E}}^n = \left(\Omega^n, \widetilde{\mathscr{F}}^n, (\widetilde{\mathsf{P}}^{n,\vartheta_0+\varphi_n\vartheta})_{\vartheta \in \mathbb{R}^k}\right)$ is AN*. Indeed, the order of factors in our experiments has not played any role up to now, so we may assume that $J_n = \{1, \ldots, j_n\}$. Then the existence of a quadratic approximation of the form (22) and nonrandomness of cluster points $\mathscr{L}(K)$ follow from the quadratic approximation (1), and it is well known that the contiguity properties of $\mathbb{E}^n$ remain valid in $\widetilde{\mathbb{E}}^n$. For more general results concerning the preservation of the AN property under information loss, see Proposition 4 in Le Cam [25, Chap. 16, Sect. 3, p. 474] and Le Cam and Yang [26].

Informally speaking, assumption (54) says that each observation has relatively little inference on the whole experiment itself. It is not surprising that this assumption is automatically satisfied in the case of identical observations within every model. Namely, assume that $(X_i^n, \mathscr{X}_i^n, (Q_i^{n,\vartheta})_{\vartheta \in \Theta})$, $i = 1, \ldots, n$ are copies of $(X^n, \mathscr{X}^n, (Q^{n,\vartheta})_{\vartheta \in \Theta})$ for all n. Then

$$\rho^2(Q_i^{n,\vartheta_0}, Q_i^{n,\vartheta_0 + \varphi_n \vartheta_n}) = \rho^2(Q^{n,\vartheta_0}, Q^{n,\vartheta_0 + \varphi_n \vartheta_n}), \quad i = 1, \ldots, n,$$

and

$$\rho^2(P^{n,\vartheta_0}, P^{n,\vartheta_0 + \varphi_n \vartheta_n}) = 1 - \left(1 - \rho^2(Q^{n,\vartheta_0}, Q^{n,\vartheta_0 + \varphi_n \vartheta_n})\right)^n.$$

Hence, assumption (54) is satisfied if $\lim \sup_{n \to \infty} \rho^2(P^{n,\vartheta_0}, P^{n,\vartheta_0 + \varphi_n \vartheta_n}) < 1$, which is, of course, true if the sequence $(\Omega^n, \mathscr{F}^n, (P^{n,\vartheta_0 + \varphi_n \vartheta})_{\vartheta \in \mathbb{R}^k})$ is asymptotically normal.

This means that if our experiments have a product structure and every factor in the nth experiment is a copy of each other for every n, then the following assumptions are necessary and sufficient for the local asymptotic normality at ϑ_0: there is a sequence $\{\varphi_n\}$ of nonsingular $k \times k$ matrices such that $\varphi_n \to 0$ as $n \to \infty$ and there is a sequence $\{H^n\}$ of matrices in $\mathbb{M}_+^k$ such that

$$\lim_{n \to \infty} \inf \det H^n > 0, \quad \lim_{n \to \infty} \sup \operatorname{tr} H^n < \infty,$$

and, with the above notation,

$$\lim_{n \to \infty} \left[n E^n \left(1 - \sqrt{\alpha_i^{n,\eta_n} \alpha_i^{n,\vartheta_n}}\right) - (\vartheta_n - \eta_n)^\top H^n (\vartheta_n - \eta_n) \right] = 0$$

for all $\{\vartheta_n\}$ and $\{\eta_n\}$ in $\mathscr{S}$, and

$$\lim_{n \to \infty} n \left[E^n \left(\sqrt{\alpha_i^{n,\vartheta_n}} - 1\right)^2 \mathbb{1}_{\left\{ \left| \sqrt{\alpha_i^{n,\vartheta_n}} - 1 \right| > \varepsilon \right\}} \right] = 0 \quad \text{for all } \varepsilon > 0$$

for each $\{\vartheta_n\} \in \mathscr{S}$.

Let us mention here that this result uses essentially the Euclidean structure of the parameter set. Le Cam [24], see also Le Cam and Yang [27], considers Gaussian approximations to experiments formed by independent identical distributions with an arbitrary parameter set.

Finally, let us consider the case of i.i.d. observations. That is, we have an experiment $(X, \mathscr{X}, (Q^\vartheta)_{\vartheta \in \Theta})$, where Θ is an open subset of $\mathbb{R}^k$. Define the infinite product experiment

$$\Omega = \prod_{i=1}^{\infty} X, \quad \mathscr{F} = \bigotimes_{i=1}^{\infty} \mathscr{X}, \quad P^\vartheta = \prod_{i=1}^{\infty} Q^\vartheta,$$

and introduce the filtrations $\mathbb{F}^n = (\mathscr{F}_t^n)_{t \in \mathbb{R}_+}$ and the stopping times T_n by

$$\mathscr{F}_t^n = \mathscr{G}_{[nt] \wedge n}, \quad T_n = 1,$$

where $\mathscr{G}_m$ is the sub-σ-field of $\mathscr{F}$ generated by the projections of Ω onto the first m coordinates: $\omega = (\omega_1, \omega_2, \dots) \rightsquigarrow \omega_i$, $i = 1, \dots, m$. We are interested in establishing the LAN property for the sequence of experiments

$$(\Omega, \mathscr{F}^n, \mathbb{F}^n, (\mathsf{P}^{n,\vartheta})_{\vartheta \in \Theta})$$

at some point $\vartheta_0 \in \Theta$, where $\mathscr{F}^n = \mathscr{G}_n$, $\mathsf{P}^{n,\vartheta} = \mathsf{P}^\vartheta|_{\mathscr{F}^n}$.

Put $\mathsf{Q} := \mathsf{Q}^{\vartheta_0}$. From the above considerations, the sequence $(\Omega, \mathscr{F}^n, \mathbb{F}^n, (\mathsf{P}^{n,\vartheta})_{\vartheta \in \Theta})$ is locally asymptotically normal at ϑ_0 if and only if there are a sequence $\{\varphi_n\}$ of nonsingular $k \times k$ matrices and a sequence of measurable mappings $g_n = (g_{n1}, \dots, g_{nk})^\top : X \to \mathbb{R}^k$ such that $\varphi_n \to 0$ as $n \to \infty$,

$$\int g_{ni}^2 \, d\mathsf{Q} < \infty \quad \text{and} \quad \int g_{ni} \, d\mathsf{Q} = 0, \quad \text{for all} \quad i = 1, \dots, k, \ n = 1, 2, \dots,$$
(56)

$$\liminf_{n \to \infty} n \det \int g_n g_n^\top \, d\mathsf{Q} > 0, \quad \limsup_{n \to \infty} n \int \|g_n\|^2 \, d\mathsf{Q} < \infty,$$
(57)

$$\lim_{n \to \infty} n \int_{\|g_n\| > \varepsilon} \|g_n\|^2 \, d\mathsf{Q} < \infty \quad \text{for all} \quad \varepsilon > 0,$$
(58)

$$\lim_{n \to \infty} n \int \left[\left(\frac{d\mathsf{Q}^{\vartheta_0 + \varphi_n \vartheta_n}}{d\mathsf{Q}} \right)^{1/2} - 1 - \frac{1}{2} \vartheta_n^\top g_n \right]^2 = 0 \quad \text{for all} \quad \{\vartheta_n\} \in \mathscr{S},$$
(59)

and

$$\lim_{n \to \infty} n \int \left(1 - \frac{d\mathsf{Q}^{\vartheta_0 + \varphi_n \vartheta_n}}{d\mathsf{Q}} \right) d\mathsf{Q} = 0 \quad \text{for all} \quad \{\vartheta_n\} \in \mathscr{S},$$
(60)

and then we have (1) with

$$w_t^n = \sum_{i=1}^{[nt] \wedge n} g_n(\omega_i), \quad \langle w^n, w^n \rangle_t = ([nt] \wedge n) \int g_n g_n^\top \, d\mathsf{Q}.$$

In particular, if LAN holds, then vectors V_n and matrices K_n satisfying

$$\log \frac{d\mathsf{P}^{\vartheta_0 + \varphi_n \vartheta_n}}{d\mathsf{P}^{\vartheta_0}} - \left(\vartheta_n^\top V_n - \frac{1}{2} \vartheta_n^\top K_n \vartheta_n \right) \xrightarrow{\mathsf{P}^n} 0, \quad n \to \infty,$$
(61)

cf. (22), can be always chosen of the form

$$V_n = \sum_{i=1}^{n} g_n(\omega_i), \quad K_n = \int V_n V_n^\top \, d\mathsf{Q},$$
(62)

where g_n satisfy (56)–(58).

It is interesting to compare the above remark with some known results dealing with the case where normalizing matrices are of the form $\varphi_n = \delta_n I_k$, where $\delta_n > 0$ and I_k is the identity matrix. Then the LAN property is possible only if $\delta_n = n^{-1/2} L(n)$ with a slowly varying sequence $L(n)$, see Strasser [36]. If the family $(Q^\vartheta)_{\vartheta \in \mathbb{R}^k}$ is continuous and translation invariant (in particular, a location parameter family), then necessary and sufficient conditions for the LAN property with rescaling by scalars are given by Janssen [17] in terms of the Hellinger distances $\rho^2(Q^0, Q^\vartheta)$.

The reader can easily check that relations (56)–(60) with

$$\varphi_n = n^{-1/2} I_k \quad \text{and} \quad g_n = n^{-1/2} v \tag{63}$$

are equivalent to the L^2-differentiability of the family $\{Q^\vartheta\}$ at ϑ_0 with the score function v and a nonsingular Fisher information matrix $J = \int vv^\top dQ$, see e.g. [10, Chap. 4] for the definition of L^2-differentiable models. L^2-differentiability is a classical sufficient condition for LAN. The converse statement (if

$$\log \frac{d\mathsf{P}^{\vartheta_0 + \varphi_n \vartheta_n}}{d\mathsf{P}^{\vartheta_0}} - \left(n^{-1/2} \vartheta_n^\top \sum_{i=1}^n v(\omega_i) - \frac{1}{2} \vartheta_n^\top J \vartheta_n\right) \xrightarrow{\mathsf{P}^n} 0, \quad n \to \infty,$$

for every $\{\vartheta_n\}$ in $\mathscr{S}$, where $\int \|v\|^2 dQ < \infty$ and $\int v\, dQ = 0$, then the family $\{Q^\vartheta\}$ is L^2-differentiable at ϑ_0) is also known, see e.g. Le Cam [25, Proposition 2, p. 584].

However, even in the one-dimensional case ($k = 1$), LAN may hold with a different choice of φ_n and/or g_n than in (63). Le Cam [25, pp. 583–584] provides an example of a family which satisfies LAN with the rate $\varphi_n = n^{-1/2}$ but is not L^2-differentiable, hence g_n cannot be represented as in (63). Janssen [19] introduces a number of models which satisfy (61) with

$$V_n = \varphi_n \sum_{i=1}^n v(\omega_i), \tag{64}$$

where v is the score function in some sense and has zero mean with respect to Q; however, v is not square integrable with respect to Q, and its law belongs to the domain of attraction of the normal law. Our choice of V_n as in (62) is definitely different from (64). On the other hand, Pfanzagl [34] constructs an example of a location parameter family $Q^\vartheta(\cdot) = Q(\cdot - \vartheta)$ on the line which satisfies LAN but it is not possible to choose V_n in (61) of the form $V_n = a_n \sum_{i=1}^n v(\omega_i)$ with some a_n and v.

Let us also mention that Janssen [18] describes experiments that appear as limit models if only LAMN holds in the considered i.i.d. case.

6 Proofs

We start with a general remark. In our proofs, we refer many times to different results in [6], in particular, to Theorems 2.1 and 3.1 and Propositions 2.5, 2.6 and 2.8, which are proved for $T_n \equiv t$, where $t \in \mathbb{R}_+$. However, they are still true (with evident modifications) for an arbitrary sequence $\{T_n\}$ of stopping times, since the general case reduces to the case $T_n \equiv 1$ by replacing the original filtrations $\mathscr{F}_t^n$ by $\widehat{\mathscr{F}}_t^n := \mathscr{F}_{\tau(t)\wedge T_n}^n$, $t \in [0, 1]$, where τ is a deterministic continuous strictly increasing function from $[0, 1]$ onto $[0, \infty]$.

6.1 Auxiliary Results

For simplicity of notation, we omit the index n everywhere in this subsection.

The next lemma generalizes relation (4.1) in [6, Lemma 4.1].

Lemma 1 *For all ϑ, $\eta \in \Theta$*

$$\overline{h}^{\vartheta,\eta} = h^\vartheta + h^\eta - \langle m^\vartheta, m^\eta \rangle - [h^\vartheta, h^\eta] \quad \text{P-a.s. } \text{ on } \Gamma^\vartheta \cap \Gamma^\eta. \tag{65}$$

Proof Recall that $Y^\vartheta = Y_0^\vartheta \mathscr{E}(m^\vartheta - h^\vartheta)$ on Γ^ϑ and $Y^\eta = Y_0^\eta \mathscr{E}(m^\eta - h^\eta)$ on Γ^η. By Yor's formula, on $\Gamma^\vartheta \cap \Gamma^\eta$

$$\overline{Y}^{\vartheta,\eta} = Y^\vartheta Y^\eta = \overline{Y}_0^{\vartheta,\eta} \mathscr{E}(m^\vartheta + m^\eta - h^\vartheta - h^\eta + [m^\vartheta - h^\vartheta, m^\eta - h^\eta])$$
$$= \overline{Y}_0^{\vartheta,\eta} \mathscr{E}\big(\{m^\vartheta + m^\eta - (\Delta h^\vartheta)\cdot m^\eta - (\Delta h^\eta)\cdot m^\eta + [m^\vartheta, m^\eta] - \langle m^\vartheta, m^\eta\rangle\}$$
$$-\{h^\vartheta + h^\eta - \langle m^\vartheta, m^\eta\rangle - [h^\vartheta, h^\eta]\}\big).$$

The expression in the first braces is a P^η-local martingale on $\Gamma^\vartheta \cap \Gamma^\eta$, and the expression in the second braces is a predictable process with finite variation on $\Gamma^\vartheta \cap \Gamma^\eta$. The claim follows from the definition of $\overline{h}^{\vartheta,\eta}$. $\qquad\square$

The next lemma can be deduced from statement (b) of Lemma 5.8 in [15]. However, the proof of that statement contains a small inaccuracy, so we give a full proof.

Lemma 2 *For all ϑ, $\eta \in \Theta$, the processes*

$$\overline{h}^{\vartheta,\eta} - h^{\vartheta,\eta} \quad \text{and} \quad \frac{1}{2}(\iota^\vartheta + \iota^\eta) - (\overline{h}^{\vartheta,\eta} - h^{\vartheta,\eta})$$

are P-a.s. increasing on $\Gamma^\vartheta \cap \Gamma^\eta$.

Proof Let Q be a probability measure that dominates P, P^ϑ, and P^η. The density processes of these measures with respect to Q are denoted by $\mathfrak{z}$, $\mathfrak{z}^\vartheta$, and $\mathfrak{z}^\eta$, respectively. Then $Z^\vartheta = \mathfrak{z}^\vartheta/\mathfrak{z}$ P- and P^ϑ-a.s., and $Z^\eta = \mathfrak{z}^\eta/\mathfrak{z}$ P- and P^η-a.s. Put also

$$S_k = \inf\{t : \mathfrak{z}_t \wedge \mathfrak{z}_t^{\vartheta} \wedge \mathfrak{z}_t^{\eta} < 1/k\}.$$

Let $\{R_k\}$ be a sequence of stopping times such that $\mathsf{P}(\lim_k R_k = \infty) = 1$ and $\left(\overline{Y}^{\vartheta,\eta} + \overline{Y}_-^{\vartheta,\eta} \cdot \overline{h}^{\vartheta,\eta}\right)^{R_k}$ is a P-martingale for every k. Since

$$\bigcup_k [\![0, S_k \wedge R_k]\!] = \left(\bigcup_k [\![0, R_k]\!]\right) \bigcap \left([\![0]\!] \cup \{\mathfrak{z}_-\mathfrak{z}_-^{\vartheta}\mathfrak{z}_-^{\eta} > 0\}\right) \quad \mathsf{Q}\text{-a.s.}$$

and $\mathsf{P}(\inf_t \mathfrak{z}_t > 0) = 1$, we have

$$\bigcup_k [\![0, S_k \wedge R_k]\!] = [\![0]\!] \cup \{Z_-^{\vartheta} Z_-^{\eta} > 0\} = \Gamma^{\vartheta} \cap \Gamma^{\eta} \quad \mathsf{P}\text{-a.s.}$$

Therefore, it is enough to prove the statement of the lemma on an interval $[\![0, R]\!]$, where $R = R_k \wedge S_k$ for some k.

Since $\left(\overline{Y}^{\vartheta,\eta} + \overline{Y}_-^{\vartheta,\eta} \cdot \overline{h}^{\vartheta,\eta}\right)^R$ is a P-martingale, $(\mathfrak{z}(\overline{Y}^{\vartheta,\eta})^R + \mathfrak{z}^R(\overline{Y}_-^{\vartheta,\eta} \cdot \overline{h}^{\vartheta,\eta})^R$ is a Q-martingale, see e.g. [16, Proposition III.3.8]. By Itô's formula,

$$\mathfrak{z}^R(\overline{Y}_-^{\vartheta,\eta} \cdot \overline{h}^{\vartheta,\eta})^R - (\mathfrak{z}_-^R \overline{Y}_-^{\vartheta,\eta}) \cdot (\overline{h}^{\vartheta,\eta})^R = \mathfrak{z}^R(\overline{Y}_-^{\vartheta,\eta} \cdot \overline{h}^{\vartheta,\eta})^R - \mathfrak{z}_-^R \cdot (\overline{Y}_-^{\vartheta,\eta} \cdot \overline{h}^{\vartheta,\eta})^R$$
$$= (\overline{Y}_-^{\vartheta,\eta} \cdot \overline{h}^{\vartheta,\eta})^R \cdot \mathfrak{z}^R$$

is a Q-local martingale. Note that $\mathfrak{z}_-^{\vartheta}\mathfrak{z}_-^{\eta} > 0$ on $]\!]0, R]\!]$, hence $\mathfrak{z}_- \overline{Y}_-^{\vartheta,\eta} = Y_-^{\vartheta,\eta}$ on $]\!]0, R]\!]$ and $\mathfrak{z}\overline{Y}^{\vartheta,\eta} = Y^{\vartheta,\eta} - Y^{\vartheta,\eta}\mathbf{1}_{\{\mathfrak{z}=0\}\cap[\![R]\!]}$ on $[\![0, R]\!]$, where $Y^{\vartheta,\eta} = \sqrt{\mathfrak{z}^{\vartheta}\mathfrak{z}^{\eta}}$. Furthermore, $Y^{\vartheta,\eta} + Y_-^{\vartheta,\eta} \cdot h^{\vartheta,\eta}$ is a Q-martingale by the definition of $h^{\vartheta,\eta}$. Combining these relations together, we obtain that

$$Y^{\vartheta,\eta}\mathbf{1}_{\{\mathfrak{z}=0\}\cap[\![R]\!]} - Y_-^{\vartheta,\eta} \cdot (\overline{h}^{\vartheta,\eta} - h^{\vartheta,\eta})^R \quad \text{is a } \mathsf{Q}\text{-local martingale.}$$

In other words, $(\overline{h}^{\vartheta,\eta} - h^{\vartheta,\eta})^R$ is the Q-compensator of $(Y^{\vartheta,\eta}/Y_-^{\vartheta,\eta})\mathbf{1}_{\{\mathfrak{z}=0\}\cap[\![R]\!]}$. Now recall that ι^{ϑ} is defined, see [16, Chap. IV, Sect. 1 d], as the Q-compensator of $(\mathfrak{z}^{\vartheta}/\mathfrak{z}_-^{\vartheta})\mathbf{1}_{\{\mathfrak{z}/\mathfrak{z}_-=0\}}$ (with the convention $0/0 = 0$), more precisely, this is true on the set $[\![0]\!] \cup \{\mathfrak{z}_-\mathfrak{z}_-^{\vartheta} > 0\}$, ι^{η} is defined similarly. It is clear that

$$\frac{Y^{\vartheta,\eta}}{Y^{\vartheta,\eta_-}} = \sqrt{1 + \frac{\Delta\mathfrak{z}^{\vartheta}}{\mathfrak{z}_-^{\vartheta}}}\sqrt{1 + \frac{\Delta\mathfrak{z}^{\eta}}{\mathfrak{z}_-^{\eta}}} \le \frac{1}{2}\left(1 + \frac{\Delta\mathfrak{z}^{\vartheta}}{\mathfrak{z}_-^{\vartheta}}\right) + \frac{1}{2}\left(1 + \frac{\Delta\mathfrak{z}^{\eta}}{\mathfrak{z}_-^{\eta}}\right)$$

on $\Gamma^{\vartheta} \cap \Gamma^{\eta}$, and the second statement of the lemma follows. $\qquad\qquad\square$

6.2 Proofs of Theorems 1–6

Proof of Theorem 1 (a) Condition (H) applied with $\eta_n \equiv 0$ implies that

$$\text{the sequence}\quad (h_{T_n}^{n,\vartheta_n}|\mathbf{P}^n)\quad\text{is }\mathbb{R}\text{-tight.}\tag{66}$$

(Note that the same is true if we consider h^{n,ϑ_n,η_n} instead of $\overline{h}^{n,\vartheta_n,\eta_n}$ in (H).) Thus, for every $\{\vartheta_n\}\in\mathscr{S}$ we are in a position to apply Theorem 2.1 in [6] obtaining (16),

$$\text{Var}\left(h^{n,\vartheta_n}-\frac{1}{2}\langle m^{n,\vartheta_n},m^{n,\vartheta_n}\rangle\right)_{T_n}\xrightarrow{\mathbf{P}^n}0,\quad n\to\infty,\tag{67}$$

and

$$\sup_{s\leq T_n}\left|\log Z_s^{n,\vartheta_n}-\log Z_0^{n,\vartheta_n}-\left(2m_s^{n,\vartheta_n}-2\langle m^{n,\vartheta_n},m^{n,\vartheta_n}\rangle_s\right)\right|\xrightarrow{\mathbf{P}^n}0,\quad n\to\infty.\tag{68}$$

We also have

$$\sup_{s\leq T_n}\Delta h_s^{n,\vartheta_n}\xrightarrow{\mathbf{P}^n}0,\quad n\to\infty,$$

see Proposition 2.6 in [6], and it follows from (66) that

$$\text{Var}\left([h^{n,\vartheta_n},h^{n,\eta_n}]\right)_{T_n}\xrightarrow{\mathbf{P}^n}0,\quad n\to\infty,\tag{69}$$

for all $\{\vartheta_n\},\{\eta_n\}\in\mathscr{S}$.

Now take two sequences $\{\vartheta_n\}$ and $\{\eta_n\}$ in $\mathscr{S}$. Combining (H), (65), and (69), and taking into account (5), we obtain that

$$\langle m^{n,\vartheta_n},m^{n,\eta_n}\rangle_{T_n}-2\vartheta_n^\top H^n\eta_n\xrightarrow{\mathbf{P}^n}0,\quad n\to\infty.\tag{70}$$

Moreover, m^{n,ϑ_n} and m^{n,η_n} can be replaced by $\widetilde{m}^{n,\vartheta_n}$ and $\widetilde{m}^{n,\eta_n}$ in (67), (68) and (70) in view of (4).

Define now the process $w^n=(w^{n,1},\ldots,w^{n,k})$ according to (20), $n=1,2,\ldots$. Each $w^{n,i}$ is a $\mathbf{P}^n$-locally square-integrable martingale, condition (10) holds in view of (66) and (67), and (11) follows from (L) and the inequality

$$(a_1^2+\cdots+a_k^2)\mathbf{1}_{\{a_1^2+\cdots+a_k^2>\varepsilon^2\}}\leq k\{a_1^2\mathbf{1}_{\{|a_1|>\varepsilon/\sqrt{k}\}}+\cdots+a_k^2\mathbf{1}_{\{|a_k|>\varepsilon/\sqrt{k}\}}\}.$$

Hence $\{w^n\}\in\mathscr{W}(\{T_n\})$.

After direct calculations based on (70), we obtain that for every $\{\vartheta_n\}\in\mathscr{S}$, $\vartheta_n=(\vartheta_{n1},\ldots,\vartheta_{nk})$,

$$\left\langle \widetilde{m}^{n,\vartheta_n} - \sum_{i=1}^{k} \vartheta_{ni}\widetilde{m}^{n,e_i}, \widetilde{m}^{n,\vartheta_n} - \sum_{i=1}^{k} \vartheta_{ni}\widetilde{m}^{n,e_i} \right\rangle_{T_n} \xrightarrow{\mathbf{P}^n} 0, \quad n \to \infty,$$

which means (15), i.e. condition (W) holds.

Applying (65), (67), (69) and (5), we obtain

$$\mathrm{Var}\left(\overline{h}^{n,\vartheta_n,\eta_n} - \frac{1}{2}\langle m^{n,\vartheta_n} - m^{n,\eta_n}, m^{n,\vartheta_n} - m^{n,\eta_n}\rangle\right)_{T_n} \xrightarrow{\mathbf{P}^n} 0, \quad n \to \infty, \quad (71)$$

for all $\{\vartheta_n\}, \{\eta_n\} \in \mathscr{S}$. Now (17) follows from (71), (15), and the Kunita–Watanabe inequality.

(b) Since $\langle \vartheta_n^\top w^n, \vartheta_n^\top w^n \rangle_{T_n} \leq \|\vartheta_n\|^2 \sum_{i=1}^{k} \langle w^{n,i}, w^{n,i} \rangle_{T_n}$ $\mathbf{P}^n$-a.s., we obtain from (10) and (15) that

$$\text{the sequence} \quad \left(\mathbf{1}_{\Gamma^{n,\vartheta_n}} \cdot \langle m^{n,\vartheta_n}, m^{n,\vartheta_n} \rangle_{T_n} \middle| \mathbf{P}^n\right) \quad \text{is } \mathbb{R}\text{-tight}$$

for any $\{\vartheta_n\} \in \mathscr{S}$. Taking into account that $0 \leq \Delta h^{n,\vartheta_n} \leq 1$ and hence $[h^{n,\vartheta_n}, h^{n,\vartheta_n}] \leq h^{n,\vartheta_n}$ $\mathbf{P}^n$-a.s. on Γ^{n,ϑ_n}, we obtain from Lemma 4.1 in [6] that

$$\text{the sequence} \quad (h_{T_n}^{\prime n,\vartheta_n} | \mathbf{P}^n) \quad \text{is } \mathbb{R}\text{-tight},$$

where $h^{\prime n,\vartheta_n} = \mathbf{1}_{\Gamma^{n,\vartheta_n}} \cdot h^{n,\vartheta_n}$ is a 'strict' version of h^{n,ϑ_n}.

It is obvious from (11) that every component $w^{n,i}$ satisfies the Lindeberg-type condition for its jumps. The same is true for $\vartheta_{ni} w^{n,i}$, where ϑ_{ni} are bounded. Using the inequality

$$(a_1 + \cdots + a_k)^2 \mathbf{1}_{\{|a_1+\cdots+a_k|>\varepsilon\}} \leq k^2 \{a_1^2 \mathbf{1}_{\{|a_1|>\varepsilon/k\}} + \cdots + a_k^2 \mathbf{1}_{\{|a_k|>\varepsilon/k\}}\},$$

we deduce that the sequence $\vartheta_n^\top w^n$ satisfies the Lindeberg-type condition, and now we obtain from (15) that

$$x^2 \mathbf{1}_{\{|x|>\varepsilon\}} \mathbf{1}_{\Gamma^{n,\vartheta_n}} \star \nu_{T_n}^{m^{n,\vartheta_n}} \xrightarrow{\mathbf{P}^n} 0, \quad n \to \infty, \quad \text{for all } \varepsilon > 0.$$

This is enough to apply Theorem 2.1 in [6] to obtain contiguity (16) and hence condition (L) for every version of the integral in (14). We also have (67) and (69) for any versions of the Hellinger processes.

Finally, we use Lemma 1, (67), and (69) to show (71). Combining it with (15) and the Kunita–Watanabe inequality, we get (17), in particular (H) with $H^n = \frac{1}{8}\langle w^n, w^n \rangle_{T_n}$ is satisfied.

(c) Part (b) of the theorem shows that the hypotheses of part (a) are satisfied, hence (68) holds true. It remains to replace $2\langle m^{n,\vartheta_n}, m^{n,\vartheta_n}\rangle$ by $\frac{1}{2}\vartheta_n^\top \langle w^n, w^n\rangle \vartheta_n$, and $2m^{n,\vartheta_n}$ by $\vartheta_n^\top w^n$. The former is possible due to (15) and the Kunita–Watanabe inequality, and the latter is due to (15) and Lenglart's inequality. □

Proof of Theorem 2 According to Theorem 1, (16) and condition (W) are satisfied, and there is a sequence $\{w^n\} \in \mathcal{W}(\{T_n\})$ such that (17) and (18) are true. Since $\Theta = \mathbb{R}^k$, (17) combined with (13) yields (27). Now (26) follows from the central limit theorem for locally square-integrable martingales, see e.g. Liptser and Shiryayev [29, Theorem 5.5.4 and Problem 5.5.6]. Contiguity $(\mathsf{P}_{T_n}^{n,\vartheta_n}) \lhd (\mathsf{P}_{T_n}^n)$ follows from Remark 6.   □

Proof of Theorem 3 Applying Theorem 1, we obtain (16) and find a sequence $\{w^n\} \in \mathcal{W}(\{T_n\})$ such that (17) and (18) hold. Combining (29) and (17) with $\vartheta_n \equiv \vartheta$ and $\eta_n \equiv 0$, we get

$$\langle w^n, w^n \rangle_t \xrightarrow{\mathsf{P}^n} 8H_t, \quad n \to \infty, \quad t \in S. \tag{72}$$

By the functional central limit theorem for locally square-integrable martingales, see e.g. Jacod and Shiryaev [16, Theorem VIII.3.22] or Liptser and Shiryayev [29, Theorem 7.1.4 and Problem 7.1.4], we have (30). The relation (31) follows directly from (72). Remaining assertions follow from Theorem 2.   □

Proof of Theorem 4 As in the proof of Theorem 2, we obtain (16) and find a sequence $\{w^n\} \in \mathcal{W}$ such that (17) and (18) are satisfied, and we obtain from (17) and (13) that

$$\langle w^n, w^n \rangle_T \xrightarrow{\mathsf{P}} C_T$$

and

$$\langle w^n, w^n \rangle_{S_n} \xrightarrow{\mathsf{P}} 0,$$

$n \to \infty$. Now (33) follows from Liptser and Shiryayev [29, Theorem 5.5.5 and Problem 5.5.6]. Contiguity $(\mathsf{P}_{T_n}^{n,\vartheta_n}) \lhd (\mathsf{P}_{T_n}^n)$ is checked using Remark 6.   □

Proof of Theorem 5 Similar to that of Theorem 3.   □

Proof of Theorem 6 (i) It follows from Theorem IX.3.27 in Jacod and Shiryaev [16] that (B), (35) and (36) imply the weak convergence

$$\mathscr{L}(B^n | \mathsf{P}^n) \xrightarrow{d} \mathscr{L}(B | \mathsf{P}), \quad n \to \infty, \quad \text{in } \mathbb{D}([0, T], \mathbb{R}^q).$$

Let $\alpha_n \to \alpha \in \mathbb{C}(\mathbb{R}^q)$ in the Skorokhod topology on $\mathbb{D}(\mathbb{R}^q)$. Then, due to (G) (b), $G^n(\alpha_n) \to G(\alpha)$ in the Skorokhod topology on $\mathbb{D}(\mathbb{R}^{k \times q})$ and, since α is continuous, $(\alpha_n, G^n(\alpha_n)) \to (\alpha, G(\alpha))$ in the Skorokhod topology on $\mathbb{D}(\mathbb{R}^{q+k \times q})$. Hence

$$\mathscr{L}(B^n, K^n | \mathsf{P}^n) = \mathscr{L}(B^n, G^n \circ B^n | \mathsf{P}^n) \xrightarrow{d} \mathscr{L}(B, G \circ B | \mathsf{P})$$
$$= \mathscr{L}(B, G | \mathsf{P}), \quad n \to \infty, \quad \text{in } \mathbb{D}([0, T], \mathbb{R}^{q+k \times q}),$$

see e.g. Theorem 4.27 in Kallenberg [20].

It can be easily seen from Jacod and Shiryaev [16, Theorem VI.6.21] that the Lindeberg-type condition (36) guarantees that the sequence $(B^n | \mathsf{P}^n)$ is predictably uniformly tight (P-UT). By Theorem VI.6.22 in Jacod and Shiryaev [16],

$$\mathscr{L}(w^n|\mathsf{P}^n) = \mathscr{L}(K_-^n \cdot B^n|\mathsf{P}^n) \xrightarrow{d} \mathscr{L}(G_- \cdot B|\mathsf{P}), \quad n \to \infty, \quad \text{in } \mathbb{D}([0, T], \mathbb{R}^k).$$

The sequence $(w^n|\mathsf{P}^n)$ is also P-UT, see Jacod and Shiryaev [16, Corollary VI.6.20], and, applying Theorem VI.6.26 in Jacod and Shiryaev [16], we obtain that

$$\mathscr{L}(w^n, [w^n, w^n]|\mathsf{P}^n) \xrightarrow{d} \mathscr{L}(G_- \cdot B, (G_- c G_-^\top) \cdot F|\mathsf{P}), \quad n \to \infty, \quad \text{in } \mathbb{D}([0, T], \mathbb{R}^{k+k^2}). \tag{73}$$

Moreover, w^n are P^n-locally square-integrable martingales satisfying (11). Indeed,

$$\|x\|^2 \mathbf{1}_{\{\|x\|>\varepsilon\}} \star v_T^{w^n} = \|K_-^n x\|^2 \mathbf{1}_{\{\|K_-^n x\|>\varepsilon\}} \star v_T^{B^n},$$

hence

$$\mathsf{P}^n\left(\|x\|^2 \mathbf{1}_{\{\|x\|>\varepsilon\}} \star v_T^{w^n} > \delta\right) \le \mathsf{P}^n\left(\|x\|^2 \mathbf{1}_{\{\|x\|>\varepsilon c^{-1}\}} \star v_T^{B^n} > \delta c^{-2}\right) + \mathsf{P}^n(\sup_t |K_t^n| > c),$$

and the claim follows from (36) and the tightness of (K^n).

It follows, in particular, from (73) that the sequence $([w^n, w^n]_T|\mathsf{P}^n)$ is $\mathbb{R}$-tight. This property combined with the Lindeberg-type condition (11) implies

$$\sup_{s \le T} \left|[w^n, w^n]_s - \langle w^n, w^n \rangle_s\right| \xrightarrow{\mathsf{P}^n} 0, \quad n \to \infty,$$

see e.g. the proof of Lemma 5.5.5 in Liptser and Shiryayev [29]. In particular, (10) and (39) hold, $\{w^n\} \in \mathscr{W}$, and we have (W) due to (37). The rest follows from Theorem 1.

(ii) For the first statement use (38) and Remark 6. Let G be a Gaussian process. Our arguments are similar to the ones used in Example 3 in Liptser and Shiryaev [30, Chap. VI, pp. 233–234]. To simplify the notation, put $\beta = G^\top \vartheta$ and $Z = \mathscr{E}(\beta \cdot B)$. Then β is a k-dimensional Gaussian process. Let us note that the quadratic characteristic $(\beta^\top c \beta) \cdot F$ of the local martingale $\beta \cdot B$ is majorized by the process $\|\beta\|^2 \cdot F$. Using the inequality

$$\exp(\delta \|\beta_t\|^2) \le \frac{1}{k} \sum_{i=1}^k \exp(k\delta(\beta_t^i)^2)$$

and following the arguments in [30], we can find $\delta > 0$ such that

$$\sup_{t \le T} \mathsf{E} \exp(\delta \|\beta_t\|^2) < \infty. \tag{74}$$

Now take a partition $0 = t_0 < t_1 < \cdots < t_n = T$ such that $\max_{j \le n}(F_{t_j} - F_{t_{j-1}}) \le 2\delta$. By Jensen's inequality,

$$\exp\left(\frac{1}{2}\int_{t_{j-1}}^{t_j}\|\beta_t\|^2\,dF_t\right) \leq \frac{1}{F_{t_j}-F_{t_{j-1}}}\int_{t_{j-1}}^{t_j}\exp\left(\delta\|\beta_t\|^2\right)dF_t, \quad j=1,\ldots,n,$$

hence, due to (74),

$$\mathsf{E}\exp\left(\frac{1}{2}\int_{t_{j-1}}^{t_j}(\beta^\top c\beta)\,dF_t\right) \leq \mathsf{E}\exp\left(\frac{1}{2}\int_{t_{j-1}}^{t_j}\|\beta_t\|^2\,dF_t\right) < \infty, \quad j=1,\ldots,n.$$

By Novikov's criterion, $\mathscr{E}\left((1_{(t_{j-1},t_j]}\beta)\cdot B\right) = Z^{t_j}/Z^{t_{j-1}}$ is a martingale. Hence $\mathsf{E}(Z_{t_j}\mid \mathscr{F}_{t_{j-1}}) = Z_{t_{j-1}}, j=1,\ldots,n$, which implies $\mathsf{E}Z_T = 1$.

(iii) The statement follows from Definition 2. $\square$

6.3   Proofs of Theorems 7–9

Proof of Theorem 7 The first part of Condition (O) is obvious and the second part is a simple consequence of (41), see e.g. [6, p. 226]. Propositions 2.8 and 2.6 in [6] show that (41) and (42) imply (L). Moreover, it follows from (41) and Proposition 2.5 in [6] that for each $\{\vartheta_n\}\in\mathscr{S}$

$$\text{the sequence} \quad (h_{T_n}^{n,\vartheta_n}\mid\mathsf{P}^n) \quad \text{is } \mathbb{R}\text{-tight.} \tag{75}$$

Thus, we are in a position to apply Theorem 2.1 in [6] to obtain

$$\text{Var}\left(\overline{h}^{n,\vartheta_n} - \frac{1}{2}\langle m^{n,\vartheta_n}, m^{n,\vartheta_n}\rangle\right)_{T_n} \xrightarrow{\mathsf{P}^n} 0, \quad n\to\infty, \tag{76}$$

and

$$\sup_{s\leq T_n}\left|\log Z_s^{n,\vartheta_n} - \log Z_0^{n,\vartheta_n} - \left(2m_s^{n,\vartheta_n} - 2\langle m^{n,\vartheta_n}, m^{n,\vartheta_n}\rangle_s\right)\right| \xrightarrow{\mathsf{P}^n} 0, \quad n\to\infty, \tag{77}$$

for every $\{\vartheta_n\}\in\mathscr{S}$. Moreover, we can replace m^{n,ϑ_n} by $\widetilde{m}^{n,\vartheta_n}$ in (76) and (77) due to (4).

Now define $w^n = (w^{n,1},\ldots,w^{n,k})$ according to (20). As in the proof of Theorem 1, it follows from (75), (76), and (14) that $\{w^n\}\in\mathscr{W}(\{T_n\})$.

It follows from (44) and (77) that

$$\sup_{s\leq T_n}\left|\left(2\widetilde{m}_s^{n,\vartheta_n} - 2\langle\widetilde{m}^{n,\vartheta_n}, \widetilde{m}^{n,\vartheta_n}\rangle_s\right) - \left(\vartheta_n^\top X_s^n - B_s^{n,\vartheta_n}\right)\right| \xrightarrow{\mathsf{P}^n} 0, \quad n\to\infty.$$

Combining it with the same relation for $\vartheta_n\equiv e_i, i=1,\ldots,k$, we get

$$\sup_{s \leq T_n} |l_s^n - b_s^n| \xrightarrow{\mathsf{P}^n} 0, \quad n \to \infty, \tag{78}$$

where

$$l^n := 2\widetilde{m}^{n,\vartheta_n} - \vartheta_n^\top w^n$$

is a P^n-locally square-integrable martingale, and

$$b^n := 2\langle \widetilde{m}^{n,\vartheta_n}, \widetilde{m}^{n,\vartheta_n} \rangle - B^{n,\vartheta_n} - \frac{1}{2}\sum_i \vartheta_{n,i}\langle w^{n,i}, w^{n,i} \rangle + \sum_i \vartheta_{n,i} B^{n,e_i}$$

is a predictable process with finite variation.

We have that

$$\text{the sequence} \quad \left(\text{Var}\,(b^n)_{T_n} \big| \mathsf{P}^n\right) \quad \text{is } \mathbb{R}\text{-tight} \tag{79}$$

due to (43), (75) and (76). Moreover,

$$x^2 \mathbf{1}_{\{|\mathsf{x}|>\varepsilon\}} \star v_{T_n}^{l^n} \xrightarrow{\mathsf{P}^n} 0, \quad n \to \infty, \quad \text{for all } \varepsilon > 0, \tag{80}$$

in view of (L). In particular,

$$\lim_{a\uparrow\infty}\lim_{n\to\infty}\sup \mathsf{P}^n\left(|x|\mathbf{1}_{\{|x|>a\}} \star v_{T_n}^{l^n} > \varepsilon\right) = 0 \quad \text{for all } \varepsilon > 0. \tag{81}$$

According to Corollary 4 in Gushchin [3], conditions (79) and (81) are sufficient to deduce from (78) that

$$\sup_{s\leq T_n} |l_s^n| \xrightarrow{\mathsf{P}^n} 0, \quad n \to \infty. \tag{82}$$

(In [3] all the processes are defined on the same filtered probability space which is not a restriction since we can take the tensor product of all stochastic bases. Alternatively, a direct proof of (82) can be given following the same lines as in [3].) Now Corollary VIII.3.24 in [16] allows us to deduce from (82) and (80) that $\langle l^n, l^n \rangle_{T_n} \xrightarrow{\mathsf{P}^n} 0$. Thus we have proved (W), and the rest of the claim follows from Theorem 1. □

Proof of Theorem 8 Condition (O) is an immediate consequence of the contiguity $(\mathsf{P}_T^{n,\vartheta_n}) \lhd \rhd (\mathsf{P}_T^n)$, $\{\vartheta_n\} \in \mathscr{S}$, see the beginning of the previous proof.

Let $\{\vartheta_n\}$ and $\{\eta_n\}$ be sequences from $\mathscr{S}$ converging to ϑ and η respectively. (Of course, it is sufficient to prove (H), (L) and (W) only for such sequences.) Let Z^{n,ϑ_n,η_n} be the generalized density process of $\mathsf{P}^{n,\vartheta_n}$ with respect to P^{n,η_n}. It is well known that asymptotic normality* of $\mathbb{E}_t^n$, $t \in S$, implies

$$\mathscr{L}\left(\log Z_t^{n,\vartheta_n,\eta_n} \Big| \mathsf{P}^{n,\eta_n}\right) \Rightarrow \mathscr{N}\left(-\frac{1}{2}(\vartheta - \eta)^\top K_t(\vartheta - \eta), (\vartheta - \eta)^\top K_t(\vartheta - \eta)\right)$$

as $n \to \infty$. In other words,

$$\mathscr{L}\left(Z^{n,\vartheta_n,\eta_n}\middle|\mathsf{P}^{n,\eta_n}\right) \xrightarrow{d_f(S)} \mathscr{L}\left(e^{(\vartheta-\eta)^\top N - \frac{1}{2}(\vartheta-\eta)^\top K(\vartheta-\eta)}\middle|\mathsf{P}\right), \quad n \to \infty.$$

The latter relation allows us to apply Theorem 4.6 in [6] to the processes Z^{n,ϑ_n,η_n} under the measures P^{n,η_n}. First, we obtain (L) (with $\eta_n \equiv 0$). Second, we get all the assumptions of Theorem 2.1 in [6]. Combining relation (2.9) in [6] with statement (v) of [6, Theorem 4.6], we obtain, in particular,

$$\sup_{s \le T}\left|h_s^{n,\vartheta_n,\eta_n} - \frac{1}{8}(\vartheta_n - \eta_n)^\top(K_s - K_0)(\vartheta_n - \eta_n)\right| \xrightarrow{\mathsf{P}^{n,\eta_n}} 0, \quad n \to \infty. \tag{83}$$

Convergence in P^{n,η_n}-probability can be replaced by convergence in P^n-probability due to contiguity, and the processes h^{n,ϑ_n,η_n} can be replaced by $\overline{h}^{n,\vartheta_n,\eta_n}$ due to Proposition 1. This shows that (H) is satisfied. By Theorem 1 condition (W) also holds. Let $\{w^n\}$ be a sequence satisfying (W). Then (46) follows from (83) and (17), and (47) is a consequence of (18) and asymptotic normality* of $\mathbb{E}_0^n$.

Finally, we again apply Theorem 4.6 in [6] in the above situation with $\vartheta_n \equiv \vartheta$ and $\eta_n \equiv 0$ and obtain

$$\mathscr{L}\left(\log Z^{n,\vartheta}\middle|\mathsf{P}^n\right) \xrightarrow{d} \mathscr{L}\left(\vartheta^\top N - \frac{1}{2}\vartheta^\top K\vartheta\middle|\mathsf{P}\right), \quad n \to \infty, \quad \text{in } \mathbb{D}([0,T]).$$

Combined with (18), (46), and asymptotic normality* of $\mathbb{E}_0^n$, the last relation reduces to

$$\mathscr{L}\left(\vartheta^\top(V_0^n + w^n)\middle|\mathsf{P}^n\right) \xrightarrow{d} \mathscr{L}\left(\vartheta^\top N\middle|\mathsf{P}\right), \quad n \to \infty, \quad \text{in } \mathbb{D}([0,T])$$

for every $\vartheta \in \mathbb{R}^k$. Since the limiting process N is continuous, the components $w^{n,i}$ are $\mathbb{C}$-tight in $\mathbb{D}([0,T])$. Therefore, the sequence w^n is $\mathbb{C}$-tight in $\mathbb{D}([0,T],\mathbb{R}^k)$. The Cramér–Wold device allows us to identify the limit, and we obtain

$$\mathscr{L}\left(V_0^n + w^n\middle|\mathsf{P}^n\right) \xrightarrow{d} \mathscr{L}\left(N\middle|\mathsf{P}\right), \quad n \to \infty, \quad \text{in } \mathbb{D}([0,T],\mathbb{R}^k),$$

which implies (45) and asymptotic independence of V_0^n and $(w^n)_{t \in [0,T]}$ under P^n. □

Proof of Theorem 9 Take an arbitrary $\{\vartheta_n\} \in \mathscr{S}$, and assume without loss of generality that $\vartheta_n \to \vartheta$. We proceed as in the beginning of the proof of Theorem 7. We have $Z_0^{n,\vartheta_n} \xrightarrow{\mathsf{P}^n} 1$ by the assumptions and deduce (12) from contiguity $(\mathsf{P}_{T_n}^{n,\vartheta_n}) \lhd \rhd (\mathsf{P}_{T_n}^n)$, hence condition (O) holds. Contiguity combined with (42) yields (L) and (75). Using condition (D) and asymptotic normality of $\{\mathbb{E}_{T_n}^n\}$, given an arbitrary subsequence $\{n'\} \subseteq \{n\}$, we can extract a further subsequence $\{n''\} \subseteq \{n'\}$ such that the matrices K_n from (22) and $h_{T_n}^{n,\vartheta_n}$ converge in P^n-probability along this subsequence $\{n''\}$ to deterministic limits, say, $K \in \mathbb{M}_+^k$ and $h \in \mathbb{R}_+$, respectively. Applying Theorem 3.1 in [6] to the subsequence $\{n''\}$ of Z^{n,ϑ_n}, we obtain that $(\log Z_{T_n}^{n,\vartheta_n}|\mathsf{P}^n)$ converges in law to $\mathscr{N}(-4h, 8h)$ along $\{n''\}$. On the other hand, asymptotic normality of $\{\mathbb{E}_{T_n}^n\}$

gives convergence in law of $(\log Z_{T_n}^{n,\vartheta_n}|\mathsf{P}^n)$ to $\mathscr{N}(-\frac{1}{2}\vartheta^\top K\vartheta, \vartheta^\top K\vartheta)$ along $\{n''\}$, hence $h = \frac{1}{8}\vartheta^\top K\vartheta$. As a conclusion, we obtain

$$h_{T_n}^{n,\vartheta_n} - \frac{1}{8}\vartheta^\top K_n \vartheta \xrightarrow{\mathsf{P}^n} 0, \quad n \to \infty.$$

Now, we want to show that for two sequences $\{\vartheta_n\}$ and $\{\eta_n\}$ in $\mathscr{S}$ with limits ϑ and η respectively,

$$h_{T_n}^{n,\vartheta_n,\eta_n} - \frac{1}{8}(\vartheta - \eta)^\top K_n(\vartheta - \eta) \xrightarrow{\mathsf{P}^{n,\eta_n}} 0, \quad n \to \infty. \tag{84}$$

To repeat the previous arguments, we must show that $(\mathsf{P}_{T_n}^{n,\vartheta_n}) \lhd \rhd (\mathsf{P}_{T_n}^{n,\eta_n})$, $Z_0^{n,\vartheta_n,\eta_n} \xrightarrow{\mathsf{P}^{n,\eta_n}} 1$, and

$$\sup_{s \le T_n} |\Delta Z_s^{n,\vartheta_n,\eta_n}| \xrightarrow{\mathsf{P}^{n,\eta_n}} 0, \quad n \to \infty, \tag{85}$$

where Z^{n,ϑ_n,η_n} is the generalized density process of $\mathsf{P}^{n,\vartheta_n}$ with respect to P^{n,η_n}. The first two claims are easy. To prove (85), let us note that

$$Z^{n,\vartheta_n,\eta_n} = \frac{Z^{n,\vartheta_n}}{Z^{n,\eta_n}} \quad \mathsf{P}^n\text{-a.s.}$$

at least on the set $\{Z_{T_n}^{n,\vartheta_n} > 0, Z_{T_n}^{n,\eta_n} > 0\}$, whose P^n-probability tends to 1. Hence, on this set

$$\frac{\Delta Z^{n,\vartheta_n,\eta_n}}{Z_-^{n,\vartheta_n,\eta_n}} = \left(\frac{\Delta Z^{n,\vartheta_n}}{Z_-^{n,\vartheta_n}} - \frac{\Delta Z^{n,\eta_n}}{Z_-^{n,\eta_n}} \right) \frac{Z_-^{n,\eta_n}}{Z^{n,\eta_n}}.$$

Using (42), (3) and (2), we have

$$\sup_{s \le T_n} \left| \frac{\Delta Z_s^{n,\vartheta_n,\eta_n}}{Z_{s-}^{n,\vartheta_n,\eta_n}} \right| \xrightarrow{\mathsf{P}^n} 0, \quad n \to \infty.$$

Convergence in P^n-probability can be replaced by convergence in P^{n,η_n}-probability due to contiguity, and inequality (2) (applied to P^{n,η_n} and Z^{n,ϑ_n,η_n}) allows us to get rid of the denominator. Thus, we have proved (85) and consequently (84). Replacing in (84) convergence in P^{n,η_n}-probability by convergence in P^n-probability and the processes h^{n,ϑ_n,η_n} by $\overline{h}^{n,\vartheta_n,\eta_n}$ due to Proposition 1, we obtain condition (H). The final claim follows from Theorem 1. $\qquad\square$

Acknowledgements This research was supported by Suomalainen Tiedeakatemia (A.A. Gushchin), by Academy of Finland grants 210465 and 212875 (E. Valkeila), and by the program Tête-à-tête in Russia (Euler International Mathematical Institute; both authors). For the first author, this work has been funded by the Russian Academic Excellence Project '5-100'. The first author is deeply grateful to the referees for a number of comments aimed at improving the exposition.

References

1. Fabian, V., Hannan, J.: Local asymptotic behavior of densities. Stat. Decis. **5**, 105–138 (1987)
2. Greenwood, P.E., Shiryayev, A.N.: Contiguity and the Statistical Invariance Principle. Gordon and Breach, New York (1985)
3. Gushchin, A.A.: On taking limits under the compensator sign. In: Ibragimov, I.A., Zaitsev, A.Yu. (eds.) Probability Theory and Mathematical Statistics (St. Petersburg 1993), pp. 185–192. Gordon and Breach, Amsterdam (1996)
4. Gushchin, A.A., Küchler, U.: Asymptotic inference for a linear stochastic differential equation with time delay. Bernoulli **5**, 1059–1098 (1999)
5. Gushchin, A.A., Valkeila, E.: Exponential approximation of statistical experiments. In: Balakrishnan, N., et al. (eds.) Asymptotic Methods in Probability and Statistics with Applications (St. Petersburg 1998), pp. 409–423. Birkhäuser, Boston (2001)
6. Gushchin, A.A., Valkeila, E.: Approximations and limit theorems for likelihood ratio processes in the binary case. Stat. Decis. **21**, 219–260 (2003)
7. Hallin, M., Van Den Akker, R., Werker, B.J.: On quadratic expansions of log-likelihoods and a general asymptotic linearity result. In: Hallin, M., et al. (eds.) Mathematical Statistics and Limit Theorems, pp. 147–165. Springer, Cham (2015)
8. Höpfner, R.: Asymptotic inference for continuous-time Markov chains. Probab. Theory Relat. Fields **77**, 537–550 (1988)
9. Höpfner, R.: On statistics of Markov step processes: representation of log-likelihood ratio processes in filtered local models. Probab. Theory Relat. Fields **94**, 375–398 (1988)
10. Höpfner, R.: Asymptotic Statistics. Walter de Gruyter, Berlin (2014)
11. Höpfner, R., Jacod, J.: Some remarks on the joint estimation of the index and the scale parameter for stable processes. In: Mandl, P., Hušková, M. (eds.) Asymptotic Statistics: Proceedings of the 5th Prague Symposium 1993, pp. 273–284. Physica Verlag, Heidelberg (1994)
12. Jacod, J.: Calcul Stochastique et Problèmes de Martingales. Lecture Notes in Mathematics, vol. 714. Springer, Berlin (1979)
13. Jacod, J.: Filtered statistical models and Hellinger processes. Stoch. Process. Appl. **32**, 3–45 (1989)
14. Jacod, J.: Convergence of filtered statistical models and Hellinger processes. Stoch. Process. Appl. **32**, 47–68 (1989)
15. Jacod, J.: Une application de la topologie d'Emery: le processus information d'un modèle statistique filtré. Séminaire de Probabilités XXIII. Lecture Notes in Mathematics, vol. 1372, pp. 448–474. Springer, Berlin (1989)
16. Jacod, J., Shiryaev, A.N.: Limit Theorems for Stochastic Processes, 2nd edn. Springer, Berlin (2003)
17. Janssen, A.: Limits of translation invariant experiments. J. Multivar. Anal. **20**, 129–142 (1986)
18. Janssen, A.: Asymptotically linear and mixed normal sequences of statistical experiments. Sankhya: Ser. A **53**, 1–26 (1991)
19. Janssen, A.: Asymptotic relative efficiency of tests at the boundary of regular statistical models. J. Stat. Plan. Inference **126**, 461–477 (2004)
20. Kallenberg, O.: Foundations of Modern Probability, 2nd edn. Springer, New York (2002)
21. Kutoyants, Yu.: Identification of Dynamical Systems with Small Noise. Kluwer, Dordrecht (1994)
22. Le Cam, L.: Locally asymptotically normal families of distributions. Univ. Calif. Publ. Stat. **3**, 37–98 (1960)
23. Le Cam, L.: Likelihood functions for large numbers of independent observations. In: David, F.N. (ed.) Research Papers in Statistics (Festschrift J. Neyman), pp. 167–187. Wiley, London (1966)
24. Le Cam, L.: Sur l'approximation de familles de mesures par des familles gaussiennes. Annales de l'I.H.P. Probabilités et statistiques **21**, 225–287 (1985)
25. Le Cam, L.: Asymptotic Methods in Statistical Decision Theory. Springer, New York (1986)

26. Le Cam, L., Yang, G.L.: On the preservation of local asymptotic normality under information loss. Ann. Stat. **16**, 483–520 (1988)
27. Le Cam, L., Yang, G.L.: Asymptotics in Statistics: Some Basic Concepts, 2nd edn. Springer, New York (2000)
28. Lin'kov, Yu.N.: Asymptotic Statistical Methods for Stochastic Processes. Translations of Mathematical Monographs, vol. 196. American Mathematical Society, Providence (2001) Russian original: Kiev, Naukova Dumka (1993)
29. Liptser, R.Sh, Shiryayev, A.N.: Theory of Martingales. Kluwer, Dordrecht (1989)
30. Liptser, R.S., Shiryaev, A.N.: Statistics of Random Processes. I. General Theory, 2nd edn. Springer, Berlin (2001)
31. Luschgy, H.: Local asymptotic mixed normality for semimartingale experiments. Probab. Theory Relat. Fields **92**, 151–176 (1992)
32. Luschgy, H.: Asymptotic inference for semimartingale models with singular parameter points. J. Stat. Plan. Inference **39**, 155–186 (1994)
33. Luschgy, H.: Local asymptotic quadraticity of stochastic process models based on stopping times. Stoch. Process. Appl. **57**, 305–317 (1995)
34. Pfanzagl, J.: On distinguished LAN-representations. Math. Methods Stat. **11**, 477–488 (2002)
35. Shiryaev, A.N., Spokoiny, V.G.: Statistical Experiments and Decisions: Asymptotic Theory. World Scientific, Singapore (2000)
36. Strasser, H.: Scale invariance of statistical experiments. Probab. Math. Stat. **5**, 1–20 (1985)
37. Strasser, H.: Stability of filtered experiments. In: Sendler, W. (ed.) Contributions to Stochastics, pp. 202–213. Physica Verlag, Heidelberg (1987)
38. Vostrikova, L.: Functional limit theorems for the likelihood ratio processes. Ann. Univ. Sci. Budapest. Sect. Comput. **6**, 145–182 (1985)
39. Vostrikova, L.: On the weak convergence of likelihood ratio processes of general statistical parametric models. Stochastics **23**, 277–298 (1988)

Part V
Fractional Brownian Motion

Noise Sensitivity of Functionals of Fractional Brownian Motion Driven Stochastic Differential Equations: Results and Perspectives

Alexandre Richard and Denis Talay

Abstract We present an innovating sensitivity analysis for stochastic differential equations: We study the sensitivity, when the Hurst parameter H of the driving fractional Brownian motion tends to the pure Brownian value, of probability distributions of smooth functionals of the trajectories of the solutions $\{X_t^H\}_{t \in \mathbb{R}_+}$ and of the Laplace transform of the first passage time of X^H at a given threshold. Our technique requires to extend already known Gaussian estimates on the density of X_t^H to estimates with constants which are uniform w.r.t. t in the whole half-line $\mathbb{R}_+ - \{0\}$ and H when H tends to $\frac{1}{2}$.

Keywords Fractional Brownian motion · First hitting time · Malliavin calculus

1 Introduction

Recent statistical studies show memory effects in biological, financial, physical data: see e.g. [18] for a statistical evidence in climatology and [6] and citations therein for an evidence and important applications in finance. For such data the Markov structure of Lévy-driven stochastic differential equations makes such models questionable. It seems worth proposing new models driven by noises with long-range memory such as fractional Brownian motions.

In practice the accurate estimation of the Hurst parameter H of the noise is difficult (see e.g. [4]) and therefore one needs to develop sensitivity analysis w.r.t. H of probability distributions of smooth and non-smooth functionals of the solutions (X_t^H) to stochastic differential equations. Similar ideas were developed in [11] for symmetric integrals of the fractional Brownian motion.

A. Richard · D. Talay (✉)
INRIA, 2004 Route des Lucioles,
06902 Sophia-Antipolis, France
e-mail: denis.talay@inria.fr

A. Richard
e-mail: alexandre.richard@inria.fr

© Springer International Publishing AG 2017

V. Panov (ed.), *Modern Problems of Stochastic Analysis and Statistics*,
Springer Proceedings in Mathematics & Statistics 208,
DOI 10.1007/978-3-319-65313-6_9

Here, we review and illustrate by numerical experiments our theoretical results obtained in [17] for two extreme situations in terms of Malliavin regularity: on the one hand, expectations of smooth functions of the solution at a fixed time; on the other hand, Laplace transforms of first passage times at prescribed thresholds. Our motivation to consider first passage times comes from their many use in various applications: default risk in mathematical finance or spike trains in neuroscience (spike trains are sequences of times at which the membrane potential of neurons reach limit thresholds and then are reset to a resting value, are essential to describe the neuronal activity), stochastic numerics (see e.g. [3, Sect. 3]) and physics (see e.g. [13]). Long-range dependence leads to analytical and numerical difficulties: see e.g. [10].

In a Markovian setting the simplest partial differential equations characterizing the probability distributions of first hitting times are those satisfied by their Laplace transforms. In some circumstances they even have explicit solutions. It is, thus, natural to concentrate our study on Laplace transforms. We have a second motivation. Laplace transforms of first hitting times are expectations of singular functionals on the Wiener space. It seemed worth to us showing that a sensitivity analysis can be developed in such singular situations.

Our theoretical estimates and numerical results tend to show that the Markov Brownian model is a good proxy model as long as the Hurst parameter remains close to $\frac{1}{2}$. This robustness property, even for probability distributions of singular functionals (in the sense of Malliavin calculus) of the paths such as first hitting times, is an important information for modeling and simulation purposes: when statistical or calibration procedures lead to estimated values of H close to $\frac{1}{2}$, then it is reasonable to work with Brownian SDEs, which allows to analyze the model by means of PDE techniques and stochastic calculus for semimartingales, and to simulate it by means of standard stochastic simulation methods.

Our Main Results
The fractional Brownian motion $\{B_t^H\}_{t\in\mathbb{R}_+}$ with Hurst parameter $H \in (0, 1)$ is the centred Gaussian process with covariance

$$R_H(s, t) = \frac{1}{2}\left(s^{2H} + t^{2H} - |t - s|^{2H}\right), \quad \forall s, t \in \mathbb{R}_+.$$

Given $H \in (\frac{1}{2}, 1)$, we consider the process $\{X_t^H\}_{t\in\mathbb{R}_+}$ solution to the following stochastic differential equation driven by $\{B_t^H\}_{t\in\mathbb{R}_+}$:

$$X_t^H = x_0 + \int_0^t b(X_s^H)\, ds + \int_0^t \sigma(X_s^H) \circ dB_s^H, \tag{1}$$

where the last integral is a pathwise Stieltjes integral in the sense of [19]. For $H = \frac{1}{2}$ the process X solves the following SDE in the classical Stratonovich sense:

$$X_t = x_0 + \int_0^t b(X_s)\, ds + \int_0^t \sigma(X_s) \circ dB_s. \tag{2}$$

Below we use the following set of hypotheses:

(H1) There exists $\gamma \in (0, 1)$ such that $b, \sigma \in C^{1+\gamma}(\mathbb{R})$;
(H2) $b, \sigma \in C^2(\mathbb{R})$;
(H3) The function σ satisfies a strong ellipticity condition: $\exists \sigma_0 > 0$ such that $|\sigma(x)| \geq \sigma_0, \forall x \in \mathbb{R}$.

Our first theorem is elementary. It describes the sensitivity w.r.t. H around the critical Brownian parameter $H = \frac{1}{2}$ of time marginal probability distributions of $\{X_t^H\}_{t \in \mathbb{R}_+}$.

Theorem 1 *Let $H \in (\frac{1}{2}, 1)$, and let X^H and X be as before. Suppose that b and σ satisfy (H1) and (H3), and φ is bounded and Hölder continuous of order $2 + \beta$ for some $\beta > 0$. Then, for any $T > 0$ there exists $C_T > 0$ such that*

$$\forall H \in [\tfrac{1}{2}, 1), \quad \sup_{t \in [0,T]} \left| \mathbb{E}\varphi(X_t^H) - \mathbb{E}\varphi(X_t) \right| \leq C_T \, (H - \tfrac{1}{2}).$$

Our next theorem concerns the first passage time at threshold 1 of X^H issued from $x_0 < 1$: $\tau_H^X := \inf\{t \geq 0 : X_t^H = 1\}$. The probability distribution of the first passage time τ_H of a fractional Brownian motion is not explicitly known. [14] obtained the asymptotic behaviour of its tail distribution function and [7] obtained an upper bound on the Laplace transform of τ_H^{2H}. The recent work of [8] proposes an asymptotic expansion (in terms of $H - \frac{1}{2}$) of the density of τ_H formally obtained by perturbation analysis techniques.

Theorem 2 *Suppose that b and σ satisfy Hypotheses (H2) and (H3) and let $x_0 < 1$. There exist constants $\lambda_0 \geq 1$, $\mu \geq 0$ (both depending on b and σ only), $\alpha > 0$ and $0 < \eta_0 < \frac{1-x_0}{2}$ such that: for all $\varepsilon \in (0, \frac{1}{4})$ and $0 < \eta \leq \eta_0$, there exists $C_{\varepsilon,\eta} > 0$ such that*

$$\forall \lambda \geq \lambda_0, \ \forall H \in [\tfrac{1}{2}, 1), \quad \left| \mathbb{E}\left(e^{-\lambda \tau_H^X}\right) - \mathbb{E}\left(e^{-\lambda \tau_{\frac{1}{2}}^X}\right) \right|$$

$$\leq C_{\varepsilon,\eta}(H - \tfrac{1}{2})^{\frac{1}{2}-\varepsilon} \, e^{-\alpha S(1-x_0-2\eta)(\sqrt{2\lambda+\mu^2}-\mu)},$$

where $S(x) = x \wedge x^{\frac{1}{2H}}$. In the pure fBm case (where $b \equiv 0$ and $\sigma \equiv 1$), the result holds with $\lambda_0 = 1$ and $\mu = 0$.

Remark 1 In [17], we extend the preceding result to the case $H < \frac{1}{2}$. The statement, the definition of the stochastic integrals, and technical arguments in the proofs are substantially different from the case $H > \frac{1}{2}$.

In addition to the preceding theorems, we provide accurate estimates on the density of X^H with constants which are uniform w.r.t. small and long times and w.r.t. H in $[\frac{1}{2}, 1)$. Our next theorem improves estimates in [2, 5]. Our contributions consists in getting constants which are uniform w.r.t. t in the whole half-line $\mathbb{R}_+ - \{0\}$ and H when H tends to $\frac{1}{2}$.

Theorem 3 *Assume that b and σ satisfy the conditions (H2) and (H3). Then for every $H \in [\frac{1}{2}, 1)$, the density of X^H satisfies: there exists $C(b, \sigma) \equiv C > 0$ such that, for all $t \in \mathbb{R}_+$ and $H \in [\frac{1}{2}, 1)$,*

$$\forall x \in \mathbb{R}, \quad p_t^H(x) \leq \frac{e^{Ct}}{\sqrt{2\pi t^{2H}}} \exp\left(-\frac{(x - x_0)^2}{2Ct^{2H}}\right). \tag{3}$$

Theorems 1–2 are proved in [17]. We do not address the proof of Theorem 3 here.

We sketch the proofs of Theorems 1 and 2 in Sect. 2. In Sect. 3 we consider a case which was not tackled in [17], that is, the case $\lambda < 1$. Finally, in Sect. 4 we show numerical experiment results which illustrate Theorem 2 and suggest that the $(H - \frac{1}{2})^{\frac{1}{2}-}$ rate is sub-optimal.

2   Sketch of the Proofs

Under Assumption (H3), the Lamperti transform F is a map such that $F(X^H)$ solves Eq. (1) with coefficients $\tilde{b} = \frac{b \circ F^{-1}}{\sigma \circ F^{-1}}$ and $\sigma(x) \equiv 1$. Since F is one-to-one, we may and do assume in the rest of this paper that $\sigma(x) \equiv 1$. See [17] for more details.

2.1   Reminders on Malliavin Calculus

We denote by D and δ, the classical derivative and Skorokhod operators of Malliavin calculus w.r.t. Brownian motion on the time interval $[0, T]$ (see e.g. [15]). In the fractional Brownian motion framework, the Malliavin derivative D^H is defined as an operator on the smooth random variables with values in the Hilbert space $\mathcal{H}_H$ defined as the completion of the space of step functions on $[0, T]$ with the following scalar product:

$$\langle \varphi, \psi \rangle_{\mathcal{H}_H} := \alpha_H \int_0^T \int_0^T \varphi_s \, \psi_t \, |s - t|^{2H-2} \, ds dt < \infty,$$

where $\alpha_H = H(2H - 1)$.

The domain of D^H in $L^p(\Omega)$ $(p > 1)$ is denoted by $\mathbb{D}^{1,p}$ and is the closure of the space of smooth random variables with respect to the norm:

$$\|F\|_{1,p}^p = \mathbb{E}(|F|^p) + \mathbb{E}\left(\|D^H F\|_{\mathcal{H}_H}^p\right).$$

Equivalently, D^H and δ_H are defined as $D^H := (K_H^*)^{-1} D$ and $\delta_H(u) := \delta(K_H^* u)$ for $u \in (K_H^*)^{-1}(\mathrm{dom}\,\delta)$ (cf. [15, p. 288]), where for any $H \in (\frac{1}{2}, 1)$ the operator K_H^* is defined as follows: for any φ with suitable integrability properties,

$$K_H^* \varphi(s) = (H - \tfrac{1}{2}) c_H \int_s^T \left(\frac{\theta}{s}\right)^{H - \frac{1}{2}} (\theta - s)^{H - \frac{3}{2}} \varphi(\theta)\, d\theta$$

with

$$c_H := \left(\frac{2H\,\Gamma(3/2 - H)}{\Gamma(H + \frac{1}{2})\,\Gamma(2 - 2H)}\right)^{\frac{1}{2}}.$$

We denote by $\|\cdot\|_{\infty,[0,T]}$ the sup norm and $\|\cdot\|_\alpha$ the Hölder norm for functions on the interval $[0, T]$.

Let X^H be the solution to (1) with $\sigma(x) \equiv 1$. There exist modifications of the processes X^H and $D^H X^H$ such that for any $\alpha < H$ it a.s. holds that

$$
\begin{cases}
\|X^H\|_{\infty,[0,T]} \le C_T (1 + |x_0| + \|B^H\|_{\infty,[0,T]}), \\
\|X^H\|_\alpha \le \|B^H\|_\alpha + C_T (1 + |x_0| + \|B^H\|_{\infty,[0,T]}), \\
\|D^H X^H\|_{\infty,[0,T]^2} \le C_T, \\
\sup_{r \le t} \frac{|D_r^H X_t^H - 1|}{t - r} \le C_T, \ \forall t \in [0, T].
\end{cases}
\tag{4}
$$

These inequalities are simple consequences of the definition of X^H, assumptions (H1) and (H3), and the equality: $D_r^H X_t^H = \mathbf{1}_{\{r \le t\}} \left(1 + \int_r^t D_r^H X_s^H b'(X_s^H)\,ds\right)$ (see Sect. 3 in [17] for more details).

2.2 Sketch of the Proof of Theorem 1

Proving Theorem 1 is easy. A first technique consists in using pathwise estimates on $B^H - B^{1/2}$ with B^H and $B^{1/2}$ defined on the same probability space. A second technique, which we present here in order to introduce the reader to the method of proof for Theorem 2, consists in differentiating $u(t, X_t^H)$ where

$$u(s, x) := \mathbb{E}_x\left(\varphi(X_{t-s})\right),$$

which leads to

$$u(t, X_t^H) = u(0, x_0) + \int_0^t \left(\partial_s u(s, X_s^H) + \partial_x u(s, X_s^H) b(X_s^H)\right) ds + \delta_H\left(\mathbf{1}_{[0,t]}\partial_x u(\cdot, X_\cdot^H)\right)$$

$$+ \alpha_H \int_0^t \int_0^s |r - s|^{2H-2} D_r^H X_s^H\, \partial_{xx}^2 u(s, X_s^H)\, dr\, ds.$$

As u solves a parabolic PDE driven by the generator of (X_t) and as the Skorokhod integral has zero mean we get

$$
\mathbb{E}\varphi(X_t^H) - \mathbb{E}_{x_0}\varphi(X_t) = \mathbb{E}u(t, X_t^H) - u(0, x_0)
$$

$$
= \mathbb{E}\int_0^t \partial_{xx}^2 u(s, X_s^H)\left(Hs^{2H-1} - \tfrac{1}{2}\right)ds
$$

$$
+ \alpha_H \mathbb{E}\int_0^t \int_0^s |r - s|^{2H-2}(D_r^H X_s^H - 1)\partial_{xx}^2 u(s, X_s^H)\,dr ds.
$$

It then remains to use the estimates (4).

2.3 Sketch of the Proof of Theorem 2

We now sketch the proof of Theorem 2. We will soon limit ourselves to the pure fBm case ($b(x) \equiv 0$ and $\sigma \equiv 1$) in order to show the main ideas used in the proof and avoid too heavy technicalities. Recall that, after having used the Lamperti transform, we are reduced to the case $\sigma(x) \equiv 1$.

Our Laplace transform's sensititivity analysis is based on a PDE representation of first hitting time Laplace transforms in the case $H = \frac{1}{2}$.

For $\lambda > 0$ it is well known that

$$
\forall x_0 \in (-\infty, 1], \ \mathbb{E}_{x_0}\left(e^{-\lambda \tau_{\frac{1}{2}}}\right) = u_\lambda(x_0),
$$

where the function u_λ is the classical solution with bounded continuous first and second derivatives to

$$
\begin{cases}
2b(x)u_\lambda'(x) + u_\lambda''(x) = 2\lambda u_\lambda(x), \ x < 1, \\
u_\lambda(1) = 1, \\
\lim_{x \to -\infty} u_\lambda(x) = 0.
\end{cases} \tag{5}
$$

For any $t \in [0, T]$ the process $\mathbf{1}_{[0,t]}u_\lambda'(B^H)\,e^{-\lambda \cdot}$ is in dom $\delta_H^{(T)}$. One thus can apply Itô's formula to $e^{-\lambda t}u_\lambda(X_t^H)$ (see [17, Sect. 2] and [15]). As u_λ satisfies (5), for any $t \leq T \wedge \tau_H$ we get

$$
e^{-\lambda t}u_\lambda(X_t^H) = u_\lambda(x_0) + \int_0^t e^{-\lambda s}\left(u_\lambda'(X_s^H)b(X_s^H) - \lambda u_\lambda(X_s^H)\right)ds
$$

$$
+ \delta_H^{(T)}\left(\mathbf{1}_{[0,t]}(\cdot)e^{-\lambda \cdot}u_\lambda'(X_\cdot^H)\right)
$$

$$
+ \alpha_H \int_0^t \int_0^t D_v^H\left(e^{-\lambda s}u_\lambda'(X_s^H)\right)|s - v|^{2H-2}\,dv ds,
$$

where the last term corresponds to the Itô term. Using

$$D_v^H X_s^H = \mathbf{1}_{[0,s]}(v) \left(1 + \int_0^s b'(X_\theta^H) \, D_v^H X_\theta^H \, d\theta \right)$$

and the ODE (5) satisfied by u_λ, we get

$$e^{-\lambda t} u_\lambda(X_t^H) = u_\lambda(x_0) + \int_0^t \left(\alpha_H \int_0^s |s-v|^{2H-2} dv - \frac{1}{2} \right) e^{-\lambda s} u_\lambda''(X_s^H) \, ds$$
$$+ \delta_H^{(T)} \left(\mathbf{1}_{[0,t]}(\cdot) e^{-\lambda \cdot} u_\lambda'(X_\cdot^H) \right)$$
$$+ \alpha_H \int_0^t \int_0^s e^{-\lambda s} w_\lambda''(X_s^H) \, I(v,s) \, |s-v|^{2H-2} \, dvds,$$

where $I(v,s) = \mathbf{1}_{\{v \le s\}} \int_v^s b'(X_\theta^H) \, D_v^H X_\theta^H \, d\theta$. Observe that the last term vanishes for H close to $\frac{1}{2}$, since $\alpha_H |s-v|^{2H-2}$ is an approximation of the identity and $I(v,s)$ converges to 0 as $|v-s| \to 0$. This argument is made rigorous in [17].

We now limit ourselves to the pure fBm case ($b(x) \equiv 0$ and $\sigma \equiv 1$) to make the rest of the computations more understandable, although the differences will be essentially technical. Given that now, $u_\lambda'(x) = \sqrt{2\lambda} u_\lambda(x)$, the previous equality becomes

$$u_\lambda(B_t^H) \, e^{-\lambda t} = u_\lambda(x_0) + \sqrt{2\lambda} \delta_H^{(T)} \left(\mathbf{1}_{[0,t]} u_\lambda(B_\cdot^H) \, e^{-\lambda \cdot} \right)$$
$$+ 2\lambda \int_0^t \left(H s^{2H-1} - \tfrac{1}{2} \right) u_\lambda(B_s^H) \, e^{-\lambda s} \, ds.$$

Evaluate the previous equation at $T \wedge \tau_H$, take expectations and let T tend to infinity. For any $\lambda \ge 0$ it comes:

$$\mathbb{E}\left(e^{-\lambda \tau_H} \right) - \mathbb{E}\left(e^{-\lambda \tau_{\frac{1}{2}}} \right) = \mathbb{E}\left[2\lambda \int_0^{\tau_H} (H s^{2H-1} - \tfrac{1}{2}) u_\lambda(B_s^H) \, e^{-\lambda s} \, ds \right] \quad (6)$$
$$+ \sqrt{2\lambda} \lim_{T \to \infty} \mathbb{E}\left[\delta_H^{(T)} \left(\mathbf{1}_{[0,t]} u_\lambda(B_\cdot^H) \, e^{-\lambda \cdot} \right) \Big|_{t=\tau_H \wedge T} \right]$$
$$=: I_1(\lambda) + I_2(\lambda). \quad (7)$$

Proposition 1 *Let T be the function of $\lambda \in \mathbb{R}_+$ defined by $T(\lambda) = (2\lambda)^{1-\frac{1}{4H}}$ if $\lambda \le 1$ and $T(\lambda) = \sqrt{2\lambda}$ if $\lambda > 1$. There exists a constant $C > 0$ such that*

$$|I_1(\lambda)| \le C \, (H - \tfrac{1}{2}) \, e^{-\frac{1}{4} S(1-x_0) T(\lambda)},$$

where S is the function defined in Theorem 2.

Proof (*Sketch of proof*) From Fubini's theorem, we get

$$I_1(\lambda) = 2\lambda \int_0^{+\infty} (H s^{2H-1} - \tfrac{1}{2}) \mathbb{E}\left[\mathbf{1}_{\{\tau_H \ge s\}} u_\lambda(B_s^H) \right] e^{-\lambda s} \, ds.$$

The inequalities

$$\forall H \in (\tfrac{1}{2}, 1), \ \forall s \in (0, \infty), \ |Hs^{2H-1} - \tfrac{1}{2}| \le (H - \tfrac{1}{2})\,(1 \vee s^{2H-1})(1 + 2H|\log s|)$$

and

$$\mathbb{E}\left[\mathbf{1}_{\{\tau_H \ge s\}} u_\lambda(B_s^H)\right] \le \int_{-\infty}^1 u_\lambda(x) \frac{e^{-\frac{x^2}{2s^{2H}}}}{\sqrt{2\pi s^{2H}}} dx = \int_{-\infty}^1 e^{-(1-x)\sqrt{2\lambda}} \frac{e^{-\frac{x^2}{2s^{2H}}}}{\sqrt{2\pi s^{2H}}} dx$$

lead to the desired result.

The above calculation can be extended to diffusions but then accurate estimates on the density of X^H are needed: They are provided by our Theorem 3.

Compared to the proof of Theorem 1, an important difficulty appears when estimating $|I_2(\lambda)|$: as the optional stopping theorem does not hold for Skorokhod integrals of the fBm one has to carefully estimate expectations of stopped Skorokhod integrals and obtain estimates which decrease infinitely fast when λ goes to infinity. We obtained the following result.

Proposition 2

$$\forall \lambda > 1, \ |I_2(\lambda)| \le C(H - \tfrac{1}{2})^{\frac{1}{2} - \varepsilon} e^{-\alpha S(1 - x_0 - 2\eta)\sqrt{2\lambda}}. \tag{8}$$

Proof Proposition 13 of [16] shows that

$$\forall T > 0, \quad \mathbb{E}\left(\delta^{(T)}(\mathbf{1}_{[0,t]}(\cdot) u_\lambda(B_\cdot^H) e^{-\lambda\cdot})\big|_{t=T\wedge\tau_H}\right) = 0.$$

Thus $I_2(\lambda)$ satisfies

$$\begin{aligned}
|I_2(\lambda)| &= \sqrt{2\lambda} \left| \lim_{N\to\infty} \mathbb{E}\left[\delta_H^{(N)}\left(\mathbf{1}_{[0,t]}(\cdot) u_\lambda(B_\cdot^H) e^{-\lambda\cdot}\right)\big|_{t=\tau_H\wedge N} \right.\right.\\
&\qquad\qquad \left.\left. - \delta^{(N)}\left(\mathbf{1}_{[0,t]}(\cdot) u_\lambda(B_\cdot^H) e^{-\lambda\cdot}\right)\big|_{t=\tau_H\wedge N}\right]\right| \\
&= \sqrt{2\lambda}\left| \lim_{N\to\infty} \mathbb{E}\left[\delta^{(N)}\left(\{K_H^* - \mathrm{Id}\}(\mathbf{1}_{[0,t]}(\cdot) u_\lambda(B_\cdot^H) e^{-\lambda\cdot})\right)\big|_{t=\tau_H\wedge N}\right]\right| \\
&\le \sqrt{2\lambda} \lim_{N\to\infty} \mathbb{E} \sup_{t\in[0,\tau_H\wedge N]} |\delta^{(N)}\left(\{K_H^* - \mathrm{Id}\}(\mathbf{1}_{[0,t]}(\cdot) u_\lambda(B_\cdot^H) e^{-\lambda\cdot})\right)| \\
&\le \sqrt{2\lambda} \lim_{N\to\infty} \mathbb{E} \sup_{t\in[0,N]} \left[\mathbf{1}_{\{\tau_H \ge t\}}|\delta^{(N)}\left(\{K_H^* - \mathrm{Id}\}(\mathbf{1}_{[0,t]}(\cdot) u_\lambda(B_\cdot^H) e^{-\lambda\cdot})\right)|\right].
\end{aligned}$$

Define the field $\{U_t(v), t \in [0, N], v \ge 0\}$ and the process $\{\Upsilon_t, t \in [0, N]\}$ by

$$\forall t \in [0, N], \ U_t(v) = \{K_H^* - \mathrm{Id}\}\left(\mathbf{1}_{[0,t]}(\cdot)\, u_\lambda(B_\cdot^H)\, e^{-\lambda\cdot}\right)(v),$$

and

$$\Upsilon_t = \delta^{(N)}(U_t(\cdot)).$$

For any real-valued function f with $f(0) = 0$ one has

$$\mathbf{1}_{\{\tau_H \geq t\}}|f(t)| \leq \mathbf{1}_{\{\tau_H \geq t\}} \sum_{n=0}^{[t]} \sup_{s \in [n, n+1]} \mathbf{1}_{\{\tau_H \geq s\}}|f(s) - f(n)|$$

$$\leq \sum_{n=0}^{[t]} \sup_{s \in [n, n+1]} \mathbf{1}_{\{\tau_H \geq s\}}|f(s) - f(n)|.$$

Therefore,

$$|I_2(\lambda)| \leq \sqrt{2\lambda} \lim_{N \to \infty} \mathbb{E} \sup_{t \in [0, N]} \left[\mathbf{1}_{\{\tau_H \geq t\}}|\Upsilon_t|\right] \tag{9}$$

$$\leq \sqrt{2\lambda} \lim_{N \to \infty} \sum_{n=0}^{N-1} \mathbb{E} \sup_{t \in [n, n+1]} \left[\mathbf{1}_{\{\tau_H \geq t\}}|\Upsilon_t - \Upsilon_n|\right].$$

Suppose for a while that we have proven: there exists $\eta_0 \in (0, \frac{1-x_0}{2})$ such that for all $\eta \in (0, \eta_0]$ and all $\varepsilon \in (0, \frac{1}{4})$, there exist constants $C, \alpha > 0$ such that

$$\mathbb{E} \sup_{t \in [n, n+1]} \left[\mathbf{1}_{\{\tau_H \geq t\}}|\Upsilon_t - \Upsilon_n|\right] \leq C (H - \tfrac{1}{2})^{\frac{1}{2} - \varepsilon} e^{-\frac{1}{3(2+4\varepsilon)}\lambda n} e^{-\alpha S(1 - x_0 - 2\eta)\sqrt{2\lambda}}. \tag{10}$$

We would then get:

$$|I_2(\lambda)| \leq C \sqrt{2\lambda} \sum_{n=0}^{\infty} e^{-\frac{\lambda n}{3(2+4\varepsilon)}} (H - \tfrac{1}{2})^{\frac{1}{4} - \varepsilon} e^{-\alpha S(1 - x_0 - 2\eta)\sqrt{2\lambda}}$$

$$\leq C (H - \tfrac{1}{2})^{\frac{1}{2} - \varepsilon} e^{-\alpha S(1 - x_0 - 2\eta)\sqrt{2\lambda}},$$

which is the desired result (8).

In order to estimate the left-hand side of Inequality (10) we aim to apply Garsia–Rodemich–Rumsey's lemma (see below). However, it seems hard to get the desired estimate by estimating moments of increments of $\mathbf{1}_{\{\tau_H \geq t\}}|\Upsilon_t - \Upsilon_n|$, in particular because $\mathbf{1}_{\{\tau_H \geq t\}}$ is not smooth in the Malliavin sense. We thus proceed by localization and construct a continuous process $\bar{\Upsilon}_t$ which is smooth on the event $\{\tau_H \geq t\}$ and is close to 0 on the complementary event. To this end we introduce the following new notations.

For some small $\eta > 0$ to be fixed set

$$\forall t \in [0, N], \ \bar{U}_t(v) = \{K_H^* - \mathrm{Id}\} \left(\mathbf{1}_{[0,t]}(\cdot) \, u_\lambda(B_\cdot^H) \phi_\eta(B_\cdot^H) \, e^{-\lambda \cdot}\right)(v)$$

and

$$\bar{\Upsilon}_t = \delta^{(N)}(\bar{U}_t),$$

where ϕ_η is a smooth function taking values in $[0, 1]$ such that $\phi_\eta(x) = 1$, $\forall x \leq 1$, and $\phi_\eta(x) = 0$, $\forall x > 1 + \eta$.

The crucial property of $\tilde{\Upsilon}_t$ is the following: For all $n \in \mathbb{N}$ and $n \leq r \leq t < n+1$, $\mathbf{1}_{\{\tau_H \geq t\}} \Upsilon_r = \mathbf{1}_{\{\tau_H \geq t\}} \tilde{\Upsilon}_r$ a.s. This is a consequence of the local property of δ [15, p. 47]. Therefore, for any $n \leq N - 1$,

$$\mathbb{E}\left(\sup_{t \in [n,n+1]} \mathbf{1}_{\{\tau_H \geq t\}} |\Upsilon_t - \Upsilon_n|\right) = \mathbb{E}\left(\sup_{t \in [n,n+1]} \mathbf{1}_{\{\tau_H \geq t\}} |\tilde{\Upsilon}_t - \tilde{\Upsilon}_n|\right) \leq \mathbb{E}\left(\sup_{t \in [n,n+1]} |\tilde{\Upsilon}_t - \tilde{\Upsilon}_n|\right).$$
(11)

Recall the Garsia–Rodemich–Rumsey lemma: if X is a continuous process, then for $p \geq 1$ and $q > 0$ such that $pq > 2$, one has

$$\mathbb{E}\left(\sup_{t \in [a,b]} |X_t - X_a|\right) \leq C \frac{pq}{pq-2} (b-a)^{q-\frac{2}{p}} \mathbb{E}\left[\left(\int_a^b \int_a^b \frac{|X_s - X_t|^p}{|t-s|^{pq}} \, ds \, dt\right)^{\frac{1}{p}}\right]$$

$$\leq C \frac{pq}{pq-2} (b-a)^{q-\frac{2}{p}} \left(\int_a^b \int_a^b \frac{\mathbb{E}(|X_s - X_t|^p)}{|t-s|^{pq}} \, ds \, dt\right)^{\frac{1}{p}}$$
(12)

provided the right-hand side in each line is finite. In order to apply (12), we thus need to estimate moments of $\tilde{\Upsilon}_t - \tilde{\Upsilon}_s$. Lemmas 1 and 2 below give bounds on the moments of $\tilde{\Upsilon}_t - \tilde{\Upsilon}_s$ in terms of a power of $|t - s|$. Thus Kolmogorov's continuity criterion implies that $\tilde{\Upsilon}$ has a continuous modification, which justifies to apply the GRR lemma to $\tilde{\Upsilon}$.

In addition, we can easily obtain bounds on the norm $\|\tilde{\Upsilon}_t - \tilde{\Upsilon}_s\|_{L^2(\Omega)}$ in terms of $(H - \frac{1}{2})$. This observation leads us to notice that

$$\mathbb{E}\left(|\tilde{\Upsilon}_s - \tilde{\Upsilon}_t|^{2+4\varepsilon}\right) \leq \|\tilde{\Upsilon}_t - \tilde{\Upsilon}_s\|_{L^2(\Omega)} \times \mathbb{E}\left(|\tilde{\Upsilon}_t - \tilde{\Upsilon}_s|^{2+8\varepsilon}\right)^{\frac{1}{2}}.$$

We then combine Lemmas 1 and 2 below to obtain: For every $[n \leq s \leq t \leq n+1]$,

$$\mathbb{E}\left(|\tilde{\Upsilon}_s - \tilde{\Upsilon}_t|^{2+4\varepsilon}\right) \leq C \, (H - \tfrac{1}{2})(t-s)^{\frac{1}{2}-\varepsilon} \, e^{-\alpha S(1-x_0-2\eta)\sqrt{2\lambda}}$$

$$\times (t-s)^{\frac{1}{2}+2\varepsilon} \, e^{-\frac{1}{3}\lambda s} e^{-\alpha S(1-x_0-2\eta)\sqrt{2\lambda}}$$

$$\leq C \, (H - \tfrac{1}{2}) \, (t-s)^{1+\varepsilon} \, e^{-\frac{1}{3}\lambda s} e^{-\alpha S(1-x_0-2\eta)\sqrt{2\lambda}}.$$

Choosing $p = 2 + 4\varepsilon$ and $q = \frac{2+\varepsilon/2}{2+4\varepsilon}$ we thus get

$$\mathbb{E}\left(\sup_{t \in [n,n+1]} \mathbf{1}_{\{\tau_H \geq t\}} |\Upsilon_t - \Upsilon_n|\right) \leq C \, (H - \tfrac{1}{2})^{\frac{1}{2+4\varepsilon}} \, e^{-\frac{\alpha}{2+4\varepsilon} S(1-x_0-2\eta)\sqrt{2\lambda}}$$

$$\left(\int_n^{n+1} \int_s^{n+1} e^{-\frac{1}{3}\lambda s} (t-s)^{\frac{\varepsilon}{2}-1} \, dt \, ds\right)^{\frac{1}{2+4\varepsilon}}$$

$$\leq C \, (H - \tfrac{1}{2})^{\frac{1}{2+4\varepsilon}} \, e^{-\alpha S(1-x_0-2\eta)\sqrt{2\lambda}} e^{-\frac{1}{3(2+4\varepsilon)}\lambda n},$$

from which Inequality (10) follows.

It now remains to prove the above estimates on $\left\| \bar{\Upsilon}_t - \bar{\Upsilon}_s \right\|_{L^2(\Omega)}$ and $\mathbb{E}\left(|\bar{\Upsilon}_t - \bar{\Upsilon}_s|^{2+8\varepsilon} \right)^{\frac{1}{2}}$: These estimates are provided by Lemmas 1 and 2 below whose proofs are very technical.

Lemma 1 *There exists* $\eta_0 \in (0, \frac{1-x_0}{2})$ *such that: for all* $0 < \eta \leq \eta_0$, *for all* $H \in [\frac{1}{2}, 1)$ *and for all* $0 < \varepsilon < \frac{1}{4}$, *there exist* $C, \alpha > 0$ *such that*

$$\forall \lambda \geq 1, \ \forall 0 \leq n \leq s \leq t \leq n+1 \leq N,$$

$$\mathbb{E}\left(|\bar{\Upsilon}_t - \bar{\Upsilon}_s|^{2+8\varepsilon} \right)^{\frac{1}{2}} \leq C \, (t-s)^{\frac{1}{2}+2\varepsilon} \, e^{-\frac{1}{3}\lambda s} e^{-\alpha S(1-x_0-2\eta)\sqrt{2\lambda}} \,,$$

where the function S is defined as in Theorem 2.

Lemma 2 *There exists* $\eta_0 \in (0, \frac{1-x_0}{2})$ *such that: For all* $0 < \eta \leq \eta_0$ *and* $0 < \varepsilon < \frac{1}{4}$, *there exist* $C, \alpha > 0$ *such that*

$$\forall n \in [0, N], \ \forall H \in [\tfrac{1}{2}, 1), \ \forall n \leq s \leq t \leq n+1, \ \forall \lambda \geq 1,$$

$$\left\| \bar{\Upsilon}_t - \bar{\Upsilon}_s \right\|_{L^2(\Omega)} \leq C \, (H - \tfrac{1}{2})(t-s)^{\frac{1}{2}-\varepsilon} \, e^{-\alpha S(1-x_0-2\eta)\sqrt{2\lambda}}.$$

3 Discussion on the fBm Case with $\lambda < 1$

We believe that Theorem 2 also holds true for $\lambda \in (0, 1]$. One of the main issues consists in getting accurate enough bounds on the right-hand side of Inequality (9).

For $a_\lambda = \lambda^{-\frac{1}{2H}}$ and $b_\lambda = \frac{-\log \sqrt{\lambda}}{\lambda}$ $(\lambda < 1)$ we have

$$|I_2(\lambda)| \leq \sqrt{2\lambda} \, \mathbb{E}\left[\sup_{t \in [0, a_\lambda]} \mathbf{1}_{\{\tau_H \geq t\}} \left| \delta \left(\{K_H^* - \mathrm{Id}\}(\mathbf{1}_{[0,t]} u_\lambda(B_\cdot^H) e^{-\lambda \cdot}) \right) \right| \right]$$

$$+ \sqrt{2\lambda} \, \mathbb{E}\left[\sup_{t \in [a_\lambda, b_\lambda]} \mathbf{1}_{\{\tau_H \geq t\}} \left| \delta \left(\{K_H^* - \mathrm{Id}\}(\mathbf{1}_{[a_\lambda,t]} u_\lambda(B_\cdot^H) e^{-\lambda \cdot}) \right) \right| \right]$$

$$+ \sqrt{2\lambda} \, \lim_{N \to +\infty} \mathbb{E}\left[\sup_{t \in [b_\lambda, N]} \mathbf{1}_{\{\tau_H \geq t\}} \left| \delta \left(\{K_H^* - \mathrm{Id}\}(\mathbf{1}_{[b_\lambda,t]} u_\lambda(B_\cdot^H) e^{-\lambda \cdot}) \right) \right| \right].$$

We here limit ourselves to examine the second summand on the right-hand side and we denote it by $I_2^{(2)}(\lambda)$. The two other terms (corresponding to $t < a_\lambda$ and $t > b_\lambda$) are easier to study.

Compared to Sect. 2.3, we localize the Skorokhod integral in a slightly different manner by using $\phi_\eta(S_t^H)$ instead of $\phi_\eta(B_t^H)$, where S_t^H denotes the running supremum of the fBm up to time t. Hence

$$\mathbf{1}_{\{\tau_H \geq t\}} \delta \left(\{K_H^* - \mathrm{Id}\} \left(\mathbf{1}_{[0,t]} u_\lambda(B_\cdot^H) e^{-\lambda \cdot} \right) \right)$$
$$= \mathbf{1}_{\{\tau_H \geq t\}} \delta \left(\{K_H^* - \mathrm{Id}\} \left(\mathbf{1}_{[0,t]} u_\lambda(B_\cdot^H) \phi_\eta(S_\cdot^H) e^{-\lambda \cdot} \right) \right) \quad \text{a.s.}$$

Set $\bar{V}_\lambda(s) := u_\lambda(B_s^H) \phi_\eta(S_s^H)$ and

$$\tilde{\Upsilon}_t := \delta \left(\{K_H^* - \mathrm{Id}\} \left(\mathbf{1}_{[0,t]} \bar{V}_\lambda(\cdot) e^{-\lambda \cdot} \right) \right).$$

Proceeding as from Eq.(11) to Eq.(12) we get for some $p > 1$ and $m > 0$ (chosen later):

$$\mathbb{E} \left(\sup_{t \in [a_\lambda, b_\lambda]} \mathbf{1}_{\{\tau_H \geq t\}} | \delta_H \left(\mathbf{1}_{[0,t]} u_\lambda(B_\cdot^H) e^{-\lambda \cdot} \right) | \right) \leq \mathbb{P} \left(\tau_H \geq a_\lambda \right)^{\frac{p-1}{p}} C (b_\lambda - a_\lambda)^{\frac{m}{p}}$$

$$\times \left(\int_{a_\lambda}^{b_\lambda} \int_{a_\lambda}^{b_\lambda} \frac{\mathbb{E} \left(|\tilde{\Upsilon}_t - \tilde{\Upsilon}_s|^p \right)}{|t - s|^{m+2}} \, ds dt \right)^{\frac{1}{p}}. \tag{13}$$

We then use the Proposition 3.2.1 in [15] to bound $\mathbb{E} |\tilde{\Upsilon}_t - \tilde{\Upsilon}_s|^p$:

$$\mathbb{E} |\tilde{\Upsilon}_t - \tilde{\Upsilon}_s|^p \leq C(t-s)^{\frac{p}{2}-1} \int_s^t |\mathbb{E} \left(\bar{V}_\lambda(r) e^{-\lambda r} \right)|^p$$
$$+ \mathbb{E} \left[\left(\int_0^{b_\lambda} |D_\theta \bar{V}_\lambda(r) e^{-\lambda r}|^2 \, d\theta \right)^{\frac{p}{2}} \right] dr. \tag{14}$$

The Malliavin derivative of the supremum of the fBm is obtained for example in [7]. Denoting by ϑ_r the first time at which B^H reaches S_r^H on the interval $[0, r]$ we have $D_\theta^H S_r^H = \mathbf{1}_{\{\vartheta_r > \theta\}}$. It follows that $D_\theta S_r^H = K_H(\vartheta_r, \theta)$. Since $D_\theta \bar{V}_\lambda(r) = \phi_\eta(S_r^H) D_\theta u_\lambda(B_r^H) + u_\lambda(B_r^H) D_\theta \phi_\eta(S_r^H)$, we are led to study the three following terms (for $p > 2$):

(i) $\mathbb{E} \left(\bar{V}_\lambda(r) e^{-\lambda r} \right) \leq \mathbb{E} \left(\phi_\eta(S_r^H) \right) \leq \mathbb{P}(S_r^H \leq 1 + \eta).$

(ii) $e^{-p\lambda r} \mathbb{E} \left[\left(\int_0^{b_\lambda} |\phi_\eta(S_r^H) D_\theta u_\lambda(B_r^H)|^2 \, d\theta \right)^{\frac{p}{2}} \right]$
$$\leq \mathbb{E} \left[\mathbf{1}_{\{S_r^H \leq 1+\eta\}} \left(\int_0^r |\sqrt{2\lambda} K_H(r, \theta) u_\lambda(B_r^H)|^2 \, d\theta \right)^{\frac{p}{2}} \right]$$
$$= (\sqrt{2\lambda})^p \, r^{pH} \, \mathbb{E}(\mathbf{1}_{\{S_r^H \leq 1+\eta\}} u_\lambda(B_r^H)^p).$$

(iii) $e^{-p\lambda r} \mathbb{E} \left[\left(\int_0^{b_\lambda} |u_\lambda(B_r^H) D_\theta \phi_\eta(S_r^H)|^2 \, d\theta \right)^{\frac{p}{2}} \right]$
$$\leq \mathbb{E} \left[\phi_\eta'(S_r^H)^p \, \vartheta_r^{Hp} \right] \leq \|\phi_\eta'\|_\infty^p \mathbb{E} \left[\mathbf{1}_{\{S_r^H \leq 1+\eta\}} \vartheta_r^{Hp} \right].$$

We do not know any accurate estimate on the joint law of either $(S_\cdot^H, B_\cdot^H)$ or $(S_\cdot^H, \vartheta_\cdot)$. We thus can only use the rough bounds $\mathbf{1}_{\{S_r^H \leq 1+\eta\}} u_\lambda(B_r^H) \leq C \mathbf{1}_{\{S_r^H \leq 1+\eta\}}$ for (ii) and

$\vartheta_r \leq r$ for (iii). Then one is in a position to use the following refinement of Molchan's asymptotic [14] obtained by Aurzada [1]: $\mathbb{P}(\tau_H \geq t) \leq t^{-(1-H)} (\log t)^c$ for some constant $c > 0$. However, when plugged into (14) and then into (13), these bounds lead us to an upper bound for $|I_2^{(2)}(\lambda)|$ which diverges when $\lambda \to 0$.

Hence, the preceding rough bounds on (ii) and (iii) must be improved. In the Brownian motion case, the joint laws of $(B_r, S_r^{\frac{1}{2}})$ and $(\vartheta_r, S_r^{\frac{1}{2}})$ are known (see e.g. [12, p. 96–102]). In particular, for $p \in (2, 3)$ the term (iii) leads to

$$\forall r \geq 0, \quad \mathbb{E}\left[\mathbf{1}_{\{S_r^{1/2} \leq 1+\eta\}} \vartheta_r^{\frac{p}{2}}\right] \leq C \tag{15}$$

instead of the bound $r^{\frac{p}{2}-\frac{1}{2}} (\log t)^c$ when one uses the previous rough method.

From numerical simulations and an incomplete mathematical analysis using arguments developed by [1, 14], we believe that Inequality (15) remains true for $H > \frac{1}{2}$. If so, the bound on $|I_2^{(2)}(\lambda)|$ would become

$$|I_2^{(2)}(\lambda)| \leq C\sqrt{2\lambda} a_\lambda^{-(1-H)\frac{p-1}{p}} (b_\lambda - a_\lambda)^{\frac{1}{2}},$$

which, in view of $a_\lambda = \lambda^{-\frac{1}{2H}}$ and $b_\lambda = \frac{-\log\sqrt{\lambda}}{\lambda}$, can now be bounded as $\lambda \to 0$.

4 Optimal Rate of Convergence in Theorem 2: Comparison with Numerical Results

In this section, we numerically approximate the quantity $\mathcal{L}(H, \lambda) = \mathbb{E}\left[e^{-\lambda\tau_H}\right]$, where τ_H is the first time a fractional Brownian motion started from 0 hits 1.

As already recalled this Laplace transform is explicitly known in the Brownian case: $\mathcal{L}(\frac{1}{2}, \lambda) = e^{-\sqrt{2\lambda}}$, $\forall \lambda \geq 0$. Our simulations suggest that the convergence of $\mathcal{L}(H, \lambda)$ towards $\mathcal{L}(\frac{1}{2}, \lambda)$ is faster than what we were able to prove. We also show numerical experiments which concern the convergence of hitting time densities.

Although several numerical schemes permit to decrease the weak error when estimating $\tau_{\frac{1}{2}}$, none seem to be available in the fractional Brownian motion case. We thus propose a heuristic extension of the bridge correction of Gobet [9] (valid in the Markov case) and compare this procedure to the standard Euler scheme.

Convergence of $\mathbb{E}\left[e^{-\lambda\tau_H}\right]$ to $\mathbb{E}\left[e^{-\lambda\tau_{\frac{1}{2}}}\right]$.
Let us fix a time horizon T and N points on each trajectory. Let $\delta = \frac{T}{N}$ be the time step. Denote by M the number of Monte-Carlo samples. For each $m \in \{1, \ldots, M\}$, we simulate $\{B_{n\delta}^{H,N}(m)\}_{1 \leq n \leq N}$, from which we obtain $\tau_H^{\delta,T}(m) = \inf\{n\delta : B_{n\delta}^{H,N}(m) > 1\}$. We then approximate $\mathcal{L}(H, \lambda)$ as follows:

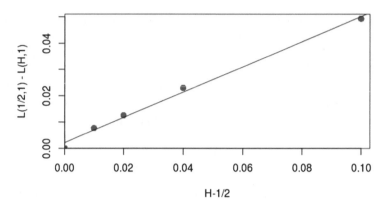

Fig. 1 Regression of $\mathcal{L}(\frac{1}{2}, 1) - \mathcal{L}(H, 1)$ against $H - \frac{1}{2}$ using the values from Table 1

$$\mathcal{L}(H, \lambda) \approx \frac{1}{M} \sum_{m=1}^{M} e^{-\lambda \tau_H^{\delta,T}(m)} =: \mathcal{L}^{\delta,T,M}(H, \lambda) .$$

The bias $\tau_H^{\delta,T}(m) \geq \tau_H(m)$ due to the time discretization implies

$$\lim_{M \to \infty} \mathcal{L}^{\delta,T,M}(H, \lambda) \leq \mathcal{L}(H, \lambda)$$

.

In view of Theorem 2 we have

$$\log \left| \mathcal{L}(H, \lambda) - \mathcal{L}(\tfrac{1}{2}, \lambda) \right| \leq C_\lambda + \beta \, \log(H - \frac{1}{2}) ,$$

with $\beta = (\frac{1}{4} - \varepsilon)$. We approximate $\log \left| \mathcal{L}(H, \lambda) - \mathcal{L}(\frac{1}{2}, \lambda) \right|$ by $\log \left| \mathcal{L}^{\delta,T,M}(H, \lambda) - \mathcal{L}(\frac{1}{2}, \lambda) \right|$ for several values of H close to $\frac{1}{2}$ and then perform a linear regression analysis around $\log(H - \frac{1}{2})$. The slope of the regression line provides a hint on the optimal value of β.

The global error $|\mathcal{L}(H, 1) - \mathcal{L}^{\delta,T,M}(H, 1)|$ results from the discretization error $\mathrm{err}(\delta)$ and the statistical error $\mathrm{err}(M)$. For $M = 2^{13}$ and $\delta = 3.10^{-4}$ the estimator of the standard deviation of $\mathcal{L}^{\delta,T,M}(H, \lambda)$ is 0.259. This allows to decrease the number of simulations to 100,000 to have a statistical error of order 0.0016.

The numerical results are presented in Table 1 for several values of $\lambda(= 1, 2, 3, 4)$ and of the parameter $H \in \{0, 5; 0, 51; 0, 52; 0, 54; 0, 6\}$. These results suggest that $|\mathcal{L}^{\delta,T,M}(\frac{1}{2}, \lambda) - \mathcal{L}^{\delta,T,M}(H, \lambda)|$ is linear w.r.t. $(H - \frac{1}{2})$. For each λ we thus perform a linear regression on these quantities (without the above log transformation). The regression line is plotted in Fig. 1.

Our numerical results suggest that Theorem 2 is not optimal but the optimal convergence rate seems hard to get. An even more difficult result to obtain concerns

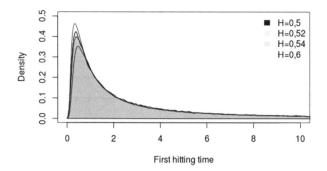

Fig. 2 Density of τ_H for several values of H

the convergence rate of the density of the first hitting time of fBm to the density of the first hitting time of Brownian motion. We analyze it numerically: See Fig. 2.

Brownian Bridge Correction. We apply the following rule (which is only heuristic when $H > \frac{1}{2}$): at each time step, if the threshold has not yet been hit and if $B_{(n-1)\delta}^{H,N}(m) < 1$ and $B_{n\delta}^{H,N}(m) < 1$, we sample a uniform random variable U on $[0, 1]$ and compare it to

$$
p_H = \exp\left\{ -2\frac{\left(1 - B_{(n-1)\delta}^{H,N}(m)\right)\left(1 - B_{n\delta}^{H,N}(m)\right)}{\delta^{2H}} \right\}.
$$

If $U < p_H$ then decide $\tau_H^{\delta,T}(m) = n\delta$. Otherwise let the algorithm continue. In the sequel we denote by $\widetilde{\mathcal{L}}^{\delta,T,M}(H, \lambda)$ the corresponding Laplace transform. This algorithm is an adaptation to our non-Markovian framework of the algorithm of [9] which is fully justified when $H = \frac{1}{2}$. In particular $p_{\frac{1}{2}}$ is the exact probability that a Brownian motion conditioned by its values at time $(n - 1)\delta$ and $n\delta$ crosses 1 in the time interval $[(n - 1)\delta, n\delta]$. Here, we approximate the unknown value of p_H by a heuristic value which coincides with $p_{\frac{1}{2}}$ when $H = \frac{1}{2}$.

Table 2 shows the corresponding results for the simple estimator $\mathcal{L}^{\delta_0,T,M}(\frac{1}{2}, \lambda)$ and the Brownian Bridge estimator $\widetilde{\mathcal{L}}^{\delta_1,T,M}(\frac{1}{2}, \lambda)$ with $\delta_0 < \delta_1$ in the Brownian case (we kept $M = 10^5$). Consistently with theoretical results, Table 2 shows that the estimator $\widetilde{\mathcal{L}}^{\delta,T,M}(H, \lambda)$ allows to substantially reduce the number of discretization steps (thus the computational time) to get a desired accuracy. The figure also shows a reasonable choice of δ_1 which we actually keep when tackling the fractional Brownian motion case.

The exact value $\mathcal{L}(H, \lambda)$ is unknown. Our reference value is the lower bound $\mathcal{L}^{\delta_0,T,M}(H, \lambda)$. The parameter δ_1 used in Table 3 allows to conjecture that the Brownian bridge correction is useful even in the non-Markovian case. Although the approximation errors of the estimators $\mathcal{L}^{\delta_1,T,M}$ and $\widetilde{\mathcal{L}}^{\delta_1,T,M}$ are similar when compared to

$\mathcal{L}^{\delta_0,T,M}(H,\lambda)$, we recommend to use the latter because we have $\mathcal{L}^{\delta_1,T,M}(H,\lambda) \leq \mathcal{L}^{\delta_0,T,M}(H,\lambda) \leq \mathcal{L}(H,\lambda)$ whereas $\mathcal{L}^{\delta_0,T,M}(H,\lambda) \leq \widetilde{\mathcal{L}}^{\delta_1,T,M}(H,\lambda)$.

Appendix: Tables

Table 1 Values of $\Delta_H = \mathbb{E}\left[e^{-\lambda\tau_{\frac{1}{2}}}\right] - \mathbb{E}\left[e^{-\lambda\tau_H}\right]$ when $H \to \frac{1}{2}$. Set of parameters: $T = 20$, $N = 2^{16}$ ($\delta \approx 3.10^{-4}$), $M = 10^5$

H	$\lambda = 1$		$\lambda = 2$		$\lambda = 3$		$\lambda = 4$	
	$\mathcal{L}^{\delta,T,M}(H,\lambda)$	Δ_H	$\mathcal{L}^{\delta,T,M}(H,\lambda)$	Δ_H	$\mathcal{L}^{\delta,T,M}(H,\lambda)$	Δ_H	$\mathcal{L}^{\delta,T,M}(H,\lambda)$	Δ_H
0,50	0,2400	–	0,1329	–	0,0846	–	0,0578	–
0,51	0,2323	0,0077	0,1271	0,0059	0,0800	0,0046	0,0542	0,0037
0,52	0,2275	0,0125	0,1232	0,0098	0,0769	0,0077	0,0517	0,0061
0,54	0,2171	0,0229	0,1149	0,0180	0,0703	0,0143	0,0464	0,0114
0,60	0,1907	0,0493	0,0958	0,0372	0,0560	0,0286	0,0354	0,0224

Table 2 Test case: Error estimation of our procedure in the Brownian case ($H = \frac{1}{2}$). Set of parameters: $T = 20$, $N = 2^{16}$ ($\delta_0 \approx 3.10^{-4}$), $M = 10^5$ for the simple estimator $T = 20$, $N = 2^{15}$ ($\delta_1 \approx 6.10^{-4}$), $M = 10^5$ for the bridge estimator

λ	$\mathcal{L}(\frac{1}{2},\lambda)$	$\mathcal{L}^{\delta,T,M}(\frac{1}{2},\lambda)$	Error (%)	$\widetilde{\mathcal{L}}^{\delta,T,M}(\frac{1}{2},\lambda)$	Error (%)
1	0,2431	0,2400	1,3	0,2438	0,3
2	0,1353	0,1329	1,7	0,1358	0,4
3	0,0863	0,0846	2,0	0,0867	0,5
4	0,0591	0,0578	2,2	0,0594	0,5

Table 3 Comparison of estimators in the fractional case ($H = 0,54$). Set of parameters: $T = 20$, $N = 2^{16}$ ($\delta_0 \approx 3.10^{-4}$), $M = 10^5$ for the simple estimator $T = 20$, $N = 2^{15}$ ($\delta_1 \approx 6.10^{-4}$), $M = 10^5$ for the simple estimator $T = 20$, $N = 2^{15}$ ($\delta_1 \approx 6.10^{-4}$), $M = 10^5$ for the bridge estimator

λ	$\mathcal{L}^{\delta_0,T,M}(H,\lambda)$	$\mathcal{L}^{\delta_1,T,M}(H,\lambda)$	Error (%)	$\widetilde{\mathcal{L}}^{\delta_1,T,M}(H,\lambda)$	Error (%)
1	0,2171	0,2147	1,1	0,2186	0,7
2	0,1149	0,1131	1,6	0,1165	1,4
3	0,07003	0,0689	2,0	0,0717	1,9
4	0,0464	0,0453	2,3	0,0476	2,5

References

1. Aurzada, F.: On the one-sided exit problem for fractional Brownian motion. Electron. Commun. Probab. **16**, 392–404 (2011)
2. Baudoin, F., Ouyang, C., Tindel, S.: Upper bounds for the density of solutions to stochastic differential equations driven by fractional Brownian motions. Ann. Inst. Henri Poincaré Probab. Stat. **50**(1), 111–135 (2014)
3. Bernardin, F., Bossy, M., Chauvin, C., Jabir, J.-F., Rousseau, A.: Stochastic Lagrangian method for downscaling problems in meteorology. M2AN Math. Model. Numer. Anal. **44**(5), 885–920 (2010)
4. Berzin, C., Latour, A., León, J.R.: Inference on the Hurst Parameter and the Variance of Diffusions Driven by Fractional Brownian Motion. Springer, Berlin (2014)
5. Besalú, M., Kohatsu-Higa, A., Tindel, S.: Gaussian type lower bounds for the density of solutions of SDEs driven by fractional Brownian motions. Ann. Probab. **44**(1), 399–443 (2016)
6. Comte, F., Coutin, L., Renault, É.: Affine fractional stochastic volatility models. Ann. Financ. **8**, 337–378 (2012)
7. Decreusefond, L., Nualart, D.: Hitting times for Gaussian processes. Ann. Probab. **36**(1), 319–330 (2008)
8. Delorme, M., Wiese, K.J.: Maximum of a fractional Brownian motion: analytic results from perturbation theory. Phys. Rev. Lett. **115**, 210601 (2015)
9. Gobet, E.: Weak approximation of killed diffusion using Euler schemes. Stoch. Process. Appl. **87**(2), 167–197 (2000)
10. Jeon, J.-H., Chechkin, A.V., Metzler, R.: First passage behaviour of multi-dimensional fractional Brownian motion and application to reaction phenomena. In: Metzler, R., Redner, S., Oshani, G. (eds.) First-Passage Phenomena and their Applications. World Scientific
11. Jolis, M., Viles, N.: Continuity in the hurst parameter of the law of the symmetric integral with respect to the fractional Brownian motion. Stoch. Process. Appl. **120**(9), 1651–1679 (2010)
12. Karatzas, I., Shreve, S.: Brownian Motion and Stochastic Calculus. Springer, New York (1988)
13. Metzler, R., Redner, S., Oshani, G. (eds.): First-Passage Phenomena and their Applications. World Scientific
14. Molchan, G.M.: Maximum of a fractional Brownian motion: probabilities of small values. Commun. Math. Phys. **205**(1), 97–111 (1999)
15. Nualart, D.: The Malliavin Calculus and Related Topics. Springer, Berlin (2006)
16. Peccati, G., Thieullen, M., Tudor, C.: Martingale structure of Skorohod integral processes. Ann. Probab. **34**(3), 1217–1239 (2006)
17. Richard, A., Talay, D.: Hölder continuity in the Hurst parameter of functionals of stochastic differential equations driven by fractional Brownian motion (2016). arXiv:1605.03475
18. Rypdal, M., Rypdal, K.: Testing hypotheses about sun-climate complexity linking. Phys. Rev. Lett. **104**(12), 128501 (2010)
19. Young, L.C.: An inequality of the Hölder type, connected with Stieltjes integration. Acta Math. **67**(1), 251–282 (1936)

Drift Parameter Estimation in the Models Involving Fractional Brownian Motion

Yuliya Mishura and Kostiantyn Ralchenko

Abstract This paper is a survey of existing estimation techniques for an unknown drift parameter in stochastic differential equations driven by fractional Brownian motion. We study the cases of continuous and discrete observations of the solution. Special attention is given to the fractional Ornstein–Uhlenbeck model. Mixed models involving both standard and fractional Brownian motion are also considered.

Keywords Fractional Brownian motion · Stochastic differential equation
Drift parameter estimation · Fractional Ornstein-Uhlenbeck process

1 Introduction

Stochastic differential equations driven by fractional Brownian motion (fBm) have been the subject of an active research for the last two decades. The main reason is that these equations seem to be one of the most suitable tools to model the so-called long-range dependence in many applied areas, such as physics, finance, biology, network studies, etc. In modeling, the problem of statistical estimation of model parameters is of a particular importance, so the growing number of papers devoted to statistical methods for equations with fractional noise is not surprising.

In this paper, we concentrate on the estimation of an unknown drift parameter θ in the fractional diffusion process given as the solution to the equation

$$X_t = X_0 + \theta \int_0^t a(s, X_s)\, ds + \int_0^s b(s, X_s)\, dB_s^H, \tag{1}$$

Y. Mishura · K. Ralchenko (✉)
Taras Shevchenko National University, 64 Volodymyrska,
Kyiv 01601, Ukraine
e-mail: k.ralchenko@gmail.com

Y. Mishura
e-mail: myus@univ.kiev.ua

© Springer International Publishing AG 2017
V. Panov (ed.), *Modern Problems of Stochastic Analysis and Statistics*,
Springer Proceedings in Mathematics & Statistics 208,
DOI 10.1007/978-3-319-65313-6_10

where B^H is a fBm with known Hurst index H. The integral with respect to fBm is understood in the path-wise sense. Special attention is given to the fractional Ornstein–Uhlenbeck process, which is a solution of the following Langevin equation

$$X_t = X_0 + \theta \int_0^t X_s \, ds + B_s^H, \qquad (2)$$

and to its generalizations. This model has been studied since the early 2000s, and comparing to the general case, it has been well developed for now. The asymptotic and explicit distributions for various estimators were obtained, and almost sure limit theorems, large deviation principles, and Berry–Esséen bounds were established for this model. In the general case, only strong consistency results are known, up to our knowledge.

Note that when $H = 1/2$ we obtain a diffusion model driven by standard Brownian motion. The statistical inference for such models has been thoroughly studied by now, presented in many papers, and summarized in several books, see, e.g., [11, 28, 33, 35, 44, 46, 66, 70] and references cited therein. At the same time, we can mention only the book [67] devoted to fractional diffusions (some fractional models are also considered in [11, 51]). In the present article, we try to present the most recent achievements in this field focusing on rather general models.

We also study the following mixed model

$$X_t = X_0 + \theta \int_0^t a(s, X_s) \, ds + \int_0^s b(s, X_s) \, dB_s^H + \int_0^s c(s, X_s) \, dW_s, \qquad (3)$$

which contains both standard and fractional Brownian motion. The motivation to consider such equations comes, in particular, from financial mathematics. When it is necessary to model randomness on a financial market, it is useful to distinguish between two main sources of this randomness. The first source is the stock exchange itself with thousands of agents. The noise coming from this source can be assumed white and is best modeled by a Wiener process. The second source has the financial and economic background. The random noise coming from this source usually has a long-range dependence property, which can be modeled by a fBm B^H with the Hurst parameter $H > 1/2$. As examples of the Eq. (3), we consider linear and mixed Ornstein–Uhlenbeck models.

Note that in the present paper the parameter H is considered to be known. The problem of the Hurst parameter estimation in stochastic differential equations driven by fBm was studied in [9, 40, 41], for mixed models see [21].

Let us mention briefly some related models that are not considered in this article. First note that if $a = b = c \equiv 1$, then we get simple models $X_t = \theta t + B_t^H$ and $X_t = \theta t + B_t^H + W_t$. They were studied in [8, 16, 32], respectively. Recently, a similar mixed model with two fractional Brownian motions was considered in [52, 56]. Prakasa Rao [67] investigated the equation $dX_t = [a(t, X_t) + \theta b(t, X_t)] \, dt + \sigma(t) \, dB_t^H$. He studied maximum likelihood, Bayes, and instrumental variable estimation in this model. Multiparameter equations with additive fractional noise were considered in [18, 71]. Multidimensional model was investigated [60]. In [19, 50], the so-called sub-fractional Ornstein–Uhlenbeck process was studied, where the process B_t^H in (2) was replaced with a sub-fractional Brownian motion. A model with more general Gaussian noise was considered in [22]. For the parameter estimation in the so-called fractional Ornstein–Uhlenbeck process of the second kind, see [1, 2]. Linear and Ornstein–Uhlenbeck models with multifractional Brownian motion were studied in [20]. The parameter estimation for partially observed fractional models related to fractional Ornstein–Uhlenbeck process was investigated in [7, 14, 15, 23].

The paper is organized as follows. In Sect. 2 the basic facts about fBm, path-wise stochastic integration, pure and mixed stochastic differential equations with fBm are given. Section 3 is devoted to the case of estimation by continuous-time observations in the fractional model (1), when the whole trajectory of the solution is observed. In Sect. 4, we consider the discrete-time versions of this model. Mixed models are discussed in Sect. 5.

2 Basic Facts

In this section, we review basic properties of the fBm (Sect. 2.1), consider the path-wise integration using the fractional calculus (Sect. 2.2), and give the existence and uniqueness theorems for stochastic differential equations driven by fBm with $H > 1/2$ (Sect. 2.3) and for mixed stochastic differential equations with long-range dependence, involving both Wiener process and fBm with $H > 1/2$ (Sect. 2.4).

2.1 Fractional Brownian Motion

Let $(\Omega, \mathcal{F}, \overline{\mathcal{F}}, \mathbf{P})$ be a complete probability space with filtration $\overline{\mathcal{F}} = \{\mathcal{F}_t, t \in \mathbb{R}^+\}$ satisfying the standard assumptions. It is assumed that all processes under consideration are adapted to filtration $\overline{\mathcal{F}}$.

Definition 2.1 *Fractional Brownian motion (fBm)* with Hurst index $H \in (0, 1)$ is a Gaussian process $B^H = \{B_t^H, t \in \mathbb{R}^+\}$ on $(\Omega, \mathcal{F}, \mathbf{P})$ featuring the properties

(a) $B_0^H = 0$;
(b) $\mathbf{E} B_t^H = 0, t \in \mathbb{R}^+$;
(c) $\mathbf{E} B_t^H B_s^H = \frac{1}{2} \left(t^{2H} + s^{2H} - |t - s|^{2H} \right), s, t \in \mathbb{R}^+$.

It is not hard to see that for $H = 1/2$ fBm is a Brownian motion. For $H \neq 1/2$ the fBm is neither a semimartingale nor a Markov process.

The fBm was first considered in [37]. Stochastic calculus for fBm was developed by Mandelbrot and van Ness [48], who obtained the following integral representation:

$$B_t^H = a_H \left\{ \int_{-\infty}^0 \left[(t - s)^{H - \frac{1}{2}} - (-s)^{H - \frac{1}{2}} \right] dW_s + \int_0^t (t - s)^{H - \frac{1}{2}} dW_s \right\},$$

where $W = \{W_t,\ t \in \mathbb{R}\}$ is a Wiener process, and $a_H = \sqrt{\dfrac{2H\Gamma(\frac{3}{2}-H)}{\Gamma(H+\frac{1}{2})\Gamma(2-2H)}}$, Γ denotes the Gamma function.

Another representation of the fBm was obtained in [61]:

$$B_t^H = \int_0^t g_H(t,s)\,dW_s, \quad t \in [0, T],$$

where $W = \{W_t,\ t \geq 0\}$ is a Wiener process, and

$$g_H(t,s) = a_H \left[\left(\frac{t}{s}\right)^{H-\frac{1}{2}} (t-s)^{H-\frac{1}{2}} - \left(H - \frac{1}{2}\right) s^{\frac{1}{2}-H} \int_s^t (v-s)^{H-\frac{1}{2}} v^{H-\frac{3}{2}}\, dv \right].$$

For $H > 1/2$ this expression can be slightly simplified:

$$g_H(t,s) = \left(H - \frac{1}{2}\right) a_H s^{\frac{1}{2}-H} \int_s^t (v-s)^{H-\frac{3}{2}} v^{H-\frac{1}{2}}\, dv.$$

Definition 2.1 implies that the fBm is self-similar with the self-similarity parameter H, that is, $\{B_H(ct)\} \overset{\mathcal{D}}{=} \{c^H B^H(t)\}$ for any $c > 0$, where $\overset{\mathcal{D}}{=}$ denotes the distributional equivalence.

The fBm has stationary increments in the sense that $\mathbf{E}\left(B_t^H - B_s^H\right)^2 = |t-s|^{2H}$. Taking into account that the process B^H is Gaussian, one can deduce from the Kolmogorov theorem that it has the continuous (and even Hölder continuous up to order H) modification. In what follows, we consider this modification of fBm.

The increments of the fBm are independent only in the case $H = 1/2$. They are negatively correlated for $H \in (0, 1/2)$ and positively correlated for $H \in (1/2, 1)$. Moreover, for $H \in (1/2, 1)$ the fBm has the property of long-range dependence. This means that $\sum_{n=1}^{\infty} |r(n)| = \infty$, where $r(n) = \mathbf{E} B_1^H \left(B_{n+1}^H - B_n^H\right)$ is the autocovariance function.

Jost [34] established the formula for the transformation of an fBm with positively correlated increments into an fBm with negatively correlated increments, and vice versa. Let $B^H = \{B_t^H, t \in [0, T]\}$ be an fBm with Hurst index $H \in (0, 1)$. Then there exists a unique (up to modification) fBm $B^{1-H} = \{B_t^{1-H}, t \in [0, T]\}$ with Hurst index $1 - H$ such that

$$B_t^H = \left(\frac{2H}{\Gamma(2H)\Gamma(3-2H)}\right)^{\frac{1}{2}} \int_0^t (t-s)^{2H-1}\, dB_s^{1-H},$$

where the integral with respect to fBm is a fractional Wiener integral.

For more details on fBm we refer to the books [10, 51, 62].

2.2 Elements of Fractional Calculus and Fractional Integration

In this subsection, we describe a construction of the path-wise integral following the approach developed by Zähle [76–78]. We start by introducing fractional integrals and derivatives, see [69] for the details on the concept of fractional calculus.

Definition 2.2 Let $f \in L_1(a, b)$. *The Riemann–Liouville left- and right-sided fractional integrals of order* $\alpha > 0$ *are defined for almost all* $x \in (a, b)$ *by*

$$\mathcal{I}_{a+}^\alpha f(x) := \frac{1}{\Gamma(\alpha)} \int_a^x (x - y)^{\alpha-1} f(y)\, dy,$$

$$\mathcal{I}_{b-}^\alpha f(x) := \frac{(-1)^{-\alpha}}{\Gamma(\alpha)} \int_x^b (y - x)^{\alpha-1} f(y)\, dy,$$

respectively, where $(-1)^{-\alpha} = e^{-i\pi\alpha}$.

Definition 2.3 *For a function* $f : [a, b] \to \mathbb{R}$ *the Riemann–Liouville left- and right-sided fractional derivatives of order* α $(0 < \alpha < 1)$ *are defined by*

$$\mathcal{D}_{a+}^\alpha f(x) := \mathbb{1}_{(a,b)}(x) \frac{1}{\Gamma(1-\alpha)} \frac{d}{dx} \int_a^x \frac{f(y)}{(x-y)^\alpha}\, dy,$$

$$\mathcal{D}_{b-}^\alpha f(x) := \mathbb{1}_{(a,b)}(x) \frac{(-1)^{1+\alpha}}{\Gamma(1-\alpha)} \frac{d}{dx} \int_x^b \frac{f(y)}{(y-x)^\alpha}\, dy.$$

Denote by $\mathcal{I}_{a+}^\alpha(L_p)$ (resp. $\mathcal{I}_{b-}^\alpha(L_p)$) the class of functions f that can be presented as $f = \mathcal{I}_{a+}^\alpha \varphi$ (resp. $f = \mathcal{I}_{b-}^\alpha \varphi$) for $\varphi \in L_p(a, b)$. For $f \in \mathcal{I}_{a+}^\alpha(L_p)$ (resp. $f \in \mathcal{I}_{b-}^\alpha(L_p)$), $p \geq 1$, the corresponding Riemann–Liouville fractional derivatives admit the following *Weyl representation*

$$\mathcal{D}_{a+}^\alpha f(x) = \frac{1}{\Gamma(1-\alpha)} \left(\frac{f(x)}{(x-a)^\alpha} + \alpha \int_a^x \frac{f(x) - f(y)}{(x-y)^{\alpha+1}}\, dy \right) \mathbb{1}_{(a,b)}(x),$$

$$\mathcal{D}_{b-}^\alpha f(x) = \frac{(-1)^\alpha}{\Gamma(1-\alpha)} \left(\frac{f(x)}{(b-x)^\alpha} + \alpha \int_x^b \frac{f(x) - f(y)}{(y-x)^{\alpha+1}}\, dy \right) \mathbb{1}_{(a,b)}(x),$$

where the convergence of the integrals holds pointwise for a. a. $x \in (a, b)$ for $p = 1$ and in $L_p(a, b)$ for $p > 1$.

Let $f, g : [a, b] \to \mathbb{R}$. Assume that the limits

$$f(u+) := \lim_{\delta \downarrow 0} f(u + \delta) \quad \text{and} \quad g(u-) := \lim_{\delta \downarrow 0} f(u - \delta)$$

exist for $a \leq u \leq b$. Denote

$$f_{a+}(x) = (f(x) - f(a+))\mathbb{1}_{(a,b)}(x),$$
$$g_{b-}(x) = (g(b-) - g(x))\mathbb{1}_{(a,b)}(x).$$

Definition 2.4 ([76]) Assume that $f_{a+} \in \mathcal{I}_{a+}^{\alpha}(L_p)$, $g_{b-} \in \mathcal{I}_{b-}^{1-\alpha}(L_q)$ for some $1/p + 1/q \le 1$, $0 < \alpha < 1$. *The generalized (fractional) Lebesgue–Stieltjes integral of f with respect to g is defined by*

$$\int_a^b f(x)\,dg(x) := (-1)^{\alpha} \int_a^b \mathcal{D}_{a+}^{\alpha} f_{a+}(x)\,\mathcal{D}_{b-}^{1-\alpha} g_{b-}(x)\,dx + \tag{4}$$
$$+ f(a+)\big(g(b-) - g(a+)\big).$$

Note that this definition is correct, i.e. independent of the choice of α ([76, Proposition 2.1]). If $\alpha p < 1$, then (4) can be simplified to

$$\int_a^b f(x)\,dg(x) := (-1)^{\alpha} \int_a^b \mathcal{D}_{a+}^{\alpha} f(x)\,\mathcal{D}_{b-}^{1-\alpha} g_{b-}(x)\,dx.$$

In particular, Definition 2.4 allows us to integrate Hölder continuous functions.

Definition 2.5 Let $0 < \lambda \le 1$. A function $f: \mathbb{R} \to \mathbb{R}$ belongs to $C^{\lambda}[a, b]$, if there exists a constant $C > 0$ such that for all $s, t \in [a, b]$

$$|f(s) - f(t)| \le C\,|s - t|^{\lambda}, \quad s, t \in [a, b].$$

Proposition 2.6 ([76, Theorem 4.2.1]) *Let $f \in C^{\lambda}[a, b]$, $g \in C^{\mu}[a, b]$ with $\lambda + \mu > 1$. Then the assumptions of Definition 2.4 are satisfied with any $\alpha \in (1 - \mu, \lambda)$ and $p = q = \infty$. Moreover, the generalized Lebesgue–Stieltjes integral $\int_a^b f(x)\,dg(x)$ defined by (4) coincides with the Riemann–Stieltjes integral*

$$\{R - S\} \int_a^b f(x)\,dg(x) := \lim_{|\pi| \to 0} \sum_i f(x_i^*)(g(x_{i+1}) - g(x_i)),$$

where $\pi = \{a = x_0 \le x_0^* \le x_1 \le \ldots \le x_{n-1} \le x_{n-1}^* \le x_n = b\}$, $|\pi| = \max_i |x_{i+1} - x_i|$.

Recall that for any $\mu \in (0, H)$ the trajectories of the fBm B^H are μ-Hölder continuous. Therefore, if $Z = \{Z_t, t \ge 0\}$ is a stochastic process whose trajectories are λ-Hölder continuous with $\lambda > 1 - H$, then the path-wise integral $\int_0^T Z_t\,dB_t^H$ is well defined and coincides with the Riemann–Stieltjes integral.

Remark 2.7 There are many papers devoted to stochastic differential equations with fBm with different definitions of the stochastic integral. In the present paper, we concentrate only on the path-wise definition proposed in [76] for $H > 1/2$. We refer to the book [10] (see also [51]) for the extended survey on various approaches on stochastic integration with respect to fBm and the relations between different types of integrals.

2.3 Stochastic Differential Equations Driven by fBm

Consider a stochastic differential equation driven by fBm $B^H = \{B_t^H, \ t \in [0, T]\}$, $H \in (1/2, 1)$ on a complete probability space $(\Omega, \mathcal{F}, \mathbf{P})$:

$$X_t = X_0 + \int_0^t a(s, X_s)ds + \int_0^t b(s, X_s)dB_s^H, \quad t \in [0, T]. \tag{5}$$

Let the function $b = b(t, x) \colon [0, T] \times \mathbb{R} \to \mathbb{R}$ satisfy the assumptions: b is differentiable in x, there exist $M > 0$, $0 < \gamma, \kappa \le 1$ and for any $R > 0$ there exists $M_R > 0$ such that

(A$_1$) b is Lipschitz continuous in x:

$$|b(t, x) - b(t, y)| \le M|x - y|, \quad \forall t \in [0, T], x, y \in \mathbb{R};$$

(A$_2$) x-derivative of b is locally Hölder in x:

$$|b_x(t, x) - b_x(t, y)| \le M_R|x - y|^\kappa, \quad \forall |x|, |y| \le R, t \in [0, T];$$

(A$_3$) b and its spatial derivative are Hölder in time:

$$|b(t, x) - b(s, x)| + |b_x(t, x) - b_x(s, x)| \le M|t - s|^\gamma, \quad \forall x \in \mathbb{R}, t, s \in [0, T].$$

Let the function $a = a(t, x) \colon [0, T] \times \mathbb{R} \to \mathbb{R}$ satisfy the assumptions

(A$_4$)   for any $R \ge 0$ there exists $L_R > 0$ such that

$$|a(t, x) - a(t, y)| \le L_R|x - y|, \quad \forall |x|, |y| \le R, \forall t \in [0, T];$$

(A$_5$)   there exists the function $a_0 \in L_p[0, T]$ and $L > 0$ such that

$$|a(t, x)| \le L|x| + a_0(t), \quad \forall (t, x) \in [0, T] \times \mathbb{R}.$$

Fix a parameter $\alpha \in (0, 1/2)$. Let $W_\infty^\alpha[0, T]$ be the space of real-valued measurable functions $f \colon [0, T] \to \mathbb{R}$ such that

$$\|f\|_{\infty,\alpha;T} = \sup_{s \in [0,T]} \left(|f(s)| + \int_0^s |f(s) - f(u)| (s - u)^{-1-\alpha} du \right) < \infty.$$

Theorem 2.8 ([65]) *Let the coefficients a and b satisfy* (A_1)–(A_5) *with* $p = (1 - H + \varepsilon)^{-1}$ *with some* $0 < \varepsilon < H - 1/2$, $\gamma > 1 - H$, $\kappa > H^{-1} - 1$ *(the constants* M, M_R, R, L_R, *and the function* a_0 *may depend on* ω*). Then there exists the unique solution* $X = \{X_t, t \in [0, T]\}$ *of Eq. (5),* $X \in L_0(\Omega, \mathcal{F}, \mathbf{P}, W_\infty^{1-H+\varepsilon}[0, T])$ *with a.a. trajectories from* $C^{H-\varepsilon}[0, T]$.

Remark 2.9 Here we restrict ourselves to the one-dimensional case, but it is worth mentioning that Theorem 2.8 was proved in [65] for the case of multidimensional processes. It also admits multiparameter [54] and multifractional [68] generalizations.

When $b(t, x) \equiv 1$, we obtain the following equation:

$$X_t = X_0 + \int_0^t a(s, X_s)ds + B_t^H, \quad t \in [0, T]. \tag{6}$$

Since this equation does not contain integration with respect to fractional Brownian motion, it can be considered for all $H \in (0, 1)$. Nualart and Ouknine [63] proved the existence and uniqueness of a strong solution to Eq. (6) under the following weak regularity assumptions on the coefficient $a(t, x)$.

Theorem 2.10 ([63])

(i) *If* $H \leq 1/2$ *(singular case), we assume the linear growth condition*

$$|a(t, x)| \leq C(1 + |x|).$$

(ii) *If* $H > 1/2$ *(regular case), we assume that a is Hölder continuous of order* $\alpha \in (1 - 1/2H, 1)$ *in x and of order* $\gamma > H - 1/2$ *in time:*

$$|a(t, x) - a(s, y)| \leq C\left(|x - y|^\alpha + |t - s|^\gamma\right).$$

Then the Eq. (6) has a unique strong solution.

Remark 2.11 The existence and uniqueness of a strong solution to (6) can be obtained under weaker conditions on $a(t, x)$. In particular, the equations with locally unbounded drift for $H < 1/2$ were studied in [64]. For $H > 1/2$ Hu et al. [31] considered the case when the coefficient $a(t, x)$ has a singularity at $x = 0$.

2.4 Mixed Stochastic Differential Equations with Long-Range Dependence

Let $(\Omega, \mathcal{F}, \{\mathcal{F}_t\}_{t \in [0, T]}, \mathbf{P})$ be a complete probability space equipped with a filtration satisfying standard assumptions, and $W = \{W_t, t \in [0, T]\}$ be a standard $\mathcal{F}_t$-Wiener process. In this subsection, we investigate more general model than (3): instead of the fBm we consider an $\mathcal{F}_t$-adapted stochastic process $Z = \{Z_t, t \in [0, T]\}$, which is almost surely Hölder continuous with exponent $\gamma > 1/2$. The processes W and Z can be dependent. We study a mixed stochastic differential equation

$$X_t = X_0 + \int_0^t a(s, X_s)\, ds + \int_0^t b(s, X_s)\, dZ_s + \int_0^t c(s, X_s)\, dW_s, \quad t \in [0, T].$$
$$(7)$$

The integral w.r.t. Wiener process W is the standard Itô integral, and the integral w.r.t. Z is path-wise generalized Lebesgue–Stieltjes integral, see Definition 2.4.

We will assume that for some $K > 0, \beta > 1/2$, and for any $t, s \in [0, T], x, y \in \mathbb{R}$,

(B$_1$) $|a(t, x)| + |b(t, x)| + |c(t, x)| \leq K(1 + |x|)$,
(B$_2$) $|a(t, x) - a(t, y)| + |c(t, x) - c(t, y)| \leq K|x - y|$,
(B$_3$) $|a(s, x) - a(t, x)| + |b(s, x) - b(t, x)| + |c(s, x) - c(t, x)|$
   $+ |\partial_x b(s, x) - \partial_x b(t, x)| \leq K|s - t|^{\beta}$,
(B$_4$) $|\partial_x b(t, x) - \partial_x b(t, y)| \leq K|x - y|$,
(B$_5$) $|\partial_x b(t, x)| \leq K$,

Theorem 2.12 ([53]) *Let $\alpha \in (1 - \gamma, \frac{1}{2} \wedge \beta)$ If the coefficients of equation (7) satisfy conditions (B$_1$)–(B$_5$), then it has a unique solution X such that $\|X\|_{\infty, \alpha, T} < \infty$ a.s.*

Remark 2.13 It was proved in [58] that Eq. (7) is uniquely solvable when assumptions (B$_1$)–(B$_5$) hold and if additionally c is bounded as follows:

(B$_6$) $|c(t, x)| \leq K_1$ for some $K_1 > 0$.

Later, in [53] the existence and uniqueness theorem without assumption (B$_6$) was obtained. Equation (7) with $Z = B^H$, a fractional Brownian motion, was first considered in [39], where existence and uniqueness of solution were proved for time-independent coefficients and zero drift. For inhomogeneous coefficients, unique solvability was established in [51] for $H \in (3/4, 1)$ and bounded coefficients, in [27] for any $H > 1/2$, but under the assumption that W and B^H are independent.

3   Drift Parameter Estimation by Continuous Observations

This section is devoted to the drift parameter estimation in the model (1) by continuous observations of the process X. We discuss the construction of the maximum likelihood estimator based on the Girsanov transform. Then we study a non-standard estimator. These results are applied to linear models. In the last subsection of this section, the various estimators in fractional Ornstein–Uhlenbeck model are considered.

3.1 General Fractional Model

Assume that $H > \frac{1}{2}$ and consider the equation

$$X_t = x_0 + \theta \int_0^t a(s, X_s)ds + \int_0^t b(s, X_s)dB_s^H, \quad t \in \mathbb{R}^+, \tag{8}$$

where $x_0 \in \mathbb{R}$ is the initial value, θ is the unknown parameter to be estimated, the first integral in the right-hand side of (8) is the Lebesgue–Stieltjes integral, and the second integral is the generalized Lebesgue–Stieltjes integral introduced in Definition 2.4.

3.1.1 The Standard Maximum Likelihood Estimator

Let the following assumptions hold:

(C₁)   *Linear growth of a, b in space:* for any $t \in [0, T]$ and $x \in \mathbb{R}$

$$|a(t, x)| + |b(t, x)| \le K(1 + |x|),$$

(C₂)   *Lipschitz continuity of a, b in space:* for any $t \in [0, T]$ and $x, y \in \mathbb{R}$

$$|a(t, x) - a(t, y)| + |b(t, x) - b(t, y)| \le K|x - y|,$$

(C₃)   *Hölder continuity of $a, b, \partial_x b$ in time:* there exists $\beta > 1/2$ such that for any $t, s \in [0, T]$ and $x \in \mathbb{R}$

$$|a(s, x) - a(t, x)| + |b(s, x) - b(t, x)| + |\partial_x b(s, x) - \partial_x b(t, x)| \le K|s - t|^{\beta},$$

(C₄)   *Hölder continuity of $\partial_x b$ in space:* there exists such $\rho \in (3/2 - H, 1)$ that for any $t \in [0, T]$ and $x, y \in \mathbb{R}$

$$|\partial_x b(t, x) - \partial_x b(t, y)| \le D|x - y|^{\rho},$$

Then, according to Theorem 2.8, solution for Eq. (8) exists on any interval $[0, T]$ and is unique in the class of processes satisfying

$$\|X\|_{\infty, \alpha, T} < \infty \quad \text{a.s.} \tag{9}$$

for some $\alpha > 1 - H$.

In addition, suppose that the following assumption holds:

(D₁) $b(t, X_t) \ne 0, t \in [0, T]$ and $\frac{a(t, X_t)}{b(t, X_t)}$ is a.s. Lebesgue integrable on $[0, T]$ for any $T > 0$.

Denote $\psi(t, x) = \frac{a(t,x)}{b(t,x)}$, $\varphi(t) := \psi(t, X_t)$. Also, let the kernel

$$l_H(t, s) = c_H s^{\frac{1}{2}-H}(t - s)^{\frac{1}{2}-H} \mathbb{1}_{\{0<s<t\}},$$

with $c_H = \left(\frac{\Gamma(3-2H)}{2H\Gamma(\frac{3}{2}-H)^3\Gamma(H+\frac{1}{2})} \right)^{\frac{1}{2}}$, and introduce the integral

$$J_t = \int_0^t l_H(t, s)\varphi(s)ds = c_H \int_0^t (t - s)^{\frac{1}{2}-H}s^{\frac{1}{2}-H}\varphi(s)ds. \tag{10}$$

Finally, let $M_t^H = \int_0^t l_H(t, s)dB_s^H$ be Gaussian martingale with square bracket $\langle M^H \rangle_t = t^{2-2H}$ (Molchan martingale, see [61]).
Consider the following two processes:

$$Y_t = \int_0^t b^{-1}(s, X_s)dX_s = \theta \int_0^t \varphi(s)ds + B_t^H$$

and

$$Z_t = \int_0^t l_H(t, s)dY_s = \theta J_t + M_t^H.$$

Remark 3.1 Note that the transformation from X to Z does not lead to loss of information since we can present Y (consequently, X) via Z and Volterra kernel introduced in Theorem 5.2 [61]. So, these processes generate the same filtration.

Also, note that we can rewrite process Z as

$$Z_t = \int_0^t l_H(t, s)b^{-1}(s, X_s)dX_s,$$

so Z is a functional of the observable process X. The following smoothness condition for the function ψ (Lemma 6.3.2 [51]) ensures the semimartingale property of Z.

Lemma 3.2 *Let* $\psi = \psi(t, x) \in C^1(\mathbb{R}^+) \times C^2(\mathbb{R})$. *Then for any* $t > 0$

$$J'(t) = (2 - 2H)C_H\psi(0, x_0)t^{1-2H}$$

$$+ \int_0^t l_H(t, s)\left(\frac{\partial\psi}{\partial t}(s, X_s) + \theta\frac{\partial\psi}{\partial x}(s, X_s)a(s, X_s) \right)ds$$

$$- \left(H - \frac{1}{2}\right)c_H \int_0^t s^{-\frac{1}{2}-H}(t - s)^{\frac{1}{2}-H} \int_0^s \left(\frac{\partial\psi}{\partial t}(u, X_u) + \theta\frac{\partial\psi}{\partial x}(u, X_u)a(u, X_u) \right)duds$$

$$+ (2 - 2H)c_H t^{1-2H} \int_0^t s^{2H-3} \int_0^s u^{\frac{3}{2}-H}(s - u)^{\frac{1}{2}-H}\frac{\partial\psi}{\partial x}(u, X_u)b(u, X_u)dB_u^H ds$$

$$+ c_H t^{-1} \int_0^t u^{\frac{3}{2}-H}(t - u)^{\frac{1}{2}-H}\frac{\partial\psi}{\partial x}(u, X_u)b(u, X_u)dB_u^H, \tag{11}$$

where $C_H = B(\frac{3}{2} - H, \frac{3}{2} - H)c_H = \left(\frac{\Gamma(\frac{3}{2}-H)}{2H\Gamma(H+\frac{1}{2})\Gamma(3-2H)}\right)^{\frac{1}{2}}$, and all of the involved integrals exists a.s.

Remark 3.3 Suppose that $\psi(t, x) \in C^1(\mathbb{R}^+) \times C^2(\mathbb{R})$ and limit $\varsigma(0) = \lim_{s \to 0} \varsigma(s)$ exists a.s., where $\varsigma(s) = s^{\frac{1}{2}-H}\varphi(s)$. In this case $J(t)$ can be presented as

$$J(t) = c_H \int_0^t (t-s)^{\frac{1}{2}-H}\varsigma(s)ds = \frac{c_H t^{\frac{3}{2}-H}}{\frac{3}{2}-H}\varsigma(0) + c_H \int_0^t \frac{(t-s)^{\frac{3}{2}-H}}{\frac{3}{2}-H}\varsigma'(s)ds,$$

and $J'(t)$ from (11) can be simplified to

$$J'(t) = c_H t^{\frac{1}{2}-H}\varsigma(0) + \int_0^t l_H(t, s)\left(\left(\frac{1}{2} - H\right)s^{-1}\varphi(s) + \frac{\partial\psi}{\partial t}(s, X_s)\right.$$

$$\left. + \theta\frac{\partial\psi}{\partial x}(s, X_s)a(s, X_s)\right)ds + \int_0^t l_H(t, s)\frac{\partial\psi}{\partial x}(s, X_s)b(s, X_s)dB_s^H.$$

Same way as Z, processes J and J' are functionals of X. It is more convenient to consider process $\chi(t) = (2 - 2H)^{-1}J'(t)t^{2H-1}$, so that

$$Z_t = (2 - 2H)\theta\int_0^t \chi(s)s^{1-2H}ds + M_t^H = \theta\int_0^t \chi(s)d\langle M^H\rangle_s + M_t^H.$$

Suppose that the following conditions hold:

(D$_2$) $\mathbf{E}I_T := \mathbf{E}\int_0^T \chi_s^2 d\langle M^H\rangle_s < \infty$ for any $T > 0$,
(D$_3$) $I_\infty := \int_0^\infty \chi_s^2 d\langle M^H\rangle_s = \infty$ a.s.

Then we can consider the maximum likelihood estimator (MLE)

$$\theta_T^{(1)} = \frac{\int_0^T \chi_s dZ_s}{\int_0^T \chi_s^2 d\langle M^H\rangle_s} = \theta + \frac{\int_0^T \chi_s dM_s^H}{\int_0^T \chi_s^2 d\langle M^H\rangle_s}.$$

Condition (D$_2$) ensures that process $\int_0^t \chi_s dM_s^H, t > 0$ is a square integrable martingale, and condition (D$_3$) alongside with the law of large numbers for martingales ensure that $\frac{\int_0^T \chi_s dM_s^H}{\int_0^T \chi_s^2 d\langle M^H\rangle_s} \to 0$ a.s. as $T \to \infty$. Summarizing, we arrive at the following result.

Theorem 3.4 ([51]) *Let* $\psi(t, x) \in C^1(\mathbb{R}^+) \times C^2(\mathbb{R})$ *and assumptions* (C_1)–(C_4) *and* (D_1)–(D_3) *hold. Then the estimator* $\theta_T^{(1)}$ *is strongly consistent as* $T \to \infty$.

Remark 3.5 In [57] the explicit form of the likelihood ratio was established. It was shown that MLE can be presented as a function of the observed process X_t, namely

$$
\widehat{\theta}_t^{(1)} = \frac{\int_0^t \left(\varphi(s) + (H - \frac{1}{2})s^{2H-1} \int_0^s \frac{s^{\frac{1}{2}-H}\varphi(s) - u^{\frac{1}{2}-H}\varphi(u)}{(s-u)^{H+\frac{1}{2}}} du \right) d\widetilde{Y}_s}{\int_0^t s^{2H-1} \left(\frac{\varphi(s)}{s^{2H-1}} + (H - \frac{1}{2}) \int_0^s \frac{s^{\frac{1}{2}-H}\varphi(s) - u^{\frac{1}{2}-H}\varphi(u)}{(s-u)^{H+\frac{1}{2}}} du \right)^2 ds},
$$

where $\widetilde{Y}_s = \int_0^s v^{\frac{1}{2}-H}(s-v)^{\frac{1}{2}-H} b^{-1}(v, X_v) dX_v$.

Remark 3.6 Tudor and Viens [74] constructed the MLE for the following model

$$
X_t = \int_0^t a(X_s) ds + B_t^H, \quad X_0 = 0.
$$

Under some regularity conditions on the coefficient $a(x)$ they proved the strong consistency of the MLE in both cases $H < 1/2$ and $H > 1/2$.

3.1.2 A Nonstandard Estimator

It is possible to construct another estimator for parameter θ, preserving the structure of the standard MLE. Similar approach was applied in [29] to the fractional Ornstein–Uhlenbeck process with constant coefficients (see the estimator (19) below). We shall use process Y to define the estimator as follows:

$$
\widehat{\theta}_T^{(2)} = \frac{\int_0^T \varphi_s dY_s}{\int_0^T \varphi_s^2 ds} = \theta + \frac{\int_0^T \varphi_s dB_s^H}{\int_0^T \varphi_s^2 ds}. \tag{12}
$$

Theorem 3.7 ([38]) *Let assumptions* (C_1)–(C_4), (D_1), *and* (D_2) *hold and let function* φ *satisfy the following assumption:*

(D_4) *There exists such* $\alpha > 1 - H$ *and* $p > 1$ *that*

$$
\rho_{\alpha, p, T} := \frac{T^{H+\alpha-1}(\log T)^p \int_0^T |(\mathcal{D}_{0+}^\alpha \varphi)(s)| ds}{\int_0^T \varphi_s^2 ds} \to 0 \quad a.s. \ as \ T \to \infty. \tag{13}
$$

Then estimator $\widehat{\theta}_T^{(2)}$ *is correctly defined and strongly consistent as* $T \to \infty$.

Relation (13) ensures convergence $\frac{\int_0^T \varphi_s dB_s^H}{\int_0^T \varphi_s^2 ds} \to 0$ a.s. in the general case. In a particular case when function φ is nonrandom and integral $\int_0^T \varphi_s dB_s^H$ is a Wiener integral w.r.t. the fractional Brownian motion, conditions for existence of this integral are simpler since assumption (13) can be simplified.

Theorem 3.8 ([38]) *Let assumptions* (C_1)–(C_4), (D_1), *and* (D_2) *hold and let function* φ *be nonrandom and satisfy the following assumption:*

(D_5) *There exists such $p > 0$ that*

$$\limsup_{T\to\infty} \frac{T^{2H-1+p}}{\int_0^T \varphi^2(t)dt} < \infty.$$

Then estimator $\widehat{\theta}_T^{(2)}$ is strongly consistent as $T \to \infty$.

In the next subsection, we consider some examples of φ and establish not only the convergence to zero but the rate of convergence as well.

3.1.3   Examples of the Remainder Terms with the Estimation of the Rate of Convergence to Zero

We start with the simplest case when φ is a power function, $\varphi(t) = t^a$, $a \geq 0$, $t \geq 0$. It means that $a(t, x) = b(t, x)t^a$. If the coefficient $b(t, x)$ satisfies assumptions (C_1)–(C_4) and $b(t, X_t) \neq 0, t \in [0, T]$, then $a(t, x)$ satisfies assumptions (C_1)–(C_4) on any interval $[0, T]$, condition (D_1) holds, then the Eq. (8) has the unique solution, the estimator $\widehat{\theta}_T^{(2)}$ is correctly defined and we can study the properties of the remainder term $\rho_{\alpha,p,T}$.

Lemma 3.9 ([3]) *Let $\varphi(t) = t^a$, $a \geq 0, t \geq 0$. Then $\rho_{\alpha,p,T} = C_a T^{H-a-1} \times (\log T)^p \to 0$ as $T \to \infty$, where*

$$C_a = \frac{(2a+1)\Gamma(a+1)}{\Gamma(a-\alpha+2)}.$$

Remark 3.10 As to the rate of convergence to zero, we can say that

$$\rho_{\alpha,p,T} = O\left(T^{H-1-a+\varepsilon}\right)$$

as $T \to \infty$ for any $\varepsilon > 0$.

Now, we can consider φ that is a polynomial function. In this case, similar to monomial case, the solution of the Eq. (7) exists and is unique, and the estimator is correctly defined. As an immediate generalization of the Lemma 3.9, we get the following statement.

Lemma 3.11 ([3]) *Let $N \in \mathbb{N} \setminus \{0\}$ and $\varphi_N(t) = \sum_{k=0}^{N} \alpha_k t^{a_k}, t \geq 0, (a_k)$ be a sequence of nonnegative power coefficients, $0 \leq a_0 < a_1 < \ldots < a_N$, and (α_k) be a sequence of nonnegative coefficients, $\alpha_N > 0$. Then $\rho_{\alpha,p,T} \to 0$ as $T \to \infty$, and the rate of convergence to zero is $\rho_{\alpha,p,T} = O\left(T^{H-1-a_N+\varepsilon}\right)$ for any $\varepsilon > 0$.*

Now consider the case of the trigonometric function.

Lemma 3.12 ([3]) *Let* $\varphi(t) = \sin(\lambda t)$, $\lambda \geq 0$. *Then estimator* $\widehat{\theta}_T^{(2)}$ *is strongly consistent as* $T \to \infty$.

Remark 3.13 We see that in the case of power and polynomial functions (Remark 3.10 and Lemma 3.11) we can get not only convergence to zero but also the rate of convergence, but in the case of the trigonometric function, we only get convergence. The difference can be seen from the following result.

Lemma 3.14 ([3]) *Let* $\varphi(t) = \sin(\lambda t)$, $\lambda \geq 0$. *Then*

$$\lim_{T \to +\infty} \rho_{\alpha, p, T} = \lim_{T \to +\infty} \frac{T^{H + \alpha - 1} (\log T)^p \int_0^T |(\mathcal{D}_{0+}^\alpha \varphi)(x)| dx}{\int_0^T \varphi^2(x) dx} = +\infty.$$

Remark 3.15 Note for completeness that for $\dfrac{T^{H + \alpha - 1} (\log T)^p \int_0^T (\mathcal{D}_{0+}^\alpha \varphi)(x) dx}{\int_0^T \varphi_x^2 dx}$ situation is different, more precisely,

$$\lim_{T \to +\infty} \frac{T^{H + \alpha - 1} (\log T)^p \int_0^T (\mathcal{D}_{0+}^\alpha \varphi)(x) dx}{\int_0^T \varphi^2(x) dx} = 0.$$

Lemma 3.16 ([3]) *Let* $\varphi(t) = \exp(-\lambda t)$, $\lambda > 0$. *Then*

$$\lim_{T \to +\infty} \rho_{\alpha, p, T} = \lim_{T \to +\infty} \frac{T^{H + \alpha - 1} (\log T)^p \int_0^T |(\mathcal{D}_{0+}^\alpha \varphi)(x)| dx}{\int_0^T \varphi^2(x) dx} = 0.$$

Remark 3.17 It is easy to deduce from the previous calculations that in the latter case

$$\rho_{\alpha, p, T} = O\left(T^{H - 1 + \varepsilon}\right)$$

as $T \to \infty$ for any $\varepsilon > 0$.

Lemma 3.18 ([3]) *Let* $\varphi(t) = \exp(\lambda t)$, $\lambda > 0$. *Then*

$$\lim_{T \to +\infty} \rho_{\alpha, p, T} = \lim_{T \to +\infty} \frac{T^{H + \alpha - 1} (\log T)^p \int_0^T |(\mathcal{D}_{0+}^\alpha \varphi)(x)| dx}{\int_0^T \varphi^2(x) dx} = 0.$$

Remark 3.19 In this case

$$\rho_{\alpha, p, T} = O\left(e^{-(\lambda - \varepsilon)T}\right) = o\left(T^{-\varepsilon}\right)$$

as $T \to \infty$ for any $\varepsilon > 0$.

Lemma 3.20 ([3]) *Let* $\varphi(t) = \log(1 + t)$. *Then*

$$\lim_{T \to +\infty} \rho_{\alpha,p,T} = \lim_{T \to +\infty} \frac{T^{H+\alpha-1}(\log T)^p \int_0^T |(\mathcal{D}_{0+}^\alpha \varphi)(x)| dx}{\int_0^T \varphi^2(x) dx} = 0.$$

Remark 3.21 In this case

$$\rho_{\alpha,p,T} = O\left(T^{H-1+\varepsilon}\right)$$

as $T \to \infty$ for any $\varepsilon > 0$.

3.1.4 Sequential Estimators

Suppose that conditions (D_1)–(D_3) hold. For any $h > 0$ consider the stopping time

$$\tau(h) = \inf \left\{ t > 0 : \int_0^t \chi_s^2 d\langle M^H \rangle_s = h \right\}.$$

Under conditions (D_1)–(D_2) we have $\tau(h) < \infty$ a.s. and $\int_0^{\tau(h)} \chi_s^2 d\langle M^H \rangle_s = h$. The sequential MLE has a form

$$\widehat{\theta}_{\tau(h)}^{(1)} = \frac{\int_0^{\tau(h)} \chi_s dZ_s}{h} = \theta + \frac{\int_0^{\tau(h)} \chi_s dM_s^H}{h}.$$

A sequential version of the estimator $\widehat{\theta}_T^{(2)}$ has a form

$$\widehat{\theta}_{\upsilon(h)}^{(2)} = \theta + \frac{\int_0^{\upsilon(h)} \varphi_s dB_s^H}{h},$$

where

$$\upsilon(h) = \inf \left\{ t > 0 : \int_0^t \varphi^2(s) ds = h \right\}.$$

Theorem 3.22 ([38])

(a) *Let assumptions (D_1)–(D_3) hold. Then the estimator $\widehat{\theta}_{\tau(h)}^{(1)}$ is unbiased, efficient, strongly consistent, $\mathbf{E}\left(\widehat{\theta}_{\tau(h)}^{(1)} - \theta\right)^2 = \frac{1}{h}$, and for any estimator of the form*

$$\widehat{\theta}_\tau = \frac{\int_0^\tau \chi_s dZ_s}{\int_0^\tau \chi_s^2 d\langle M^H \rangle_s} = \theta + \frac{\int_0^\tau \chi_s dM_s^H}{\int_0^\tau \chi_s^2 d\langle M^H \rangle_s}$$

with $\tau < \infty$ a.s. and $\mathbf{E} \int_0^\tau \chi_s^2 d\langle M^H \rangle_s \leq h$ we have that

$$\mathbf{E}\left(\widehat{\theta}_{\tau(h)}^{(1)} - \theta\right)^2 \leq \mathbf{E}(\widehat{\theta}_\tau - \theta)^2.$$

(b) *Let function φ be separated from zero, $|\varphi(s)| \geq c > 0$ a.s. and satisfy the assumption: for some $1 - H < \alpha < 1$ and $p > 0$*

$$\frac{\int_0^{\upsilon(h)} |(\mathcal{D}_{0+}^{\alpha}\varphi)(s)|ds}{(\upsilon(h))^{2-\alpha-H-p}} \to 0 \quad a.s. \tag{14}$$

as $h \to \infty$. Then estimator $\widehat{\theta}_{\upsilon(h)}^{(2)}$ is strongly consistent.

Remark 3.23 The assumption (14) holds, for example, for a bounded and Lipschitz function φ.

3.2 Linear Models

Consider the linear version of model (8):

$$dX_t = \theta a(t)X_t dt + b(t)X_t dB_t^H,$$

where a and b are locally bounded nonrandom measurable functions. In this case solution X exists, it is unique and can be presented in the integral form

$$X_t = x_0 + \theta \int_0^t a(s)X_s ds + \int_0^t b(s)X_s dB_s^H = x_0 \exp\left\{\theta \int_0^t a(s)ds + \int_0^t b(s)dB_s^H\right\}.$$

Suppose that function b is nonzero and note that in this model

$$\varphi(t) = \frac{a(t)}{b(t)}.$$

Suppose that $\varphi(t)$ is also locally bounded and consider maximum likelihood estimator $\widehat{\theta}_T^{(1)}$. According to (10), to guarantee existence of process J', we have to assume that the fractional derivative of order $\frac{3}{2} - H$ for function $\varsigma(s) := \varphi(s)s^{\frac{1}{2}-H}$ exists and is integrable. The sufficient conditions for the existence of fractional derivatives can be found in [69]. One of these conditions states the following:

(D$_6$)   Functions φ and ς are differentiable and their derivatives are locally integrable.

So, it is hard to conclude what is the behavior of the MLE for an arbitrary locally bounded function φ. Suppose that condition (D$_6$) holds and limit $\varsigma_0 = \lim_{s \to 0} \varsigma(s)$ exists. In this case, according to Lemma 3.2 and Remark 3.3, process J' admits both of the following representations:

$$J'(t) = (2 - 2H)C_H\varphi(0)t^{1-2H} + \int_0^t l_H(t, s)\varphi'(s)ds$$

$$- \left(H - \frac{1}{2}\right)c_H \int_0^t s^{-\frac{1}{2}-H}(t - s)^{\frac{1}{2}-H} \int_0^s \varphi'(u)du\, ds$$

$$= c_H\varsigma_0 t^{\frac{1}{2}-H} + c_H \int_0^t (t - s)^{\frac{1}{2}-H} \varsigma'(s)ds,$$

and assuming (D$_3$) also holds true, the estimator $\widehat{\theta}_T^{(1)}$ is strongly consistent. Let us formulate some simple conditions sufficient for the strong consistency.

Lemma 3.24 ([38]) *If function φ is nonrandom, locally bounded, satisfies (D$_6$), limit $\varsigma(0)$ exists, and one of the following assumptions hold:*

(a) function φ is not identically zero and φ' is nonnegative and nondecreasing;
(b) derivative ς' preserves the sign and is separated from zero;
(c) derivative ς' is nondecreasing and has a nonzero limit,

then the estimator $\widehat{\theta}_T^{(1)}$ is strongly consistent as $T \to \infty$.

Example 3.25 If the coefficients are constant, $a(s) = a \neq 0$ and $b(s) = b \neq 0$, then the estimator has a form $\widehat{\theta}_T^{(1)} = \theta + \frac{bM_T^H}{aC_HT^{2-2H}}$ and is strongly consistent. In this case assumption (a) holds. In addition, power functions $\varphi(s) = s^\rho$ are appropriate for $\rho > H - 1$: this can be verified directly from (10).

Let us now apply estimator $\widehat{\theta}_T^{(2)}$ to the same model. It has a form (12). We can use Theorem 3.8 directly and under assumption (D$_5$) estimator $\widehat{\theta}_T^{(2)}$ is strongly consistent. Note that we do not need any assumptions on the smoothness of φ, which is a clear advantage of $\widehat{\theta}_T^{(2)}$. We shall consider two more examples.

Example 3.26 If the coefficients are constant, $a(s) = a \neq 0$ and $b(s) = b \neq 0$, then the estimator has a form $\widehat{\theta}_T^{(2)} = \theta + \frac{bB_T^H}{aT}$. In this case both estimators $\widehat{\theta}_T^{(1)}$ and $\widehat{\theta}_T^{(2)}$ are strongly consistent and $\mathbf{E}\left(\theta - \widehat{\theta}_T^{(1)}\right)^2 = \frac{\gamma^2 T^{2H-2}}{a^2 C_H^2}$ has the same asymptotic behavior as $\mathbf{E}\left(\theta - \widehat{\theta}_T^{(2)}\right)^2 = \frac{\gamma^2 T^{2H-2}}{a^2}$.

Example 3.27 If nonrandom functions φ and ς are bounded on some fixed interval $[0, t_0]$ but ς is sufficiently irregular on this interval and has no fractional derivative of order $\frac{3}{2} - H$ or higher then we cannot even calculate $J'(t)$ on this interval and it is hard to analyze the behavior of the maximum likelihood estimator. However, if we assume that $\varphi(t) \sim t^{H-1+\rho}$ at infinity with some $\rho > 0$, then assumption (D$_5$) holds and estimator $\widehat{\theta}_T^{(2)}$ is strongly consistent as $T \to \infty$. In this sense, the estimator $\widehat{\theta}_T^{(2)}$ is more flexible. The estimator $\widehat{\theta}_T^{(1)}$ was considered in [45].

3.3 Fractional Ornstein–Uhlenbeck Model

3.3.1 General Case

Consider the fractional Ornstein–Uhlenbeck, or Vasicek, model with nonconstant coefficients. It has a form

$$dX_t = \theta(a(t)X_t + b(t))dt + \gamma(t)dB_t^H, \ t \geq 0,$$

where a, b, and γ are nonrandom measurable functions. Suppose they are locally bounded and $\gamma = \gamma(t) > 0$. The solution for this equation is a Gaussian process and has a form

$$X_t = e^{\theta A(t)}\left(x_0 + \theta\int_0^t b(s)e^{-\theta A(s)}ds + \int_0^t \gamma(s)e^{-\theta A(s)}dB_s^H\right) := E(t) + G(t),$$

where $A(t) = \int_0^t a(s)ds$, $E(t) = e^{\theta A(t)}\left(x_0 + \theta\int_0^t b(s)e^{-\theta A(s)}ds\right)$ is a nonrandom function, $G(t) = e^{\theta A(t)}\int_0^t \gamma(s)e^{-\theta A(s)}dB_s^H$ is a Gaussian process with zero mean.

Denote $c(t) = \frac{a(t)}{\gamma(t)}, d(t) = \frac{b(t)}{\gamma(t)}$. Now we shall state the conditions for strong consistency of the maximum likelihood estimator.

Theorem 3.28 ([38]) *Let functions a, c, d, and γ satisfy the following assumptions:*

(D_7) $-a_1 \leq a(s) \leq -a_2 < 0, -c_1 \leq c(s) \leq -c_2 < 0, 0 < \gamma_1 \leq \gamma(s) \leq \gamma_2$, *functions c and d are continuously differentiable, c' is bounded, $c'(s) \geq 0$, and $c'(s) \to 0$ as $s \to \infty$.*

Then estimator $\widehat{\theta}_T^{(1)}$ is strongly consistent as $T \to \infty$.

Remark 3.29 The assumptions of the theorem are fulfilled, for example, if $a(s) = -1$, $b(s) = b \in \mathbb{R}$ and $\gamma(s) = \gamma > 0$. In this case we deal with a standard Ornstein–Uhlenbeck process X with constant coefficients that satisfies the equation

$$dX_t = \theta(b - X_t)dt + \gamma dB_t^H, \ t \geq 0.$$

3.3.2 The Case of Constant Coefficients

Consider a simple version of the Ornstein–Uhlenbeck model where $a = \gamma = 1$, $b = x_0 = 0$. Corresponding stochastic differential equation has a form

$$dX_t = \theta X_t dt + dB_t^H, \ t \geq 0$$

with evident solution $X_t = e^{\theta t}\int_0^t e^{-\theta s}dB_s^H$. We start with maximum likelihood estimator $\widehat{\theta}_T^{(1)}$. According to [36], it has the following form

$$\widehat{\theta}_T^{(1)} = \frac{\int_0^T Q(s)\,dZ_s}{\int_0^T Q^2(s)\,dw_s^H}, \tag{15}$$

where $w_t^H = \frac{t^{2-2H}\Gamma(3/2-H)}{2H\Gamma(3-2H)\Gamma(H+1/2)}$, $Q(t) = \frac{d}{dw_t^H}\int_0^t k_H(t,s)X_s\,ds$, $Z_t = \int_0^t k_H(t,s)\,dX_s$, $k_H(t,s) = \frac{s^{1/2-H}(t-s)^{1/2-H}}{2H\Gamma(3/2-H)\Gamma(H+1/2)}$.

Theorem 3.30 ([14, 36, 72, 73]) *Let $H \in [\frac{1}{2}, 1)$.*

1. *For any $\theta \in \mathbb{R}$ the estimator $\widehat{\theta}_T^{(1)}$ defined by (15) is strongly consistent.*
2. *Denote $B(\theta, T) = \mathbf{E}\left(\widehat{\theta}_T^{(1)} - \theta\right)$, $V(\theta, T) = \mathbf{E}\left(\widehat{\theta}_T^{(1)} - \theta\right)^2$. The following properties hold:*

    (i) *If $\theta < 0$, then, as $T \to \infty$,*
    $$B(\theta, T) \sim -2T^{-1}; \quad V(\theta, T) \sim 2\,|\theta|\,T^{-1}, \tag{16}$$

    (ii) *If $\theta = 0$, then, for all T,*
    $$B(0, T) = B(0, 1)T^{-1}; \quad V(0, T) = V(0, 1)T^{-2},$$

    (iii) *If $\theta > 0$, then, as $T \to \infty$,*
    $$B(\theta, T) \sim -2\sqrt{\pi \sin \pi H}\theta^{3/2}e^{-\theta T}\sqrt{T}; \tag{17}$$
    $$V(\theta, T) \sim 2\sqrt{\pi \sin \pi H}\theta^{5/2}e^{-\theta T}\sqrt{T}. \tag{18}$$

3. (i) *If $\theta < 0$, then, as $T \to \infty$,*
    $$\sqrt{T}\left(\widehat{\theta}_T^{(1)} - \theta\right) \xrightarrow{\mathcal{L}} \mathcal{N}(0, -2\theta),$$

    (ii) *If $\theta = 0$, then, for all T,*
    $$T\widehat{\theta}_T^{(1)} \overset{\mathcal{D}}{=} \widehat{\theta}_1^{(1)}$$

    (iii) *If $\theta > 0$, then, as $T \to \infty$,*
    $$\frac{e^{\theta T}}{2\theta}\left(\widehat{\theta}_T^{(1)} - \theta\right) \xrightarrow{\mathcal{L}} \sqrt{\sin \pi H}\,\mathcal{C}(1),$$

    where $\mathcal{C}(1)$ is the standard Cauchy distribution, and $\xrightarrow{\mathcal{L}}$ denotes the convergence in law.

Remark 3.31 The MLE for fractional Ornstein–Uhlenbeck process was first studied in [36]. The authors derived the formula for MLE, proved its strong consistency, and got the asymptotic properties of the bias and the mean square error. The asymptotic normality in the case $\theta < 0$ was established in [14]. The asymptotic distributions for $\theta = 0$ and $\theta > 0$ were obtained in [72, 73]. The large deviation properties of the MLE were investigated in [5] (see also [6, 26]). The exact distribution of MLE was computed in [72, 73].

Remark 3.32 It holds that $\widehat{\theta}_{H,T}^{(1)} \overset{\mathcal{D}}{=} \widehat{\theta}_{1-H,T}^{(1)}$, where $\widehat{\theta}_{H,T}^{(1)}$ is the MLE under the Hurst parameter H and the time span T (see [14] for $\theta < 0$, [72] for $\theta = 0$, and [73] for $\theta > 0$). The MLE for $H < 1/2$ was also considered in [74], where the relations (16)–(18) was proved for $H < 1/2$.

Remark 3.33 The properties of estimators in the fractional Ornstein–Uhlenbeck model substantially depend on the sign of θ. The hypothesis testing of the drift parameter sign was studied in [43, 59, 72, 73].

Consider for $H \in (\frac{1}{2}, 1)$ the estimator $\widehat{\theta}_T^{(2)}$:

$$\widehat{\theta}_T^{(2)} = \frac{\int_0^T X_s\,dX_s}{\int_0^T X_s^2\,ds} = \theta + \frac{\int_0^T X_s\,dB_s^H}{\int_0^T X_s^2\,ds}. \tag{19}$$

It admits the following representation

$$\widehat{\theta}_T^{(2)} = \frac{X_T^2}{2\int_0^T X_s^2\,ds}. \tag{20}$$

Note that this form of the estimator is well defined for all $H \in (0, 1)$.

Theorem 3.34 ([4, 22]) *Let $\theta > 0$, $H \in (0, 1)$. Then the estimator $\widehat{\theta}_T^{(2)}$ given by (20) is strongly consistent as $T \to \infty$. Moreover,*

$$e^{\theta T}\left(\widehat{\theta}_T^{(2)} - \theta\right) \overset{\mathcal{L}}{\to} 2\theta\mathcal{C}(1),$$

as $T \to \infty$, where $\mathcal{C}(1)$ is the standard Cauchy distribution.

Remark 3.35 If $\theta < 0$, then $\widehat{\theta}_T^{(2)}$ converges to zero in $L_2(\Omega, \mathbf{P})$ ([29], see the remark at the end of Sect. 3). If the path-wise integral in (19) is replaced by the divergence-type integral, then the estimator (19) is strongly consistent and asymptotically normal [29, Theorems 3.2, 3.4]. The divergence-type integral is the limit of the Riemann sums defined in terms of the Wick product. Since it is not suitable for simulation and discretization, Hu and Nualart [29] proposed the following estimator for the ergodic case $\theta < 0$

$$\widehat{\theta}_T^{(3)} = -\left(\frac{1}{H\Gamma(2H)T}\int_0^T X_s^2\,ds\right)^{-\frac{1}{2H}}.$$

Theorem 3.36 ([29, 43]) *Let $\theta < 0$, $H \in (0, 1)$. Then the estimator $\widehat{\theta}_T^{(3)}$ is strongly consistent as $T \to \infty$. If $H \in (\frac{1}{2}, \frac{3}{4})$, then*

$$\sqrt{T}\left(\widehat{\theta}_T^{(3)} - \theta\right) \xrightarrow{\mathcal{L}} \mathcal{N}\left(0, -\theta\sigma_H^2\right),$$

as $T \to \infty$, where

$$\sigma_H^2 = \frac{4H - 1}{(2H)^2}\left(1 + \frac{\Gamma(3 - 4H)\Gamma(4H - 1)}{\Gamma(2 - 2H)\Gamma(2H)}\right). \tag{21}$$

To construct the estimator for all $\theta \in \mathbb{R}$, Moers [59] combined $\widehat{\theta}_T^{(2)}$ and $\widehat{\theta}_T^{(3)}$ as follows (assuming $x_0 \in \mathbb{R}$ is arbitrary):

$$\widehat{\theta}_T^{(4)} = \frac{X_T^2 - x_0^2}{2\int_0^T X_t^2 dt} - \left(\frac{1}{H\Gamma(2H)T}\int_0^T X_t^2 dt\right)^{-\frac{1}{2H}}.$$

Theorem 3.37 ([59]) *Let* $H \in [\frac{1}{2}, 1)$. *Then the estimator* $\widehat{\theta}_T^{(4)}$ *is strongly consistent for all* $\theta \in \mathbb{R}$. *As* $T \to \infty$,

$$\sqrt{|\theta|T}\left(\widehat{\theta}_T^{(4)} - \theta\right) \xrightarrow{\mathcal{L}} \mathcal{N}\left(0, \theta^2\sigma_H^2\right), \quad \theta < 0, \ H \in \left[\frac{1}{2}, \frac{3}{4}\right),$$

$$T\widehat{\theta}_T^{(4)} \xrightarrow{\mathcal{L}} \psi_H, \quad \theta = 0,$$

$$e^{\theta T}\left(\widehat{\theta}_T^{(4)} - \theta\right) \xrightarrow{\mathcal{L}} 2\theta\frac{\eta_1}{\eta_2 + x_0 b_H}, \quad \theta > 0,$$

where σ_H^2 *is defined in* (21), $b_H = \frac{\theta^H}{\sqrt{H\Gamma(2H)}}$,

$$\psi_H = \frac{\left(B_1^H\right)^2}{2\int_0^1 \left(B_t^H\right)^2 dt} - \left(\frac{1}{H\Gamma(2H)}\int_0^1 \left(B_t^H\right)^2 dt\right)^{-\frac{1}{2H}},$$

and η_1 *and* η_2 *are independent standard normal random variables.*

Bishwal [12] studied for $H \in (1/2, 1)$ and $\theta < 0$ the following minimum contrast estimator

$$\widehat{\theta}_T^{(5)} = -\frac{T}{2\int_0^T Q^2(s)\, dw_s^H}, \tag{22}$$

and proved the same asymptotic normality as the MLE (see statement 3(i) of Theorem 3.30). The distribution of $\widehat{\theta}_T^{(5)}$ was computed in [72].

4 Drift Parameter Estimation by Discrete Observations

4.1 General Fractional Model

Consider a stochastic differential equation

$$X_t = X_0 + \theta \int_0^t a(X_s)ds + \int_0^t b(X_s)dB_s^H, \tag{23}$$

where X_0 is a nonrandom coefficient. In [47] it is shown that this equation has a unique solution under the following assumptions: there exist constants $K > 0$, $L > 0$, $\delta \in (1/H - 1, 1]$, and for every $N > 0$ there exists $R_N > 0$ such that

(E$_1$) $|a(x)| + |b(x)| \leq K$ for all $x, y \in \mathbb{R}$,
(E$_2$) $|a(x) - a(y)| + |b(x) - b(y)| \leq L |x - y|$ for all $x, y \in \mathbb{R}$,
(E$_3$) $\left|b'(x) - b'(y)\right| \leq R_N |x - y|^\delta$ for all $x \in [-N, N]$, $y \in [-N, N]$.

Our main problem is to construct an estimator for θ based on discrete observations of X. Specifically, we will assume that for some $n \geq 1$ we observe values $X_{t_k^n}$ at the following uniform partition of $[0, 2^n]$: $t_k^n = k2^{-n}$, $k = 0, 1, \ldots, 2^{2n}$.

In order to construct consistent estimators for θ, we need another technical assumption, in addition to conditions (E$_1$)–(E$_3$):

(E$_4$) $a(x)$ and $b(x)$ are separated from zero.

We now define an estimator, which is a discretized version of a maximum likelihood estimator for $F(X)$, where $F(x) = \int_0^x b(y)^{-1}dy$:

$$\widetilde{\theta}_n^{(1)} = \frac{2^n \sum_{k=1}^{2^{2n}} \left(t_k^n\right)^{-\alpha} \left(2^n - t_k^n\right)^{-\alpha} b^{-1}\left(X_{t_{k-1}^n}\right)\left(X_{t_k^n} - X_{t_{k-1}^n}\right)}{\sum_{k=1}^{2^{2n}} \left(t_k^n\right)^{-\alpha}\left(2^n - t_k^n\right)^{-\alpha} b^{-1}\left(X_{t_{k-1}^n}\right) a\left(X_{t_{k-1}^n}\right)}.$$

Theorem 4.1 ([55]) *Under conditions* (E$_1$)–(E$_4$), $\widetilde{\theta}_n^{(1)}$ *is strongly consistent. Moreover, for any* $\beta \in (1/2, H)$ *and* $\gamma > 1/2$ *there exists a random variable* $\eta = \eta_{\beta,\gamma}$ *with all finite moments such that* $\left|\widetilde{\theta}_n^{(1)} - \theta\right| \leq \eta n^{\kappa+\gamma} 2^{-\tau n}$, *where* $\kappa = \gamma/\beta$, $\tau = (1 - H) \wedge (2\beta - 1)$.

Consider a simpler estimator:

$$\widetilde{\theta}_n^{(2)} = \frac{2^n \sum_{k=1}^{2^{2n}} b^{-1}\left(X_{t_{k-1}^n}\right)\left(X_{t_k^n} - X_{t_{k-1}^n}\right)}{\sum_{k=1}^{2^{2n}} b^{-1}\left(X_{t_{k-1}^n}\right) a\left(X_{t_{k-1}^n}\right)}.$$

This is a discretized maximum likelihood estimator for θ in Eq. (23), where B^H is replaced by Wiener process.

Theorem 4.2 ([55]) *Theorem 4.1 holds for* $\widetilde{\theta}_n^{(2)}$.

Now let us define a discretized version of $\widehat{\theta}_T^{(2)}$ defined in (12). Put

$$\widetilde{\theta}_n^{(3)} := \frac{2^n \sum_{k=1}^{2^{2n}} a\left(X_{t_{k-1}^n}\right) b^{-2}\left(X_{t_{k-1}^n}\right)\left(X_{t_k^n} - X_{t_{k-1}^n}\right)}{\sum_{k=1}^{2^{2n}} a^2\left(X_{t_{k-1}^n}\right) b^{-2}\left(X_{t_{k-1}^n}\right)}.$$

Let $\varphi(t) = \frac{a(X_t)}{b(X_t)}$,

$$\widehat{\varphi}_n(t) := \sum_{k=0}^{2^{2n}-1} \varphi(t_k^n) \mathbb{1}_{[t_k^n, t_{k+1}^n)}(t).$$

Theorem 4.3 ([57]) *Under conditions (E_1)–(E_4), assume that there exist constants $\beta > 1 - H$ and $p > 1$ such that*

$$\frac{2^{n(H+\beta)} n^p \int_0^{2^n} \left|\left(D_{0+}^\beta \widehat{\varphi}_n\right)(s)\right| ds}{\sum_{k=1}^{2^{2n}} \varphi^2(t_{k-1}^n)} \to 0 \quad a.\, s.\ at\ n \to \infty.$$

Then $\widetilde{\theta}_n^{(3)}$ is strongly consistent.

4.2 Fractional Ornstein–Uhlenbeck Model

In this subsection, we consider discretized versions of the estimators $\widehat{\theta}_T^{(2)}$ and $\widehat{\theta}_T^{(3)}$ in the fractional Ornstein–Uhlenbeck model with constant coefficients

$$dX_t = \theta X_t dt + dB_t^H, \quad t \geq 0.$$

We start with the case $\theta > 0$. Assume that a trajectory of $X = X(t)$ is observed at the points $t_{k,n} = k\Delta_n$, $0 \leq k \leq n$, $n \geq 1$, and $T_n = n\Delta_n$ denotes the length of "observation window". Let us consider the following two estimators:

$$\widetilde{\theta}_n^{(4)} = \frac{\sum_{i=1}^n X_{t_{i-1}}\left(X_{t_i} - X_{t_{i-1}}\right)}{\Delta_n \sum_{i=1}^n X_{t_{i-1}}^2},$$

$$\widetilde{\theta}_n^{(5)} = \frac{X_{t_n}^2}{2\Delta_n \sum_{i=1}^n X_{t_{i-1}}^2}.$$

These estimators are discretized versions of $\widehat{\theta}_T^{(2)}$, obtained from representations (19) and (20).

Theorem 4.4 ([24]) *Let $\theta > 0$, $H \in (\frac{1}{2}, 1)$. Suppose that $\Delta_n \to 0$ and $n\Delta_n^{1+\alpha} \to 0$ as $n \to \infty$ for some $\alpha > 0$. Then the estimators $\widetilde{\theta}_n^{(4)}$ and $\widetilde{\theta}_n^{(5)}$ are strongly consistent as $n \to \infty$.*

A similar estimator to $\widetilde{\theta}_n^{(4)}$ was considered in [42]. Let $n \geq 1$, $t_{k,n} = \frac{k}{n}$, $0 \leq k \leq n^m$, where $m \in \mathbb{N}$ is some fixed integer. Suppose that we observe X at the points $\{t_{k,n}, n \geq 1, 0 \leq k \leq n^m\}$. Consider the estimator

$$\widetilde{\theta}_n^{(6)}(m) = \frac{\sum_{k=0}^{n^m-1} X_{k,n} \Delta X_{k,n}}{\frac{1}{n} \sum_{k=0}^{n^m-1} X_{k,n}^2},$$

where $X_{k,n} = X_{t_{k,n}}$, $\Delta X_{k,n} = X_{k+1,n} - X_{k,n}$.

Theorem 4.5 ([42]) *Let* $\theta > 0$, $H \in (0, 1)$. *Then for any* $m > 1$ *the estimator* $\widetilde{\theta}_n^{(6)}(m)$ *is strongly consistent.*

Now let $\theta < 0$. In [30, 75] the following discretized version of the estimator $\widehat{\theta}_T^{(3)}$ was considered

$$\widetilde{\theta}_n^{(7)} = -\left(\frac{1}{nH\Gamma(2H)} \sum_{k=1}^{n} X_{k\Delta}^2 \right)^{-\frac{1}{2H}},$$

where the process X was observed at the points $\Delta, 2\Delta, \ldots, n\Delta$ for some fixed $\Delta > 0$.

Theorem 4.6 ([30]) *Let* $\theta < 0$, $H \in [\frac{1}{2}, 1)$. *Then the estimator* $\widetilde{\theta}_n^{(7)}$ *is strongly consistent as* $n \to \infty$. *If* $H \in [\frac{1}{2}, \frac{3}{4})$, *then*

$$\sqrt{n} \left(\widetilde{\theta}_n^{(7)} - \theta \right) \xrightarrow{\mathcal{L}} \mathcal{N}\left(0, \frac{\theta^2}{2H^2} \right),$$

as $n \to \infty$.

Remark 4.7 The discretization of MLE was considered in [74]. Discrete approximations to the minimum contrast estimator (22) were studied in [12].

Remark 4.8 For the case $\theta < 0$ the drift parameter estimator based on polynomial variations was proposed in [25].

Remark 4.9 In [13, 79], a more general situation was studied, where the equation had the form $dX_t = \theta X_t dt + \sigma dB_t^H$, $t > 0$, and $\vartheta = (\theta, \sigma, H)$ is the unknown parameter, $\theta < 0$. Consistent and asymptotically Gaussian estimators of the parameter θ were proposed using the discrete observations of the sample path $(X_{k\Delta_n}, k = 0, \ldots, n)$ for $H \in (\frac{1}{2}, \frac{3}{4})$, where $n\Delta_n^p \to \infty$, $p > 1$, and $\Delta_n \to 0$ as $n \to \infty$. In [79] the strongly consistent estimator is constructed for the scheme when $H > \frac{1}{2}$, the time interval $[0, T]$ is fixed and the process is observed at the points $h_n, 2h_n, \ldots, nh_n$, where $h_n = \frac{T}{n}$.

5 Drift Parameter Estimation in Mixed Models

5.1 General Mixed Model

Let us take a Wiener process $W = \{W_t, t \in \mathbb{R}^+\}$ on probability space $(\Omega, \mathcal{F}, \overline{\mathcal{F}}, P)$, possibly correlated with B^H. Assume that $H > \frac{1}{2}$ and consider a one-dimensional mixed stochastic differential equation involving both the Wiener process and the fractional Brownian motion

$$X_t = x_0 + \theta \int_0^t a(s, X_s)ds + \int_0^t b(s, X_s)dB_s^H + \int_0^t c(s, X_s)dW_s, \ t \in \mathbb{R}^+,$$
(24)

where $x_0 \in \mathbb{R}$ is the initial value, θ is the unknown parameter to be estimated, the first integral in the right-hand side of (24) is the Lebesgue–Stieltjes integral, the second integral is the generalized Lebesgue–Stieltjes integral introduced in Definition 2.4, and the third one is the Itô integral. From now on, we shall assume that the coefficients of equation (24) satisfy the assumptions (B_1)–(B_6) on any interval $[0, T]$. It was proved in [58] that under these assumptions there exists a solution $X = \{X_t, \mathcal{F}_t, t \in [0, T]\}$ for the Eq. (24) on any interval $[0, T]$ which satisfies (9) for any $\alpha \in (1 - H, \kappa)$, where $\kappa = \frac{1}{2} \wedge \beta$. This solution is unique in the class of processes satisfying (9) for some $\alpha > 1 - H$.

Remark 5.1 In case when components W and B^H are independent, assumptions for the coefficients can be relaxed, as it has been shown in [27]. More specifically, coefficient c can be of linear growth and $\partial_x b$ can be Hölder continuous up to some order less than 1.

If we consider general equation (24) with nonzero c, then it is impossible to construct reasonable MLE of the parameter θ. Therefore we construct the estimator of the same type as in (12). More exactly, suppose that the following assumption holds:

(F_1) $c(t, X_t) \neq 0, t \in [0, T]$, $\frac{a(t, X_t)}{c(t, X_t)}$ is a.s. Lebesgue integrable on $[0, T]$ for any $T > 0$ and there exists generalized Lebesgue–Stieltjes integral $\int_0^T \frac{b(t, X_t)}{c(t, X_t)}dB_t^H$.

Define functions $\psi_1(t, x) = \frac{a(t,x)}{c(t,x)}$ and $\psi_2(t, x) = \frac{b(t,x)}{c(t,x)}$, processes $\varphi_i(t) = \psi_i(t, X_t)$, $i = 1, 2$, and process

$$Y_t = \int_0^t c^{-1}(s, X_s)dX_s = \theta \int_0^t \varphi_1(s)ds + \int_0^t \varphi_2(s)dB_s^H + W_t.$$

Evidently, Y is a functional of X and is observable. Assume additionally that the generalized Lebesgue–Stieltjes integral $\int_0^T \varphi_1(t)\varphi_2(t)dB_t^H$ exists and

(F_2) for any $T > 0$ $\mathbf{E}\int_0^T \varphi_1^2(s)ds < \infty$.

Denote $\vartheta(s) = \varphi_1(s)\varphi_2(s)$. We can consider the following estimator of parameter θ:

$$\widehat{\theta}_T = \frac{\int_0^T \varphi_1(s)dY_s}{\int_0^T \varphi_1^2(s)ds} = \theta + \frac{\int_0^T \vartheta(s)dB_s^H}{\int_0^T \varphi_1^2(s)ds} + \frac{\int_0^T \varphi_1(s)dW_s}{\int_0^T \varphi_1^2(s)ds}. \tag{25}$$

Estimator $\widehat{\theta}_T$ preserves the traditional form of MLE for diffusion models. The right-hand side of (25) provides a stochastic representation of $\widehat{\theta}_T$.

Theorem 5.2 ([38]) *Let assumptions (F_1) and (F_2) hold, and, in addition,*

(F_3) $\int_0^T \varphi_1^2(s)ds = \infty$ *a.s.*
(F_4) *There exist such $\alpha > 1 - H$ and $p > 1$ that*

$$\frac{T^{H+\alpha-1}(\log T)^p \int_0^T |(\mathcal{D}_{0+}^\alpha \vartheta)(s)|ds}{\int_0^T \varphi_1^2(s)ds} \to 0 \quad a.s. \ as \ T \to \infty.$$

Then the estimator $\widehat{\theta}_T$ is strongly consistent as $T \to \infty$.

Similar to Theorem 3.8, conditions stated in Theorem 5.2 can be simplified in case when function ϑ is nonrandom.

Theorem 5.3 ([38]) *Let assumptions (F_1) and (F_2) hold. Then, if functions φ_1 and φ_2 are nonrandom, function φ_1 satisfies condition (D_5), function φ_2 is bounded, then estimator $\widehat{\theta}_T$ is strongly consistent as $T \to \infty$.*

Sequential version of the estimator $\widehat{\theta}_T$ has a form

$$\widehat{\theta}_{v_1(h)} = \theta + \frac{\int_0^{v_1(h)} \vartheta(s)dB_s^H}{h} + \frac{\int_0^{v_1(h)} \varphi_1(s)dW_s}{h},$$

where

$$v_1(h) = \inf \left\{ t > 0 : \int_0^t \varphi_1^2(s)ds = h \right\}.$$

Theorem 5.4 ([38])

(a) *Let function φ_1 be separated from zero, $|\varphi_1(s)| \geq c > 0$ a.s. and let function ϑ satisfy the assumption: for some $1 - H < \alpha < 1$ and $p > 0$*

$$\frac{\int_0^{v_1(h)} |(\mathcal{D}_{0+}^\alpha \vartheta)(s)|ds}{(v_1(h))^{2-\alpha-H-p}} \to 0 \quad a.s. \tag{26}$$

as $h \to \infty$. Then estimator $\widehat{\theta}_{v_1(h)}$ is strongly consistent.

(b) *Let function ϑ be nonrandom, bounded, and positive, φ_1 be separated from zero. Then estimator $\widehat{\theta}_{v(h)}$ is consistent in the following sense: for any $p > 0$,*
$$\mathbf{E}\left|\theta - \widehat{\theta}_{v_1(h)}\right|^p \to 0 \ as \ h \to \infty.$$

Remark 5.5 The assumption (26) holds, for example, for a bounded and Lipschitz function ϑ.

5.2   Linear Model

Consider a mixed linear model of the form

$$dX_t = X_t \left(\theta a(t)dt + b(t)dB_t^H + c(t)dW_t \right), \tag{27}$$

where a, b, and c are nonrandom measurable functions. Assume that they are locally bounded. In this case solution X for Eq. (27) exists, is unique and can be presented in the integral form

$$X_t = x_0 \exp \left\{ \theta \int_0^t a(s)ds + \int_0^t b(s)dB_s^H + \int_0^t c(s)dW_s - \frac{1}{2} \int_0^t c^2(s)ds \right\}.$$

Assume that $c(s) \neq 0$. We have that $\varphi_1(t) = \frac{a(t)}{c(t)}$ and $\varphi_2(t) = \frac{b(t)}{c(t)}$. The estimator $\widehat{\theta}_T$ has a form

$$\widehat{\theta}_T = \frac{\int_0^T \varphi_1(s)dY_s}{\int_0^T \varphi_1^2(s)ds} = \theta + \frac{\int_0^T \varphi_1(s)\varphi_2(s)dB_s^H}{\int_0^T \varphi_1^2(s)ds} + \frac{\int_0^T \varphi_1(s)dW_s}{\int_0^T \varphi_1^2(s)ds}.$$

In accordance with Theorem 5.3, assume that function φ_1 satisfies (D$_5$) and φ_2 is bounded. Then the estimator $\widehat{\theta}_T$ is strongly consistent. Evidently, these assumptions hold for the constant coefficients.

5.3   Mixed Fractional Ornstein–Uhlenbeck Model

Chigansky and Kleptsyna [17] considered the maximum likelihood estimation in the mixed fractional Ornstein–Uhlenbeck model

$$X_t = X_0 + \theta \int_0^t X_s \, ds + V_t$$

with $V = B + B^H$, where B and B^H, $H \in (0, 1) \setminus \{\frac{1}{2}\}$ are independent standard and fractional Brownian motions. Let $g(s, t)$ be the solution of the integro-differential Wiener–Hopf type equation:

$$g(s, t) + \frac{d}{ds} \int_0^t g(r, t) H \, |s - r|^{2H-1} \, \text{sign}(s - r) \, dr = 1, \quad 0 < s \neq t \leq T.$$

Then the process $M_t = \int_0^t g(s,t)\,dV_s$, $t \in [0,T]$, is a Gaussian martingale with quadratic variation $\langle M \rangle_t = \int_0^t g(s,t)\,ds$, $t \in [0,T]$. The MLE of θ is given by

$$\widehat{\theta}_T = \frac{\int_0^T Q_t(X)\,dZ_t}{\int_0^T Q_t(X)^2\,d\langle M \rangle_t},$$

where $Q_t(X) = \frac{d}{d\langle M \rangle_t} \int_0^t g(s,t)X_s\,ds$, and $Z_t = \int_0^t g(s,t)\,dX_s$.

Theorem 5.6 ([17]) *For $\theta < 0$ the estimator $\widehat{\theta}_T$ is asymptotically normal:*

$$\sqrt{T}\left(\widehat{\theta}_T - \theta\right) \xrightarrow{\mathcal{L}} \mathcal{N}(0, -2\theta), \quad as\ T \to \infty.$$

Large deviation properties of this estimator where investigated in [49].

References

1. Azmoodeh, E., Morlanes, J.I.: Drift parameter estimation for fractional Ornstein–Uhlenbeck process of the second kind. Statistics **49**(1), 1–18 (2015)
2. Azmoodeh, E., Viitasaari, L.: Parameter estimation based on discrete observations of fractional Ornstein–Uhlenbeck process of the second kind. Stat. Inference Stoch. Process. **18**(3), 205–227 (2015)
3. Bel Hadj Khlifa, M., Mishura, Y., Zili, M.: Asymptotic properties of non-standard drift parameter estimators in the models involving fractional Brownian motion. Theory Probab. Math. Stat. **94**, 73–84 (2016)
4. Belfadli, R., Es-Sebaiy, K., Ouknine, Y.: Parameter estimation for fractional Ornstein–Uhlenbeck processes: non-ergodic case. Front. Sci. Eng. **1**(1), 1–16 (2011)
5. Bercu, B., Gamboa, F., Rouault, A.: Large deviations for quadratic forms of stationary Gaussian processes. Stoch. Process. Appl. **71**(1), 75–90 (1997)
6. Bercu, B., Coutin, L., Savy, N.: Sharp large deviations for the fractional Ornstein–Uhlenbeck process. Theory Probab. Appl. **55**(4), 575–610 (2011)
7. Bercu, B., Proïa, F., Savy, N.: On Ornstein–Uhlenbeck driven by Ornstein–Uhlenbeck processes. Stat. Probab. Lett. **85**, 36–44 (2014)
8. Bertin, K., Torres, S., Tudor, C.A.: Drift parameter estimation in fractional diffusions driven by perturbed random walks. Stat. Probab. Lett. **81**(2), 243–249 (2011)
9. Berzin, C., León, J.R.: Estimation in models driven by fractional Brownian motion. Ann. Inst. Henri Poincaré Probab. Stat. **44**(2), 191–213 (2008)
10. Biagini, F., Hu, Y., Øksendal, B., Zhang, T.: Stochastic Calculus for Fractional Brownian Motion and Applications. Springer, London (2008)
11. Bishwal, J.P.N.: Parameter Estimation in Stochastic Differential Equations. Springer, Berlin (2008)
12. Bishwal, J.P.N.: Minimum contrast estimation in fractional Ornstein–Uhlenbeck process: continuous and discrete sampling. Fract. Calc. Appl. Anal. **14**, 375–410 (2011)
13. Brouste, A., Kleptsyna, M.: Asymptotic properties of MLE for partially observed fractional diffusion system. Stat. Inference Stoch. Process. **13**(1), 1–13 (2010)
14. Brouste, A., Iacus, S.M.: Parameter estimation for the discretely observed fractional Ornstein–Uhlenbeck process and the Yuima R package. Comput. Stat. **28**(4), 1529–1547 (2013)
15. Brouste, A., Kleptsyna, M., Popier, A.: Design for estimation of the drift parameter in fractional diffusion systems. Stat. Inference Stoch. Process. **15**(2), 133–149 (2012)

16. Cai, C., Chigansky, P., Kleptsyna, M.: Mixed Gaussian processes: a filtering approach. Ann. Probab. **44**(4), 3032–3075 (2016)
17. Chigansky, P., Kleptsyna, M.: Statistical analysis of the mixed fractional Ornstein–Uhlenbeck process. arXiv:1507.04194 (2016)
18. Clarke De la Cerda, J., Tudor, C.A.: Least squares estimator for the parameter of the fractional Ornstein–Uhlenbeck sheet. J. Korean Stat. Soc. **41**(3), 341–350 (2012)
19. Diedhiou, A., Manga, C., Mendy, I.: Parametric estimation for SDEs with additive sub-fractional Brownian motion. J. Numer. Math. Stoch. **3**(1), 37–45 (2011)
20. Dozzi, M., Mishura, Y., Shevchenko, G.: Asymptotic behavior of mixed power variations and statistical estimation in mixed models. Stat. Inference Stoch. Process. **18**(2), 151–175 (2015)
21. Dozzi, M., Kozachenko, Y., Mishura, Y., Ralchenko, K.: Asymptotic growth of trajectories of multifractional Brownian motion, with statistical applications to drift parameter estimation. Stat. Inference Stoch. Process. (2016). https://doi.org/10.1007/s11203-016-9147-z
22. El Machkouri, M., Es-Sebaiy, K., Ouknine, Y.: Least squares estimator for non-ergodic Ornstein–Uhlenbeck processes driven by Gaussian processes. J. Korean Stat. Soc. **45**, 329–341 (2016)
23. El Onsy, B., Es-Sebaiy, K., Viens, F.: Parameter estimation for a partially observed Ornstein–Uhlenbeck process with long-memory noises. arXiv:1501.04972 (2015)
24. Es-Sebaiy, K., Ndiaye, D.: On drift estimation for non-ergodic fractional Ornstein–Uhlenbeck process with discrete observations. Afr. Stat. **9**(1), 615–625 (2014)
25. Es-Sebaiy, K., Viens, F.: Optimal rates for parameter estimation of stationary Gaussian processes. arXiv:1603.04542 (2016)
26. Gamboa, F., Rouault, A., Zani, M.: A functional large deviations principle for quadratic forms of Gaussian stationary processes. Stat. Probab. Lett. **43**(3), 299–308 (1999)
27. Guerra, J., Nualart, D.: Stochastic differential equations driven by fractional Brownian motion and standard Brownian motion. Stoch. Anal. Appl. **26**(5), 1053–1075 (2008)
28. Heyde, C.C.: Quasi-Likelihood and Its Application. A General Approach to Optimal Parameter Estimation. Springer, New York (1997)
29. Hu, Y., Nualart, D.: Parameter estimation for fractional Ornstein–Uhlenbeck processes. Stat. Probab. Lett. **80**(11–12), 1030–1038 (2010)
30. Hu, Y., Song, J.: Parameter estimation for fractional Ornstein–Uhlenbeck processes with discrete observations. Malliavin Calculus and Stochastic Analysis. A Festschrift in Honor of David Nualart, pp. 427–442. Springer, New York (2013)
31. Hu, Y., Nualart, D., Song, X.: A singular stochastic differential equation driven by fractional Brownian motion. Statist. Probab. Lett. **78**(14), 2075–2085 (2008)
32. Hu, Y., Nualart, D., Xiao, W., Zhang, W.: Exact maximum likelihood estimator for drift fractional Brownian motion at discrete observation. Acta Math. Sci. Ser. B Engl. Ed. **31**(5), 1851–1859 (2011)
33. Iacus, S.M.: Simulation and Inference for Stochastic Differential Equations. With R Examples. Springer, New York (2008)
34. Jost, C.: Transformation formulas for fractional Brownian motion. Stoch. Process. Appl. **116**(10), 1341–1357 (2006)
35. Kessler, M., Lindner, A., Sørensen, M. (eds.): Statistical methods for stochastic differential equations. In: Selected Papers Based on the Presentations at the 7th séminaire Européen de statistiques on Statistics for Stochastic Differential Equations Models, La Manga del Mar Menor, Cartagena, Spain, 7–12 May 2007. CRC Press, Boca Raton (2012)
36. Kleptsyna, M.L., Le Breton, A.: Statistical analysis of the fractional Ornstein–Uhlenbeck type process. Statist. Inference Stoch. Process. **5**, 229–248 (2002)
37. Kolmogoroff, A.N.: Wienersche Spiralen und einige andere interessante Kurven im Hilbertschen Raum. C. R. (Doklady) Acad. Sci. URSS (N.S.) **26**, 115–118 (1940)
38. Kozachenko, Y., Melnikov, A., Mishura, Y.: On drift parameter estimation in models with fractional Brownian motion. Statistics **49**(1), 35–62 (2015)
39. Kubilius, K.: The existence and uniqueness of the solution of an integral equation driven by a p-semimartingale of special type. Stoch. Process. Appl. **98**(2), 289–315 (2002)

40. Kubilius, K., Melichov, D.: Quadratic variations and estimation of the Hurst index of the solution of SDE driven by a fractional Brownian motion. Lith. Math. J. **50**(4), 401–417 (2010)
41. Kubilius, K., Mishura, Y.: The rate of convergence of Hurst index estimate for the stochastic differential equation. Stoch. Process. Appl. **122**(11), 3718–3739 (2012)
42. Kubilius, K., Mishura, Y., Ralchenko, K., Seleznjev, O.: Consistency of the drift parameter estimator for the discretized fractional Ornstein–Uhlenbeck process with Hurst index $H \in (0, \frac{1}{2})$. Electron. J. Stat. **9**(2), 1799–1825 (2015)
43. Kukush, A., Mishura, Y., Ralchenko, K.: Hypothesis testing of the drift parameter sign for fractional Ornstein–Uhlenbeck process. arXiv:1604.02645 [math.PR] (2016)
44. Kutoyants, Y.A.: Statistical Inference for Ergodic Diffusion Processes. Springer, London (2004)
45. Le Breton, A.: Filtering and parameter estimation in a simple linear system driven by a fractional Brownian motion. Stat. Probab. Lett. **38**(3), 263–274 (1998)
46. Liptser, R., Shiryayev, A.: Statistics of Random Processes II. Applications. Springer, New York (1978)
47. Lyons, T.J.: Differential equations driven by rough signals. Rev. Mat. Iberoamericana **14**(2), 215–310 (1998)
48. Mandelbrot, B.B., Van Ness, J.W.: Fractional Brownian motions, fractional noises and applications. SIAM Rev. **10**, 422–437 (1968)
49. Marushkevych, D.: Large deviations for drift parameter estimator of mixed fractional Ornstein–Uhlenbeck process. Mod. Stoch. Theory Appl. **3**(2), 107–117 (2016)
50. Mendy, I.: Parametric estimation for sub-fractional Ornstein–Uhlenbeck process. J. Stat. Plan. Inference **143**(4), 663–674 (2013)
51. Mishura, Y.: Stochastic Calculus for Fractional Brownian Motion and Related Processes, vol. 1929. Springer Science & Business Media, Berlin (2008)
52. Mishura, Y.: Maximum likelihood drift estimation for the mixing of two fractional Brownian motions. Stochastic and Infinite Dimensional Analysis, pp. 263–280. Springer, Berlin (2016)
53. Mishura, Y., Shevchenko, G.: Mixed stochastic differential equations with long-range dependence: existence, uniqueness and convergence of solutions. Comput. Math. Appl. **64**(10), 3217–3227 (2012)
54. Mishura, Y., Ralchenko, K.: On drift parameter estimation in models with fractional Brownian motion by discrete observations. Austrian J. Stat. **43**(3), 218–228 (2014)
55. Mishura, Y., Voronov, I.: Construction of maximum likelihood estimator in the mixed fractional-fractional Brownian motion model with double long-range dependence. Mod. Stoch. Theory Appl. **2**(2), 147–164 (2015)
56. Mishura, Y., Ralchenko, K., Seleznev, O., Shevchenko, G.: Asymptotic properties of drift parameter estimator based on discrete observations of stochastic differential equation driven by fractional Brownian motion. Modern Stochastics and Applications. Springer Optimization and Its Applications, vol. 90, pp. 303–318. Springer, Cham (2014)
57. Mishura, Y.S., Il'chenko, S.A.: Stochastic integrals and stochastic differential equations with respect to the fractional Brownian field. Theory Probab. Math. Stat. **75**, 93–108 (2007)
58. Mishura, Y.S., Shevchenko, G.M.: Existence and uniqueness of the solution of stochastic differential equation involving Wiener process and fractional Brownian motion with Hurst index $H > 1/2$. Commun. Stat. Theory Methods **40**(19–20), 3492–3508 (2011)
59. Moers, M.: Hypothesis testing in a fractional Ornstein–Uhlenbeck model. Int. J. Stoch. Anal. Art. ID 268568, 23 pp. (2012)
60. Neuenkirch, A., Tindel, S.: A least square-type procedure for parameter estimation in stochastic differential equations with additive fractional noise. Stat. Inference Stoch. Process. **17**(1), 99–120 (2014)
61. Norros, I., Valkeila, E., Virtamo, J.: An elementary approach to a Girsanov formula and other analytical results on fractional Brownian motions. Bernoulli **5**(4), 571–587 (1999)
62. Nourdin, I.: Selected Aspects of Fractional Brownian Motion. Bocconi & Springer Series, vol. 4. Springer, Bocconi University Press, Milan (2012)
63. Nualart, D., Ouknine, Y.: Regularization of differential equations by fractional noise. Stoch. Process. Appl. **102**(1), 103–116 (2002)

64. Nualart, D., Rǎşcanu, A.: Differential equations driven by fractional Brownian motion. Collect. Math. **53**(1), 55–81 (2002)
65. Nualart, D., Ouknine, Y.: Stochastic differential equations with additive fractional noise and locally unbounded drift. Stochastic Inequalities and Applications. Progress in Probability, vol. 56, pp. 353–365. Birkhäuser, Basel (2003)
66. Prakasa Rao, B.: Asymptotic Theory of Statistical Inference. Wiley, New York (1987)
67. Prakasa Rao, B.L.S.: Statistical Inference for Fractional Diffusion Processes. Wiley, Chichester (2010)
68. Ralchenko, K.V.: Approximation of multifractional Brownian motion by absolutely continuous processes. Theory Probab. Math. Stat. **82**, 115–127 (2011)
69. Samko, S., Kilbas, A., Marichev, O.: Fractional Integrals and Derivatives: Theory and Applications. Translate from the Russian. Gordon and Breach, New York (1993)
70. Sørensen, H.: Parametric inference for diffusion processes observed at discrete points in time: a survey. Int. Stat. Rev. **72**(3), 337–354 (2004)
71. Sottinen, T., Tudor, C.A.: Parameter estimation for stochastic equations with additive fractional Brownian sheet. Stat. Inference Stoch. Process. **11**(3), 221–236 (2008)
72. Tanaka, K.: Distributions of the maximum likelihood and minimum contrast estimators associated with the fractional Ornstein–Uhlenbeck process. Stat. Inference Stoch. Process. **16**, 173–192 (2013)
73. Tanaka, K.: Maximum likelihood estimation for the non-ergodic fractional Ornstein–Uhlenbeck process. Stat. Inference Stoch. Process. **18**(3), 315–332 (2015)
74. Tudor, C.A., Viens, F.G.: Statistical aspects of the fractional stochastic calculus. Ann. Stat. **35**(3), 1183–1212 (2007)
75. Xiao, W., Zhang, W., Xu, W.: Parameter estimation for fractional Ornstein–Uhlenbeck processes at discrete observation. Appl. Math. Model. **35**, 4196–4207 (2011)
76. Zähle, M.: Integration with respect to fractal functions and stochastic calculus. I. Probab. Theory Relat. Fields **111**(3), 333–374 (1998)
77. Zähle, M.: On the link between fractional and stochastic calculus. Stochastic Dynamics (Bremen 1997), pp. 305–325. Springer, New York (1999)
78. Zähle, M.: Integration with respect to fractal functions and stochastic calculus. II. Math. Nachr. **225**, 145–183 (2001)
79. Zhang, P., Xiao, W., Zhang, X., Niu, P.: Parameter identification for fractional Ornstein–Uhlenbeck processes based on discrete observation. Econ. Model. **36**, 198–203 (2014)

Part VI
Particle Systems

Convergence to Equilibrium for Many Particle Systems

Alexander Lykov and Vadim Malyshev

Abstract The goal of this paper is to give a short review of recent results of the authors concerning classical Hamiltonian many-particle systems. We hope that these results support the new possible formulation of Boltzmann's ergodicity hypothesis which sounds as follows. For almost all potentials, the minimal contact with external world, through only one particle of N, is sufficient for ergodicity. But only if this contact has no memory. Also new results for quantum case are presented.

Keywords Markov processes · Boltzmann hypothesis · Quantum controllability

1 Introduction

The goal of this paper is to give a short review of recent results [13–18] of the authors. In these results, classical Hamiltonian many-particle systems were considered from new point of view: they have minimal contact with external world, for example, only one particle of N can have this contact. Thus, we consider Hamiltonian systems with minimal possible randomness. In despite of this, ergodicity can be proved for almost all potentials of a wide natural class.

Also we present some new results concerning quantum situation and discuss common points and difference of our results with other research in mathematical physics and Markov chains theory, for example with [1–3, 10–12, 19, 20, 22, 23, 25, 26].

A. Lykov (✉) · V. Malyshev
Lomonosov Moscow State University,
Vorobyevy Gory 1, Moscow 119991, Russia
e-mail: alekslyk@yandex.ru

© Springer International Publishing AG 2017
V. Panov (ed.), *Modern Problems of Stochastic Analysis and Statistics*,
Springer Proceedings in Mathematics & Statistics 208,
DOI 10.1007/978-3-319-65313-6_11

1.1 Intro to Intro

To start with, we give very simple intuition. Let finite set X be given, and let $M(X)$ be the set of probability measures on X. Stochastic matrix P defines linear map $P : M(X) \rightarrow M(X)$, and discrete time Markov chain ξ_k depending on the initial distribution μ_0 of ξ_0.

It is known that if the matrix P^k, for some k, has all elements positive, then there exists unique P-invariant measure π, and moreover for any initial measure μ_0 as $n \rightarrow \infty$

$$P^n \mu_0 \rightarrow \pi, \tag{1}$$

that is for any $A \subset X$ the sequence of real numbers $(P^n \mu_0)(A)$ converges to $\pi(A)$. We will call this property strong ergodicity. A weaker ergodicity property (we will call it Cesaro ergodicity)

$$\frac{1}{n} \sum_{k=1}^{n} P^k \mu \rightarrow \pi \tag{2}$$

follows. It can be formulated differently: for any real function $f(x)$ on X and for any initial state ξ_0, time averages are approximately equal to space averages (this was Boltzmann's formulation of his famous hypothesis in statistical physics). Exact formulation for this could be the following:

$$\frac{1}{n} \sum_{k=1}^{n} f(\xi_k) \rightarrow \sum_{x \in X} f(x) \pi(x) \tag{3}$$

as $n \rightarrow \infty$, with L_1-convergence, or in some other sense.

Deterministic map $U : X \rightarrow X$ is a particular case of Markov chains - when any element of matrix P is either 0 or 1. We will consider only one-to-one maps U. Then it is clear that

1. if $N = |X| > 1$ then strong convergence never holds because any U defines a partition $X = X_1 \cup \ldots \cup X_m$ such that U is cyclic on any X_i;
2. convergence of

$$\frac{1}{n} \sum_{k=1}^{n} f(U^k x)$$

   holds for any U and any x (this is a trivial case of the famous Birkhoff–Khinchin ergodicity theorem) but Cesaro ergodicity (the limit is the unique invariant measure) holds iff there is only one cycle;
3. note that there are N^N deterministic maps, among them $N!$ one-to-one maps, and among the latter only $(N-1)!$ maps with unique cycle. Thus, Cesaro ergodicity is also a rare event but not so rare as strong ergodicity.

If the set X is not finite, for example, a smooth manifold, the situation becomes enormously more complicated. Ludwig Boltzmann did not give exact mathematical formulations. Later on, various formulations of the problem appeared. For some history of ergodicity theory we refer to [24] and references therein. What could be the ways to avoid extreme complexity? First of all, one must find wider and possibly alternative exact formulations of the problem.

1.2 Classical Ergodicity

We will consider N-particle systems with arbitrary but finite N. Namely, N point particles in (coordinate) space R^d with coordinate vectors $q_i = (q_{i1}, \ldots, q_{id})$, velocities $v_i = (v_{i1}, \ldots, v_{id})$, momenta $p_i = m_i v_i$, and with the interaction defined by smooth symmetric potentials $V_{ij}(q_i, q_j)$. To avoid double indices we write further N instead of dN (thus the index i should be considered as a pair (particle number, coordinate number)). Then the dynamics in the phase space $R^{2N} = \{\psi = (q_1, \ldots, q_N, p_1, \ldots, p_N)\}$ is defined by the following system of Hamiltonian equations

$$\frac{dq_k}{dt} = \frac{\partial H}{\partial p_k} = v_k, \quad \frac{dp_k}{dt} = -\frac{\partial H}{\partial q_k}, k = 1, \ldots, N, \tag{4}$$

with the Hamiltonian

$$H = H(\psi) = \sum_{k=1}^{N} \frac{p_k^2}{2m_k} + Q, \quad Q = \sum_{1 \le k \le l \le N} V_{kl}(q_k, q_l).$$

This dynamics defines a one parameter group of one-to-one transformations $U^t : R^{2N} \to R^{2N}$ of the phase space. We assume that $Q \to +\infty$ as $\max_k |q_k| \to \infty$, so that no particle could escape to infinity. This assumption is similar to assuming the system to be in some finite volume (system in the box) Λ with reflecting boundary $\partial \Lambda$. Then the energy surface $M_h = \{\psi : H(\psi) = h\} \subset R^{2N}$ is bounded for any h and (by the energy conservation law) is invariant with respect to this dynamics.

Liouville's theorem says that on any M_h there exists finite probability measure λ_h (Liouville's measure—normalized restriction of the Lebesgue measure λ on the phase space), invariant with respect to this dynamics.

We say that for a given H the system is ergodic if for any $\psi \in M_h$

$$\lim_{T \to \infty} \frac{1}{T} \int_0^T f(U^t \psi) dt = \int_{M_h} f(\psi) d\lambda_h(\psi) \tag{5}$$

in some space of measurable functions. It can be L_2, L_1-convergence, or uniform convergence with respect to ψ.

Possible problems could be the following:

1. Give examples of V_{kl} or, better, classes of V_{kl} such that ergodicity holds for all sufficiently large N. We do not know any such example, but there are many counterexamples: linear (due to invariant tori) and nonlinear integrable systems;

2. prove the contrary: for typical (or almost any) Q, from interesting classes of potentials, ergodicity does not hold. Of course, one should define what means <<almost all>>;

3. instead of problems 1 and 2 one could look for more natural problems. What are the reasons for this:

(a) the N-particle systems discussed above are closed systems, but it is not known whether closed systems exist in nature. More realistic is to assume that any system always has some contact with external world. Then the first natural question is: how weak can be this contact for the system to be ergodic;

(b) this does not contradict to the recent development of theoretical physics, where the notion of space point itself becomes an approximation. Namely, in quantum physics the dynamics is defined not as a transformation of the phase space, but of L_2 space of functions on the coordinate space. Moreover, in modern physics the notion of space itself is being reconsidered: discrete space, quantum space, or no space at all.

1.3   Systems with Minimal Randomness

We consider three types of models with minimum randomness, or combinations of them.

1. Only one degree of freedom open to external influence Namely, we change only one equation (for $k = 1$) of the system (4)

$$\frac{dq_1}{dt} = \frac{\partial H}{\partial p_1} = p_1, \quad \frac{dp_1}{dt} = -\frac{\partial H}{\partial q_1} + F(x_1, p_1, t), \tag{6}$$

where we assume unit masses. All other Eq. (4) are left unchanged. This is used in part III.

2. Two deterministic evolutions with switching at random time moments Let $U_i^t, i = 1, 2, t \in [0, \infty)$, be two semigroups of deterministic transformations (of some set X). For example, when X is the phase space of N-particle system, and the equations are of the type (4). Consider the sequence

$$0 = t_0 < t_1 < t_2 < \dots \tag{7}$$

of time moments and denote $\tau_n = t_n - t_{n-1}$. For any integer $m \geqslant 1$ and nonnegative real $\tau_1, \tau_2, \ldots \tau_{2m+1} \geqslant 0$ consider the following transformations

$$J_0 = E, \quad J_1 = U_1^{\tau_1},$$

$$J_{2m}(\tau_1, \ldots, \tau_{2m}) = U_2^{\tau_{2m}} U_1^{\tau_{2m-1}} \ldots U_2^{\tau_2} U_1^{\tau_1}, \tag{8}$$

$$J_{2m+1}(\tau_1, \ldots, \tau_{2m+1}) = U_1^{\tau_{2m+1}} J_{2m}(\tau_1, \ldots, \tau_{2m}), \tag{9}$$

and define the evolution $W(t)$:

$$W(t) = U_1^{t-t_{2m}} J_{2m}(\tau_1, \ldots, \tau_{2m}), \, t_{2m} \leq t < t_{2m+1}, \tag{10}$$

$$W(t) = U_2^{t-t_{2m+1}} J_{2m+1}(\tau_1, \ldots, \tau_{2m+1}), \, t_{2m+1} \leq t < t_{2m+2}.$$

Define also the following sets of transformations:

$$\mathcal{J}_n(U_1^t, U_2^t) = \{J_n(\tau_1, \ldots, \tau_n) : \tau_1, \tau_2, \ldots, \tau_n \geqslant 0\}.$$

We say that the triple (U_1^t, U_2^t, x) satisfies the covering (or contrallability) condition if there exists n such that

$$\mathcal{J}_n(x) = \mathcal{J}_n^x(U_1^t, U_2^t) = \mathcal{J}_n(U_1^t, U_2^t)x = X, \tag{11}$$

that is, starting from x, n transformations cover all the set X. The triple satisfies strong covering (strong controllability) condition if n does not depend on x.

Below we always assume **Condition D**: τ_k are independent identically distributed positive random variables with $E\tau_1 < \infty$, having some density $p(s) = p_\tau(s)$ with respect to Lebesgue measure, positive for all $s \geq 0$. However, in some cases weaker assumptions are possible.

This model is used in Sect. 2.2.

3. One deterministic evolution with external deterministic intrusion at random time moments Let be given semigroup U_1^t and fixed transformation U_2. We put $J(t) = U_2 U_1^t$ and for $t_n \leq t < t_{n+1}$ put

$$W(t) = U_1^{t-t_n} J(\tau_n) \ldots J(\tau_1). \tag{12}$$

This model is used in Sect. 2.1. Note that in case 2 the trajectories are continuous, and here not.

2 Convergence and Covering (Controllability) Property

2.1 Classical Dynamics with Random Time Velocity Flips

On the phase space

$$L = L_{2N} = \mathbb{R}^{2N} = \left\{ \psi = \begin{pmatrix} q \\ p \end{pmatrix}, q = (q_1, \ldots, q_N)^T, p = (p_1, \ldots, p_N)^T \in \mathbb{R}^N \right\}$$
(13)

(T denotes transposition, thus q, p, ψ are the column vectors) we consider quadratic Hamiltonian

$$H = H(\psi) = \frac{1}{2} \sum_{i=1}^{N} p_i^2 + \frac{1}{2} \sum_{i,j} V(i, j) q_i q_j = \frac{1}{2} \left(\begin{pmatrix} V & 0 \\ 0 & E \end{pmatrix} \psi, \psi \right)_2$$
(14)

with (symmetric) positive-definite matrix V, and the corresponding Hamiltonian system of linear ODE with $k = 1, \ldots, N$

$$\dot{q}_k = p_k, \ \dot{p}_k = - \sum_{l=1}^{N} V_{kl} q_l.$$
(15)

Note that here the energy surface $\mathcal{M}_h$ is a smooth manifold (ellipsoid) in L of codimension 1.

With $(2N \times 2N)$-matrix

$$A = \begin{pmatrix} 0 & E \\ -V & 0 \end{pmatrix}$$

the system (15) can be rewritten as follows:

$$\dot{\psi} = A\psi,$$
(16)

and the solution of (16) defines the transformation group

$$U_1^t = e^{tA}$$

Now define the transformation U_2. Assume that at time moments (7) the following deterministic transformation $U_2 : L \to L$ occurs: all q_k, p_k are left unchanged, except for p_1, the sign of which becomes inverted

$$p_1(t_m - 0) \to p_1(t_m) = -p_1(t_m - 0), m \geq 1.$$

One can say that U_2 is the velocity flip of the first coordinate of particle 1. Note that the Liouville measure π is invariant w.r.t. Hamiltonian dynamics and also w.r.t. velocity flips.

For any $t_n \leq t < t_{n+1}$ define linear transformations $L \rightarrow L$, putting as in (12)

$$W(t)\psi = e^{(t-t_n)A} U_2 e^{\tau_n A} \ldots U_2 e^{\tau_1 A} \psi, \ \psi \in L.$$

Thus, we are in the situation of 1.3.3. It is clear that $\mathcal{M}_h$ is invariant w.r.t. $W(t)$ for any $h > 0$ and $t \geq 0$.

What means "almost all" Define the mixing subspace

$$L_- = L_-(V) = \left\{ \begin{pmatrix} q \\ p \end{pmatrix} \in L : q, p \in l_V \right\}, \tag{17}$$

where $l_V = l_{V,1}$ is the subspace of $\mathbb{R}^N$, generated by the vectors $V^k e_1$, $k = 0, 1, 2 \ldots$, where $e_1, \ldots, e_N$ is the standard basis in $\mathbb{R}^N$.

Let $\mathbf{V}$ be the set of all positive-definite $(N \times N)$-matrices, and let $\mathbf{V}^+ \subset \mathbf{V}$ be the subset of matrices for which

$$L_-(V) = L. \tag{18}$$

Note that $\mathbf{V}$ can be considered as subset of $R^{\frac{N(N+1)}{2}}$, thus (the restriction of) Lebesgue measure is defined on it. Let $\omega_1^2, \ldots, \omega_N^2$ be the eigenvalues of V, and let $\mathbf{V}_{ind}$ be the set of $V \in \mathbf{V}$ such that the square roots $\omega_1, \ldots, \omega_N$ of the eigenvalues are independent over the field of rational numbers.

Lemma 1 *(1) The set $\mathbf{V}^+$ is open and everywhere dense (assuming topology of $R^{\frac{N(N+1)}{2}}$) in $\mathbf{V}$,*

(2) The set $\mathbf{V}^+ \cap \mathbf{V}_{ind}$ is dense both in $\mathbf{V}^+$ and in $\mathbf{V}$, and the Lebesgue measures on $\mathbf{V}$, $\mathbf{V}^+$, $\mathbf{V} \cap \mathbf{V}_{ind}$ are all equal.

Covering Theorem

Theorem 1 *Assume that $V \in \mathbf{V}^+ \cap \mathbf{V}_{ind}$, then there exists $m \geq 1$ such that for any $\psi \in L$ we have*

$$\mathcal{J}_m(\psi) = \mathcal{M}_h$$

Moreover, there is the following upper bound on m

$$m \leq \frac{2}{\min_k \beta_k^2} + 2$$

where $\beta_k = (v_k, e_1)$ and $v_1, \ldots, v_N$ are the eigenvectors of V. Moreover, from the properties of L_- it follows that all β_k are not zero.

Similar property was called pure state controllability in quantum case, see for example [5, 12, 25, 26].

Convergence Theorem

Theorem 2 *Assume that $V \in \mathbf{V}^+ \cap \mathbf{V}_{ind}$. Then, under condition D, for any initial $\psi(0)$ and any bounded measurable real function f on $\mathcal{M}_h$ we have a.s.*

$$M_f(T) =^{def} \frac{1}{T} \int_0^T f(\psi(t))dt \to_{T \to \infty} \pi(f) =^{def} \int_{\mathcal{M}_h} f \, d\pi$$

If, for example, τ_i have exponential distribution with the density $\lambda \exp(-\lambda \tau)$, $\lambda > 0$, then it defines Markov process $\psi(t)$ with right continuous deterministic trajectories and random jumps. Such processes are often called piecewise deterministic Markov processes, see for example [2]. At the same time, this can be considered as an example from random perturbation theory, see [11] where the problem of invariant measures is studied.

2.2 Finite Quantum Dynamics with Random Time Switching

Here we consider the situation of the Sect. 1.3.2̇, and assume both groups U_i^t to be unitary evolutions in C^N. Examples could be quantum walks on finite lattices.

2.2.1 Definitions and Results

We consider $\mathcal{H} = C^N$, $N > 1$, as the Hilbert space with the scalar product (Hermitian form)

$$(\psi, \psi') = \sum_{k=1}^N \psi_k \bar{\psi}'_k, \quad \psi, \psi' \in \mathcal{H}.$$

Let $\mathcal{O}$ be the set of all Hermitian (self adjoint) operators on $\mathcal{H}$. Lie algebra structure on $\mathcal{O}$ is introduced as follows:

$$\{A, B\} = i[A, B] = i(AB - BA) \in \mathcal{O}. \tag{19}$$

Let $U(N)$ be the group of unitary transformations of $\mathcal{H}$. Consider two its one-parametric subgroups $U_k^t = e^{-itH_k}$, $k = 1, 2$, $t \geq 0$, where $H_1, H_2 \in \mathcal{O}$. For any integer $m \geq 1$ and any real $s_1, s_2, \ldots s_{2m+1} \geq 0$ consider the transformations (8) and (9) and define the following sets of unitary matrices

$$\mathcal{J}_n(H_1, H_2) = \{J_n(s_1, \ldots, s_n) : s_1, s_2, \ldots, s_n \geq 0\}.$$

U-**controllability** We say that the pair (H_1, H_2) of Hermitian operators satisfies the U-controllability condition, if there exists n such that

$$\mathcal{J}_n(H_1, H_2) = U(N).$$

Theorem 3 *For the pair of Hermitian operators* (H_1, H_2) *the U-controllability condition holds iff the linear span* $\mathcal{L} = \mathcal{L}(H_1, H_2)$ *(over the field of real numbers) of the operators*

$$H_1, H_2, \{H_1, H_2\}, \{H_1, \{H_1, H_2\}\}, \{H_2, \{H_1, H_2\}\}, \ldots \qquad (20)$$

coincides with $\mathcal{O}$.

The proof of this assertion can be found in many sources: see [25], also Theorem 3.2.1, p. 82 in the book [5], also many references in [26]. Then $\mathcal{L}$ is a subalgebra of $\mathcal{O}$ with respect to the operation (19), and $i\mathcal{L}$ is called the dynamical Lie algebra in [5].

Denote $\Sigma \subset \mathcal{O} \times \mathcal{O}$ the set of all pairs of Hermitian operators (H_1, H_2), for which the U-controllability property holds. For any $H_1 \in \mathcal{O}$ define the set $\Sigma(H_1)$ of all $H_2 \in \mathcal{O}$ such that the pair (H_1, H_2) is U-controllable. We shall say that the operator H_1 is **almost U-controllable**, if the set $\Sigma(H_1)$ is open and everywhere dense in $\mathcal{O}$.

Theorem 4 (almost all theorem) *The following assertions hold:*
(1) Σ is open and everywhere dense in $\mathcal{O} \times \mathcal{O}$.
(2) the set of almost U-controllable operators is open and everywhere dense in $\mathcal{O}$.

One can find the formulations of Theorem 4 in the papers [10, 12, 25]. We provide below formal rigorous proof. But first we want to give more constructive criteria. Let $\lambda_1, \ldots, \lambda_N$ be the eigenvalues of H_2 and $\psi_1, \ldots, \psi_N$ be the corresponding eigenvectors.

Theorem 5 *Assume that the following two conditions hold:*

1. $(H_1\psi_k, \psi_j) \neq 0$ *for all $k \neq j$;*
2. $\lambda_k - \lambda_l \neq \lambda_{k'} - \lambda_{l'}$ *for any ordered pairs* $(k, l) \neq (k', l') \in \{1, \ldots, N\}^2$.

Then for $\mathcal{L} = \mathcal{L}(H_1, H_2)$ the following assertions hold:

1. *if* $\mathrm{Tr}(H_1) = \mathrm{Tr}(H_2) = 0$, *then $\mathcal{L}$ coincides with the subalgebra of all Hermitian operators with zero trace;*
2. *otherwise $\mathcal{L}$ coincides with $\mathcal{O}$.*

Corollary 1 *If the operator H has all eigenvalues different, then H is almost U-controllable.*

Note that for the second condition of this theorem to hold it is sufficient that $\lambda_1, \ldots, \lambda_N$ were linearly independent over $\mathbb{Z}$. One could deduce Theorem 5 from results of [1], but we will give below a direct and simple proof.

Convergence to Haar measure Consider the sequence (7) of time moments. For $t \geqslant 0$ define the following continuous time random process with values in $U(N)$: if $t_{n-1} \leq t < t_n$ then

$$X(t) = J_n(\tau_1, \tau_2, \ldots, \tau_{n-1}, t - t_{n-1}), \quad X(0) = E, \tag{21}$$

(that is $X(t) = W(t)$ from 10). Define also the discrete time <<embedded>> process

$$X_n = X(t_n) = J_n(\tau_1, \tau_2, \ldots, \tau_{n-1}, \tau_n).$$

Note that X_n is a Markov chain with values in $U(N)$, but $X(t)$ in general is not Markov. For any Borel subset $A \subset U(N)$ let $P_n(A)$ be the probability distribution of the random variable X_n.

Denote π the normed Haar measure on $U(N)$.

Theorem 6 (convergence to Haar measure) *Assume Condition D and that the pair (H_1, H_2) satisfies the U-controllability condition. Then the following assertions hold:*

1. *$P_n \to \pi$ in variation as $n \to \infty$ exponentially fast, that is for some positive constants $c > 0, q < 1$, all Borel subsets $A \subset U(N)$ and all $n \geq 1$*

$$|P_n(A) - \pi(A)| \leqslant cq^n;$$

2. *For any bounded measurable function f, defined on $U(N)$, a. s.*

$$\frac{1}{T} \int_0^T f(X(t)) \, dt \to_{T \to \infty} \int_{U(N)} f(u)\pi(du).$$

Convergence for quantum states Consider the set $\mathcal{S}$ of real valued linear functionals on the algebra $\mathcal{O}$, such that

$$F(E) = 1, \quad F(A^2) \geqslant 0,$$

for any $A \in \mathcal{O}$, where E is the identity operator. Remind that any functional $F \in \mathcal{S}$ can be written as

$$F(A) = \mathrm{Tr}(\rho A)$$

for some nonnegative definite operator ρ such that $\mathrm{Tr}(\rho) = 1$, that is

$$\rho = \rho^*, \quad (\rho\psi, \psi) \geqslant 0,$$

for all $\psi \in \mathcal{H}$.

Dynamics on the set $\mathcal{S}$ is defined by the differential (Schrodinger) equation

$$\frac{d\rho(t)}{dt} = -i[H, \rho(t)], \tag{22}$$

having the solution

$$\rho(t) = U(t)\rho(0)U^*(t),$$

where $U(t) = e^{-iHt}$ is unitary and H is Hermitian.

We will say that the function $\rho(t)$, $t \geqslant 0$, converges in Cesaro sense as $t \to \infty$ to $\rho \in \mathcal{S}$, if

$$\lim_{T \to \infty} \frac{1}{T} \int_0^T \text{Tr}(\rho(t)A) \, dt = \text{Tr}(\rho A)$$

for any $A \in \mathcal{O}$. We shall use the notation $\rho(t) \to^c \rho$.

Theorem 7 (pure state convergence)
Assume that all eigenvalues of the matrix H are different and $\rho(0) = P_\psi$ is the projector on the unit vector ψ, then

$$\rho(t) \xrightarrow{c} \sum_{k=1}^{N} |(\psi, \psi_k)|^2 P_{\psi_k}$$

as $t \to \infty$, where $\psi_1, \ldots, \psi_n$ -are the eigenvectors of H, which form the orthonormal basis on $\mathcal{H}$.

From this theorem it follows that Cesaro limit of $\rho(t)$ depends on $\rho(0)$ (thus there is no "ergodicity" in this case). Now consider the case when the Hamiltonian H is time dependent:

$$\frac{d\rho(t)}{dt} = -i[H(t), \rho(t)]. \tag{23}$$

Namely, for the time sequence (7) define $H(t)$ as follows:

$$H(t) = \begin{cases} H_1, & t_{2k} \leq t < t_{2k+1} \\ H_2, & t_{2k+1} \leq t < t_{2k+2} \end{cases},$$

for $k = 0, 1, \ldots$ and some pair of Hermitian operators H_1, H_2.

Then one can write down the solution of (23) in terms of the process $X(t)$ (see (21)):

$$\rho(t) = X(t)\rho(0)X^*(t). \tag{24}$$

Theorem 8 (mixed state convergence) *Assume that the conditions of the Theorem 6 hold. Then for any $\rho(0) \in \mathcal{S}$ with probability one we have*

$$\rho(t) \xrightarrow{c} \frac{1}{N} E, t \to \infty.$$

Generalizations for a weaker controllability condition Let us say that the pair of Hermitian operators (H_1, H_2) is pure states controllable (or controllable for short), if there exists n, such that for any $\psi \in \mathcal{H}$

$$\mathcal{J}_n^\psi(H_1, H_2) = \mathcal{H}.$$

It is obvious that this condition follows from the U-controllability condition. The inverse statement in general is not true. Moreover, in the book [5] there is a general criterion of when the pair (H_1, H_2) is controllable in terms of $\mathcal{L}$ (Theorem 3.4.7).

Define the random process $\psi(t) = X(t)\psi$ and the embedded chain $\psi_n = X_n\psi$ as $\psi \in \mathcal{H}$. Let $P_n(\psi, A)$ denote the probability that ψ_n belongs to Borel subset $A \subset \mathcal{H}$. Denote π^* the uniform measure on $S = \{\psi \in \mathcal{H} : (\psi, \psi) = 1\}$.

Theorem 9 (measure convergence for weaker controllability)

Assume condition D and that for the pair (H_1, H_2) the (pure state) controllability condition holds. Then:

1. *$P_n(\psi, \cdot)$ converges to π^* in variation as $n \to \infty$ exponentially fast and uniformly in $\psi \in S$ that is for some positive constants $c > 0$ and $q < 1$, for any Borel subsets $A \subset \mathcal{H}$ and all $\psi \in S$*

$$|P_n(\psi, A) - \pi(A)| \leqslant cq^n$$

   for all $n \geqslant 1$.
2. *For any bounded measurable function f on S and any initial $\psi(0) \in S$ a.s.*

$$\frac{1}{T}\int_0^T f(\psi(t))\,dt \to_{T\to\infty} \int_S f(\psi)d\pi^*(\psi).$$

The proof is exactly the same as the proof of Theorem 6.

Theorem on mixed states convergence holds also under controllability condition.

Theorem 10 (mixed state convergence 2)

Assume that the conditions of Theorem 9 hold. Then for any $\rho(0) \in S$ as $t \to \infty$ a.s.

$$\rho(t) \xrightarrow{c} \frac{1}{N}E.$$

2.3 Proofs

2.3.1 Proof of Theorems 4 and 5

We prove first the Theorem 5.

Further on, all matrices are considered in the basis $\psi_1, \ldots, \psi_N$. Note that the set

$$\mathcal{T} = \{H \in \mathcal{O} : (H\psi_k, \psi_k) = 0, \quad for\ all\ k = 1, \ldots, N\}$$

is a linear real space of dimension $d = N(N - 1)$.

Lemma 2 $\mathcal{T}$ *is a subset of $\mathcal{L}$.*

Proof Define the operator $T : \mathcal{O} \to \mathcal{O}$ by

$$T(H) = \{H_2, H\}.$$

To prove the lemma it is sufficient to show that the real linear space generated by the matrices

$$T(H_1), T^2(H_1), \ldots, T^d(H_1), \ldots \tag{25}$$

coincides with $\mathcal{T}$. For the (k, j)-th element of the matrix $T(H)$ we have

$$(T(H))_{k,j} = h_{k,j}(\lambda_k - \lambda_j)i,$$

where $H = (h_{k,j})$. It follows that

$$\left(T^n(H)\right)_{k,j} = h_{k,j}\left((\lambda_k - \lambda_j)i\right)^n.$$

As all elements of the matrix H_1 are non zero, then, for all n, the linear dependence of $T(H_1), T^2(H_1), \ldots, T^n(H_1)$ over $\mathbb{C}$ is equivalent to the linear dependence of the matrices $T_1, \ldots, T_n$ over $\mathbb{C}$, where

$$(T_n)_{k,j} = \left((\lambda_k - \lambda_j)i\right)^n.$$

But this is possible (due to the condition on the eigenvalues of H_2) only for $n > \frac{N(N-1)}{2} = \frac{d}{2}$. Lemma is proved.

We will need one more lemma. Denote $E_{k,j} \in \mathcal{O}$ the Hermitian operator with the matrix

$$(E_{k,j}\psi_{k'}, \psi_{j'}) = \begin{cases} 1, & k' = j' = k, \\ -1, & k' = j' = j, \\ 0, & otherwise. \end{cases} \cdot$$

Lemma 3 *For all $k \neq j = 1, \ldots, N$*

$$E_{k,j} \in \mathcal{L}.$$

Proof By symmetry it is sufficient to prove that $E_{1,N} \in \mathcal{L}$. For this we shall define the operator $S \in \mathcal{T}$, such that $\{H_1, S\} = E_{1,N}$. Lemma will follow from this. For any $\psi \in \mathcal{H}$ and $S \in \mathcal{O}$ we have the following:

$$(\{H_1, S\}\psi, \psi) = i((S\psi, H_1\psi) - (H_1\psi, S\psi)) = 2\mathrm{Im}((H_1\psi, S\psi)).$$

Denote $H_1 = (h_{k,j})$. Define now the operator $S \in \mathcal{T}$ as follows:

$$S\psi_1 = b_1\psi_2,$$

$$S\psi_k = a_k\psi_{k-1} + b_k\psi_{k+1}, \ k = 2, \ldots, N-1,$$
$$S\psi_N = a_N\psi_{N-1},$$

where $b_k = \bar{a}_{k+1}, \ k = 1, \ldots, N-1$ and

$$a_k = \frac{i}{2h_{k,k-1}}, \quad k = 2, \ldots, N.$$

We have the following:

$$(\{H_1, S\}\psi_1, \psi_1) = 2\mathrm{Im}(h_{2,1}\bar{b}_1) = 1,$$

$$(\{H_1, S\}\psi_k, \psi_k) = 2\mathrm{Im}\left(h_{k-1,k}\bar{a}_k + h_{k+1,k}\bar{b}_k\right) = \mathrm{Im}\left(-h_{k-1,k}\frac{i}{\bar{h}_{k,k-1}} + h_{k+1,k}\frac{i}{\bar{h}_{k+1,k}}\right) = 0,$$

$$(\{H_1, S\}\psi_N, \psi_N) = 2\mathrm{Im}(h_{N-1,N}\bar{a}_N) = -1,$$

where $k = 2, \ldots, N-1$. It follows that for some $T \in \mathcal{T}$ one can write $\{H_1, S\} = E_{1,N} + T \in \mathcal{L}$. This proves the Lemma.

Return now to the proof of the theorem. In the first case, $\mathrm{Tr}(H_1) = \mathrm{Tr}(H_2) = 0$, it follows from the definition of $\mathcal{L}$ that the trace of any operator $H \in \mathcal{L}$ is zero. In other words, $i\mathcal{L} \subset su(N)$, where $su(N)$ is the Lie algebra of the group of special unitary matrices. The dimension of $su(N)$ is $N^2 - 1$. Moreover, as $E_{1,k} \in \mathcal{L}$, $k = 1, \ldots, N-1$ are linearly independent and do not belong to $\mathcal{T}$, the dimension of $\mathcal{L}$ also equals $N(N-1) + N - 1 = N^2 - 1$. Thus, $i\mathcal{L} = su(N)$.

Consider now the second case of the Theorem, i.e., when for some $k = 1, 2$ the trace of H_k is not zero. Let D be the operator with diagonal matrix, having the (j, j)-th element equal to $(H_k)_{j,j}$. As $\mathcal{T} \subset \mathcal{L}$, then $D \in \mathcal{L}$. As the trace of D is not zero, then $D, E_{1,2}, \ldots, E_{N-1,N}$ are linearly independent. Then, by the arguments similar to those in the first case above, we get the proof of the Theorem.

Now we will give the **Proof of Theorem 4**.

Proof of Theorem

Proof of assertion (1) To prove the first statement of the theorem it is sufficient to prove the following two assertions:
(a) Σ is the complement to some algebraic set in $\mathcal{O} \times \mathcal{O}$, that is to the set of zeroes of some system of polynomial equations.
(b) the set Σ is not empty. This follows from Theorem 5.

Let us prove the assertion (a). Let $\mathcal{P}$ be the countable set of all operators (20). That is the algebra $\mathcal{L}$ is, by definition, the linear span of the vectors from $\mathcal{P}$. The set $\mathcal{O}$ of all Hermitian operators can be considered as N^2-dimensional linear space over reals. Then for the set $S_1, \ldots, S_{N^2} \in \mathcal{O}$ of such operators denote $F(S_1, \ldots, S_{N^2})$ the determinant of the matrix, with rows of which are these vectors. Note that if $S_1, \ldots, S_{N^2} \in \mathcal{P}$, then

$$G_{S_1,\ldots,S_{N^2}}(H_1, H_2) = F(S_1, \ldots, S_{N^2})$$

is the polynomial of the elements of the matrices H_1, H_2. Let E be the complement to Σ in $\mathcal{O} \times \mathcal{O}$. It is clear that $(H_1, H_2) \in E$ iff for any $S_1, \ldots, S_{N^2} \in \mathcal{P}$ will be

$$G_{S_1, \ldots, S_{N^2}}(H_1, H_2) = 0. \tag{26}$$

But by Hilbert's Basis theorem there exists finite set of polynomials of the elements of the pair (H_1, H_2), with the same set of zeroes as the set (26). Thus the first assertion is proved.

Proof of (2) We proved above that Σ is the complement to some algebraic set E, i.e.,

$$E = \{(H_1, H_2) : F_1(H_1, H_2) = \ldots = F_m(H_1, H_2) = 0\}$$

for some polynomials $F_1, \ldots, F_m$ of the coefficients of the matrices of operators H_1, H_2 in some fixed basis. Consider the following algebraic set in $\mathcal{O}$:

$$E(H_1) = \{H_2 : F_1(H_1, H_2) = \ldots = F_m(H_1, H_2) = 0\}.$$

It is clear that for any $H_1 \in \mathcal{O}$ the set $\Sigma(H_1)$ is the complement to $E(H_1)$ in $\mathcal{O}$. Then $\Sigma(H_1)$ is either open and everywhere dense or empty. The latter possibility can occur iff for any $k = 1, \ldots, N$ the polynomial (considered as the function of the matrix H_2) $f_k(H_2) = F_k(H_1, H_2)$ is identically zero.

Let us show first that the set of almost U-controllable H_1, i.e., for which $\Sigma(H_1)$ is open and everywhere dense, is open. Let H_1 be almost U-controllable. Then there exists H_2, such that $F_k(H_1, H_2) \neq 0$ for some $k = 1, \ldots, m$. Then for all H in some neighborhood of H_1 the inequality $F_k(H, H_2) \neq 0$ holds. We get from this that $\Sigma(H) \neq \emptyset$, then H is also almost U-controllable. Now it is sufficient to prove that the set of almost U-controllable operators from $\mathcal{O}$ is dense. Now take H_2 from Theorem 5. It is clear that the set of all H_1 for which $H_2 \in \Sigma(H_1)$ is dense. Our statement follows from this.

Proof of the Corollary

Let us prove that in some orthonormal basis all non-diagonal elements of the matrix of H are nonzero. Let $\psi_1, \ldots, \psi_N$ be the eigenvectors of H. For $t \geqslant 0$ consider the orthonormal basis

$$\psi_k(t) = e^{itS}\psi_k, \quad k = 1, \ldots, N,$$

where the Hermitian operator S is such that $(S\psi_k, \psi_j) \neq 0$ for all $k, j = 1, \ldots, N$. We have

$$(H\psi_k(t), \psi_j(t)) = (H(t)\psi_k, \psi_j), \quad H(t) = e^{-itS}He^{itS},$$

and

$$\frac{dH(0)}{dt} = i[H, S].$$

It follows that

$$\left(\frac{dH(0)}{dt}\psi_k, \psi_j\right) = (S\psi_k, \psi_j)i(\lambda_j - \lambda_k),$$

where $\lambda_1, \ldots, \lambda_N$ are the eigenvalues of H corresponding to $\psi_1, \ldots, \psi_N$. Then for $t \to 0$

$$(H\psi_k(t), \psi_j(t)) = \lambda_k \delta_{k,j} + (S\psi_k, \psi_j)i(\lambda_j - \lambda_k)t + \bar{\bar{o}}(t).$$

Using the assumptions on H and the choice of S we conclude that for some small t and all $k \neq j = 1, \ldots, N$ the following inequality holds

$$(H\psi_k(t), \psi_j(t)) \neq 0.$$

Now take any Hermitian operator H_2, satisfying the conditions of Theorem 5 with eigenvectors $\psi_1(t), \ldots, \psi_N(t)$. By this theorem (H_1, H_2) is U-controllable. In the Proof of Theorem 4 we got that there is the alternative: either $\Sigma(H_1)$ is open and everywhere dense or empty. The theorem is proved.

Note that the condition that all eigenvalues are different is important. Because one can show that there is no orthonormal basis in which the matrix elements of the operator

$$H = \begin{pmatrix} \lambda & 0 \\ 0 & E \end{pmatrix}, \quad \lambda \neq 1, \lambda > 0,$$

are nonzero. Nevertheless, from this one cannot state that this H is not almost U-controllable.

2.3.2 Mixed States Convergence: Theorem 8

By equality (24) and Theorem 6 about convergence, we have (further on $u \in U(N)$)

$$\rho(t) \xrightarrow{c} \rho = \int_{U(N)} u\rho(0)u^* \, d\pi(u).$$

For any $g \in U(N)$ we have

$$g\rho g^* = \int_{U(N)} (gu)\rho(0)(gu)^* \, d\pi(u) = \int_{U(N)} u\rho(0)u^* \, d\pi(u).$$

The last equality follows from the invariance of Haar measure with respect to left and right multiplication. Then for any $g \in U(N)$

$$g\rho g^* = \rho.$$

It follows that

$$\rho = \frac{1}{N}E.$$

The proof is finished.

2.3.3 Theorem 10 for (Pure State) Controllability Condition

One can write the initial state as follows:

$$\rho(0) = \sum_{k=1}^{N} c_k P_{\psi_k}, \quad \sum_{k=1}^{N} c_k = 1, \ c_k \geqslant 0, k = 1, \ldots, N,$$

where $\psi_1, \ldots, \psi_N$ is an orthonormal basis of $\mathcal{H}$. Then

$$\rho(t) = \sum_{k=1}^{N} c_k P_{\psi_k(t)},$$

where $\psi_k(t) = X(t)\psi_k$. By Theorem 9 concerning convergence with probability 1 we have:

$$\lim_{T \to \infty} \frac{1}{T} \int_0^T \mathrm{Tr}(P_{\psi_k(t)}A)dt = \int_S (A\psi, \psi)d\pi^*(\psi) = \mathrm{Tr}(\rho A),$$

where we put

$$\rho = \int_S \psi\psi^* d\pi^*(\psi).$$

Thus, with probability 1

$$\rho(t) \xrightarrow{c} \rho.$$

As measure π^* is invariant with respect to unitary transformations, then for any unitary matrix $u \in U(N)$ we have the following:

$$u\rho u^* = \int_S (u\psi)(u\psi)^* d\pi^*(\psi) = \rho,$$

and it follows that

$$\rho = \frac{1}{N}E.$$

2.3.4   Theorem 7: Pure State Convergence

Use the expansion of vector ψ in the eigenvectors of H:

$$\psi = \sum_{k=1}^{N} a_k \psi_k, \quad a_k = (\psi, \psi_k).$$

Then

$$\rho(t) = P_{\psi(t)}, \quad \psi(t) = e^{-iHt} \psi.$$

Let $\lambda_1, \ldots, \lambda_N$ be eigenvalues of H corresponding to eigenvectors $\psi_1, \ldots, \psi_N$ correspondingly. Then

$$\psi(t) = \sum_{k=1}^{N} a_k e^{-i\lambda_k t} \psi_k.$$

For any Hermitian operator A we have the following:

$$\mathrm{Tr}(\rho(t)A) = (A\psi(t), \psi(t)) = \sum_{k,j} a_k \bar{a}_j e^{it(\lambda_j - \lambda_k)} (A\psi_k, \psi_j).$$

As

$$\lim_{T \to \infty} \frac{1}{T} \int_0^T e^{it(\lambda_j - \lambda_k)} = \begin{cases} 1, & k = j \\ 0, & k \neq j \end{cases},$$

the theorem is proved.

2.3.5   Theorem 6

Here it is convenient to denote $U(N) = \mathcal{M}$.

Convergence for embedded chain It is necessary to do some remarks concerning possible proofs. This assertion could be examined using the general theory of Markov chains with general state space, see, for example, [19, 20, 22], as it was done in simpler cases for random walks on groups (see, for example, [7] p. 83, Theorem 3.2.6). However, our proof will be based on Theorem 4.1 in [17].

Note that X_n is a Markov process, which is not time homogeneous. But $\xi_n = X_{2n}$ will already be time homogeneous Markov process. We shall study ergodic properties of ξ_n and will understand how they could be related to ergodic properties of X_n.

Otherwise speaking ξ_n on $\mathcal{M}$ can be defined as follows:

$$\xi_n = U_2^{T_{2n}} U_1^{T_{2n-1}} \xi_{n-1} = X_{2n} g, \ n = 1, \ldots, \quad \xi_0 = g \in \mathcal{M}.$$

For $g \in \mathcal{M}$ and Borel subset $A \subset \mathcal{M}$ let $P(g, A)$ be the one step transition probability of the chain ξ_n. The probability $P_m(A)$, defined at the beginning of this section, and $P(g, A)$ are connected as follows:

$$P_{2m}(A) = P^m(e, A),$$

$$P_{2m+1}(A) = \int_{\mathcal{M}} P_1(du) P^m(u, A),$$

for all $m \geqslant 1$, where $e \in \mathcal{M}$ is the identity transformation, $P^m(\cdot, \cdot)$— m-th degree of the kernal $P(\cdot, \cdot)$.

Using Theorem 11, we get the following:

$$|P_{2m}(A) - \pi(A)| = |P^m(e, A) - \pi(A)| \leqslant cq^m,$$

$$|P_{2m+1}(A) - \pi(A)| = |\int_{\mathcal{M}} P_1(du) P^m(u, A) - \pi(A)|$$

$$\leqslant \int_{\mathcal{M}} P_1(du) |P^m(u, A) - \pi(A)| \leqslant cq^m.$$

Thus we have proved the first assertion of Theorem 6.

Theorem 11 *Assume that the conditions of Theorem 6 hold. Then $P^n(g, \cdot)$ converges to π in variation as $n \to \infty$ exponentially fast and uniformly in $g \in \mathcal{M}$, that is for some positive constants $c > 0, q < 1$, all Borel subsets $A \subset \mathcal{M}$ and all $g \in \mathcal{M}$:*

$$|P^n(g, A) - \pi(A)| \leqslant cq^n \tag{27}$$

for all $n \geqslant 1$.

To prove this theorem we shall use Theorem 4.1 from [17]. Let us check the conditions of this theorem, namely that ξ_n is a weakly Feller process, and that for some $n \geqslant 1$ the measure $P^n(g, \cdot)$ is equivalent to Haar measure π for any $g \in \mathcal{M}$.

Lemma 4 (Condition A2 from [17]) *The kernel $P(\cdot, \cdot)$ is a weak Feller that is for any open $O \subset \mathcal{M}$ the transition probability $P(g, O)$ is lower semicontinuous in $g \in \mathcal{M}$.*

For any g denote $\mathbf{1}_g(s_1, s_2)$ the indicator function on $R_+ \times R_+$, that is $\mathbf{1}_g(s_1, s_2) = 1$ if $J_2(s_1, s_2)g \in O$, and zero otherwise. Then we have

$$P(g, O) = \int_{R_+ \times R_+} \mathbf{1}_g(s_1, s_2) p(s_1) p(s_2) ds_1 ds_2.$$

Let $g_n \to g$, $g_n \in \mathcal{M}$ as $n \to \infty$. Fix $s_1, s_2 \geqslant 0$ and consider two cases:

1. $J_2(s_1, s_2)g \in O$, then starting from some n the inclusion $J_2(s_1, s_2)g_n \in O$ holds, as O is open. That is why

$$\lim_{n \to \infty} \mathbf{1}_{g_n}(s_1, s_2) = \mathbf{1}_g(s_1, s_2) = 1;$$

2. $J_2(s_1, s_2)g \notin O$. Then

$$\liminf_n \mathbf{1}_{g_n}(s_1, s_2) \geqslant \mathbf{1}_g(s_1, s_2) = 0.$$

Thus for any s_1, s_2

$$\liminf_n \mathbf{1}_{g_n}(s_1, s_2) \geqslant \mathbf{1}_g(s_1, s_2).$$

Then by Fatou lemma

$$\liminf_n P(g_n, O) \geqslant P(g, O).$$

So, the lemma is proved.

Lemma 5 (Condition A1 from [17]) *For some $m \geqslant 1$ the measures π and $P^m(g, \cdot)$ are equivalent for any g. Moreover, there is exist m-step transition density $p^m(g, u)$ measurable on $\mathcal{M} \times \mathcal{M}$ and positive almost everywhere, such that*

$$P^m(g, B) = \int_B p^m(g, u) d\pi(u)$$

for all $g \in \mathcal{M}$ and all Borel subset $B \subset \mathcal{M}$.

Let us remind that ξ_n can be presented as follows:

$$\xi_n = J_{2n}(\tau_1, \tau_2, \ldots, \tau_{2n})g,$$

where operator J_{2n} was defined above. Further, we assume that $m = 2n^2$, where n is as in the definition of U-controllability. Introduce the following set

$$\Omega_m = \{(s_1, \ldots, s_m) : s_i \geqslant 0, \ i = 1, \ldots, m\} \subset \mathbb{R}_{\geqslant 0}^m.$$

For any $g \in \mathcal{M}$ the function $J_m^g(s_1, \ldots, s_m) = J_m(s_1, \ldots, s_m)g$ acts from Ω_m to $\mathcal{M}$, then by definition of U-controllability:

$$J_m^g(\Omega_m) = \mathcal{M}.$$

Lemma 6 *For any measurable $B \subset \mathcal{M}$ its Haar measure $\pi(B) = 0$ iff the Lebesgue measure λ of the set $(J_m^g)^{-1}(B)$ in Ω_m is zero.*

(1) Assume that for some $B \subset \mathcal{M}$ we have $\pi(B) = 0$. Let us show that $\lambda((J_m^g)^{-1}$ $(B)) = 0$. Let A_{cr} be the set of critical points of the map J_m^g (that is points $\bar{\tau} = (\tau_1, \ldots, \tau_m)$ where the rank of the Jacobian is not maximal) and let $E = J_m^g(A_{cr}) \subset \mathcal{M}$ be the set of critical values of J_m^g. By Sard's theorem $\pi(E) = 0$. But as $J_m^g(\Omega_m) = \mathcal{M}$, then there exists noncritical point $\bar{\tau} = (\tau_1, \ldots, \tau_m) \in \Omega_m$, that is such that the rank of dJ_m^g at this point equals N^2. As the map J_m^g is analytic in the variables $\tau_1, \ldots, \tau_m$, the set of points A_{cr}, where the rank is less than N^2, has Lebesgue measure zero. Then the equality $\lambda((J_m^g)^{-1}(B)) = 0$ follows from Theorem 1 of [21].

(2) Assume that for some $B \subset \mathcal{M}$ we have $\pi(B) > 0$, and let us show that $\lambda((J_m^g)^{-1}(B)) > 0$. By Lebesgue differentiation theorem there exists point $g' \in \mathcal{M} \setminus E$ and its neighborhood $O(g')$ such that $\pi(O(g') \cap B) > 0$. Then there is point $\bar{\tau} = \bar{\tau}(g') \in (J_m^g)^{-1}(g')$ and some its neighborhood $O(\bar{\tau}) \subset \Omega_m$, so that the restriction of J_m^g on $O(\bar{\tau})$ is a submersion. Then $\pi(O(g') \cap B) > 0$ implies $\lambda((J_m^g)^{-1}(B) \cap O(\bar{\tau})) > 0$. So, Lemma 6 is proven.

Denote $p_{\bar{\tau}}^{(m)}$ the product of $2m$ densities p_τ, then as for any $B \subset \mathcal{M}$

$$P^m(g, B) = \int_{(J_m^g)^{-1}(B)} p_{\bar{\tau}}^{(m)}(\bar{\tau}) d\bar{\tau},$$

by Lemma 6 we get that P^m and π are equivalent measures.

The proof of measurability of the transition density one can find in Theorem 1, p. 180 of [22], and in Proposition 1.1, p. 5, of [20].

So, Lemma 5 is proven.

Let us continue the proof of the assertion of Theorem 11 concerning convergence of the embedded chain. Let us check that Haar measure is invariant with respect to ξ_n. For Borel subset $B \subset \mathcal{M}$ we have the following:

$$(\pi P)(B) = \int_{\mathcal{M}} d\pi(u) P(u, B) = \int_{\mathcal{M}} d\pi(u) \int_{R_+ \times R_+} \mathbf{1}(U_2^{s_2} U_1^{s_1} u \in B) p(s_1) p(s_2) ds_1 ds_2 =$$

$$= \int_{R_+ \times R_+} p(s_1) p(s_2) ds_1 ds_2 \int_{\mathcal{M}} d\pi(u) \mathbf{1}(U_2^{s_2} U_1^{s_1} u \in B) = \pi(B),$$

where the last equality follows from the invariance of Haar measure with respect to multiplication.

Further we shall use Theorem 4.1 from [17]. In this paper, there is no assertions concerning geometric rate convergence. However, during proof of the Theorem 4.1 in [17] (see the end of the proof) the following inequality was proved:

$$S_{n+k}(A) - I_{n+k}(A) \leqslant (1 - \delta)(S_n(A) - I_n(A)), \quad \text{for all } n = 1, 2, \ldots, \tag{28}$$

where $0 < \delta < 1, k > 1, A \subset \mathcal{M}$, and

$$I_n(A) = \inf_{g \in \mathcal{M}} P^n(g, A), \quad S_n(A) = \sup_{g \in \mathcal{M}} P^n(g, A).$$

But it is obvious that from (28) the assertion (27) holds. Thus, we have proved the first item of Theorem 6.

Cesaro convergence For any measurable bounded function f on $\mathcal{M}$ and any $T > 0$ define the followings integrals:

$$M_f(T) = \frac{1}{T} \int_0^T f(X(t)) \, dt, \quad \pi(f) = \int_{\mathcal{M}} f(u) d\pi(u).$$

Define the random time T_n as

$$T_n = \sum_{k=1}^{2n} \tau_k, \quad n = 1, 2, \ldots.$$

Lemma 7 *For any measurable bounded function f on $\mathcal{M}$ the following limit holds a.s.*

$$\lim_{n \to \infty} M_f(T_n) = \pi(f).$$

Proof Denote $Y_k = (\xi_k, \tau_{2k+1}, \tau_{2k+2})$, $k = 0, 1, \ldots$, $\xi_0 = e$ the Markov chain with values in $\mathcal{Y} = \mathcal{M} \times \mathbb{R}_+ \times \mathbb{R}_+$. Then

$$\int_{T_k}^{T_{k+1}} f(X(s)) ds = \int_{T_k}^{T_k + \tau_{2k+1}} f(U_1^{s-T_k} \xi_k) ds + \int_{T_k + \tau_{2k+1}}^{T_{k+1}} f(U_2^{s-(T_k+\tau_{2k+1})} U_1^{\tau_{2k+1}} \xi_k) ds =$$

$$(29)$$

$$= \int_0^{\tau_{2k+1}} f(U_1^s \xi_k) ds + \int_0^{\tau_{2k+2}} f(U_2^s U_1^{\tau_{2k+1}} \xi_k) ds = F(Y_k),$$

where

$$F(g, t_1, t_2) = \int_0^{t_1} f(U_1^s g) ds + \int_0^{t_2} f(U_2^s U_1^{t_1} g) ds, \quad (g, t_1, t_2) \in \mathcal{Y}.$$

Then

$$M_f(T_n) = \frac{1}{T_n} \sum_{k=0}^{n-1} \int_{T_k}^{T_{k+1}} f(X(s)) ds = \frac{1}{T_n} \sum_{k=0}^{n-1} F(Y_k). \quad (30)$$

It is easy to show that Y_k has invariant measure $\mu = \pi \times P_\tau$, $P_\tau = p_\tau(s_1) p_\tau(s_2) ds_1 ds_2$, satisfies the conditions of Theorem 4.2 in [17] as ξ_k satisfies it. Then

$$\lim_{n \to \infty} \frac{1}{n} \sum_{k=0}^{n-1} F(Y_k) = \mu(F) = \int_{\mathcal{Y}} F(g, t_1, t_2) d\mu,$$

where

$$\mu(F) = \int_{\mathbb{R}_+ \times \mathbb{R}_+} P_\tau(dt_1 dt_2) \int_{\mathcal{M}} d\pi(g) \left(\int_0^{t_1} f(U_1^s g) ds + \int_0^{t_2} f(U_2^s U_1^{t_1} g) ds \right) =$$

$$= \int_{\mathbb{R}_+ \times \mathbb{R}_+} P_\tau(dt_1 dt_2) \left(\int_0^{t_1} ds \int_{\mathcal{M}} d\pi(g) f(U_1^s g) + \int_0^{t_2} ds \int_{\mathcal{M}} d\pi(g) f(U_2^s U_1^{t_1} g) \right)$$

$$= \pi(f) \int_{\mathbb{R}_+ \times \mathbb{R}_+} P_\tau(dt_1 dt_2) \left(\int_0^{t_1} ds + \int_0^{t_2} ds \right) = 2\pi(f) E\tau_1.$$

Moreover, by strong law of large numbers for independent random variables τ_k we have

$$\lim_{n \to \infty} \frac{T_n}{n} = 2E\tau_1.$$

Then by (30) we get the proof of the lemma.

To prove the second part of Theorem 6 we have to estimate the difference between $M_f(T)$ and $M_f(T_n)$. Using the boundedness $|f(g)| \leqslant c$ we have

$$|M_f(T) - M_f(T_n)| \leqslant |\frac{1}{T} \int_{T_n}^T f(X(s)) ds| + \frac{|T - T_n|}{T} |M_f(T_n)|$$

$$\leqslant \frac{|T - T_n|}{T} (c + |M_f(T_n)|). \tag{31}$$

For any $T > 0$ define the random index $n(t)$ so that

$$T_{n(t)} \leqslant T < T_{n(T)+1},$$

and note that

$$\frac{|T - T_{n(T)}|}{T} \leqslant \frac{\tau_{2n(T)+1} + \tau_{2n(T)+2}}{T_{n(T)}} = \frac{\tau_{2n(T)+1} + \tau_{2n(T)+2}}{\sum_{k=1}^{2n(T)} \tau_k}.$$

As $E\tau_1 < \infty$, the law of large numbers, as $n \to \infty$, gives a.s.

$$\frac{\tau_{2N+1} + \tau_{2N+2}}{\sum_{k=1}^{2N} \tau_k} \to 0.$$

But $n(T) \to \infty$ as $T \to \infty$. Then the right-hand side of (31) tends to 0 a.s. as $n = n(T)$ and $T \to \infty$. Thus, we complete the proof of Theorem 6.

2.4 From Unitary to Symplectic

Here, on a general but very simple example, we show how convergence in situations with unitary transformations is related to the similar question for the symplectic transformations. More information one can find in physical literature, see [4, 8, 9].

We consider C^N as complex Hilbert space of dimension $N < \infty$ with the standard basis e_n, $n = 1, 2, \ldots, N$. Then any vector $f \in C^N$ can be presented as

$$f = \sum_n \lambda_n e_n, \quad \lambda_n = q_n + i p_n. \tag{32}$$

with real q_n, p_n. Now let $U^t = e^{it\hat{H}}$ be unitary group in C^N where $\hat{H}$ is a selfadjoint operator in C^N with matrix

$$(a_{kl} + i b_{kl}), \quad a_{kl} = a_{lk}, \quad b_{kl} = -b_{lk}.$$

For the Hamiltonian $\hat{H}$ the quantum dynamics $f(t) = e^{it\hat{H}} f(0)$ for any vector $f(0) \in C^N$ satisfies the Schrodinger equation

$$-i \frac{\partial f}{\partial t} = \hat{H} f, \tag{33}$$

or

$$-i \frac{d\lambda_k}{dt} = -i \left(\frac{dq_k}{dt} + i \frac{dp_k}{dt} \right) = \sum_l (a_{kl} + i b_{kl})(q_l + i p_l),$$

or

$$\frac{dp_k}{dt} = \sum_l (a_{kl} q_l - b_{kl} p_l), \quad \frac{dq_k}{dt} = \sum_l (-a_{kl} p_l - b_{kl} q_l). \tag{34}$$

If we introduce the quadratic Hamiltonian

$$H = -\frac{1}{2} \sum_{k,l=1}^{N} a_{kl}(q_k q_l - p_k p_l) + \sum_{k,l=1}^{N} b_{kl} q_k p_l, \tag{35}$$

then the Eq. (34) coincide with the classical Hamiltonian equations

$$\frac{dq_k}{dt} = \frac{\partial H}{\partial p_k}, \quad \frac{dp_k}{dt} = -\frac{\partial H}{\partial q_k}, \tag{36}$$

as

$$\frac{\partial(\sum_{k,l} b_{kl} q_k p_l)}{\partial p_k} = -\frac{\partial(\sum_{k,l} b_{lk} q_k p_l)}{\partial p_k} = -\frac{\partial(\sum_{l,k} b_{kl} p_l q_k)}{\partial p_k} = -\sum_{k,l} b_{kl} q_l.$$

Remark 1 It is interesting that this class of classical Hamiltonian dynamics has nothing with the standard Hamiltonian dynamics considered in Sects. II.1 and III. Possible convergence to Liouville and Gibbs measures of such (gyroscopic) dynamics we shall discuss elsewhere.

3 Gibbs Equilibrium and Memory

Here we use the notation (13)–(16) from Sect. II.1, and consider the system (15) with quadratic Hamiltonian (14). Then, the density of Gibbs measure μ_β with respect to Lebesgue measure λ on R^{2N} is given by

$$\frac{d\mu_\beta}{d\lambda} = Z_\beta^{-1} \exp(-\beta H) = Z_\beta^{-1} \exp\left(-\frac{1}{2}(C_{G,\beta}^{-1}\psi, \psi)_2\right). \tag{37}$$

So it is gaussian with covariance matrix

$$C_{G,\beta} = \frac{1}{\beta}\begin{pmatrix} V^{-1} & 0 \\ 0 & E \end{pmatrix}. \tag{38}$$

Although Gibbs distribution is invariant with respect to this dynamics, convergence (for closed system) to it is impossible due to the law of energy conservation. Thus we have to introduce some random influence, and we consider the dynamics defined by the system of $2N$ stochastic differential equations, as in (6),

$$\frac{dq_k}{dt} = p_k, \quad \frac{dp_k}{dt} = -\sum_{l=1}^{N} V(k,l)q_l + \delta_{k,1}(-\alpha p_k + f_t). \tag{39}$$

This means that only one degree of freedom, namely 1 (first coordinate of the particle 1) is subjected to damping (defined by the factor $\alpha > 0$) and to the external force f_t, which we assume to be a gaussian stationary stochastic process.

3.1 Large Time Behavior for Fixed Finite N

One can rewrite system (39) in the vector notation

$$\frac{d\psi}{dt} = A\psi + F_t, \tag{40}$$

where

$$A = \begin{pmatrix} 0 & E \\ -V & -\alpha D \end{pmatrix}, \tag{41}$$

E is the unit $(N \times N)$-matrix, D is the diagonal $(N \times N)$-matrix with all zeroes on the diagonal except $D_{11} = 1$, and F_t is the vector $(0, \ldots, 0. f_t, 0, \ldots, 0) \in R^{2N}$.

Covariance All our external forces f_t will be gaussian stationary processes with zero mean. Among them there is the white noise—the generalized stationary gaussian process having covariance $C_f(s) = \sigma^2 \delta(s)$, it is sometimes called process with independent values (without memory). All other stationary gaussian processes, which we consider here, are processes with memory. We will assume that they have continuous trajectories and integrable (short memory) covariance

$$C_f(s) = < f_t f_{t+s} > = E(f_t f_{t+s}).$$

Then the solution of (40) with arbitrary initial vector $\psi(0)$ is unique and is equal to

$$\psi(t) = e^{tA} \left(\int_0^t e^{-sA} F_s ds + \psi(0) \right). \tag{42}$$

Our goal, in particular, is to show that even weak memory, in the generic situation, prevents the limiting invariant measure (which always exists and unique) from being Gibbs. To formulate more readable results we assume more: C_f belongs to the Schwartz space $S = S(R)$. Then also the spectral density

$$a(\lambda) = \frac{1}{2\pi} \int_{-\infty}^{+\infty} e^{-it\lambda} C_f(t) \, dt$$

belongs to the space S.

We shall say that some property (for given V) holds for almost all C_f from the space S if the set $S^{(+)} \subset S$ where this property holds is open and everywhere dense in S.

Invariant subspaces The subspace $L_- \subset L$ was introduced in (17). Now we describe important properties of this set.

Lemma 8 1. L_- and its orthogonal complement denoted by L_0, are invariant with respect to the operator A.
2. The spectrum of the restriction A_- of A on the subspace L_- belongs to the left half-plane, and as $t \to \infty$
$$||e^{tA_-}||_2 \to 0$$

exponentially fast, Moreover, L_- can be defined as

$$L_- = \{\psi \in L : \ H(e^{tA}\psi) \to 0, \ t \to \infty\} \subset L$$

Role of the Memory

Theorem 12 Let f_t be either white noise or has continuous trajectories and integrable C_f. Then for any Hamiltonian H with $L_0 = \{0\}$ the following holds:

1. *there exists gaussian random $(2N)$-vector $\psi(\infty)$ such that for any initial condition $\psi(0)$ the distribution of $\psi(t)$ converges, as $t \to \infty$, to that of $\psi(\infty)$;*
2. *for the process $\psi(t)$ we have $E\psi(t) \to 0$ and the covariance -*

$$C_{\psi(\infty)}(s) = \lim_{t \to \infty} < \psi(t)\psi^T(t+s) >= \lim_{t \to \infty} C_\psi(t, t+s) = W(s)C_{G,1} + C_{G,1}W(-s)^T,$$
(43)

where

$$W(s) = \int_0^{+\infty} e^{\tau A} C_f(\tau + s) d\tau;$$
(44)

3. *For the white noise with variance σ^2 the vector $\psi(\infty)$ has Gibbs distribution (37) with the temperature*

$$\beta^{-1} = \frac{\sigma^2}{2\alpha};$$

4. *If $\alpha = 0, \sigma^2 > 0$, then for any i the mean energy EH_i, where*

$$H_i = \frac{p_i^2}{2} + \sum_j V(i, j)q_i q_j,$$

of the particle i tends to infinity. If $\alpha > 0, \sigma^2 = 0$, then it tends to zero.

We will use here the shorter notation $C_{\psi(\infty)}(0) = C_\psi$.

Theorem 13 *Let $N \geq 2$, and the Hamiltonian H is such that $L_0 = L_0(H) = \{0\}$. Then the following assertions hold:*

1. *for any $C_f \in S$ the limiting distribution does not have correlations between coordinates and velocities;*
2. *for almost any $C_f \in S$ there are non zero correlations between velocities, that is for some $i \neq j$ $C_\psi(p_i, p_j) \neq 0$. It follows that the limiting distribution cannot be Gibbs.*

Classes of Hamiltonians Here we describe classes of potentials with dim $L_0 = 0$.

Let $\Gamma = \Gamma_N$ be connected graph with N vertices $i = 1, \ldots, N$, and not more than one edge per each (unordered) pair of vertices (i, j). It is assumed that all loops (i, i) are the edges of Γ. Denote $\mathbf{H}_\Gamma$ the set of (positive-definite) V such that $V(i, j) = 0$ if (i, j) is not the edge of Γ. It is easy to see that the dimension of the set $\mathbf{H}_\Gamma$ is equal to the number of edges of Γ.

Examples can be complete graph with N vertices, or we can consider the d-dimensional integer lattice Z^d and the graph $\Gamma = \Gamma(d, \Lambda)$, the set of vertices of which is the cube

$$\Lambda = \Lambda(d, M) = \{(x_1, \ldots, x_d) \in Z^d : |x_i| \leq M, i = 1, \ldots, d\} \subset Z^d$$

and the edges (i, j), $|i - j| \leq 1$.

In general, V is called γ-local on Γ if $V(i, j) = 0$ for all pairs i, j having distance $r(i, j)$ between them greater than γ, where the distance $r(i, j)$ between two vertices i, j on a graph is the minimal length (number of edges) of paths between them.

We shall say that some property holds for almost any Hamiltonian from the set $\mathbf{H}_\Gamma$ if the set $\mathbf{H}_\Gamma^{(+)}$, where the property holds, is open and everywhere dense. Moreover, the dimension of the set $\mathbf{H}_\Gamma^{(-)} = \mathbf{H}_\Gamma \setminus \mathbf{H}_\Gamma^{(+)}$ where it does not hold, is less than the dimension of $\mathbf{H}_\Gamma$ itself.

Lemma 9 *For almost any $H \in \mathbf{H}_\Gamma$ we have* $\dim L_0 = 0$.

4 Thermodynamic Limit

We have studied above the limit $t \to \infty$ for fixed N and fixed potential $V = V_N$. Here we discuss the limit

$$\lim_{N \to \infty} \lim_{t \to \infty} .$$

First of all, it is not clear that this limit exists, and even less how it can look like. The only immediate conclusion is that, if it exists, it will be gaussian, and will depend on the covariance C_f. One of the central question is of course: how the limiting distribution will look like far away from the place of external influence that is far away from the particle 1. Will the effect of the memory disappear or not, i.e., will this limit have Gibbs covariance or not.

In the white noise case, it is easy to prove that we will get anyway the Gibbs distribution. Consider now the case when f_t is not the white noise. We will prove that for large N the matrices C_ψ become close to the simpler matrix

$$C_V = \frac{\pi}{\alpha} \begin{pmatrix} a(\sqrt{V})V^{-1} & 0 \\ 0 & a(\sqrt{V}) \end{pmatrix},$$

where $\sqrt{V}$ is the unique positive root of V. First of all note that: 1) C_V also defines an invariant measure with respect to pure (that is with $\alpha = 0$, $f_t = 0$) Hamiltonian dynamics; 2) for the white noise case C_V, corresponds to the Gibbs distribution.

We assume that some graph Γ is given with the set of vertices Λ, $|\Lambda| = N$. For any $V \in \mathbf{H}_\Gamma$ such that $L_0(V) = \{0\}$, the following representation of the limiting covariance matrix appears to be crucial

$$C_\psi = C_V + Y_V,$$

where Y_V is some remainder term.

The following theorem gives the estimates for Y_V. The norm $||V||_\infty$ of a matrix V we define by the formula

$$||V||_\infty = \max_i \sum_j |V(i, j)|.$$

Theorem 14 *Assume that V is γ-local and $||V||_\infty < B$ for some $B > 0$. Fix also some number $\eta = \eta(N) \geqslant \gamma$. Then the following assertions hold the following:*

1. *If $C_f \in S$ and has bounded support, that is $C_f(t) = 0$ if $|t| > b$ for some $b > 0$, then for any pair i, j far away from the particle 1, that is the distances $r(i, 1)$, $r(j, 1) > \eta(N)$, there is the following estimate*

$$|Y_V(q_i, q_j)|, \ |Y_V(p_i, p_j)| < K_0 \left(\frac{K}{\eta}\right)^{\eta\gamma^{-1}}$$

   for some constants $K_0 = K(C_f, B, b, \alpha, \gamma)$ and $K = K(C_f, B, b, \alpha, \gamma)$, not depending on N.
2. *For arbitrary $C_f \in S$ the estimate is*

$$|Y_V(q_i, q_j)|, \ |Y_V(p_i, p_j)| < C(k)\eta^{-k},$$

   for any $k > 0$ and some constant $C(k) = C(C_f, k, B, \alpha, \gamma)$, not depending on N.

This theorem allows to do various conclusions concerning the thermodynamic limit. We give an example.

Fix some $C_f(t) \in S$ and some connected countable graph Γ_∞ with the set of vertices Λ_∞ and an increasing sequence of subsets $\Lambda_1 \subset \Lambda_2 \subset \ldots \subset \Lambda_n \subset \ldots$ such that $\Lambda = \cup \Lambda_n$. Let Γ_n be the subgraph of Γ_∞ with the set of vertices Λ_n, i.e., Γ_n inherits all edges between vertices of Λ_n from Γ. Here it will be convenient to assume that, for any fixed n, the specified particle (the only one having contact with external world) has number $N_n = |\Lambda_n|$. We assume also that for any $i \in \Lambda_\infty$ its distance $r_n(i, N_n)$ to the particle N_n tends to ∞ as $n \to \infty$.

Let $l^\infty(\Gamma_\infty)$ be the complex Banach space of bounded functions on the set of vertices of Γ_∞:

$$l^\infty(\Gamma_\infty) = \{(x_i)_{i \in \Gamma_\infty} : \sup_{i \in \Gamma_\infty} |x_i| < \infty, \ x_i \in \mathbb{C}\}.$$

Fix some γ-local infinite matrix V on this space and such that $||V||_\infty \leqslant B$. It is clear that V defines a bounded linear operator on $l^\infty(\Gamma_\infty)$. Denote $\sigma(V)$ the spectrum of this operator. Let $V_n = (V(i, j))_{i,j \in \Lambda_n}$ be the restriction of V on Λ_n, it is a matrix of the order N_n. Assume that for all $n = 1, 2, \ldots$ the matrices V_n are positive definite. Note that the condition $L_-(V_n) = L$ may not hold for some n. However, one can choose a sequence of positive-definite matrices $V'_n \in \mathbf{H}_{\Lambda_n}$ such that $||V_n - V'_n||_\infty \to 0$ as $n \to \infty$ with $L_0(V'_n) = \{0\}$. Moreover, the convergence of V'_n to V_n can be chosen arbitrary fast. Denote $C_\psi^{(n)}$ the limiting covariance matrices corresponding to V'_n.

Corollary 2 *The following assertions hold:*

1. for any $i, j \in \Lambda_\infty$ there exists the thermodynamic limit

$$\lim_{n\to\infty} C_\psi^{(n)}(p_i, p_j) = C_\psi^{(\infty),p}(i, j),$$

that is for distribution of velocities;
2. if for any $i, j \in \Lambda_\infty$ there exists finite limits:

$$U(i, j) \doteq \lim_{n\to\infty} V_n^{-1}(i, j), \tag{45}$$

then for the coordinates we have

$$\lim_{n\to\infty} C_\psi^{(n)}(q_i, q_j) = C_\psi^{(\infty),q}(i, j);$$

3. assume that the spectral density $a(\sqrt{\lambda})$ is analytic on the open set containing the spectrum $\sigma(V)$. Then

$$C_\psi^{(\infty),p}(i, j) = a(\sqrt{V}),$$

where $a(\sqrt{V})$ is defined in terms of the operator calculus on $l^\infty(\Gamma_\infty)$ ([6], p. 568).

In [15] one can find all proofs in more general situation when more than one particle have contact with external world.

References

1. Altafini, C.: Controllability of quantum mechanical systems by root space decomposition of su(N). J. Math. Phys. **43**(5), 2051–2062 (2002)
2. Azais, R., Bardet, J.-B., Genadot, A., Krell, N., Zitt, P.-A.: Piecewise deterministic Markov process - recent results. arXiv:1309.6061 (2013)
3. Bruneau, L., Joye, A., Merkli, M.: Repeated interactions in open quantum systems. J. Math. Phys. **55**, 075204 (2014)
4. Buric, N.: Reduction of infinite-dimensional Hamiltonian system in classical and quantum mechanics
5. D'Alessandro, D.: Introduction to Quantum Control and Dynamics. Taylor & Francis, London (2008)
6. Dunford, N., Schwartz, J.: Linear Operators. Part 1. Interscience, New York (1958)
7. Grenander, U.: Probabilities on Algebraic Structures. Wiley, New York (1963)
8. Heslot, A.: Classical mechanics and the electron spin. Am. J. Phys. **51**, 1096–1102 (1983)
9. Heslot, A.: Quantum mechanics as a classical theory. Phys. Rev. D **31**(6), 1341–1348 (1985)
10. Jurdjevic, V.: Geometric Control Theory. Cambridge University Press, Cambridge (2006)
11. Kifer, Yu.: Random Perturbations of Dynamical Systems. Birkhauser, Boston (1988)
12. Lloyd, S.: Almost any quantum logic gate is universal. Phys. Rev. Lett. **75**(2), 346–349 (1995)
13. Lykov, A.A., Malyshev, V.A.: Harmonic chain with weak dissipation. Markov Process. Relat. Fields **18**(4), 721–729 (2012)

14. Lykov, A.A., Malyshev, V.A.: Role of the memory in convergence to invariant Gibbs measure. Dokl. Math. **88**(2), 513–515 (2013)
15. Lykov, A.A., Malyshev, V.A.: Convergence to Gibbs equilibrium - unveiling the mystery. Markov Process. Relat. Fields **19**, 4 (2013)
16. Lykov, A.A., Malyshev, V.A.: A new approach to Boltzmann's ergodic hypothesis. Dokl. Math. **92**(2), 624–626 (2015)
17. Lykov, A.A., Malyshev, V.A.: Liouville ergodicity of linear multi-particle Hamiltonian systems with one marked particle velocity flips. Markov Process. Relat. Fields **2**, 381–412 (2015)
18. Lykov, A.A., Malyshev, V.A., Muzychka, S.A.: Linear hamiltonian systems under microscopic random influence. Theory Probab. Appl. **57**(4), 684–688 (2013)
19. Meyn, S., Tweedie, R.: Markov Chains and Stochastic Stability. Cambridge University Press, Cambridge (2009)
20. Orey, S.: Lecture Notes on Limit Theorems for Markov Chain Transition Probabilities. Van Nostrand, London (1971)
21. Ponomarev, S.: Submersions and pre-images of sets of zero measure. Sib. Math. J. **28**(1), 199–210 (1987)
22. Portenko, N., Skorohod, A., Shurenkov, V.: Markov Processes. Itogi nauki i tehniki. VINITI, Moscow (1989)
23. Revuz, D.: Markov Chains. North Holland, New York (1984)
24. Szasz, D.: Boltzmann's Ergodicity Hypothesis, A Conjecture for Centuries? Lecture (1994)
25. Weaver, N.: On the universality of almost every quantum logic gate. J. Math. Phys. **41**(1), 240–243 (2000)
26. Weaver, N.: Time optimal control of finite quantum systems. J. Math. Phys. **41**(8), 5262–5269 (2000)

Large Deviations for the Rightmost Position in a Branching Brownian Motion

Bernard Derrida and Zhan Shi

Abstract We study the lower deviation probability of the position of the rightmost particle in a branching Brownian motion and obtain its large deviation function.

Keywords Branching Brownian motion · Lower deviation probability

2010 Mathematics Subject Classification 60F10 · 60J80

1 Introduction

The question of the distribution of the position $X_{\max}(t)$ of the rightmost particle in a branching Brownian motion (BBM) has a long history in probability theory [3–6, 9, 17, 20, 24, 26, 27] and in physics [15, 19, 22, 23].

By branching Brownian motion, we mean that the system starts with a single particle at the origin which performs a Brownian motion with variance σ^2 at time 1, and branches at rate 1 into two independent Brownian motions which themselves branch at rate 1 independently, and so on. For such a BBM, one knows since the work of McKean [20] that

$$u(x,\, t) := \mathbf{P}(X_{\max}(t) \le x),$$

satisfies the F-KPP (Fisher–Kolmogorov–Petrovskii–Piskunov) equation

---

Dedicated to Professor Valentin Konakov on the occasion of his 70th birthday.

B. Derrida
Collège de France, 11 place Marcelin Berthelot, 75231 Paris Cedex 05, France
e-mail: derrida@lps.ens.fr

Z. Shi (✉)
Université Pierre et Marie Curie, 4 place Jussieu, 75252 Paris Cedex 05, France
e-mail: zhan.shi@upmc.fr

© Springer International Publishing AG 2017   303
V. Panov (ed.), *Modern Problems of Stochastic Analysis and Statistics*,
Springer Proceedings in Mathematics & Statistics 208,
DOI 10.1007/978-3-319-65313-6_12

$$\frac{\partial u}{\partial t} = \frac{\sigma^2}{2} \frac{\partial^2 u}{\partial x^2} + u^2 - u \tag{1}$$

with the initial condition $u(x, 0) = 1_{\{x \geq 0\}}$. It is also known since the works of Bramson [5, 6] that in the long time limit

$$u(x + m(t)\sigma, t) \to F(x), \tag{2}$$

where $F(z)$ is a traveling wave solution of

$$\frac{\sigma^2}{2} F'' + \sqrt{2\sigma^2} F' + F^2 - F = 0$$

and

$$m(t) := \sqrt{2} t - \frac{3}{2\sqrt{2}} \ln t . \tag{3}$$

This implies in particular that

$$\lim_{t \to \infty} \frac{X_{\max}(t)}{t} = \sqrt{2\sigma^2} , \qquad \text{in probability.}$$

[The convergence also holds almost surely.]

In 1988, Chauvin and Rouault [9, 24] proved a large deviation result for $X_{\max}(t)/t > \sqrt{2\sigma^2}$, namely, that for $v > \sqrt{2\sigma^2}$

$$\ln \left[\mathbf{P} \left(\frac{X_{\max}(t)}{t} > v \right) \right] \sim t \left(1 - \frac{v^2}{2\sigma^2} \right). \tag{4}$$

In (4) and everywhere below, the symbol $\sim$ means that

$$\lim_{t \to \infty} \frac{\ln \mathbf{P}(X_{\max}(t) > vt)}{t(1 - \frac{v^2}{2\sigma^2})} = 1 . \tag{5}$$

Here, we are interested in the *lower deviation* probability $\mathbf{P}(X_{\max}(t) \leq vt)$ for each $v \in (-\infty, \sqrt{2\sigma^2})$. It turns out that $v/\sqrt{2\sigma^2}$ is an important parameter, so we fix $\alpha \in (-\infty, 1)$, and study

$$\mathbf{P}(X_{\max}(t) \leq \alpha\sqrt{2\sigma^2} t),$$

when $t \to \infty$.

Throughout the paper, we write

$$\rho := \sqrt{2} - 1 . \tag{6}$$

Theorem 1 *Let $X_{\max}(t)$ denote the rightmost position of the BBM at time t. Then for all $\alpha \in (-\infty, 1)$,*

Fig. 1 The large deviation function of the position of the rightmost particle of a branching Brownian motion. The expression of $\psi(\alpha)$ is nonanalytic at $\alpha = -\rho = 1 - \sqrt{2}$ and at $\alpha = 1$

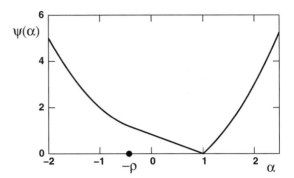

$$\ln \mathbf{P}(X_{\max}(t) \leq \alpha\sqrt{2\sigma^2 t}) \sim -t\,\psi(\alpha), \tag{7}$$

where

$$\psi(\alpha) = \begin{cases} 2\rho(1-\alpha), & \text{if } \alpha \in [-\rho,\, 1), \\ 1 + \alpha^2, & \text{if } \alpha \in (-\infty,\, -\rho]. \end{cases} \tag{8}$$

Together with Theorem 1 and the upper large deviation probability in (4), a routine argument (proof of Theorem III.3.4 in den Hollander [16], proof of Theorem 2.2.3 in Dembo and Zeitouni [11]) yields the following formalism of large deviation principle: the family of the distributions of $\frac{X_{\max}(t)}{\sqrt{2\sigma^2}\,t}$, for $t \geq 1$, satisfies the large deviation principle on $\mathbf{R}$, with speed t and with the rate function $\psi(\alpha)$ (shown in Fig. 1).

$$\psi(\alpha) = \begin{cases} 1 + \alpha^2, & \text{if } \alpha \leq -\rho, \\ 2\rho(1-\alpha), & \text{if } -\rho \leq \alpha \leq 1, \\ \alpha^2 - 1, & \text{if } \alpha \geq 1, \end{cases} \tag{9}$$

i.e., for any closed set $F \subset \mathbf{R}$ and open set $G \subset \mathbf{R}$,

$$\limsup_{t\to\infty} \frac{1}{t} \ln \mathbf{P}\left(\frac{X_{\max}(t)}{\sqrt{2\sigma^2}\,t} \in F\right) \leq -\inf_{\alpha \in F} \psi(\alpha),$$

$$\liminf_{t\to\infty} \frac{1}{t} \ln \mathbf{P}\left(\frac{X_{\max}(t)}{\sqrt{2\sigma^2}\,t} \in G\right) \geq -\inf_{\alpha \in G} \psi(\alpha).$$

Let us also mention that Proposition 2.5 of Chen [10] (recalled as Lemma 3 in Sect. 3 below) implies that for all $\alpha < 1$,

$$\psi(\alpha) \geq \frac{1-\alpha}{6},$$

which is in agreement with (8).

The reason for the nonanalyticity of $\psi(\alpha)$ in (9) at $\alpha = -\rho$ is that, as we will see it in Sects. 2 and 3, for $\alpha < -\rho$ the events which dominate are those where the initial particle does not branch or branches at a very late time (at a time τ very close to t) while in the range $-\rho < \alpha < 1$ the first branching event occurs at a time $\tau \sim (1 - \alpha)t/\sqrt{2}$.

The rest of the paper is as follows. Sections 2 and 3 are devoted to the proof of the lower bound and the upper bound, respectively, for the probability in Theorem 1. In Sect. 4, we present some further remarks.

2 Lower Bound

Fix $v \in (-\infty, \sqrt{2\sigma^2}\,)$. We prove the lower bound in the deviation probability, by considering a special event described as follows: The initial particle does not produce any offspring during time interval $[0, \tau]$ and is positioned at $y \in (-\infty, vt - \sqrt{2\sigma^2}\,(t - \tau) - 1]$ at time τ; then, at time t, the maximal position lies in $(-\infty, vt)$. As such, we get

$$\mathbf{P}(X_{\max}(t) \leq vt)$$

$$\geq \mathrm{e}^{-\tau} \int_{-\infty}^{vt - \sqrt{2\sigma^2}\,(t-\tau)-1} \frac{\mathrm{d}y}{\sqrt{2\pi\sigma^2\tau}} \, \mathrm{e}^{-\frac{y^2}{2\sigma^2\tau}} \, \mathbf{P}(X_{\max}(t - \tau) < vt - y). \quad (10)$$

Note that for $y \in (-\infty, vt - \sqrt{2\sigma^2}\,(t - \tau) - 1]$, we have $vt - y \geq \sqrt{2\sigma^2}\,(t - \tau) + 1$, so

$$\mathbf{P}(X_{\max}(t - \tau) \leq vt - y) \geq \mathbf{P}(X_{\max}(t - \tau) \leq \sqrt{2\sigma^2}\,(t - \tau) + 1).$$

Let $m(t) := \sqrt{2}\,t - \frac{3}{2\sqrt{2}} \ln t$ be as in (3). By (2), for any $z \in \mathbf{R}$, $\mathbf{P}(X_{\max}(s) \leq m(s)\sigma + z)$ converges, as $s \to \infty$, to a positive limit (which depends on z). This yields the existence of a constant $c > 0$ such that

$$\mathbf{P}(X_{\max}(t - \tau) \leq \sqrt{2\sigma^2}\,(t - \tau) + 1) \geq c,$$

for all $\tau \in [0, t]$. [The presence of $+1$ in $\sqrt{2\sigma^2}\,(t - \tau) + 1$ is only to ensure the positivity of the probability when τ equals t or is very close to t.] Going back to (10), we get that for all $\tau \in (0, t]$,

$$\mathbf{P}(X_{\max}(t) \leq vt) \geq c\,\mathrm{e}^{-\tau} \int_{-\infty}^{vt - \sqrt{2\sigma^2}\,(t-\tau)-1} \frac{1}{\sqrt{2\pi\sigma^2\tau}} \, \mathrm{e}^{-\frac{y^2}{2\sigma^2\tau}} \, \mathrm{d}y.$$

Hence,

$$P(X_{\max}(t) \le vt) \ge c \sup_{\tau \in (0, t]} \left\{ e^{-\tau} \int_{-\infty}^{vt - \sqrt{2\sigma^2}\,(t-\tau)-1} \frac{1}{\sqrt{2\pi\sigma^2\tau}} e^{-\frac{y^2}{2\sigma^2\tau}}\, dy \right\}. \quad (11)$$

We now use the following result.

Lemma 2 *For* $v < \sqrt{2\sigma^2}$ *and* $t \to \infty$,

$$\ln \left(\sup_{\tau \in (0, t]} \left\{ e^{-\tau} \int_{-\infty}^{vt - \sqrt{2\sigma^2}\,(t-\tau)-1} \frac{1}{\sqrt{2\pi\sigma^2\tau}} e^{-\frac{y^2}{2\sigma^2\tau}}\, dy \right\} \right) \sim -\varphi(v)t,$$

where

$$\varphi(v) := \begin{cases} 2\rho(1 - \alpha), & \text{if } \alpha \ge -\rho, \\ 1 + \alpha^2, & \text{if } \alpha \le -\rho, \end{cases} \quad (12)$$

with $\alpha := \frac{v}{\sqrt{2\sigma^2}} < 1$ *and* $\rho := \sqrt{2} - 1$ *as before.*

The proof of Lemma 2 is quite elementary (as $\ln(\int_{-\infty}^{z} e^{-y^2}\, dy) \sim -z^2$ for $z \to -\infty$, and $\int_{-\infty}^{z} e^{-y^2}\, dy$ is greater than a positive constant if $z \ge 0$). We only indicate the optimal value of τ:

$$\tau = \begin{cases} \frac{1-\alpha}{\sqrt{2}} t + o(t), & \text{if } \alpha \ge -\rho, \\ t + o(t), & \text{if } \alpha \le -\rho. \end{cases} \quad (13)$$

By (11) and Lemma 2, we obtain

$$\liminf_{t \to \infty} \frac{1}{t} \ln P(X_{\max}(t) \le vt) \ge -\varphi(v),$$

with $\varphi(v)$ as in (12). This yields the desired lower bound for the probability in the theorem, as $\varphi(v)$ coincides with $\psi(\alpha)$ defined in (9).

3 Upper Bound

We now look for the upper bound in the deviation probability. Fix $x = vt$ with $v < \sqrt{2\sigma^2}$. Let

$$u(x, t) := P(X_{\max}(t) \le x),$$

as before. Considering the event that the first branching time is τ, we have

$$u(x, t) = \int_{-\infty}^{x} \frac{dy}{\sqrt{2\pi\sigma^2 t}} e^{-t - \frac{y^2}{2\sigma^2 t}}$$

$$+ \int_{0}^{t} d\tau \int_{-\infty}^{\infty} \frac{dy}{\sqrt{2\pi\sigma^2 \tau}} e^{-\tau - \frac{y^2}{2\sigma^2 \tau}} u^2(x - y, t - \tau),$$

the first term on the right-hand side originating from the event that the first branching time is greater than t. [It is easy to check that this expression satisfies the F-KPP equation (1).] We also have a lower bound for $u(x, t)$ by considering only the event that there is no branching up to time τ: For any $\tau \in [0, t]$,

$$u(x, t) \geq \int_{-\infty}^{\infty} \frac{dy}{\sqrt{2\pi\sigma^2 \tau}} e^{-\tau - \frac{y^2}{2\sigma^2 \tau}} u(x - y, t - \tau).$$

Writing $(B_s, s \geq 0)$ for a standard Brownian motion (with variance of B_1 being 1), the last two displayed formulas can be expressed as follows:

$$u(x, t) = e^{-t} \mathbf{P}(\sigma B_t \leq x) + \int_{0}^{t} e^{-\tau} \mathbf{E}[u^2(x - \sigma B_\tau, t - \tau)] d\tau, \quad (14)$$

$$u(x, t) \geq e^{-\tau} \mathbf{E}[u(x - \sigma B_\tau, t - \tau)], \quad \forall \tau \in [0, t]. \quad (15)$$

Consider, for $\tau \in [0, t]$,

$$\Phi(\tau) := e^{-\tau} \mathbf{E}[u^2(x - \sigma B_\tau, t - \tau)].$$

Since Φ is a continuous function on $[0, t]$, there exists $\tau_0 = \tau_0(t, x)$ such that

$$\Phi(\tau_0) = \sup_{\tau \in [0, t]} \Phi(\tau).$$

On the other hand, since $u(\cdot, 0) = \mathbf{1}_{[0, \infty)}(\cdot)$, we have $e^{-t} \mathbf{P}(\sigma B_t \leq x) = \Phi(t)$. So (14) becomes $u(x, t) = \Phi(t) + \int_{0}^{t} \Phi(\tau) d\tau$, which is bounded by $(t + 1) \sup_{\tau \in [0, t]} \Phi(\tau)$. Taking $\tau = \tau_0$ in (15), it follows from (15) to (14) that

$$e^{-\tau_0} \mathbf{E}[u(x - \sigma B_{\tau_0}, t - \tau_0)] \leq u(x, t) \leq (t + 1)\Phi(\tau_0),$$

which can be represented as

$$e^{-\tau_0} \mathbf{E}(Y) \leq u(x, t) \leq (t + 1)e^{-\tau_0} \mathbf{E}(Y^2), \quad (16)$$

where

$$Y = Y(x, t, \sigma) := u(x - \sigma B_{\tau_0}, t - \tau_0).$$

Let us have a closer look at $\mathbf{E}(Y)$. We write

$$e^{-\tau_0} \mathbf{E}(Y) = A_1 + A_2,$$

with

$$A_1 = A_1(x,\, t,\, \sigma) := \mathrm{e}^{-T_0}\, \mathbf{E}[Y\, \mathbf{1}_{\{Y < \frac{1}{2(t+1)}\}}],$$

$$A_2 = A_2(x,\, t,\, \sigma) := \mathrm{e}^{-T_0}\, \mathbf{E}[Y\, \mathbf{1}_{\{Y \geq \frac{1}{2(t+1)}\}}].$$

Then

$$(t+1)\mathrm{e}^{-T_0}\, \mathbf{E}(Y^2)$$

$$= (t+1)\mathrm{e}^{-T_0}\, \mathbf{E}[Y^2\, \mathbf{1}_{\{Y < \frac{1}{2(t+1)}\}}] + (t+1)\mathrm{e}^{-T_0}\, \mathbf{E}[Y^2\, \mathbf{1}_{\{Y \geq \frac{1}{2(t+1)}\}}]$$

$$\leq \frac{1}{2}\mathrm{e}^{-T_0}\, \mathbf{E}[Y\, \mathbf{1}_{\{Y < \frac{1}{2(t+1)}\}}] + (t+1)\mathrm{e}^{-T_0}\, \mathbf{E}[Y\, \mathbf{1}_{\{Y \geq \frac{1}{2(t+1)}\}}],$$

where, on the right-hand side, we have used the trivial inequality $Y^2 \leq Y$ when dealing with the event $\{Y \geq \frac{1}{2(t+1)}\}$. In other words,

$$(t+1)\mathrm{e}^{-T_0}\, \mathbf{E}(Y^2) \leq \frac{1}{2}A_1 + (t+1)A_2.$$

So by (16), we obtain

$$A_1 + A_2 \leq u(x,\, t) \leq (t+1)\mathrm{e}^{-T_0}\, \mathbf{E}(Y^2) \leq \frac{1}{2}A_1 + (t+1)A_2.$$

In particular, this implies $A_1 \leq 2t\, A_2$. As a consequence,

$$A_2 \leq u(x,\, t) \leq (2t+1)A_2. \tag{17}$$

This yields that A_2 has the same asymptotic behavior as $u(x,\, t)$, as far as large deviation functions are concerned.

We now look for an upper bound for A_2, which, multiplied by $2t+1$, will be served as an upper bound for $u(x,\, t)$. Let us recall the following estimate:

Lemma 3 (Chen [10], Proposition 2.5) *Let* $m(t) := \sqrt{2}\, t - \frac{3}{2\sqrt{2}}\ln t$ *as in* (3). *There exist two constants* $c_1 > 0$ *and* $c_2 > 0$ *independent of* σ, *such that*

$$\mathbf{P}(X_{\max}(r) \leq \sigma m(r) - \sigma z\, \text{for some}\, r \leq \mathrm{e}^z) \leq c_1\, \mathrm{e}^{-c_2 z},$$

for all sufficiently large z. *Moreover, one can take* $c_2 = \frac{1}{6\sqrt{2}}$.

We apply the lemma to $z := t^{1/3}$, to see that when t is sufficiently large (say $t \geq t_0$), for any $\tau \in [0,\, t]$,

$$y < \sqrt{2\sigma^2}\, \tau - t^{1/2} \;\Rightarrow\; u(y,\, \tau) < \frac{1}{2(t+1)}.$$

As such, for $t \geq t_0$, we have

$$A_2 = e^{-T_0} \, \mathbf{E}[Y \, 1_{\{Y \geq \frac{1}{2(t+1)}\}}] \leq e^{-T_0} \, \mathbf{E}[Y \, 1_{\{x - \sigma B_{T_0} \geq \sqrt{2\sigma^2} \, (t - T_0) - t^{1/2}\}}].$$

Since $Y \leq 1$, this yields, for $t \geq t_0$,

$$
\begin{aligned}
A_2 &\leq e^{-T_0} \, \mathbf{P}(x - \sigma B_{T_0} \geq \sqrt{2\sigma^2} \, (t - T_0) - t^{1/2}) \\
&\leq \sup_{\tau \in [0, t]} \left\{ e^{-\tau} \, \mathbf{P}(x - \sigma B_\tau \geq \sqrt{2\sigma^2} \, (t - \tau) - t^{1/2}) \right\} \\
&= \sup_{\tau \in (0, t]} \left\{ \int_{-\infty}^{x - \sqrt{2\sigma^2} \, (t-\tau) + t^{1/2}} \frac{1}{\sqrt{2\pi\sigma^2\tau}} \, e^{-\tau - \frac{y^2}{2\sigma^2\tau}} \, dy \right\}.
\end{aligned}
$$

By (17), we have therefore, for all sufficiently large t,

$$u(x, t) \leq (2t + 1) \sup_{\tau \in (0, t]} \left\{ \int_{-\infty}^{x - \sqrt{2\sigma^2} \, (t-\tau) + t^{1/2}} \frac{1}{\sqrt{2\pi\sigma^2\tau}} \, e^{-\tau - \frac{y^2}{2\sigma^2\tau}} \, dy \right\}.$$

Recall that $x = vt$. The supremum on the right-hand side has already been estimated in Lemma 2 in Sect. 2: For $v < \sqrt{2\sigma^2}$ and $t \to \infty$,

$$\ln \left(\sup_{\tau \in (0, t]} \left\{ \int_{-\infty}^{x - \sqrt{2\sigma^2} \, (t-\tau) + t^{1/2}} \frac{1}{\sqrt{2\pi\sigma^2\tau}} \, e^{-\tau - \frac{y^2}{2\sigma^2\tau}} \, dy \right\} \right) \sim -\varphi(v)t,$$

where $\varphi(v)$ is defined in (12). Note that we have $t^{1/2}$ here (in $x - \sqrt{2\sigma^2} \, (t - \tau) + t^{1/2}$) instead of -1 in the lemma; this makes in practice no difference because $t^{1/2} \leq \varepsilon t$ (for any $\varepsilon > 0$ and all sufficiently large t) and we can use the continuity of the function $v \mapsto \varphi(v)$. Consequently, for $x = vt$ with $v < \sqrt{2\sigma^2}$,

$$\limsup_{t \to \infty} \frac{\ln u(x, t)}{t} \leq -\varphi(v),$$

which yields the upper bound for the probability in the theorem because $\varphi(v)$ coincides with $\psi(\alpha)$ given in (8).

4 Conclusion and Remarks

The main result stated in (8) and (9) of the present work is the expression of the (lower) large deviation function $\psi(\alpha)$ of the position of the rightmost particle of a branching Brownian motion. One remarkable feature of this large deviation function is its nonanalyticity at some particular values $\alpha = -\sqrt{2} + 1$ and $\alpha = 1$ due to a change of scenario of the dominant contribution to the large deviation function: for $\alpha < -\sqrt{2} + 1$, the dominant event is a single Brownian particle which does not branch up to time t; for $-\sqrt{2} + 1 < \alpha < 1$, it corresponds to a particle which moves to position $-(\sqrt{2} - 1)(1 - \alpha)\sigma t$ without branching up to a time $t(1 - \alpha)/\sqrt{2}$, and then behaves like a normal BBM up to time t; for $\alpha > 1$, the tree branches normally but one branch moves at the speed $\alpha\sqrt{2\sigma^2}$, faster than the normal speed $\sqrt{2\sigma^2}$.

Using more *heuristic* arguments as in [12], it is possible to determine the time dependence of the prefactor, for example, by showing [14] that for $-\rho < \alpha < 1$, there exists a constant $c \in (0, \infty)$ such that

$$\mathbf{P}(X_{\max}(t) \leq \alpha\sqrt{2\sigma^2}\,t) \sim c\,t^{\frac{3(\sqrt{2}-1)}{2}}\mathrm{e}^{-\psi(\alpha)t}\,. \tag{18}$$

The result of the present work can also be easily extended to more general branching Brownian motions, where one includes the possibility that a particle branches into more than two particles (for example, one could consider that a particle branches into k particles with probability p_k). It can also be extended to branching random walks. In all these cases, one finds [14] as in (8) and (9) three different regimes with the same scenarios as described above.

It is, however, important to notice that expressions (8) and (9) of the large deviation function $\psi(\alpha)$ for $\alpha < 1$ depend crucially on the fact that one starts initially with a single particle and that branchings occur at random times according to Poisson processes. If instead one starts at time $t = 0$ with several particles in [21] or if the distribution of the branching times is not exponential (for example in the case of a branching random walk generated by a regular binary tree where at each (integer) time step each particle branches into two particles), $\mathbf{P}(X_{\max} \leq vt)$ might decay faster than an exponential of time.

Recently, there has been a renewed interest in the understanding of the extremal process and in particular of the measure seen at the tip of the branching Brownian motion [1, 2, 7, 8, 18, 25]. We think that it would be interesting to investigate how this extremal process is modified when it is conditioned on the position of the rightmost particle, i.e., how it depends on the parameter α.

References

1. Aïdékon, E., Berestycki, J., Brunet, E., Shi, Z.: Branching Brownian motion seen from its tip. Probab. Theory Relat. Fields **157**, 405–451 (2013)
2. Arguin, L.P., Bovier, A., Kistler, N.: The extremal process of branching Brownian motion. Probab. Theory Relat. Fields **157**, 535–574 (2013)
3. Berestycki, J. Topics on Branching Brownian Motion. Lecture notes available at: http://www.stats.ox.ac.uk/~berestyc/articles.html (2015)
4. Bovier, A.: Gaussian Processes on Trees. Cambridge University Press, New York (2016)
5. Bramson, M.D.: Maximal displacement of branching Brownian motion. Comm. Pure Appl. Math. **31**, 531–581 (1978)
6. Bramson, M.D.: Convergence of solutions of the Kolmogorov equation to travelling waves. Mem. Amer. Math. Soc. **44**(285) (1983)
7. Brunet, E., Derrida, B.: Statistics at the tip of a branching random walk and the delay of traveling waves. EPL (Europhys. Lett.) **87**, 60010 (2009)

8. Brunet, E., Derrida, B.: A branching random walk seen from the tip. J. Stat. Phys. **143**, 420–446 (2011)
9. Chauvin, B., Rouault, A.: KPP equation and supercritical branching Brownian motion in the subcritical speed area. Application to spatial trees. Probab. Theory Relat. Fields **80**, 299–314 (1988)
10. Chen, X.: Waiting times for particles in a branching Brownian motion to reach the rightmost position. Stoch. Proc. Appl. **123**, 3153–3182 (2013)
11. Dembo, A., Zeitouni, O.: Large Deviations Techniques and Applications, 2nd edn. Springer, New York (1998)
12. Derrida, B., Meerson, B., Sasorov, P.V.: Large-displacement statistics of the rightmost particle of the one-dimensional branching Brownian motion. Phys. Rev. E **93**, 042139 (2016)
13. Derrida, B., Shi, Z.: Large deviations for the branching Brownian motion in presence of selection or coalescence. J. Stat. Phys. **163**, 1285–1311 (2016)
14. Derrida, B. and Shi, Z.: Slower deviations of the branching Brownian motion and of branching random walks. J. Phys. A **50**, 344001 (2017)
15. Derrida, B., Spohn, H.: Polymers on disordered trees, spin glasses, and traveling waves. J. Stat. Phys. **51**, 817–840 (1988)
16. den Hollander, F.: Large Deviations. American Mathematical Society, Providence (2000)
17. Hu, Y., Shi, Z.: Minimal position and critical martingale convergence in branching random walks, and directed polymers on disordered trees. Ann. Probab. **37**, 742–789 (2009)
18. Lalley, S.P., Sellke, T.: A conditional limit theorem for the frontier of a branching Brownian motion. Ann. Probab. **15**, 1052–1061 (1987)
19. Majumdar, S.N., Krapivsky, P.L.: Extremal paths on a random Cayley tree. Phys. Rev. E **62**, 7735 (2000)
20. McKean, H.P.: Application of Brownian motion to the equation of Kolmogorov-Petrovskii-Piskunov. Commun. Pure Appl. Math. **28**, 323–331 (1975)
21. Meerson, B., Sasorov, P.V.: Negative velocity fluctuations of pulled reaction fronts. Phys. Rev. E **84**, 030101(R) (2011)
22. Mueller, A.H., Munier, S.: Phenomenological picture of fluctuations in branching random walks. Phys. Rev. E **90**, 042143 (2014)
23. Ramola, K., Majumdar, S.N., Schehr, G.: Spatial extent of branching Brownian motion. Phys. Rev. E **91**, 042131 (2015)
24. Rouault, A.: Large deviations and branching processes. Proceedings of the 9th International Summer School on Probability Theory and Mathematical Statistics (Sozopol, 1997). Pliska Studia Math. Bulgarica **13**, 15–38 (2000)
25. Schmidt, M.A., Kistler, N.: From Derrida's random energy model to branching random walks: from 1 to 3. Electronic Commun. Prob. **20**, 1–12 (2015)
26. Shi, Z.: Branching Random Walks. École d'été Saint-Flour XLII (2012). Lecture Notes in Mathematics 2151. Springer, Berlin (2015)
27. Zeitouni, O.: Branching Random Walks and Gaussian Fields. Lecture notes available at: http://www.wisdom.weizmann.ac.il/~zeitouni/pdf/notesBRW.pdf (2012)

Part VII
Statistics

Bounds on the Prediction Error of Penalized Least Squares Estimators with Convex Penalty

Pierre Bellec and Alexandre Tsybakov

Abstract This paper considers the penalized least squares estimator with arbitrary convex penalty. When the observation noise is Gaussian, we show that the prediction error is a subgaussian random variable concentrated around its median. We apply this concentration property to derive sharp oracle inequalities for the prediction error of the LASSO, the group LASSO, and the SLOPE estimators, both in probability and in expectation. In contrast to the previous work on the LASSO-type methods, our oracle inequalities in probability are obtained at any confidence level for estimators with tuning parameters that do not depend on the confidence level. This is also the reason why we are able to establish sparsity oracle bounds in expectation for the LASSO-type estimators, while the previously known techniques did not allow for the control of the expected risk. In addition, we show that the concentration rate in the oracle inequalities is better than it was commonly understood before.

Keywords Penalized least squares · Oracle inequality · LASSO estimator SLOPE estimator · Group LASSO

1 Introduction and Notation

Assume that we have noisy observations

$$y_i = f_i + \xi_i, \qquad i = 1, \ldots, n, \tag{1}$$

where $\xi_1, \ldots, \xi_n$ are i.i.d. centered Gaussian random variables with variance σ^2, and $\mathbf{f} = (f_1, \ldots, f_n)^T \in \mathbb{R}^n$ is an unknown mean vector. In vector form, the model (1) can be rewritten as $\mathbf{y} = \mathbf{f} + \boldsymbol{\xi}$ where $\boldsymbol{\xi} = (\xi_1, \ldots, \xi_n)^T$ and $\mathbf{y} = (y_1, \ldots, y_n)^T$.

P. Bellec
Rutgers University, Piscataway, NJ 08854, USA

A. Tsybakov (✉)
ENSAE ParisTech, 3 avenue Pierre Larousse, 92245 Malakoff Cedex, France
e-mail: alexandre.tsybakov@ensae.fr

© Springer International Publishing AG 2017
V. Panov (ed.), *Modern Problems of Stochastic Analysis and Statistics*,
Springer Proceedings in Mathematics & Statistics 208,
DOI 10.1007/978-3-319-65313-6_13

Let $\mathbb{X} \in \mathbb{R}^{n \times p}$ be a matrix with p columns that we will call the design matrix. We consider the problem of estimation of $\mathbf{f}$ by $\mathbb{X}\hat{\boldsymbol{\beta}}(\mathbf{y})$ where $\hat{\boldsymbol{\beta}}(\mathbf{y})$ is an estimator valued in $\mathbb{R}^p$. Specifically, we restrict our attention to penalized least squares estimators of the form

$$\hat{\boldsymbol{\beta}}(\mathbf{y}) \in \underset{\boldsymbol{\beta} \in \mathbb{R}^p}{\operatorname{argmin}} \left(\|\mathbf{y} - \mathbb{X}\boldsymbol{\beta}\|^2 + 2F(\boldsymbol{\beta}) \right), \tag{2}$$

where $\| \cdot \|$ is the scaled Euclidean norm defined by $\|\mathbf{u}\|^2 = \frac{1}{n} \sum_{i=1}^n u_i^2$ for any $\mathbf{u} = (u_1, \dots, u_n)$, and the penalty function $F : \mathbb{R}^p \to [0, +\infty]$ is convex. If the context prevents any ambiguity, we will omit the dependence on $\mathbf{y}$ and write $\hat{\boldsymbol{\beta}}$ for the estimator $\hat{\boldsymbol{\beta}}(\mathbf{y})$.

The object of study in this paper is the prediction error of the estimator $\hat{\boldsymbol{\beta}}(\mathbf{y})$, that is, the value $\|\mathbb{X}\hat{\boldsymbol{\beta}}(\mathbf{y}) - \mathbf{f}\|$. Under the mild assumption that the penalty function F is convex, proper, and lower semicontinuous, we show that the prediction error $\|\mathbb{X}\hat{\boldsymbol{\beta}}(\mathbf{y}) - \mathbf{f}\|$ is a subgaussian random variable concentrated around its median and its expectation. This holds for any design matrix $\mathbb{X}$. Furthermore, when F is a norm, we obtain an explicit formula for the predictor $\mathbb{X}\hat{\boldsymbol{\beta}}(\mathbf{y})$ in terms of the projection on the dual ball. Finally, we apply the subgaussian concentration property around the median to derive sharp oracle inequalities for the prediction error of the LASSO, the group LASSO, and the SLOPE estimators, both in probability and in expectation. The inequalities in probability improve upon the previous work on the LASSO-type estimators (see, e.g., the papers [3, 6, 9, 11] or the monographs [5, 7, 16]) since, in contrast to the results of these works, our bounds hold at any given confidence level for estimators with tuning parameter that does not depend on the confidence level. This is also the reason why we are able to establish bounds in expectation, while the previously known techniques did not allow for the control of the expected risk. In addition, we show that the concentration rate in the oracle inequalities is better than it was commonly understood before. Similar results have been obtained quite recently in [2] by a different and somewhat more involved construction conceived specifically for the LASSO and the SLOPE estimators. The techniques of the present paper are more general since they can be used not only for these two estimators but for any penalized least squares estimators with convex penalty.

2 Notation

For any random variable Z, let Med$[Z]$ be a median of Z, i.e., any real number M such that $\mathbb{P}(Z \geq M) = \mathbb{P}(Z \leq M) = 1/2$. For a vector $\mathbf{u} = (u_1, \dots, u_n)$, the sup-norm, the Euclidean norm and the ℓ_1-norm will be denoted by $|\mathbf{u}|_\infty = \max_{i=1,\dots,n} |u_i|$, $|\mathbf{u}|_1 = \sum_{i=1}^n |u_i|$ and $|\mathbf{u}|_2 = (\sum_{i=1}^n u_i^2)^{1/2}$. The inner product in $\mathbb{R}^n$ is denoted by $\langle \cdot, \cdot \rangle$. We also denote by Supp$(\mathbf{u})$ the support of $\mathbf{u}$, and by $|\mathbf{u}|_0$ the cardinality of Supp$(\mathbf{u})$. We denote by $I(\cdot)$ the indicator function. For any $S \subset \{1, \dots, p\}$ and a vector $\mathbf{u} = (u_1, \dots, u_p)$, we set $\mathbf{u}_S = (u_j I(j \in S))_{j=1,\dots,p}$, and we denote by $|S|$ the cardinality of S.

3 The Prediction Error of Convex Penalized Estimators Is Subgaussian

The aim of this section is to show that the prediction error $\|\mathbb{X}\hat{\boldsymbol{\beta}}(\mathbf{y}) - \mathbf{f}\|$ is subgaussian and concentrates around its median for any estimator $\hat{\boldsymbol{\beta}}(\mathbf{y})$ defined by (2). The results of the present section will allow us to carry out a unified analysis of LASSO, group LASSO, and SLOPE estimators in Sects. 4–6.

Proposition 1 *Let $\hat{\boldsymbol{\mu}} : \mathbb{R}^n \to \mathbb{R}^n$ be an L-Lipschitz function, that is, a function satisfying*

$$\|\hat{\boldsymbol{\mu}}(\mathbf{y}) - \hat{\boldsymbol{\mu}}(\mathbf{y}')\| \leq L\|\mathbf{y} - \mathbf{y}'\|, \qquad \forall \mathbf{y}, \mathbf{y}' \in \mathbb{R}^n. \tag{3}$$

Let $g(\mathbf{z}) = \|\hat{\boldsymbol{\mu}}(\mathbf{f} + \sigma\mathbf{z}) - \mathbf{f}\|$ for some fixed $\mathbf{f} \in \mathbb{R}^n$ and $\mathbf{z} \sim \mathscr{N}(\mathbf{0}, I_{n\times n})$. Then, for all $t > 0$,

$$\mathbb{P}\left(g(\mathbf{z}) > \mathrm{Med}[g(\mathbf{z})] + \frac{\sigma L t}{\sqrt{n}}\right) \leq 1 - \Phi(t), \tag{4}$$

where $\Phi(\cdot)$ is the $\mathscr{N}(0, 1)$ cumulative distribution function.

Proof The result follows immediately from the Gaussian concentration inequality (cf., e.g., [10, Theorem 6.2]) and the fact that $g(\cdot)$ satisfies the Lipschitz condition

$$\left|g(\mathbf{u}) - g(\mathbf{u}')\right| \leq \|\hat{\boldsymbol{\mu}}(\mathbf{f} + \sigma\mathbf{u}) - \hat{\boldsymbol{\mu}}(\mathbf{f} + \sigma\mathbf{u}')\| \leq \frac{\sigma L}{\sqrt{n}}|\mathbf{u} - \mathbf{u}'|_2, \qquad \forall \mathbf{u}, \mathbf{u}' \in \mathbb{R}^n.$$

$\square$

We now show that $\hat{\boldsymbol{\mu}}(\mathbf{y}) = \mathbb{X}\hat{\boldsymbol{\beta}}(\mathbf{y})$ where $\hat{\boldsymbol{\beta}}(\mathbf{y})$ is estimator (2) satisfies the Lipschitz condition (3) with $L = 1$, provided that the penalty function F is convex, proper, and lower semicontinuous.

We first consider estimators penalized by a norm in $\mathbb{R}^p$, for which we get a sharper result. Namely, in this case, the explicit expression for $\mathbb{X}\hat{\boldsymbol{\beta}}(\mathbf{y})$ is available. In addition, we get a stronger property than the Lipschitz condition (3). Let $N : \mathbb{R}^p \to \mathbb{R}_+$ be a norm and let $N_\circ(\cdot)$ be the corresponding dual norm defined by $N_\circ(\mathbf{u}) = \sup_{\mathbf{v}\in\mathbb{R}^p : N(\mathbf{v})=1} \mathbf{u}^T\mathbf{v}$. For any $\mathbf{y} \in \mathbb{R}^n$, define $\hat{\boldsymbol{\beta}}(\mathbf{y})$ as a solution of the following minimization problem:

$$\hat{\boldsymbol{\beta}}(\mathbf{y}) \in \underset{\boldsymbol{\beta}\in\mathbb{R}^p}{\mathrm{argmin}} \left(\|\mathbf{y} - \mathbb{X}\boldsymbol{\beta}\|^2 + 2N(\boldsymbol{\beta})\right). \tag{5}$$

The next two propositions are crucial in proving that the concentration bounds (4) apply when $g(\mathbf{z})$ is the prediction error associated with $\hat{\boldsymbol{\beta}}(\mathbf{y})$.

Proposition 2 *Let $N : \mathbb{R}^p \to \mathbb{R}_+$ be a norm and let $\hat{\boldsymbol{\beta}}(\mathbf{y})$ be a solution of (5). For all $\mathbf{y} \in \mathbb{R}^n$ and all matrices $\mathbb{X} \in \mathbb{R}^{n\times p}$, we have*

(i) $\mathbb{X}\hat{\boldsymbol{\beta}}(\mathbf{y}) = \mathbf{y} - P_C(\mathbf{y})$ where $P_C(\cdot) : \mathbb{R}^n \to C$ is the operator of projection onto the closed convex set $C = \{\mathbf{u} \in \mathbb{R}^n : N_\circ(\mathbb{X}^T \mathbf{u}) \le 1/n\}$,

(ii) the function $\hat{\boldsymbol{\mu}}(\mathbf{y}) = \mathbb{X}\hat{\boldsymbol{\beta}}(\mathbf{y})$ satisfies

$$\|\hat{\boldsymbol{\mu}}(\mathbf{y}) - \hat{\boldsymbol{\mu}}(\mathbf{y}')\|^2 \le \|\mathbf{y} - \mathbf{y}'\|^2 - \frac{1}{n}|P_C(\mathbf{y}) - P_C(\mathbf{y}')|_2^2.$$

Proof Since C is a closed convex set, we have that $\boldsymbol{\theta} = P_C(\mathbf{y})$ if and only if

$$(\mathbf{y} - \boldsymbol{\theta})^T(\boldsymbol{\theta} - \mathbf{u}) \ge 0 \qquad \text{for all } \mathbf{u} \in C. \tag{6}$$

Thus, to prove statement (i) of the proposition, it is enough to check that (6) holds for $\boldsymbol{\theta} = \mathbf{y} - \mathbb{X}\hat{\boldsymbol{\beta}}(\mathbf{y})$. Since (6) is trivial when $\hat{\boldsymbol{\beta}}(\mathbf{y}) = 0$, we assume in what follows that $\hat{\boldsymbol{\beta}}(\mathbf{y}) \ne 0$. Any solution $\hat{\boldsymbol{\beta}}(\mathbf{y})$ of the convex minimization problem in (5) satisfies

$$\frac{1}{n}\mathbb{X}^T(\mathbb{X}\hat{\boldsymbol{\beta}}(\mathbf{y}) - \mathbf{y}) + \mathbf{v} = \mathbf{0} \tag{7}$$

where $\mathbf{v}$ is an element of the subdifferential of $N(\cdot)$ at $\hat{\boldsymbol{\beta}}(\mathbf{y})$. Recall that the subdifferential of any norm $N(\cdot)$ at $\hat{\boldsymbol{\beta}}(\mathbf{y}) \ne 0$ is the set $\{\mathbf{v} \in \mathbb{R}^p : N(\mathbf{v}) = 1 \text{ and } \mathbf{v}^T \hat{\boldsymbol{\beta}}(\mathbf{y}) = N(\hat{\boldsymbol{\beta}}(\mathbf{y}))\}$ [1, Sect. 2.6]. Therefore, taking an inner product of (7) with $\hat{\boldsymbol{\beta}}(\mathbf{y})$ yields

$$(\mathbb{X}\hat{\boldsymbol{\beta}}(\mathbf{y}))^T(\mathbf{y} - \mathbb{X}\hat{\boldsymbol{\beta}}(\mathbf{y})) = nN(\hat{\boldsymbol{\beta}}(\mathbf{y})) = n \max_{\mathbf{w} \in \mathbb{R}^p : N_\circ(\mathbf{w})=1} \hat{\boldsymbol{\beta}}(\mathbf{y})^T \mathbf{w}$$

$$\ge \max_{\mathbf{u} \in \mathbb{R}^n : N_\circ(\mathbb{X}^T \mathbf{u})=1/n} (\mathbb{X}\hat{\boldsymbol{\beta}}(\mathbf{y}))^T \mathbf{u} = \max_{\mathbf{u} \in C}(\mathbb{X}\hat{\boldsymbol{\beta}}(\mathbf{y}))^T \mathbf{u}.$$

This proves (6) with $\boldsymbol{\theta} = \mathbf{y} - \mathbb{X}\hat{\boldsymbol{\beta}}(\mathbf{y})$. Thus, we have established that $\mathbb{X}\hat{\boldsymbol{\beta}}(\mathbf{y}) = \mathbf{y} - P_C(\mathbf{y})$.

To prove part (ii) of the proposition, we use that, for any closed convex subset C of $\mathbb{R}^n$ and any $\mathbf{y}, \mathbf{y}' \in \mathbb{R}^n$,

$$|P_C(\mathbf{y}) - P_C(\mathbf{y}')|_2^2 \le \langle P_C(\mathbf{y}) - P_C(\mathbf{y}'), \mathbf{y} - \mathbf{y}' \rangle,$$

see, e.g., [8, Proposition 3.1.3]. This immediately implies

$$|\mathbf{y} - P_C(\mathbf{y}) - (\mathbf{y}' - P_C(\mathbf{y}'))|_2^2 \le |\mathbf{y} - \mathbf{y}'|_2^2 - |P_C(\mathbf{y}) - P_C(\mathbf{y}')|_2^2.$$

Part (ii) of the proposition follows now from part (i) and the last display. □

We note that Proposition 2 generalizes to any norm $N(\cdot)$ an analogous result obtained for the ℓ_1-norm in [15, Lemma 3].

We now turn to the general case assuming that F is any convex penalty.

Proposition 3 *Let the penalty function* $F : \mathbb{R}^p \rightarrow [0, +\infty]$ *be convex, proper, and lower semicontinuous. For all* $\mathbf{y} \in \mathbb{R}^n$, *let* $\hat{\boldsymbol{\beta}}(\mathbf{y})$ *be any solution of the convex minimization problem* (2). *Then the estimator* $\hat{\boldsymbol{\mu}}(\mathbf{y}) = \mathbb{X}\hat{\boldsymbol{\beta}}(\mathbf{y})$ *satisfies* (3) *with* $L = 1$.

Proof Let $\mathbf{y}, \mathbf{y}' \in \mathbb{R}^n$. The case $\mathbb{X}\hat{\boldsymbol{\beta}}(\mathbf{y}) = \mathbb{X}\hat{\boldsymbol{\beta}}(\mathbf{y}')$ is trivial so we assume in the following that $\mathbb{X}\hat{\boldsymbol{\beta}}(\mathbf{y}) \neq \mathbb{X}\hat{\boldsymbol{\beta}}(\mathbf{y}')$. The optimality condition and the Moreau–Rockafellar Theorem [14, Theorem 3.30] yield that there exists an element $\mathbf{h} \in \mathbb{R}^p$ of the subdifferential $\partial F(\hat{\boldsymbol{\beta}}(\mathbf{y}))$ of $F(\cdot)$ at $\hat{\boldsymbol{\beta}}(\mathbf{y})$ and $\mathbf{h}' \in \partial F(\hat{\boldsymbol{\beta}}(\mathbf{y}'))$ such that

$$\frac{1}{n}\mathbb{X}^T(\mathbb{X}\hat{\boldsymbol{\beta}}(\mathbf{y}) - \mathbf{y}) + \mathbf{h} = \mathbf{0}, \quad \text{and} \quad \frac{1}{n}\mathbb{X}^T(\mathbb{X}\hat{\boldsymbol{\beta}}(\mathbf{y}') - \mathbf{y}') + \mathbf{h}' = \mathbf{0}.$$

Taking the difference of these two equalities, we obtain

$$\mathbb{X}^T(\mathbb{X}\hat{\boldsymbol{\beta}}(\mathbf{y}) - \mathbb{X}\hat{\boldsymbol{\beta}}(\mathbf{y}')) - \mathbb{X}^T(\mathbf{y} - \mathbf{y}') = n(\mathbf{h}' - \mathbf{h}).$$

Let $\boldsymbol{\Delta} = \hat{\boldsymbol{\beta}}(\mathbf{y}) - \hat{\boldsymbol{\beta}}(\mathbf{y}')$. Since F is convex, proper, and lower semicontinuous, we have that $\boldsymbol{\Delta}^T(\mathbf{h} - \mathbf{h}') = \langle \mathbf{h} - \mathbf{h}', \hat{\boldsymbol{\beta}}(\mathbf{y}) - \hat{\boldsymbol{\beta}}(\mathbf{y}') \rangle \geq 0$ for any $\mathbf{h} \in \partial F(\hat{\boldsymbol{\beta}}(\mathbf{y}))$ and any $\mathbf{h}' \in \partial F(\hat{\boldsymbol{\beta}}(\mathbf{y}'))$ (see, e.g., [14, Proposition 3.22]). Therefore,

$$\boldsymbol{\Delta}^T\mathbb{X}^T\mathbb{X}\boldsymbol{\Delta} - \boldsymbol{\Delta}^T\mathbb{X}^T(\mathbf{y} - \mathbf{y}') = n\boldsymbol{\Delta}^T(\mathbf{h}' - \mathbf{h}) \leq 0.$$

This and the Cauchy–Schwarz inequality yield

$$|\mathbb{X}\boldsymbol{\Delta}|_2^2 \leq \boldsymbol{\Delta}^T\mathbb{X}^T(\mathbf{y} - \mathbf{y}') \leq |\mathbb{X}\boldsymbol{\Delta}|_2|\mathbf{y} - \mathbf{y}'|_2, \tag{8}$$

which implies $|\mathbb{X}\boldsymbol{\Delta}|_2 \leq |\mathbf{y} - \mathbf{y}'|_2$ since $\mathbb{X}\hat{\boldsymbol{\beta}}(\mathbf{y}) \neq \mathbb{X}\hat{\boldsymbol{\beta}}(\mathbf{y}')$. □

Combining the above two propositions, we obtain the following theorem.

Theorem 1 *Let* $R \geq 0$ *be a constant and* $\mathbf{f} \in \mathbb{R}^n$. *Assume that* $\boldsymbol{\xi} \sim \mathcal{N}(\mathbf{0}, \sigma^2 I_{n \times n})$ *and let* $\mathbf{y} = \mathbf{f} + \boldsymbol{\xi}$. *Let the penalty function* $F : \mathbb{R}^p \rightarrow [0, +\infty]$ *be convex, proper, and lower semicontinuous. Assume also that the estimator* $\hat{\boldsymbol{\beta}}$ *defined in* (5) *satisfies*

$$\mathbb{P}\left(\|\mathbb{X}\hat{\boldsymbol{\beta}}(\mathbf{y}) - \mathbf{f}\| \leq R\right) \geq 1/2, \tag{9}$$

or equivalently, the median of the prediction error satisfies $\text{Med}[\|\mathbb{X}\hat{\boldsymbol{\beta}}(\mathbf{y}) - \mathbf{f}\|] \leq R$. *Then, for all* $t > 0$,

$$\mathbb{P}\left(\|\mathbb{X}\hat{\boldsymbol{\beta}}(\mathbf{y}) - \mathbf{f}\| \leq R + \frac{\sigma t}{\sqrt{n}}\right) \geq \Phi(t) \tag{10}$$

and consequently, for all $x > 0$,

$$\mathbb{P}\left(\|\mathbb{X}\hat{\boldsymbol{\beta}}(\mathbf{y}) - \mathbf{f}\| \leq R + \sigma\sqrt{2x/n}\right) \geq 1 - e^{-x}. \tag{11}$$

Furthermore,

$$\mathbb{E}\|\mathbb{X}\hat{\boldsymbol{\beta}}(\mathbf{y}) - \mathbf{f}\| \leq R + \frac{\sigma}{\sqrt{2\pi n}}. \tag{12}$$

Proof Fix $\mathbf{f} \in \mathbb{R}^n$ and let $\mathbf{z} \sim \mathcal{N}(\mathbf{0}, I_{n \times n})$. Proposition 3 implies that the function $g(\mathbf{z}) = \|\mathbb{X}\hat{\boldsymbol{\beta}}(\mathbf{f} + \sigma\mathbf{z}) - \mathbf{f}\|$ satisfies (4) with $L = 1$ for all $x > 0$. Thus, we can apply Proposition 1 and (11) follows from (4). The bound (11) is a simplified version of (10) using that $1 - \Phi(t) \leq e^{-t^2/2}$, $\forall t > 0$. Finally, inequality (12) is obtained by integration of (10). □

Note that condition (9) in Theorem 1 is a weak property. To satisfy, it is enough to have a rough bound on $\|\mathbb{X}\hat{\boldsymbol{\beta}}(\mathbf{y}) - \mathbf{f}\|$. Of course, we would like to have a meaningful value of R. In the next two sections, we give examples of such R. Namely, we show that Theorem 1 allows one to derive sharp oracle inequalities for the prediction risk of such estimators as LASSO, group LASSO, and SLOPE.

Remark 1 Along with the concentration around the median, the prediction error $\|\mathbb{X}\hat{\boldsymbol{\beta}}(\mathbf{y}) - \mathbf{f}\|$ also concentrates around its expectation. Using the Lipschitz property of Proposition 1, and the theorem about Gaussian concentration with respect to the expectation (cf., e.g., [7, Theorem B.6]), we find that

$$\mathbb{P}\left(\|\mathbb{X}\hat{\boldsymbol{\beta}}(\mathbf{y}) - \mathbf{f}\| \leq \mathbb{E}\|\mathbb{X}\hat{\boldsymbol{\beta}}(\mathbf{y}) - \mathbf{f}\| + \sigma\sqrt{2x/n}\right) \geq 1 - e^{-x} \tag{13}$$

and

$$\mathbb{P}\left(\|\mathbb{X}\hat{\boldsymbol{\beta}}(\mathbf{y}) - \mathbf{f}\| \geq \mathbb{E}\|\mathbb{X}\hat{\boldsymbol{\beta}}(\mathbf{y}) - \mathbf{f}\| - \sigma\sqrt{2x/n}\right) \geq 1 - e^{-x}. \tag{14}$$

For the special case of identity design matrix $\mathbb{X} = I_{n \times n}$, these properties have been proved in [17] where they were applied to some problems of nonparametric estimation. However, the bounds (13) and (14) dealing with the concentration around the expectation are of no use for the purposes of the present paper since initially we have no control of the expectation. On the other hand, a meaningful control of the median is often easy to obtain as shown in the examples below. This is the reason why we focus on the concentration around the median.

Remark 2 The argument used to prove Theorem 1 relies on the concentration property of a Lipschitz function of the noise random vector. In the setting of the present paper, the noise vector is standard normal and such a concentration result is available, see for instance [10, Theorem 6.2]. However, to our knowledge, its analog for subgaussian random vectors is not available. For this reason, the method presented above does not readily extend to subgaussian noise.

4 Application to LASSO

The LASSO is a convex regularized estimator defined by the relation

$$\hat{\boldsymbol{\beta}} \in \underset{\boldsymbol{\beta} \in \mathbb{R}^p}{\text{argmin}} \left(\|\mathbf{y} - \mathbb{X}\boldsymbol{\beta}\|^2 + 2\lambda|\boldsymbol{\beta}|_1 \right), \tag{15}$$

where $\lambda > 0$ is a tuning parameter. Risk bounds for the LASSO estimator are established under some conditions on the design matrix $\mathbb{X}$ that measure the correlations between its columns. The Restricted Eigenvalue (RE) condition [3] is defined as follows. For any $S \subset \{1, \ldots, p\}$ and $c_0 > 0$, we define the RE constant $\kappa(S, c_0) \geq 0$ by the formula

$$\kappa^2(S, c_0) \triangleq \min_{\boldsymbol{\Delta} \in \mathbb{R}^p : |\boldsymbol{\Delta}_{S^c}|_1 \leq c_0 |\boldsymbol{\Delta}_S|_1} \frac{\|\mathbb{X}\boldsymbol{\Delta}\|^2}{|\boldsymbol{\Delta}|_2^2}. \tag{16}$$

The RE condition $RE(S, c_0)$ is said to hold if $\kappa(S, c_0) > 0$. Note that (16) is slightly different from the original definition given in [3] since we have $\boldsymbol{\Delta}$ and not $\boldsymbol{\Delta}_S$ in the denominator. However, the two definitions are equivalent up to a constant depending only on c_0, cf. [2]. In terms of the RE constant, we have the following deterministic result.

Proposition 4 *Let $\lambda > 0$ be a tuning parameter. On the event*

$$\left\{ \frac{1}{n} |\mathbb{X}^T \boldsymbol{\xi}|_\infty \leq \frac{\lambda}{2} \right\}, \tag{17}$$

the LASSO estimator (15) with tuning parameter λ satisfies

$$\|\mathbb{X}\hat{\boldsymbol{\beta}} - \mathbf{f}\|^2 \leq \min_{S \subset \{1,\ldots,p\}} \left[\min_{\boldsymbol{\beta} \in \mathbb{R}^p : \text{Supp}(\boldsymbol{\beta})=S} \|\mathbb{X}\boldsymbol{\beta} - \mathbf{f}\|^2 + \frac{9|S|\lambda^2}{4\kappa^2(S, 3)} \right] \tag{18}$$

with the convention that $a/0 = +\infty$ for any $a > 0$.

An oracle inequality as in Proposition 4 has been first established in [3] with a multiplicative constant greater than 1 in front of the right-hand side of (18). The fact that this constant can be reduced to 1, so that the oracle inequality becomes sharp, is due to [9]. For the sake of completeness, we provide below a sketch of the proof of Proposition 4.

Proof We will use the following fact [2, Lemma A.2].

Lemma 1 *Let $F : \mathbb{R}^p \to \mathbb{R}$ be a convex function, let $\mathbf{f}, \boldsymbol{\xi} \in \mathbb{R}^n$, $\mathbf{y} = \mathbf{f} + \boldsymbol{\xi}$, and let $\mathbb{X}$ be any $n \times p$ matrix. If $\hat{\boldsymbol{\beta}}$ is a solution of the minimization problem (2), then $\hat{\boldsymbol{\beta}}$ satisfies, for all $\boldsymbol{\beta} \in \mathbb{R}^p$,*

$$\|\mathbb{X}\hat{\boldsymbol{\beta}} - \mathbf{f}\|^2 - \|\mathbb{X}\boldsymbol{\beta} - \mathbf{f}\|^2 \leq 2 \left(\frac{1}{n} \boldsymbol{\xi}^T \mathbb{X}(\hat{\boldsymbol{\beta}} - \boldsymbol{\beta}) + F(\boldsymbol{\beta}) - F(\hat{\boldsymbol{\beta}}) \right) - \|\mathbb{X}(\hat{\boldsymbol{\beta}} - \boldsymbol{\beta})\|^2.$$

Let $S \subset \{1, \ldots, p\}$ and β be minimizers of the right-hand side of (18) and let $\Delta = \hat{\beta} - \beta$. We will assume that $\kappa(S, 3) > 0$ since otherwise the claim is trivial. From Lemma 1 with $F(\beta) = \lambda|\beta|_1$, we have

$$\|\mathbb{X}\hat{\beta} - \mathbf{f}\|^2 - \|\mathbb{X}\beta - \mathbf{f}\|^2 \leq 2\left(\tfrac{1}{n}\xi^T\mathbb{X}\Delta + \lambda|\beta|_1 - \lambda|\hat{\beta}|_1\right) - \|\mathbb{X}\Delta\|^2 \triangleq D.$$

On the event (17), using the duality inequality $\mathbf{x}^T\Delta \leq |\mathbf{x}|_\infty|\Delta|_1$ valid for all $\mathbf{x}, \Delta \in \mathbb{R}^p$ and the triangle inequality for the ℓ_1-norm, we find that the right-hand side of the previous display satisfies

$$D \leq 2\lambda\left[\frac{1}{2}|\Delta|_1 + |\beta|_1 - |\hat{\beta}|_1\right] - \|\mathbb{X}\Delta\|^2 \leq 2\lambda\left[\frac{3}{2}|\Delta_S|_1 - \frac{1}{2}|\Delta_{S^c}|_1\right] - \|\mathbb{X}\Delta\|^2.$$

If $|\Delta_{S^c}|_1 > 3|\Delta_S|_1$, then the claim follows trivially. Otherwise, if $|\Delta_{S^c}|_1 \leq 3|\Delta_S|_1$ we have $|\Delta|_2 \leq \|\mathbb{X}\Delta\|/\kappa(S, 3)$ and thus, by the Cauchy–Schwarz inequality,

$$3\lambda|\Delta_S|_1 \leq 3\lambda\sqrt{|S|}|\Delta_S|_2 \leq \frac{9|S|\lambda^2}{4\kappa^2(S, 3)} + \|\mathbb{X}\Delta\|^2. \tag{19}$$

Combining the above three displays yields (18). □

Theorem 2 below is a simple consequence of Proposition 4 and Theorem 1. Its proof is given at the end of the present section.

Theorem 2 *Let $p \geq 2$ and $\lambda \geq 2\sigma\sqrt{2\log(p)/n}$. Assume that the diagonal elements of matrix $\frac{1}{n}\mathbb{X}^T\mathbb{X}$ are not greater than 1. Then for any $\delta \in (0, 1)$, the LASSO estimator (15) with tuning parameter λ satisfies*

$$\|\mathbb{X}\hat{\beta} - \mathbf{f}\| \leq \min_{S \subset \{1,\ldots,p\}}\left[\min_{\beta \in \mathbb{R}^p : \mathrm{Supp}(\beta)=S}\|\mathbb{X}\beta - \mathbf{f}\| + \frac{3\lambda\sqrt{|S|}}{2\kappa(S, 3)}\right] + \frac{\sigma\Phi^{-1}(1-\delta)}{\sqrt{n}} \tag{20}$$

with probability at least $1 - \delta$, noting that $\Phi^{-1}(1-\delta) \leq \sqrt{2\log(1/\delta)}$. Furthermore,

$$\mathbb{E}\|\mathbb{X}\hat{\beta} - \mathbf{f}\| \leq \min_{S \subset \{1,\ldots,p\}}\left[\min_{\beta \in \mathbb{R}^p : \mathrm{Supp}(\beta)=S}\|\mathbb{X}\beta - \mathbf{f}\| + \frac{3\lambda\sqrt{|S|}}{2\kappa(S, 3)}\right] + \frac{\sigma}{\sqrt{2\pi n}}. \tag{21}$$

Previous works on the LASSO estimator established that for some fixed $\delta_0 \in (0, 1)$ the estimator (15) with tuning parameter $\lambda = c_1\sigma\sqrt{2\log(c_2p/\delta_0)}$, where $c_1 > 1, c_2 \geq 1$ are some constants, satisfies an oracle inequality of the form (18) with probability at least $1 - \delta_0$, see for instance [3, 6, 9] or the books on high-dimensional statistics [5, 7, 16]. Thus, such oracle inequalities were available only for one fixed confidence level $1 - \delta_0$ tied to the tuning parameter λ. Remarkably, Theorem 2 shows that the LASSO estimator with a universal (not level-dependent) tuning parameter, which can be as small as $2\sigma\sqrt{(2\log p)/n}$, satisfies (20) for all confidence levels $\delta \in (0, 1)$. As a consequence, we can obtain an oracle inequality

(21) for the expected error, while control of the expected error was not achievable with the previously known methods of proof. Furthermore, bounds for any moments of the prediction error can be readily obtained by integration of (20). Analogous facts have been shown recently in [2] using different techniques. To our knowledge, the present paper and [2] provide the first evidence of such properties of the LASSO estimator.

In addition, Theorem 2 shows that the rate of concentration in the oracle inequalities is better than it was commonly understood before. Let $S \subset \{1, \ldots, p\}, s = |S|$ and set $\delta = \exp(-2s\lambda^2 n/\sigma^2\kappa^2(S, 3))$. For this choice of δ, Theorem 2 implies that if $\lambda \geq 2\sigma\sqrt{2\log(p)/n}$ then

$$\mathbb{P}\left(\|\mathbb{X}\hat{\boldsymbol{\beta}} - \mathbf{f}\| \leq \min_{\boldsymbol{\beta} \in \mathbb{R}^p : \mathrm{Supp}(\boldsymbol{\beta}) = S} \|\mathbb{X}\boldsymbol{\beta} - \mathbf{f}\| + \frac{7\lambda\sqrt{|S|}}{2\kappa(S, 3)} \right) \geq 1 - e^{-2s\lambda^2 n/\sigma^2\kappa^2(S,3)}.$$

Since the diagonal elements of $\frac{1}{n}\mathbb{X}^T\mathbb{X}$ are at most 1, we have $\kappa(S, 3) \leq 1$. Thus, the probability on the right-hand side of the last display is at least $1 - p^{-16s}$. Interestingly, this probability depends on the sparsity s and tends to 1 exponentially fast as s grows. The previous proof techniques [3, 5, 6, 9] provided, for the same type of probability, only an estimate of the form $1 - p^{-b}$ for some fixed constant $b > 0$ independent of s.

The oracle inequality (18) holds for the error $\|\mathbb{X}\hat{\boldsymbol{\beta}} - \mathbf{f}\|$. In order to obtain an oracle inequality for the squared error $\|\mathbb{X}\hat{\boldsymbol{\beta}} - \mathbf{f}\|^2$, one can combine (20) with the basic inequality $(a + b + c)^2 \leq 3(a^2 + b^2 + c^2)$. This yields that under the assumptions of Theorem 2, the LASSO estimator with tuning parameter $\lambda \geq 2\sigma\sqrt{2\log(p)/n}$ satisfies, with probability at least $1 - \delta$,

$$\|\mathbb{X}\hat{\boldsymbol{\beta}} - \mathbf{f}\|^2 \leq \min_{S \subset \{1, \ldots, p\}} \left[\min_{\boldsymbol{\beta} \in \mathbb{R}^p : \mathrm{Supp}(\boldsymbol{\beta}) = S} 3\|\mathbb{X}\boldsymbol{\beta} - \mathbf{f}\|^2 + \frac{27\lambda^2|S|}{4\kappa^2(S, 3)} \right] + \frac{6\log(1/\delta)}{n}.$$

The constant 3 in front of the $\|\mathbb{X}\boldsymbol{\beta} - \mathbf{f}\|^2$ can be reduced to 1 using the techniques developed in [2].

Proof of Theorem 2. The random variable $|\mathbb{X}^T\boldsymbol{\xi}|_\infty/\sqrt{n}$ is the maximum of p-centered Gaussian random variables with variance at most σ^2. If $\eta \sim \mathcal{N}(0, 1)$, a standard approximation of the Gaussian tail gives $\mathbb{P}(|\eta| > x) \leq \sqrt{2/\pi}(e^{-x^2/2}/x)$ for all $x > 0$. This approximation with $x = \sqrt{2\log p}$ together with and the union bound imply that the event (17) with $\lambda \geq 2\sigma\sqrt{(2\log p)/n}$ has probability at least $1 - 1/\sqrt{\pi \log p}$, which is greater than $1/2$ for all $p \geq 3$. For $p = 2$, the probability of this event is bounded from below by $1 - 2\mathbb{P}(|\eta| > \sqrt{2\log 2}) > 1/2$. Thus, Proposition 4 implies that condition (9) is satisfied with R being the square root of the right-hand side of (18). Let S and $\boldsymbol{\beta}$ be minimizers of the right-hand side of (20). Applying Theorem 1 and the inequality $\sqrt{a + b} \leq \sqrt{a} + \sqrt{b}$ with $\sqrt{a} = \|\mathbb{X}\boldsymbol{\beta} - \mathbf{f}\|$ and $\sqrt{b} = 3\lambda\sqrt{|S|}/(2\kappa(S, 3))$ completes the proof.

5   Application to Group LASSO and Related Penalties

The above arguments can be used to establish oracle inequalities for the group LASSO estimator similar to those obtained in Sect. 4 for the usual LASSO. The improvements as compared to the previously known oracle bounds (see, e.g., [11] or the books [5, 7, 16]) are the same as above—independent of the tuning parameter on the confidence level, better concentration, and derivation of bounds in expectation.

Let $G_1, \ldots, G_M$ be a partition of $\{1, \ldots, p\}$. The group LASSO estimator is a solution of the convex minimization problem

$$\hat{\boldsymbol{\beta}} \in \underset{\boldsymbol{\beta} \in \mathbb{R}^p}{\operatorname{argmin}} \left(\|\mathbf{y} - \mathbb{X}\boldsymbol{\beta}\|^2 + 2\lambda \sum_{k=1}^{M} |\boldsymbol{\beta}_{G_k}|_2 \right), \tag{22}$$

where $\lambda > 0$ is a tuning parameter. In the following, we assume that the groups G_k have the same cardinality $|G_k| = T = p/M, k = 1, \ldots, M$.

We will need the following group analog of the RE constant introduced in [11]. For any $S \subset \{1, \ldots, M\}$ and $c_0 > 0$, we define the group RE constant $\kappa_G(S, c_0) \geq 0$ by the formula

$$\kappa_G^2(S, c_0) \triangleq \min_{\boldsymbol{\Delta} \in \mathscr{C}(S, c_0)} \frac{\|\mathbb{X}\boldsymbol{\Delta}\|^2}{|\boldsymbol{\Delta}|_2^2}, \tag{23}$$

where $\mathscr{C}(S, c_0)$ is the cone

$$\mathscr{C}(S, c_0) \triangleq \{\boldsymbol{\Delta} \in \mathbb{R}^p : \sum_{k \in S^c} |\boldsymbol{\Delta}_{G_k}|_2 \leq c_0 \sum_{k \in S} |\boldsymbol{\Delta}_{G_k}|_2\}.$$

Denote by $\mathbb{X}_{G_k}$ the $n \times |G_k|$ submatrix of $\mathbb{X}$ composed from all the columns of $\mathbb{X}$ with indices in G_k. For any $\boldsymbol{\beta} \in \mathbb{R}^p$, set $\mathscr{K}(\boldsymbol{\beta}) = \{k \in \{1, \ldots, M\} : \boldsymbol{\beta}_{G_k} \neq \mathbf{0}\}$. The following deterministic result holds.

Proposition 5 *Let $\lambda > 0$ be a tuning parameter. On the event*

$$\left\{ \max_{k=1,\ldots,M} \frac{1}{n} |\mathbb{X}_{G_k}^T \boldsymbol{\xi}|_2 \leq \frac{\lambda}{2} \right\}, \tag{24}$$

the group LASSO estimator (22) *with tuning parameter λ satisfies*

$$\|\mathbb{X}\hat{\boldsymbol{\beta}} - \mathbf{f}\|^2 \leq \min_{S \subset \{1,\ldots,M\}} \left[\min_{\boldsymbol{\beta} \in \mathbb{R}^p : \mathscr{K}(\boldsymbol{\beta}) = S} \|\mathbb{X}\boldsymbol{\beta} - \mathbf{f}\|^2 + \frac{9|S|\lambda^2}{4\kappa_G^2(S, 3)} \right] \tag{25}$$

with the convention that $a/0 = +\infty$ for any $a > 0$.

Proof We follow the same lines as in the proof of Proposition 4. The difference is that we replace the ℓ_1 norm by the group LASSO norm $\sum_{k=1}^{M} |\boldsymbol{\beta}_{G_k}|_2$, and the value D now has the form

$$D = 2\left(\frac{1}{n}\boldsymbol{\xi}^T \mathbb{X}\boldsymbol{\Delta} + \lambda \sum_{k=1}^{M} |\boldsymbol{\beta}_{G_k}|_2 - \lambda \sum_{k=1}^{M} |\hat{\boldsymbol{\beta}}_{G_k}|_2 \right) - \|\mathbb{X}\boldsymbol{\Delta}\|^2.$$

Then, on the event (24), we obtain

$$D \leq 2\lambda \left(\frac{1}{2}\sum_{k=1}^{M} |\boldsymbol{\Delta}_{G_k}|_2 + \sum_{k=1}^{M} |\boldsymbol{\beta}_{G_k}|_2 - \sum_{k=1}^{M} |\hat{\boldsymbol{\beta}}_{G_k}|_2 \right) - \|\mathbb{X}\boldsymbol{\Delta}\|^2$$

$$\leq 2\lambda \left(\frac{3}{2}\sum_{k\in S} |\boldsymbol{\Delta}_{G_k}|_2 - \frac{1}{2}\sum_{k\in S^c} |\boldsymbol{\Delta}_{G_k}|_2 \right) - \|\mathbb{X}\boldsymbol{\Delta}\|^2,$$

where the last inequality uses the fact that $\mathcal{K}(\boldsymbol{\beta}) = S$. The rest of the proof is quite analogous to that of Proposition 4 if we replace there $\kappa(S, 3)$ by $\kappa_G(S, 3)$. □

To derive the oracle inequalities for group LASSO, we use the same argument as in the case of LASSO. In order to apply Theorem 1, we need to find a "weak bound" R on the error $\|\mathbb{X}\hat{\boldsymbol{\beta}} - \mathbf{f}\|$, i.e., a bound valid with probability at least $1/2$. The next lemma gives a range of values of λ such that the event (24) holds with probability at least $1/2$. Then, due to Proposition 5, we can take as R the square root of the right-hand side of (25).

Denote by $\|\mathbb{X}_{G_k}\|_{sp} \triangleq \sup_{|\mathbf{x}|_2 \leq 1} |\mathbb{X}_{G_k}\mathbf{x}|_2$ the spectral norm of matrix $\mathbb{X}_{G_k}$, and set $\psi^* = \max_{k=1,\dots,M} \|\mathbb{X}_{G_k}\|_{sp}/\sqrt{n}$.

Lemma 2 *Let the diagonal elements of matrix $\frac{1}{n}\mathbb{X}^T\mathbb{X}$ be not greater than 1. If*

$$\lambda \geq \frac{2\sigma}{\sqrt{n}}\left(\sqrt{T} + \psi^*\sqrt{2\log(2M)} \right), \tag{26}$$

then the event (24) has probability at least $1/2$.

Proof Note that the function $\mathbf{u} \mapsto |\mathbb{X}_{G_k}\mathbf{u}|_2$ is $\psi^*\sqrt{n}$-Lipschitz with respect to the Euclidean norm. Therefore, the Gaussian concentration inequality, cf., e.g., [7, Theorem B.6], implies that, for all $x > 0$,

$$\mathbb{P}\left(|\mathbb{X}_{G_k}\boldsymbol{\xi}|_2 \geq \mathbb{E}|\mathbb{X}_{G_k}\boldsymbol{\xi}|_2 + \sigma\psi^*\sqrt{2xn} \right) \leq e^{-x}, \qquad k = 1, \dots, M.$$

Here, $\mathbb{E}|\mathbb{X}_{G_k}\boldsymbol{\xi}|_2 \leq \left(\mathbb{E}|\mathbb{X}_{G_k}\boldsymbol{\xi}|_2^2 \right)^{1/2} = \sigma\|\mathbb{X}_{G_k}\|_F$, where $\|\cdot\|_F$ is the Frobenius norm. By the assumption of the lemma, all columns of $\mathbb{X}$ have the Euclidean norm at most $\sqrt{n}$. Since $\mathbb{X}_{G_k}$ is composed from T columns of $\mathbb{X}$ we have $\|\mathbb{X}_{G_k}\|_F^2 \leq nT$, so that $\mathbb{E}|\mathbb{X}_{G_k}\boldsymbol{\xi}|_2 \leq \sigma\sqrt{nT}$ for $k = 1, \dots, M$. Thus, for all $x > 0$,

$$\mathbb{P}\left(|\mathbb{X}_{G_k}\boldsymbol{\xi}|_2 \geq \sigma(\sqrt{nT} + \psi^*\sqrt{2xn}) \right) \leq e^{-x}, \qquad k = 1, \dots, M,$$

and the result of the lemma follows by application of the union bound. □

Combining Proposition 5, Lemma 2, and Theorem 1, we get the following result.

Theorem 3 *Assume that the diagonal elements of matrix $\frac{1}{n}\mathbb{X}^T\mathbb{X}$ are not greater than 1. Let λ be such that (26) holds. Then for any $\delta \in (0, 1)$, the group LASSO estimator (22) with tuning parameter λ satisfies, with probability at least $1 - \delta$, the oracle inequality (20) with $\kappa(S, 3)$ replaced by $\kappa_G(S, 3)$, and $\mathrm{Supp}(\boldsymbol{\beta})$ replaced by $\mathscr{K}(\boldsymbol{\beta})$. Furthermore, it satisfies (21) with the same modifications.*

We can consider in a similar way a more general class of penalties generated by cones [13]. Let $\mathscr{A}$ be a convex cone in $(0, +\infty)^p$. For any $\beta \in \mathbb{R}^p$, set

$$\|\beta\|_{\mathscr{A}} \triangleq \inf_{a \in \mathscr{A}} \frac{1}{2} \sum_{j=1}^{p} \left(\frac{\beta_j^2}{a_j} + a_j \right) = \inf_{a \in \mathscr{A}: |a|_1 \leq 1} \sqrt{\sum_{j=1}^{p} \frac{\beta_j^2}{a_j}} \qquad (27)$$

and consider the penalty $F(\beta) = \lambda \|\beta\|_{\mathscr{A}}$ where $\lambda > 0$. The function $\|\cdot\|_{\mathscr{A}}$ is convex since it is a minimum of a convex function of the couple (β, a) over a in a convex set [8, Corollary 2.4.5]. In view of its positive homogeneity, it is also a norm. The group LASSO penalty is a special case of (27) corresponding to the cone of all vectors a with positive components that are constant on the blocks G_k of the partition. Many other interesting examples are given in [12, 13], see also [16, Sect. 6.9].

Such penalties induce a class of admissible sets of indices $S \subset \{1, \ldots, p\}$. This is a generalization of the sets of indices corresponding to vectors β that vanish on entire blocks in the case of group LASSO. Roughly speaking, the set of indices S would be suitable for our construction if, for any $a \in \mathscr{A}$, the vectors a_S and a_{S^c} belong to $\mathscr{A}$. However, this is not possible since, by definition, the elements of $\mathscr{A}$ must have positive components. Thus, we slightly modify this condition on S. A set $S \subset \{1, \ldots, p\}$ will be called *admissible* with respect to $\mathscr{A}$ if, for any $a \in \mathscr{A}$ and any $\epsilon > 0$, there exist vectors $b_{S^c} \in \mathbb{R}^p$ and $b_S \in \mathbb{R}^p$ supported on S^c and S, respectively, with all components in $(0, \epsilon)$ and such that $a_S + b_{S^c} \in \mathscr{A}$, and $a_{S^c} + b_S \in \mathscr{A}$.

The following lemma shows that, for admissible S, the norm $\|\cdot\|_{\mathscr{A}}$ has the same decomposition property as the ℓ_1 norm.

Lemma 3 *If $S \subset \{1, \ldots, p\}$ is an admissible set of indices with respect to $\mathscr{A}$, then*

$$\|\beta\|_{\mathscr{A}} = \|\beta_S\|_{\mathscr{A}} + \|\beta_{S^c}\|_{\mathscr{A}}.$$

Proof As $\|\cdot\|_{\mathscr{A}}$ is a norm, we have to show only that $\|\beta\|_{\mathscr{A}} \geq \|\beta_S\|_{\mathscr{A}} + \|\beta_{S^c}\|_{\mathscr{A}}$. Obviously,

$$\|\beta\|_{\mathscr{A}} \geq \inf_{a \in \mathscr{A}} \frac{1}{2} \sum_{j \in S} \left(\frac{\beta_j^2}{a_j} + a_j \right) + \inf_{a \in \mathscr{A}} \frac{1}{2} \sum_{j \in S^c} \left(\frac{\beta_j^2}{a_j} + a_j \right). \qquad (28)$$

Since S is admissible, adding the sum $\sum_{j \in S^c} a_j$ under the infimum in the first term on the right-hand side does not change the result:

$$\inf_{a\in\mathscr{A}} \frac{1}{2}\sum_{j\in S}\left(\frac{\beta_j^2}{a_j}+a_j\right) = \inf_{a\in\mathscr{A}} \frac{1}{2}\left[\sum_{j\in S}\left(\frac{\beta_j^2}{a_j}+a_j\right)+\sum_{j\in S^c}a_j\right] = \|\beta_S\|_{\mathscr{A}}.$$

The second term on the right-hand side of (28) is treated analogously. □

Next, for any $S \subset \{1,\ldots,p\}$ and $c_0 > 0$, we need an analog of the RE constant corresponding to the penalty $\|\cdot\|_{\mathscr{A}}$, cf. [16]. We define $q_{\mathscr{A}}(S,c_0) \geq 0$ by the formula

$$q_{\mathscr{A}}^2(S,c_0) \triangleq \min_{\Delta\in\mathscr{C}'(S,c_0)} \frac{\|\mathbb{X}\Delta\|^2}{\|\Delta_S\|_{\mathscr{A}}^2}, \tag{29}$$

where $\mathscr{C}'(S,c_0)$ is the cone

$$\mathscr{C}'(S,c_0) \triangleq \{\Delta\in\mathbb{R}^p : \|\Delta_{S^c}\|_{\mathscr{A}} \leq c_0\|\Delta_S\|_{\mathscr{A}}\}.$$

As in the previous examples, our starting point will be a deterministic bound that holds on a suitable event. This result is analogous to Propositions 4 and 5. To state it, we define

$$\|\beta\|_{\mathscr{A},\circ} = \sup_{a\in\mathscr{A}:|a|_1\leq 1} \sqrt{\sum_{j=1}^{p}a_j\beta_j^2}$$

which is the dual norm to $\|\cdot\|_{\mathscr{A}}$.

Proposition 6 *Let $\mathscr{A}$ be a convex cone in $(0,+\infty)^p$, and let $\mathbb{S}_{\mathscr{A}}$ be set of all $S \subset \{1,\ldots,p\}$ that are admissible with respect to $\mathscr{A}$. Let $\lambda > 0$ be a tuning parameter. On the event*

$$\left\{\|\tfrac{1}{n}\mathbb{X}^T\xi\|_{\mathscr{A},\circ} \leq \frac{\lambda}{2}\right\}, \tag{30}$$

the estimator (2) with penalty $F(\cdot) = \lambda\|\cdot\|_{\mathscr{A}}$ satisfies

$$\|\mathbb{X}\hat{\beta} - \mathbf{f}\|^2 \leq \min_{S\in\mathbb{S}_{\mathscr{A}}}\left[\min_{\beta\in\mathbb{R}^p:\mathrm{Supp}(\beta)=S} \|\mathbb{X}\beta - \mathbf{f}\|^2 + \frac{9\lambda^2}{4q_{\mathscr{A}}^2(S,3)}\right] \tag{31}$$

with the convention that $a/0 = +\infty$ for any $a > 0$.

Proof In view of Lemma 3, we can follow exactly the lines of the proof of Proposition 4 by replacing there the ℓ_1 norm by the norm $\|\cdot\|_{\mathscr{A}}$ and taking into account the duality bound $\frac{1}{n}\xi^T\mathbb{X}\Delta \leq \|\frac{1}{n}\mathbb{X}^T\xi\|_{\mathscr{A},\circ}\|\Delta\|_{\mathscr{A}}$. At the end, instead of (19), we use that

$$3\lambda\|\Delta_S\|_{\mathscr{A}} \leq 3\lambda\frac{\|\mathbb{X}\Delta\|}{q_{\mathscr{A}}(S,3)} \leq \frac{9\lambda^2}{4q_{\mathscr{A}}^2(S,3)} + \|\mathbb{X}\Delta\|^2.$$

□

Our next step is to find a range of values of λ such that the event (30) holds with probability at least 1/2. We will consider only the case when $\mathscr{A}$ is a polyhedral cone, which corresponds to many examples considered in [12, 13]. We will denote by $\mathscr{A}'$ the closure of the set $\mathscr{A} \cap \{a : |a|_1 \leq 1\}$.

Lemma 4 *Let the diagonal elements of matrix $\frac{1}{n}\mathbb{X}^T\mathbb{X}$ be not greater than 1. Let $\mathscr{A}$ be a polyhedral cone, and let $\mathscr{E}_{\mathscr{A}'}$ be the set of extremal points of $\mathscr{A}'$. If*

$$\lambda \geq \frac{2\sigma}{\sqrt{n}}\left(1 + \sqrt{2\log(2|\mathscr{E}_{\mathscr{A}'}|)}\right), \tag{32}$$

then the event (30) has probability at least 1/2.

Proof Denote by $\eta_j = \frac{1}{n}e_j^T\mathbb{X}^T\boldsymbol{\xi}$ the jth component of $\frac{1}{n}\mathbb{X}^T\boldsymbol{\xi}$. We have

$$\left\|\frac{1}{n}\mathbb{X}^T\boldsymbol{\xi}\right\|_{\mathscr{A},\circ} = \sup_{a\in\mathscr{A}:|a|_1\leq 1}\sqrt{\sum_{j=1}^p a_j\eta_j^2} = \max_{a\in\mathscr{E}_{\mathscr{A}'}}\sqrt{\sum_{j=1}^p a_j\eta_j^2}, \tag{33}$$

where the last equality is due to the fact that $\mathscr{A}'$ is a convex polytope. Let $\mathbf{z} = \boldsymbol{\xi}/\sigma$ be a standard normal $\mathcal{N}(\mathbf{0}, I_{n\times n})$ random vector. Note that, for all a such that $|a|_1 \leq 1$, the function $f_a(\mathbf{z}) = \sigma\sqrt{\sum_{j=1}^p a_j(\frac{1}{n}e_j^T\mathbb{X}^T\mathbf{z})^2}$ is $\sigma/\sqrt{n}$-Lipschitz with respect to the Euclidean norm. Indeed,

$$|f_a(\mathbf{z}) - f_a(\mathbf{z}')| \leq \sigma\sqrt{\sum_{j=1}^p a_j(\frac{1}{n}e_j^T\mathbb{X}^T(\mathbf{z}-\mathbf{z}'))^2} \leq \frac{\sigma}{\sqrt{n}}\sqrt{\sum_{j=1}^p a_j\|\mathbb{X}e_j\|^2|\mathbf{z}-\mathbf{z}'|_2^2}$$

$$\leq \frac{\sigma}{\sqrt{n}}|\mathbf{z}-\mathbf{z}'|_2, \quad \forall |a|_1 \leq 1,$$

since $\max_j\|\mathbb{X}e_j\|^2 \leq 1$ by the assumption of the lemma. Therefore, the Gaussian concentration inequality, cf., e.g., [7, Theorem B.6], implies that, for all $x > 0$,

$$\mathbb{P}\left(f_a(\mathbf{z}) \geq \mathbb{E}f_a(\mathbf{z}) + \sigma\sqrt{\frac{2x}{n}}\right) \leq e^{-x}.$$

Here, $f_a(\mathbf{z}) = \sqrt{\sum_{j=1}^p a_j\eta_j^2}$ and $\mathbb{E}\sqrt{\sum_{j=1}^p a_j\eta_j^2} \leq \left(\mathbb{E}\sum_{j=1}^p a_j\eta_j^2\right)^{1/2} \leq \sigma/\sqrt{n}$ for all a in the positive orthant such that $|a|_1 \leq 1$ where we have used that $\mathbb{E}\eta_j^2 \leq \sigma^2/n$ for $j = 1,\ldots,p$. Thus, for all a in the positive orthant such that $|a|_1 \leq 1$ and all $x > 0$, we have

$$\mathbb{P}\left(\sqrt{\sum_{j=1}^p a_j\eta_j^2} \geq \frac{\sigma}{\sqrt{n}}(1+\sqrt{2x})\right) \leq e^{-x}.$$

The result of the lemma follows immediately from this inequality, (33) and the union bound.   □

Finally, from Proposition 6, Lemma 4, and Theorem 1, we get the following theorem.

Theorem 4 *Assume that the diagonal elements of matrix $\frac{1}{n}\mathbb{X}^T\mathbb{X}$ are not greater than 1. Let λ be such that (32) holds. Then for any $\delta \in (0, 1)$, the estimator (2) with penalty $F(\cdot) = \lambda \|\cdot\|_{\mathscr{A}}$ satisfies*

$$\|\mathbb{X}\hat{\boldsymbol{\beta}} - \mathbf{f}\| \leq \min_{S \in \mathbb{S}_{\mathscr{A}}} \left[\min_{\boldsymbol{\beta} \in \mathbb{R}^p : \mathrm{Supp}(\boldsymbol{\beta}) = S} \|\mathbb{X}\boldsymbol{\beta} - \mathbf{f}\| + \frac{3\lambda}{2q_{\mathscr{A}}(S, 3)} \right] + \frac{\sigma \Phi^{-1}(1 - \delta)}{\sqrt{n}}$$

with probability at least $1 - \delta$. Furthermore,

$$\mathbb{E}\|\mathbb{X}\hat{\boldsymbol{\beta}} - \mathbf{f}\| \leq \min_{S \in \mathbb{S}_{\mathscr{A}}} \left[\min_{\boldsymbol{\beta} \in \mathbb{R}^p : \mathrm{Supp}(\boldsymbol{\beta}) = S} \|\mathbb{X}\boldsymbol{\beta} - \mathbf{f}\| + \frac{3\lambda}{2q_{\mathscr{A}}(S, 3)} \right] + \frac{\sigma}{\sqrt{2\pi n}}.$$

Note that, in contrast to Theorems 2 and 3, Theorem 4 is a less explicit result. Indeed, the form of the oracle inequalities depends on the value $q_{\mathscr{A}}(S, 3)$ and, through λ, on the value $|\mathscr{E}_{\mathscr{A}'}|$. Both quantities are solutions of nontrivial geometric problems depending on the form of the cone $\mathscr{A}$. Little is known about them. Note also that the knowledge of $|\mathscr{E}_{\mathscr{A}'}|$ (or of an upper bound on it) is required to find the appropriate λ.

6 Application to SLOPE

This section studies the SLOPE estimator introduced in [4], which is yet another convex regularized estimator. Define the norm $|\cdot|_*$ in $\mathbb{R}^p$ by the relation

$$|\mathbf{u}|_* \triangleq \max_{\phi} \sum_{j=1}^p \mu_j u_{\phi(j)}, \qquad \mathbf{u} = (u_1, \ldots, u_p) \in \mathbb{R}^p,$$

where the maximum is taken over all permutations ϕ of $\{1, \ldots, p\}$ and $\mu_j > 0$ are some weights. In what follows, we assume that

$$\mu_j = \sigma \sqrt{\log(2p/j)/n}, \qquad j = 1, \ldots, p.$$

For any $\mathbf{u} = (u_1, \ldots, u_p) \in \mathbb{R}^p$, let $u_1^* \geq u_2^* \geq \cdots \geq u_p^* \geq 0$ be a nonincreasing rearrangement of $|u_1|, \ldots, |u_p|$. Then the norm $|\cdot|_*$ can be equivalently defined as

$$|\mathbf{u}|_* = \sum_{j=1}^p \mu_j u_j^*, \qquad \mathbf{u} = (u_1, \ldots, u_p) \in \mathbb{R}^p.$$

Given a tuning parameter $A > 0$, we define the SLOPE estimator $\hat{\boldsymbol{\beta}}$ as a solution of the optimization problem

$$\hat{\boldsymbol{\beta}} \in \underset{\boldsymbol{\beta} \in \mathbb{R}^p}{\mathrm{argmin}} \left(\|\mathbf{y} - \mathbb{X}\boldsymbol{\beta}\|^2 + 2A|\boldsymbol{\beta}|_* \right). \tag{34}$$

As $|\cdot|_*$ is a norm, it is a convex function so Proposition 3 and Theorem 1 apply. For any $s \in \{1, \ldots, p\}$ and any $c_0 > 0$, the Weighted Restricted Eigenvalue (WRE) constant $\vartheta(s, c_0) \geq 0$ is defined as follows:

$$\vartheta^2(s, c_0) \triangleq \min_{\boldsymbol{\Delta} \in \mathbb{R}^p : \sum_{j=s+1}^p \mu_j \delta_j^* \leq c_0 (\sum_{j=1}^s \mu_j^2)^{1/2} |\boldsymbol{\Delta}|_2} \frac{\|\mathbb{X}\boldsymbol{\Delta}\|^2}{|\boldsymbol{\Delta}|_2^2}.$$

The $WRE(s, c_0)$ condition is said to hold if $\vartheta(s, c_0) > 0$.

We refer the reader to [2] for a comparison of this RE-type constant with other restricted eigenvalue constants such as (16). A high-level message is that the WRE condition is only slightly stronger than the RE condition. It is also established in [2] that a large class of random matrices $\mathbb{X}$ with independent and possibly anisotropic rows satisfies the condition $\vartheta(s, c_0) > 0$ with high probability provided that $n > Cs \log(p/s)$ for some absolute constant $C > 0$.

For $j = 1, \ldots, p$, let $g_j = \frac{1}{\sqrt{n}} e_j \mathbb{X}^T \boldsymbol{\xi}$, where e_j is the jth canonical basis vector in $\mathbb{R}^p$, and let $g_1^* \geq g_2^* \geq \cdots \geq g_p^* \geq 0$ be a nonincreasing rearrangement of $|g_1|, \ldots, |g_p|$. Consider the event

$$\Omega_* \triangleq \cap_{j=1}^p \left\{ g_j^* \leq 4\sigma \sqrt{\log(2p/j)} \right\}. \tag{35}$$

The next proposition establishes a deterministic result for the SLOPE estimator on the event (35).

Proposition 7 *On the event* (35), *the SLOPE estimator* $\hat{\boldsymbol{\beta}}$ *defined by* (34) *with* $A \geq 8$ *satisfies*

$$\|\mathbb{X}\hat{\boldsymbol{\beta}} - \mathbf{f}\|^2 \leq \min_{s \in \{1,\ldots,p\}} \left[\min_{\boldsymbol{\beta} \in \mathbb{R}^p : |\boldsymbol{\beta}|_0 \leq s} \|\mathbb{X}\boldsymbol{\beta} - \mathbf{f}\|^2 + \frac{9A^2\sigma^2 s \log(2ep/s)}{4n\vartheta^2(s, 3)} \right] \tag{36}$$

with the convention that $a/0 = +\infty$ *for any* $a > 0$.

Proof Let $s \in \{1, \ldots, p\}$ and $\boldsymbol{\beta}$ be minimizers of the right-hand side of (36) and let $\boldsymbol{\Delta} \triangleq \hat{\boldsymbol{\beta}} - \boldsymbol{\beta}$. We will assume that $\vartheta(s, 3) > 0$ since otherwise the claim is trivial. From Lemma 1 with $F(\boldsymbol{\beta}) = A|\boldsymbol{\beta}|_*$, we have

$$\|\mathbb{X}\hat{\boldsymbol{\beta}} - \mathbf{f}\|^2 - \|\mathbb{X}\boldsymbol{\beta} - \mathbf{f}\|^2 \leq 2 \left(\frac{1}{n} \boldsymbol{\xi}^T \mathbb{X}\boldsymbol{\Delta} + A|\boldsymbol{\beta}|_* - A|\hat{\boldsymbol{\beta}}|_* \right) - \|\mathbb{X}\boldsymbol{\Delta}\|^2 \triangleq D.$$

On the event (35), the right-hand side of the previous display satisfies

$$D \leq 2A \left[\frac{1}{2}|\boldsymbol{\Delta}|_* + |\boldsymbol{\beta}|_* - |\hat{\boldsymbol{\beta}}|_* \right] - \|\mathbb{X}\boldsymbol{\Delta}\|^2.$$

By [2, Lemma A.1], $\frac{1}{2}|\boldsymbol{\Delta}|_* + |\boldsymbol{\beta}|_* - |\hat{\boldsymbol{\beta}}|_* \leq \frac{3}{2}(\sum_{j=1}^{s}\mu_j^2)^{1/2}|\boldsymbol{\Delta}|_2 - \frac{1}{2}\sum_{j=s+1}^{p}\mu_j\delta_j^*$. If $3(\sum_{j=1}^{s}\mu_j^2)^{1/2}|\boldsymbol{\Delta}|_2 \leq \sum_{j=s+1}^{p}\mu_j\delta_j^*$, then the claim follows trivially. If the reverse inequality holds, we have $|\boldsymbol{\Delta}|_2 \leq \|\mathbb{X}\boldsymbol{\Delta}\|/\vartheta(s,3)$. This implies

$$3A(\sum_{j=1}^{s}\mu_j^2)^{1/2}|\boldsymbol{\Delta}|_2 \leq \frac{9A^2\sum_{j=1}^{s}\mu_j^2}{4\vartheta^2(s,3)} + \|\mathbb{X}\boldsymbol{\Delta}\|^2 \leq \frac{9A^2\sigma^2 s \log(2ep/s)}{4n\vartheta^2(s,3)} + \|\mathbb{X}\boldsymbol{\Delta}\|^2,$$

where for the last inequality we have used that, by Stirling's formula, $\log(1/s!) \leq s\log(e/s)$ and thus $\sum_{j=1}^{s}\mu_j^2 \leq \sigma^2 s \log(2ep/s)/n$. Combining the last three displays yields the result.   □

We now follow the same argument as in Sects. 4 and 5. In order to apply Theorem 1, we need to find a "weak bound" R on the error $\|\mathbb{X}\hat{\boldsymbol{\beta}} - \mathbf{f}\|$, i.e., a bound valid with probability at least $1/2$. If the event Ω_* holds with probability at least $1/2$ then, due to Proposition 7, we can take as R the square root of the right-hand side of (36). Since $\boldsymbol{\xi} \sim \mathcal{N}(\mathbf{0}, \sigma^2 I_{n \times n})$ and the diagonal elements of $\frac{1}{n}\mathbb{X}^T\mathbb{X}$ are bounded by 1, the random variables $g_1, \ldots, g_p$ are centered Gaussian with variance at most σ^2. The following proposition from [2] shows that the event (35) has probability at least $1/2$.

Proposition 8 *[2] If $g_1, \ldots, g_p$ are centered Gaussian random variables with variance at most σ^2, then the event* (35) *has probability at least* $1/2$.

Proposition 8 cannot be substantially improved without additional assumptions. To see this, let $\eta \sim \mathcal{N}(0, 1)$ and set $g_j = \sigma\eta$ for all $j = 1, \ldots, p$. The random variables $g_1, \ldots, g_p$ satisfy the assumption of Proposition 8. In this case, the event (35) satisfies $\mathbb{P}(\Omega_*) = \mathbb{P}(|\eta| \leq 4\sqrt{\log 2})$ so that $\mathbb{P}(\Omega_*)$ is an absolute constant. Thus, without additional assumptions on the random variables $g_1, \ldots, g_p$, there is no hope to prove a lower bound better than $\mathbb{P}(\Omega_*) \geq c$ for some fixed numerical constant $c \in (0, 1)$ independent of p.

By combining Propositions 7 and 8, we obtain that the oracle bound (36) holds with probability at least $1/2$. At first sight, this result is uninformative as it cannot even imply the consistency, i.e., the convergence of the error $\|\mathbb{X}\hat{\boldsymbol{\beta}} - \mathbf{f}\|$ to 0 in probability. But the SLOPE estimator is a convex regularized estimator and the argument of Sect. 3 yields that a risk bound with probability $1/2$ is in fact very informative: Theorem 1 immediately implies the following oracle inequality for any confidence level $1 - \delta$ as well as an oracle inequality in expectation.

Theorem 5 *Assume that the diagonal elements of the matrix $\frac{1}{n}\mathbb{X}^T\mathbb{X}$ are not greater than 1. Then for all $\delta \in (0, 1)$, the SLOPE estimator $\hat{\boldsymbol{\beta}}$ defined by* (34) *with tuning parameter $A \geq 8$ satisfies*

$$\|\mathbb{X}\hat{\boldsymbol{\beta}} - \mathbf{f}\| \leq \min_{s \in \{1,\dots,p\}} \left[\min_{\boldsymbol{\beta} \in \mathbb{R}^p : |\boldsymbol{\beta}|_0 \leq s} \|\mathbb{X}\boldsymbol{\beta} - \mathbf{f}\| + \frac{3\sigma A}{2\vartheta(s,3)} \sqrt{\frac{s \log(2ep/s)}{n}} \right]$$
$$+ \frac{\sigma \Phi^{-1}(1-\delta)}{\sqrt{n}}$$

with probability at least $1 - \delta$. Furthermore,

$$\mathbb{E}\|\mathbb{X}\hat{\boldsymbol{\beta}} - \mathbf{f}\| \leq \min_{s \in \{1,\dots,p\}} \left[\min_{\boldsymbol{\beta} \in \mathbb{R}^p : |\boldsymbol{\beta}|_0 \leq s} \|\mathbb{X}\boldsymbol{\beta} - \mathbf{f}\| + \frac{3\sigma A}{2\vartheta(s,3)} \sqrt{\frac{s \log(2ep/s)}{n}} \right] + \frac{\sigma}{\sqrt{2\pi n}}.$$

The proof is similar to that of Theorem 2, and thus it is omitted. Remarks analogous to the discussion after Theorem 2 apply here as well.

7 Generalizations and Extensions

The list of applications of Theorem 1 considered in the previous sections can be further extended. For instance, the same techniques can be applied when, instead of prediction by $\mathbb{X}\boldsymbol{\beta}$ for $\mathbf{f}$, one uses a trace regression prediction. In this case, the estimator $\hat{\boldsymbol{\beta}} \in \mathbb{R}^{m_1 \times m_2}$ is a matrix satisfying

$$\hat{\boldsymbol{\beta}}(\mathbf{y}) \in \operatorname*{argmin}_{\boldsymbol{\beta} \in \mathbb{R}^{m_1 \times m_2}} \left(\frac{1}{n} \sum_{i=1}^{n} (y_i - \operatorname{trace}(X_i^T \boldsymbol{\beta}))^2 + 2F(\boldsymbol{\beta}) \right), \tag{37}$$

where $X_1, \dots, X_n$ are given deterministic matrices in $\mathbb{R}^{m_1 \times m_2}$, $F : \mathbb{R}^{m_1 \times m_2} \to \mathbb{R}$ is a convex penalty. A popular example of $F(\boldsymbol{\beta})$ in this context is the nuclear norm of $\boldsymbol{\beta}$. The methods of this paper apply for such an estimator as well, and we obtain analogous bounds. Indeed, (37) can be rephrased as (2) by vectorizing $\boldsymbol{\beta}$ and defining a new matrix $\mathbb{X}$. Thus, Theorem 1 can be applied. Next, note that the examples of application of Theorem 1 considered above required only two ingredients: a deterministic oracle inequality and a weak bound on the probability of the corresponding random event. The deterministic bound is obtained here quite analogously to the previous sections or following the same lines as in [9] or in [16, Corollary 12.8]. A bound on the probability of the random event can be also borrowed from [9]. We omit further details.

Finally, we observe that Proposition 3 and Theorem 1 generalize to Hilbert space setting. Let H, H' be two Hilbert spaces and $\mathbb{X} : H' \to H$ a bounded linear operator. If H is equipped with a norm $\| \cdot \|_H$, and $F : H' \to [0, +\infty]$ is convex, proper, and lower semicontinuous, consider for any $\mathbf{y} \in H$ a solution

$$\hat{\boldsymbol{\beta}}(\mathbf{y}) \in \operatorname*{argmin}_{\boldsymbol{\beta} \in H'} \left(\|\mathbf{y} - \mathbb{X}\boldsymbol{\beta}\|_H^2 + 2F(\boldsymbol{\beta}) \right). \tag{38}$$

Proposition 9 *Under the above assumptions, any solution* $\hat{\boldsymbol{\beta}}(\mathbf{y})$ *of* (38) *satisfies* $\|\mathbb{X}(\hat{\boldsymbol{\beta}}(\mathbf{y}) - \hat{\boldsymbol{\beta}}(\mathbf{y}'))\|_H \leq \|\mathbf{y} - \mathbf{y}'\|_H$.

The proof of this proposition is completely analogous to that of Proposition 3. It suffices to note that the properties of convex functions used in the proof of Proposition 3 are valid when these functions are defined on a Hilbert space, cf. [14]. This and the fact that the Gaussian concentration property extends to Hilbert space valued Gaussian variables [10, Theorem 6.2] immediately imply a Hilbert space analog of Theorem 1.

Acknowledgements This work was supported by GENES and by the French National Research Agency (ANR) under the grants IPANEMA (ANR-13-BSH1-0004-02) and Labex Ecodec (ANR-11-LABEX-0047). It was also supported by the "Chaire Economie et Gestion des Nouvelles Donné es", under the auspices of Institut Louis Bachelier, Havas-Media and Paris-Dauphine.

References

1. Alekseev, V.M., Tikhomirov, V.M., Fomin, S.V.: Optimal Control. Consultants Bureau, New York (1987)
2. Bellec, P.C., Lecué, G., Tsybakov, A.B.: Slope Meets Lasso: Improved Oracle Bounds and Optimality (2016). arXiv:1605.08651
3. Bickel, P.J., Ritov, Y., Tsybakov, A.B.: Simultaneous analysis of Lasso and Dantzig selector. Ann. Stat. **37**(4), 1705–1732 (2009)
4. Bogdan, M., van den Berg, E., Sabatti, C., Su, W., Candès, E.J.: SLOPE-adaptive variable selection via convex optimization. Ann. Appl. Stat. **9**(3), 1103–1140 (2015)
5. Bühlmann, P., van de Geer, S.: Statistics for High-dimensional Data: Methods, Theory and Applications. Springer, Berlin (2011)
6. Dalalyan, A.S., Hebiri, M., Lederer, J.: On the Prediction Performance of the Lasso (2014). arXiv:1402.1700
7. Giraud. C.: Introduction to High-dimensional Statistics, vol. 138. CRC Press, Boca Raton (2014)
8. Hiriart-Urruty, J.-B., Lemaréchal, C.: Convex Analysis and Minimization Algorithms I: Fundamentals. Springer, Berlin (1993)
9. Koltchinskii, V., Lounici, K., Tsybakov, A.B.: Nuclear-norm penalization and optimal rates for noisy low-rank matrix completion. Ann. Stat. **39**(5), 2302–2329 (2011)
10. Lifshits, M.: Lectures on Gaussian Processes. Springer, Berlin (2012)
11. Lounici, K., Pontil, M., Tsybakov, A.B., van de Geer, S.: Oracle inequalities and optimal inference under group sparsity. Ann. Stat. **39**, 2164–2204 (2011)
12. Maurer, A., Pontil, M.: Structured sparsity and generalization. J. Mach. Learn. Res. **13**, 671–690 (2012)
13. Micchelli, C.A., Morales, J.M., Pontil, M.: A family of penalty functions for structured sparsity. Adv. Neural. Inf. Process. Syst. NIPS **23**, 2010 (2010)
14. Peypouquet, J.: Convex Optimization in Normed Spaces: Theory, Methods and Examples. Springer, Berlin (2015)
15. Tibshirani, R.J., Taylor, J.: Degrees of freedom in lasso problems. Ann. Stat. **40**(2), 1198–1232 (2012)
16. van de Geer, S.: Estimation and Testing under Sparsity. Springer, Berlin (2016)
17. van de Geer, S., Wainwright, M.: On Concentration for (Regularized) Empirical Risk Minimization (2015). arXiv:1512.00677

Structured Nonparametric Curve Estimation

Enno Mammen

Abstract In this note, we discuss structured nonparametric models. Under a structured nonparametric model, we understand a non- or semiparametric model with several nonparametric components where one of the nonparametric components lies in the focus of statistical interest but where all other nonparametric components are nuisance parameters. In structured nonparametrics, the focus of the statistical analysis is inference on this component whereas the goodness of fit of the whole model is only of secondary interest. This creates new challenging problems in the theory of nonparametrics. We will outline this in this note by discussing two classes of models from structured nonparametrics and by highlighting the theoretical questions arising in these classes of models.

Keywords Structured nonparametrics · Kernel smoothing
Nonparametric additive models · Chain ladder mode

1 Introduction

Structured nonparametrics is a class of models in non- or semiparametrics with several nonparametric components $f_1,\ldots,f_q$. In structured nonparametrics, the focus of statistical inference is directed to only one nonparametric component, f_1 say. One is interested in the shape or other characteristics of f_1. All other nonparametric components $f_2,\ldots,f_q$ and all parametric components of the model are nuisance parameters that are of no specific interest. Examples are applications where one wants to construct confidence bands or pointwise confidence sets for f_1 or where one wants to test hypothesis on the component f_1 but where the other components $f_2,\ldots,f_q$ are nuisance components.

Dedicated to Valentin Konakov on the occasion of his 70th birthday.

E. Mammen (✉)
Heidelberg University, Heidelberg, Germany
e-mail: mammen@math.uni-heidelberg.de

© Springer International Publishing AG 2017
V. Panov (ed.), *Modern Problems of Stochastic Analysis and Statistics*,
Springer Proceedings in Mathematics & Statistics 208,
DOI 10.1007/978-3-319-65313-6_14

This is related to semiparametrics where one is interested in one finite-dimensional parameter and where the nonparametric components are nuisance. But there is a big difference. For a finite-dimensional parameter, optimality in estimation and testing can be easily described. This is the case under regularity conditions that allow asymptotic central limit theorems with Gaussian limits for asymptotically linear statistics. Studies of optimality reduce then to the comparison of asymptotic covariance matrices. In structured nonparametrics, infinite-dimensional objects are estimated. Often, the estimators do not have a global distributional limit. And typically, there exists no unique optimal estimator. Typically, there are several ways to judge optimality and each criterion leads to another optimal statistical procedure. An example is classical nonparametric curve estimation problems. Here, the performance of the estimators can be tuned by looking for estimators with small bias and large variance, by choosing estimators with low bias, large variance or by balancing bias and variance of the estimator. Thus, it cannot be expected to get an asymptotic optimality theory in structured nonparametrics as it is available in semiparametrics.

There exist a lot of examples of models in structured nonparametrics. A first class of examples is structured nonparametric regression where one observes i.i.d. $\mathbb{R}^q \times \mathbb{R}$-valued random variables (X^i, Y^i) $(i = 1, .., n)$ with

$$Y^i = G[\theta, f_1, \ldots, f_q](X^i) + \varepsilon_i$$

for some $f_1, \ldots, f_q$ belonging to some specified function classes and for a finite-dimensional parameter θ and with error variables ε_i that fulfill:

$$\mathbb{E}[\varepsilon_i | X^i] = 0.$$

In structured nonparametrics, one is interested in a good fit of only one of the nonparametric components $f_1, \ldots, f_q$. This differs from prediction where the focus is a good fit of the composed regression function $G[\theta, f_1, \ldots, f_q]$. Many tools in mathematical statistics answer the question how a good fit can be achieved for the full model. But an analysis for estimation of one component of the model needs novel tools and approaches.

Perhaps, the simplest example of structured nonparametric regression is the additive model where

$$G[c, f_1, \ldots, f_q](x) = c + f_1(x_1) + \cdots + f_q(x_q).$$

Here, we observe $(X_1^i, \ldots, X_q^i, Y^i)$ $(i = 1, .., n)$ with

$$Y^i = c + f_1(X_1^i) + \cdots + f_q(X_q^i) + \varepsilon_i$$

for functions $f_1, \ldots, f_q$ belonging to some specified function classes and some constant c. For the error variables ε_i, it is assumed that:

$$\mathbb{E}[\varepsilon_i | X_1^i, \ldots, X_q^i] = 0.$$

Other examples in structured nonparametric regression include:

- additive models with monotone component functions,
- additive models with increasing number of additive components and sparsity,
- generalized additive models with unknown link function

$$G[f_0, \ldots, f_q](x) = f_0(f_1(x_1) + \cdots + f_q(x_q)),$$

- varying coefficient models

$$G[f_{j,k} : j \in \{1, \ldots, d\}, k \in I_j](x) = \sum_{j=1}^{d} x_j \sum_{k \in I_j} f_{j,k}(x_k),$$

- index models

$$G[f_1, \ldots, f_q, \theta_1, \ldots, \theta_q](x) = \sum_{j=1}^{d} f_j(\theta_j^\mathsf{T} x),$$

- age-cohort-period models: $G[f_1, f_2, f_3](x) = f_1(x_1) + f_2(x_2) + f_3(x_1 + x_2)$,
- age-cohort-period models with operational time: $G[f_1, f_2, f_3, f_4](x) = f_1(x_1) + f_2(f_4(x_1)x_2) + f_3(x_1 + x_2)$.

In structured nonparametric density estimation, one observes i.i.d. $\mathbb{R}^q$-valued random variables X^i $(i = 1, .., n)$ with density

$$G[\theta, f_1, \ldots, f_q](x)$$

for some $f_1, \ldots, f_q$ belonging to some specified function classes. A specification that we will discuss below is the nonparametric chain-ladder model where

$$G[f_1, f_2](x) = f_1(x_1)f_2(x_2)\mathbb{I}_{x_1+x_2 \leq 1; x_1, x_2 \geq 0}.$$

In this note, we will start with a short discussion of some general theoretical questions in structured nonparametrics. Then, we will report on some ongoing research projects with Young Kyung Lee (Seoul), María Dolores Martínez Miranda (Granada, London), Jens Perch Nielsen (London), Byeong Park (Seoul) where we discussed the chain-ladder model and some of its modifications. In the last part of this note, we will state some asymptotic oracle results for high-dimensional additive models. For the additive model

$$Y^i = c + f_1(X_1^i) + \cdots + f_q(X_q^i) + \varepsilon_i$$

with $q \to \infty$ we show under sparsity constraints: A component f_1 in the additive model can be estimated asymptotically as well as f_1 in the model

$$Z^i = c + f_1(X_1^i) + \varepsilon_i.$$

This means that not knowing $f_2, \ldots, f_q$ does not lead to a loss of statistical information on f_1, asymptotically up to first order. This result was obtained in a project with Karl Gregory (University of South Carolina) and Martin Wahl (Berlin).

2 Theoretical Questions

There are some theoretical questions that naturally arise in structured nonparametrics.

I. Does the global function $x \to G[\theta, f_1, \ldots, f_q](x)$ identify $\theta, f_1, \ldots, f_q$?
II. What are the optimal rates for the estimation of a component f_j. Is it the same rate as for $G[\theta, f_1, \ldots, f_q]$?
III. How can one construct an estimator for a component f_j? Is an asymptotic distribution theory available for the estimator?
IV. Can theory be developed for optimal estimation of a component f_j? Does there exist a concept like efficiency in semiparametrics?

We conjecture that there exist no general answers to all these questions that work for all models in structured nonparametrics. For this reason, we think that one has to consider these questions separately for each class of models in structured nonparametrics. In this note, we will do this for two classes of models. In the next section, we will discuss Questions I–III for age-cohort-period models with and without operational time. In Sect. 4, we will discuss Question IV for additive nonparametric models. There we will show that one can show that in an additive model a component can be estimated with the same asymptotic limit as it would be the case if the other additive nonparametric would be known. We formalize this statement and we interpret this as an optimality theory. Clearly, it cannot be expected that such an optimality result is available for all classes of models in structured nonparametrics.

3 A Worked Out Applied Model: Chain-ladder Model

In the simplest version of the chain-ladder model, one observes n i.i.d. tuples $\{(X_i, Y_i), i = 1, \ldots, n\}$ with density

$$f(x, y) = c_f f_1(x) f_2(y)$$

and support $\mathcal{I}_f$ that is contained in the set

$$\mathcal{S}_f = \{(x, y) : 0 \le x \le T_1, 0 \le y \le T_2\}$$

with $T_1, T_2 > 0$, see [5, 8]. Discrete versions of this model are used in claims reserving in non-life insurance where an important aim is to forecast the function $f(x, y)$ in $\mathcal{S}_f \setminus \mathcal{I}_f$. There the data arrange is a triangle support defined as

$\mathcal{I}_f = \{(x, y) : 0 \leq x, y \leq T, x + y \leq T\}$, where x is the underwriting time, y is the claims development time and $[0, T]$ (with $T > 0$) is the time observation window. Claims were paid at $x + y$.

There exist other examples for such data structures. In all these models, the covariate X represents the start of something. This could be the start of unemployment for an employee, onset of some infection, the reporting of an insurance claim, birth of a new member of a cohort or, as is the case in the above example underwriting of an insurance contract. The variable Y measures the time passed until some specified event occurs. It could be the duration of unemployment, incubation period of some disease, age of a cohort member, or development of an insurance claim. In all these cases, $X + Y$ is the calendar time of the relevant event. The functions f_1 and f_2 are interesting by themselves. Inference on their values gives insight about the future development of the data under consideration.

To simplify things, we here restrict our theory to the triangular support $\mathcal{I}_f = \{(x, y) : 0 \leq x, y \leq 1, x + y \leq 1\} \subset \mathcal{S}_f = [0, 1]^2$, where for simplicity, we transform the time into the interval $[0, 1]$. Thus, we observe n i.i.d. observations (X_i, Y_i) with density f on the triangle $\mathcal{I}_f$ where f is of the form: $f(x, y) = c_f f_1(x) f_2(y)$, with probability densities f_1 and f_2 on $[0, 1]$ and constant c_f such that $\int_{\mathcal{I}_f} c_f f_1(x) f_2(y) dx\, dy = 1$.

We now define

$$g_1(x) = \int_0^{1-x} f(x, y)w(x, y)\, dy,$$

$$g_2(y) = \int_0^{1-y} f(x, y)w(x, y)\, dx$$

with some weight function $w(x, y) > 0$. For the choice $w(x, y) \equiv 1$ we get that g_1 is the marginal density of X and g_2 is the marginal density of Y. But we allow also for other choices of w. We will consider estimators of f_1 and f_2 that are based on pilot estimators $\hat{g}_1$ and $\hat{g}_2$ of g_1 and g_2. The functions g_1 and g_2 can be estimated by kernel smoothing:

$$\hat{g}_1(x) = \frac{1}{nh_1} \sum_{i=1}^{n} K\left(\frac{X_i - x}{h_1}\right) w(X_i, Y_i),$$

$$\hat{g}_2(y) = \frac{1}{nh_2} \sum_{i=1}^{n} K\left(\frac{Y_i - y}{h_2}\right) w(X_i, Y_i),$$

where the kernel function K is a probability density function and where the bandwidths h_1, h_2 are positive sequences that converge to zero.

Our estimators $\hat{c}_f$, $\hat{f}_1$ and $\hat{f}_2$ of c_f, f_1 and f_2 are given as solutions of the equation

$$\hat{\mathcal{F}}(\hat{c}_f, \hat{f}_1, \hat{f}_2) \equiv 0$$

under the constraint $\int_0^1 \hat{f}_1(u)du = 1$ and $\int_0^1 \hat{f}_2(v)dv = 1$, with

$$\hat{\mathcal{F}}(c, r_1, r_2)(x, y) = \begin{pmatrix} c\, r_1(x) \frac{1}{\hat{g}_1(x)} \int_0^{1-x} r_2(v) w(x, v) dv - 1 \\ c\, r_2(y) \frac{1}{\hat{g}_2(y)} \int_0^{1-y} r_1(u) w(u, y) du - 1 \end{pmatrix}.$$

Note that $\hat{\mathcal{F}}(\hat{c}_f, \hat{f}_1, \hat{f}_2) \equiv 0$ is equivalent to

$$\hat{g}_1(x) = \int_0^{1-x} \hat{c}_f \hat{f}_1(x) \hat{f}_2(y) w(x, y)\, dy,$$

$$\hat{g}_2(y) = \int_0^{1-y} \hat{c}_f \hat{f}_1(x) \hat{f}_2(y) w(x, y)\, dx.$$

Under regularity assumptions, one gets the following result, see [5].

Theorem 1 *The following expansions hold*

$$\hat{f}_1(x) = f_1(x) - \frac{\frac{1}{nh_1} \sum_{i=1}^n K\left(\frac{X_i-x}{h_1}\right) w(X_i, Y_i) - \mathbb{E}\left[K\left(\frac{X_i-x}{h_1}\right) w(X_i, Y_i)\right]}{g_1(x)}$$

$$+ h_1^2 b_1(x) + o_P(\frac{1}{\sqrt{nh_1}} + h_1^2),$$

$$\hat{f}_2(y) = f_2(y) - \frac{\frac{1}{nh_2} \sum_{i=1}^n K\left(\frac{Y_i-y}{h_2}\right) w(X_i, Y_i) - \mathbb{E}\left[K\left(\frac{Y_i-y}{h_2}\right) w(X_i, Y_i)\right]}{g_2(y)}$$

$$+ h_2^2 b_2(y) + o_P(\frac{1}{\sqrt{nh_2}} + h_2^2),$$

uniformly for $\delta \le x, y \le 1 - \delta$ for $\delta > 0$ with b_1, b_2 given as solutions of deterministic linear integral equations.

We shortly outline how this result can be achieved. In the proof, one can make use of the following theorem.

Newton–Kantorovich Theorem. *Suppose that there exist constants α, β, k, r and a value ξ_0 such that a functional T has a derivative $T'(\xi)$ for $\|\xi - \xi_0\| \le r$, $T'(\xi)$ is invertible,*

$$\|T'(\xi_0)^{-1} T(\xi_0)\| \le \alpha,$$
$$\|T'(\xi_0)^{-1}\| \le \beta,$$
$$\|T'(\xi) - T'(\xi')\| \le k\|\xi - \xi'\|,$$

for all ξ, ξ' with $\|\xi - \xi_0\| \le r, \|\xi' - \xi_0\| \le r, 2k\alpha\beta < 1$ and $2\alpha < r$. Then $T(\xi) = 0$ has a unique solution ξ^* in $\{\xi : \|\xi - \xi_0\| \le 2\alpha\}$.

The main point in the proof of our theorem is to show that the random operator $\hat{\mathcal{F}}$ is differentiable with a derivative that has a bounded inverse. This allows to apply the Newton–Kantorovich Theorem with the choice $\mathcal{T} = \hat{\mathcal{F}}$. The choice $\xi_0 = (c_f, f_1, f_2)$ can be used to show consistency of $(\hat{c}_f, \hat{f}_1, \hat{f}_2)$. The choice $\xi_0 = (c_f, f_1, f_2) - \mathcal{T}'(c_f, f_1, f_2)^{-1} \mathcal{T}(c_f, f_1, f_2)$ leads to the stochastic expansion of $(\hat{c}_f, \hat{f}_1, \hat{f}_2)$ presented in our theorem.

The stochastic expansion in the theorem shows that f_1 and f_2 can be estimated with the same rate as in kernel smoothing in classical nonparametric regression or density estimation. We have a stochastic term that is mean zero and has the same structure as known from kernel smoothing in classical nonparametric regression or density estimation. As there, the stochastic terms are of order $(nh_1)^{-1/2}$ or $(nh_2)^{-1/2}$, respectively. Additionally, there is a bias term that is of order h_1^2 or h_2^2, respectively. Again, this is the same order as in classical nonparametric regression or density estimation. Furthermore, the expansions of our theorem allow to construct point wise confidence intervals or confidence bands for f_1 and f_2 and to construct testing procedures for their shape. This answers questions I–III for this model. It also shows that the optimal rate for estimation of f_1 and f_2 is equal to $n^{-2/5}$. This rate can be achieved by choosing h_1 and h_2 of order $n^{-1/5}$. Furthermore, no better rate can be achieved because we cannot do better than in the model where one of the two functions, f_1 or f_2, is known. But our theorem does not answer questions of optimality that go beyond rate optimality.

There exist several extensions of the chain-ladder model. We will discuss a version of the chain-ladder model that contains a varying time scale $\phi(x)$ (operational time)

$$f(x, y) = f_1(x) f_2(y\phi(x)), \quad (x, y) \in \mathcal{I}_f,$$

with unknown functions f_1, f_2 and ϕ. We choose this model as an example to discuss issues of identification. We will discuss why ϕ is identifiable. One can show that:

$$\frac{\phi'(x)}{\phi(x)} = \frac{\int_0^{1-x} \left(\frac{\partial}{\partial x} \log f(x, y) \right) w(y; x) \, dy}{\int_0^{1-x} \left(\frac{\partial}{\partial y} \log f(x, y) \right) y w(y; x) \, dy},$$

where $w(\cdot; x) : \mathbb{R} \to \mathbb{R}$ is a contrast function for each $x \in [0, 1)$, having the property that $\int_0^{1-x} w(y; x) \, dy = 0$. This motivates use of a plug-in estimator $\hat{\phi}$ using kernel estimators of (derivatives of) f.

We have the following result for this estimator, see [6].

Theorem 2 *Suppose that the bandwidths h_1 and h_2 are of order $n^{-1/5}$. Then under some regularity conditions for $x \in [0, 1)$ it holds that*

$$\hat{\phi}(x) - \phi(x) = O_p(n^{-2/5}). \tag{1}$$

Furthermore, for an arbitrarily small $\epsilon > 0$, it holds that

$$\int_0^{1-\epsilon} (\hat{\phi}(x) - \phi(x))^2 \, dx = O_p(n^{-4/5}), \tag{2}$$

$$\sup_{x \in [0, 1-\epsilon]} |\hat{\phi}(x) - \phi(x)| = O_p(n^{-2/5}\sqrt{\log n}). \tag{3}$$

Under additional assumptions, one can proceed now as if $\hat{\phi}$ would be the true time transform and one can apply similar methods as above for the estimation of f_1 and f_2. For the resulting estimators $\hat{f}_1$ and $\hat{f}_2$, one can show the following results. Under regularity conditions, it holds that the estimators $\hat{f}_1$ and $\hat{f}_2$ differ asymptotically from oracle estimators in the model where ϕ is known by a random and by a deterministic term of order $n^{-2/5}$. In particular, one gets that

$$\hat{f}_j(x) - f_j(x) = O_p(n^{-2/5}) \tag{4}$$

for $j = 1, 2$. Again, we arrive at results that show rate optimality of the estimators ϕ, f_1 and f_2. This can be seen by looking at the oracle models where two of the three functions are known. Asymptotic distribution theory in this model turns out to be more complex. But one can also develop asymptotic expansions for the estimators of f_1, f_2 and ϕ, that allow for such a theory. In particular, this theory allows the construction of statistical methods for testing and confidence intervals. For details see [6].

The theory can also be generalized to other shapes of the region where the density is observed and to the inclusion of a multiplicative factor of seasonal effects see again [6]. This is an important extension because seasonal effects are present in many actuarial, biostatistical, econometric, and statistical studies.

4 Asymptotic Oracle Results for High-dimensional Additive Models

In the last part of this note, we compare estimation of f_1 in the additive model

$$Y^i = c + f_1(X_1^i) + \cdots + f_q(X_q^i) + \varepsilon_i$$

with estimation of f_1 in the **oracle model**

$$Z^i = c + f_1(X_1^i) + \varepsilon_i.$$

For identification, we assume that $\mathbf{E}[f_j(X_j^i)] = 0$. We will show that f_1 can be estimated in an additive model asymptotically as well as f_1 in the oracle model. This means that not knowing $f_2, \ldots, f_q$ does not lead to a loss of statistical information on f_1, at least asymptotically up to first order. This can be judged as an answer to our question IV. At least it answers this question for the additive model. It reduces statistical questions on optimal estimation and testing in the additive model to the same questions in classical nonparametric regression model where these issues are well understood.

We now give a more precise formulation of this asymptotic equivalence result. Suppose that a smoothing estimator

$$\hat{f}_1^{oracle}(x_1) = SMOOTH_{X_1^i \to Z^i}(x_1)$$

of f_1 in the **oracle model** $Z^i = c + f_1(X_1^i) + \varepsilon_i$ is given. We now ask: can we construct an estimator $\hat{f}_1(x_1)$ of f_1 in the additive model

$$Y^i = c + f_1(X_1^i) + \cdots + f_q(X_q^i) + \varepsilon_i$$

with

$$\|\hat{f}_1 - \hat{f}_1^{oracle}\|_\infty = o_P(\delta_n),$$

where δ_n is the rate of convergence of $\hat{f}_1^{oracle}$ to f_1?

The answer is: Yes!

For an additive model with a fixed number q of functions, this has been shown in [2]. For a sparse high-dimensional additive model, this has been shown in [1]. There it has been allowed that the number q of functions may grow with n, even with $q >> n$, but that the number s_0 of nonzero functions may grow, but only with $s_0 << n$.

The basic idea of the construction in these papers is the observation that for a nonparametric estimator $\tilde{f}_1^{oracle}$ with low bias and high variance (undersmoothing) it holds that

$$\hat{f}_1^{oracle}(x_1)(= SMOOTH_{X_1^i \to Z^i}(x_1)) = SMOOTH_{X_1^i \to \tilde{Z}^i}(x_1) + o_P(\delta_n), \quad (5)$$

where $\tilde{Z}^i = \tilde{f}_1^{oracle}(X_1^i)$. This means that the application of one smoothing step leads to asymptotically the same result as if one applies the smoothing after one undersmoothing of the data: "smoothing $\approx$ smoothing $\circ$ undersmoothing". This asymptotic equivalence can be easily checked for many smoothing estimators such as kernel estimators, smoothing splines, orthogonal series estimators, Pinsker estimator, etc. It is a natural property because a negligible increase of a smoothing parameter typically does not lead to an asymptotically different result of the smoothing operation.

For a fixed choice of the undersmoothing estimator $\tilde{f}_1^{oracle}$ in the oracle model, [1, 2] state conditions under which it is possible to construct undersmoothing estimators $\tilde{f}_1, \ldots, \tilde{f}_q$ in the additive model such that:

$$\tilde{Z}^i = \tilde{f}_1^{oracle}(X_1^i) = \tilde{f}_1(X_1^i) + o_P(\delta_n). \quad (6)$$

This means that using the original data one can construct values that are asymptotically equivalent to the undersmoothed oracle data. This asymptotic equivalence has an important consequence. If one applies a smoothing operator with property (5) to the undersmoothed oracle data or to the data constructed from the original data then one gets the same asymptotic output. For the estimator $\hat{f}_1(x_1) = SMOOTH_{X_1^i \to \tilde{Y}^i}(x_1)$ with $\tilde{Y}^i = \tilde{f}_1(X_1^i)$ it holds that:

$$\hat{f}_1(x_1) = SMOOTH_{X_1^i \to \tilde{Z}^i}(x_1) + o_P(\delta_n) = SMOOTH_{X_1^i \to Z^i}(x_1) + o_P(\delta_n) \quad (7)$$
$$= \hat{f}_1^{oracle}(x_1) + o_P(\delta_n).$$

This means that we have constructed an estimator $\hat{f}_1$ based on the original data that is asymptotically equivalent to the oracle estimator $\hat{f}_1^{oracle}$.

Here is the argument again: For *one* simple undersmoothing estimator $\tilde{f}_1^{oracle}$ in the oracle model, one shows the existence of an estimator $\tilde{f}_1$ with (6). Then one gets for *all* estimators $\hat{f}_1^{oracle}$ in the oracle model with (5) that (7) holds for the estimator $\hat{f}_1(x_1) = SMOOTH_{X_1^i \to \tilde{Y}^i}(x_1)$ with $\tilde{Y}^i = \tilde{f}_1(X_1^i)$. This is the oracle result for additive models with a fixed number of additive components and for sparse high-dimensional additive model.

This gives an answer to our Question IV for additive models. It has to be studied to which extent the oracle results of additive models carry over to other nonparametric models.

The results of this section complement recent results that only discuss optimal rates in additive models, see [11] for additive models of additive components belonging to function classes with differing complexity, and see [4, 7, 9, 10] for additive models with an increasing number of components.

References

1. Gregory, K., Mammen, E., Wahl, M: Optimal estimation of sparse high-dimensional additive models, Preprint (2016)
2. Horowitz, J., Klemelä, J., Mammen, E.: Optimal estimation in additive regression models. Bernoulli **12**, 271–298 (2006)
3. Horowitz, J., Mammen, E.: Rate-optimal estimation for a general class of nonparametric regression models with unknown link functions. Ann. Statist. **35**, 2589–2619 (2007)
4. Koltchinskii, V., Yuan, M.: Sparse recovery in large ensembles of kernel machines. In: Servedio, R.A., Zhang, T. (eds.) Colt, pp. 229–238. Omnipress, Madison (2008)
5. Lee, Y.K., Mammen, E., Nielsen, J.P., Park, B.U.: Asymptotics for In-Sample Density Forecasting. Ann. Statist. **43**, 620–645 (2015)
6. Lee, Y.K., Mammen, E., Nielsen, J.P., Park, B.U.: Operational time and in-sample density forecasting, Ann. Statist. **45**, 1312–1341 (2017)
7. Lu, J., Kolar,M., Liu, H.: Post-regularization confidence bands for high dimensional nonparametric models with local sparsity, Technical Report (2015) arXiv:1503.02978
8. Mammen, E., Martínez Miranda, M.D., Nielsen, J.P.: In-sample forecasting applied to reserving and mesothelioma. Insur.: Math. Econ. **61**, 76–86 (2015)

9. Meier, L., van de Geer, S., Bühlmann, P.: High-dimensional additive modeling. Ann. Statist. **37**, 3779–3821 (2009)
10. Raskutti, G., Wainwright, M.J., Yu, B.: Minimax-optimal rates for sparse additive models over kernel classes via convex programming. J. Mach. Learn. Res. **13**, 389–427 (2012)
11. van de Geer, S., Muro, A.: Penalized least squares estimation in the additive model with different smoothness for the components. J. Statist. Planning and Inf. **162**, 43–61 (2015)

Part VIII
Acturial Science

New Research Directions in Modern Actuarial Sciences

Ekaterina Bulinskaya

Abstract The aim of the paper is to outline the new trends in modern actuarial sciences in order to help the researchers to find new domains of activity and university professors teaching future actuaries to prepare special courses. The paper begins by description of actuarial profession and a brief historical sketch. After recalling the main achievements of the first two periods in actuarial sciences, we describe the new research directions of the third and fourth periods characterized by interplay of insurance and finance, unification of reliability and cost approaches, as well as, consideration of complex systems. Sophisticated mathematical tools are used for analysis and optimization of insurance systems including dividend payment, reinsurance, and investment. Discrete-time models turned out to be more realistic in some situations for investigation of insurance problems.

Keywords Risk · Dividends · Reinsurance · Investment · Ruin · Bankruptcy

1 Introduction

Web site CareerCast.com has ranked actuary the fourth-best job of 2014 taking into account environment, income, hiring outlook, and stress. Data from the U.S. Department of Labor and the Bureau of Labor Statistics, as well as other government agencies, trade associations, and private survey firms were used to evaluate the 200 jobs included in its annual Jobs Rated report. The top three jobs, according to the report, are mathematician, tenured university professor, and statistician.

Math skills are key in landing some of the best jobs in the nation, according to CareerCast's 2015 Jobs Rated report, with four of the nation's ten best jobs focusing on mathematics. An actuary—who uses mathematics, statistics, and financial theory to assess the risk that an event will occur—came in at No. 1 on the list, just ahead of mathematician (No. 3), statistician (No. 4), and data scientist (No. 6).

E. Bulinskaya (✉)
Lomonosov Moscow State University, Moscow, Russia
e-mail: ebulinsk@yandex.ru

© Springer International Publishing AG 2017   349
V. Panov (ed.), *Modern Problems of Stochastic Analysis and Statistics*,
Springer Proceedings in Mathematics & Statistics 208,
DOI 10.1007/978-3-319-65313-6_15

Thus, it is natural to ask the following questions. What is an actuary? What is actuarial science? One of the answers is given below.

Actuarial science is the discipline that applies mathematical and statistical methods to assess risk in insurance, finance, and other industries and professions. Actuaries are professionals who are qualified in this field through intense education and experience. In many countries, actuaries must demonstrate their competence by passing a series of thorough professional examinations.

Actuarial profession was formally established in 1848, with the formation of Institute of Actuaries, London. The Faculty of Actuaries, Edinburgh, was organized in 1856, and in 2010 it merged with Institute of Actuaries. The International Actuarial Association (IAA) is a worldwide association of local professional actuarial associations. It was established in 1895 as an association of individuals under the name the "Comité Permanent des Congrés d'Actuaires", renamed IAA in 1968 and restructured at the 26th International Congress of Actuaries, held in Birmingham on 7–12 June 1998. Nowadays IAA includes 69 Full Member Associations, representing 98% of qualified actuaries worldwide, and 28 Associate Member Associations. It has seven sections.

ASTIN, the section for **A**ctuarial **ST**udies **I**n **N**on-life insurance, was created in 1957 as the first section of the IAA. ASTIN's main objective is to promote actuarial research, particularly in non-life insurance. ASTIN is continually working to further develop the mathematical foundation of non-life insurance and reinsurance.

Another section of the IAA, created in 1986, was **AFIR**, which stands for **A**ctuarial Approach for **FI**nancial **R**isks. Its objective was defined as promotion of actuarial research in financial risks and problems, see, e.g., [407]. Effective from 2011, the section mandate was extended to formally include **E**nterprise **R**isk **M**anagement (ERM), hence, the section was named **AFIR/ERM**. The purpose of this change was to expand the discussion beyond market risk issues and provide a strong home for international discussion and research on ERM topics. It is a reflection of the expanding and developing role of ERM in actuarial practice and the IAA efforts to provide support for this growing area of actuarial practice. It is a natural extension and many ERM papers and topics have been presented at past AFIR colloquia, see, e.g., [135] and references therein.

In November 2009, a group of actuarial professional bodies took the unprecedented step of agreeing to collaborate to develop and administer a new qualification in enterprise risk management (ERM)—the Chartered Enterprise Risk Actuary (CERA)—a ground breaking achievement, and the birth of the Global CERA Treaty. The first nine actuaries received this certificate in July 2010.

We do not consider in this paper the scientific activity of such important IAA Sections as the Health Section (IAAHS) created in 2003, the Pensions, Benefits and Social Security Section (PBSS) also started in 2003, and Life Section (IAALS) created in 2005, although these branches of research deserve a special consideration, see, e.g., [398].

The Russian Actuarial Society was organized on September 14, 1994, the first President was Professor A.N. Shiryaev, see [381]. The Russian Guild of Actuaries was founded in 2002 on the basis of the Society of actuaries, established in 1994.

On November 4, 2008, the Russian Guild of Actuaries became the full member of the IAA and was acknowledged as an integral part of international actuarial community.

Actuarial education at the Moscow State University was initiated by Professor B.V. Gnedenko in 1993, see [91]. It is necessary to mention the achievements of Russian actuarial science before 1917. The most well-known person is S.E. Savitsch (1864–1936) who was a vice-president of the first four International Congresses of Actuaries and a member of Organizing Committee of the 8th Congress which was planned to take place in St. Petersburg in 1915 (however canceled due to war). He was a permanent member of the Insurance Committee at the Ministry of Internal Affairs, which carried out insurance supervision in the Russian Empire. For the most part, he was interested in life insurance, health and pensions (see, e.g., his book [367]). However, there also exists his paper [368] dealing with premiums in fire insurance. The worldwide known specialists in probability theory, V.Ya. Bunyakovski [97] and A.A. Markov ([297], chap. VIII) have also contributed to the development of life insurance.

This paper is organized as follows. Historical background is provided in Sect. 2. In particular, we sketch the main steps in the history of actuarial sciences and describe what is actuary of the fourth kind. General description of applied probability models is given in Sect. 3. This description clearly demonstrates the similarity of models arising in different research domains. It is also useful for models classification. New research directions in modern actuarial sciences are presented in Sect. 4 (for continuous-time models) and in Sect. 5 (for discrete-time models). Three examples are treated in Sect. 6. Conclusion is given in Sect. 7.

2   Historical Background

The keyword in all definitions of actuarial sciences is risk. According to the Concise Oxford English Dictionary, "risk is a hazard, a chance of bad consequences, loss or exposure to mischance" (see also [330]).

There exists the following classification of risks. First of all, risk can be pure or speculative. Pure risk entails loss only, whereas speculative one can provide gain, as well as loss. The most known sources of the latter risks are gambling and stock exchange. In its turn, pure risk is subdivided into physical and moral. Both are typical for insurance. Insurance is a means of protection from financial loss. It is a form of risk management primarily used to hedge against the risk of a contingent, uncertain loss. Not all pure risks can be insured. To be insurable a risk must be random, not depend entirely on the will of insured and materialize in the future. Randomness can be of two types. Either the event under consideration (insured's death) will happen with certainty sometimes, however the occurrence time is random, or the event (e.g., theft of auto) may not occur at all. In the latter case, the occurrence time is also a random variable however its distribution is improper. That is one of the reasons for different approaches in life insurance and non-life insurance.

Risk is present whenever the outcome is uncertain, whether favorable or unfavorable. Traditional actuarial mathematics work best on hazard risks, as they are generally independent and discontinuous. Actuaries and other risk professionals have done a remarkably good job assessing and evaluating hazard risks. Organizations rarely become insolvent due to failure to manage hazard risks.

Financial risks are those that affect assets, including interest rates, inflation, equity values, and foreign exchange rate. These risks are correlated, continuous, and require an understanding of stochastic calculus to be measured appropriately. Unlike hazard risks, financial risks provide the possibility of a gain, not just a loss. The techniques for managing financial risks—financial derivatives such as forwards, futures, options, and swaps—are relatively new. Misuse of these techniques and the resulting financial debacles they caused have actually led to the need for enterprise risk management (ERM), see [133].

According to the Casualty Actuarial Society (CAS), enterprise risk management is defined as: "The process by which organizations in all industries assess, control, exploit, finance and monitor risks from all sources for the purpose of increasing the organization's short and long term value to its stakeholders."

In other words, ERM is the systematic evaluation of all the significant risks facing an organization and how they affect the organization in an aggregate way. Hence, categorizing risks as hazard, financial, operational, or strategic is most useful. Operational risks represent the failure of people, processes, or systems. Strategic risk reflects the business decisions of an organization or the impact of competition or regulation. Examples of strategic risk for insurance are the benefits produced for those first to use credit scoring (see, e.g., [359]) as a rating variable, and the market share losses of those companies that were slow to adopt this approach. ERM originally focused on loss prevention, controlling negative surprises, and reducing downside risk. Now ERM deals with the entire range of potential outcomes, not just downside risk. Accepting risks where it has a comparative advantage, and transferring or avoiding risks where it does not, a company is adding value by efficient risk treatment.

Methods for transferring or distributing risk were practiced by Chinese and Babylonian traders as long ago as the 3rd and 2nd millennia BC, respectively. Chinese merchants traveling treacherous river rapids would redistribute their wares across many vessels to limit the loss due to any single vessel's capsizing. The Babylonians developed a system which was recorded in the famous Code of Hammurabi, c. 1750 BC, and practiced by early Mediterranean sailing merchants. If a merchant received a loan to fund his shipment, he would pay the lender an additional sum in exchange for the lender's guarantee to cancel the loan should the shipment be stolen or lost at sea. Further history of insurance development is described, e.g., in [381].

Why actuarial science emerged significantly later (in the 17th century) one can read in the interesting book by P.L. Bernstein [64] written in 1996 about the risk history.

According to classification given in 1987 by H. Bühlmann [82], there were three periods in actuarial sciences. However less than two decades later, in 2005, P. Embrechts declared the beginning of the fourth period, namely, appearance of actuaries of the fourth kind. S. D'Arcy, in his Presidential address [133] to CAS

(Casualty Actuarial Society), has told that such a term is applied to actuaries working in ERM (enterprise risk management) and explained how to become an actuary of the fourth kind.

Actuaries of the first kind are life actuaries. According to Bühlmann, the primary methods of life actuaries involve deterministic calculations. Actuaries of the second kind, the casualty actuaries, develop probabilistic methods for dealing with risky situations. The actuaries of the third kind deal with the investment side of insurance and incorporate stochastic processes into actuarial calculations. Nowadays, almost all aspects of insurance product development and pricing involve a combination of investment and insurance characteristics. This change requires all actuaries to become actuaries of the third kind. How to reach this goal one can read in [134]. The actuaries of the third kind, who were the object of Bühlmann's editorial, were the investment actuaries applying stochastic processes, contingent claims, and derivatives to assets and liabilities. This specialty developed in the 1980s as financial risk became more important and tools to manage financial risk were created. In order to become the actuary of the fourth kind, one has to learn to deal not only with hazard and financial risks but with operational and strategic risks as well, see [130].

According to [133], in ERM, as in traditional risk management, the first step is *risk identification*. Focus on the most significant risks an organization faces. Deal with those first, then in future iterations expand the focus to the next level of risk elements, as advised one of ERM pioneers, J. Lam (see [248]).

Step two in ERM, as in traditional risk management, is to *quantify the risks*. Actuaries are well skilled in this area, at least for hazard risks, but ERM also requires the quantification of the correlations among different risks. Two risks can be generally uncorrelated, but, if an extreme event were to occur, then they could be highly correlated. Techniques for evaluating these forms of correlations, filters, tail dependency, copulas, and other numerical techniques must be incorporated. Much needs to be done to be able to quantify operational and strategic risk to the standards common in hazard and financial risk (see, e.g., [130, 131]).

Step three of the risk management process involves *evaluating the different methods for handling risk*. Risks can be assumed, transferred, or reduced. A variety of methods exist for transferring (subcontracting, insurance, or securitization) or reducing risk (loss control, contract, or reinsurance).

Step four is to *select the best method for handling the risk*, which in most cases will involve a combination of different techniques. Moreover, the organization wants to make consistent choices about all the risks it faces, how much risk it will accept, and what return it would require for accepting a particular level of risk.

Step five is to *monitor and adjust the risk management approach* selected. It is an iterative process that entails identifying additional significant risks, quantifying those risks, and improving the quantification of previously identified risks based on additional information and improved mathematical techniques. It also entails reevaluating the different approaches to handle risk, implementing an improved strategy, and then, once more, monitoring the result.

In addition to references in [133], the following papers and books may be helpful: [51, 105, 107, 135, 136, 140, 151, 164, 194, 196, 228, 233, 302, 317, 323, 365, 384, 392, 396, 419].

Thus, the first period in actuarial science development was deterministic, see, e.g., [398]. It is characterized by E. Haley's mortality tables which appeared in 1693 and D. Bernoulli's utility functions introduced in 1738. Although some researchers claim that idea of mortality tables belongs to Roman juror Ulpian, the first life tables appeared in the seventeeth century. They were issued by John Graunt in 1662 (some historians attribute them to William Petty, who introduced the new subject named "political arithmetic") and Johan de Witt, 1671. However, E. Halley "was the first individual to describe the principles of actuarial mathematics on scientifically accurate lines" (see [200]).

The second (stochastic) period is marked by the application of probability theory and stochastic processes to solving the actuarial problems. The main achievement of this period is the collective risk theory, in particular, a well-known Cramér–Lundberg model, see, e.g. [299]. It is worth mentioning that one of widely used in practice stochastic processes with independent increments, namely, Poisson process was introduced for the first time in the dissertation of F. Lundberg in 1903, see, e.g. [129]. The other process with independent increments called Brownian motion or Wiener process appeared as a model for stock exchange performance in dissertation of L. Bachelier "Theory of speculation" in 1900. The results of Lundberg were explained and further developed by H. Cramér in 1930s. It is said that the reason for Swedish insurance companies successes was the attention paid to actuarial sciences. Thus, in 1929, a special chair of Statistics and Actuarial Sciences was created at Stockholm university for H. Cramér.

The science has gone through revolutionary changes during the last 40 years due to the proliferation of high-speed computers and the union of stochastic actuarial models with modern financial theory. Thus, one can call the third period financial. It was very short, not more than three decades. The fourth (modern) period has brought, in addition to achievements of previous periods, development of enterprise risk management.

Hence, the modern period is characterized by strong interaction of insurance and finance, investigation of complex systems and employment of sophisticated mathematical tools. The aim of the paper is to outline the new research directions which emerged during the last two decades. Further on, we are going to focus on non-life (general) insurance, mentioning in passing that life insurance is thoroughly treated in the book [234] by M. Koller, see also [165]. The models used in health insurance can be found in [347] by E. Pitacco. Those interested in the famous Wilkie's investment model and its generalizations are referred to [420] and original papers [362, 363, 406, 408, 409].

It is important to underline that the books [127, 158, 195, 217, 232, 237, 241, 326, 329, 341, 348, 352, 361, 383, 413, 421] demonstrate the similarity between the models arising in insurance, finance, and other research fields. Thus, methods used in one research field may turn out fruitful in others. The books [71, 73, 83, 126, 141, 142, 145, 208, 221, 231, 300, 304, 349, 370, 375, 380, 420] also can be useful, along with traditional textbooks such as [56, 75, 81, 138, 173, 371], for professors planning the special courses for actuarial students.

Although the bibliography of this paper contains 446 papers and books, almost all of them published in this century, the list is far from being complete. Further references can be found in the mentioned books and reviews [8, 28, 40, 202, 272, 379]. The last review was published during the preparation of this paper, so the material was rearranged in order not to repeat [379]. Thus, the taxation problems (see, e.g., the loss-carry-forward tax model for Lundberg risk process in [7], or [245] where general tax processes are investigated for Lévy insurance model, as well as [305] dealing with a compound Poisson process under absolute ruin) and statistical estimation (see, e.g., [436] where nonparametric estimation for ruin probability in Lévy risk model is treated) are only mentioned, the interested reader is referred to [379].

3 General Description of Applied Probability Models

Not only insurance, but other applied probability research domains such as inventory and dams, finance, queueing theory, reliability, and some others can be considered as special cases of decision-making under uncertainty (or risk management) aimed at the systems performance optimization, thus eliminating or minimizing risk, see, e.g., [85, 301]. "The capacity to manage risk, and with it appetite to take risk and make forward-looking choices, are key elements of the energy that drives the economic system forward"—one reads in [64]. The ability of businesses to survive and thrive often requires unconventional thinking and calculated risk taking. The key is to make the right decisions—even under the most risky, uncertain, and turbulent conditions, see, e.g., [168].

For correct decision-making, one needs an appropriate mathematical model. For several centuries, mathematics has been the language of the exact sciences. Only in the twentieth century has mathematics become predominant in other fields, particularly economics and finance. Obviously, it is possible to construct a lot of models describing the same real-life event or process more or less precisely. Furthermore, the same mathematical model can arise in different research domains.

Constructing an insurance company model one has to take into account its twofold nature. Originally all insurance societies were designed for risk sharing. Hence, their primary task is policyholders indemnification. Nowadays, for the most part, they are joint-stock companies. Thus, the secondary but very important task is dividend payments to shareholders.

It is well known that insurance company performance generates two cash flows. Namely, the inflow consists of premiums paid by insureds and outflow is determined by claim process. Premiums are paid by all policyholders (insureds) however reimbursement is obtained only by those who suffered from risk realization. Clearly, the insurance company models are of input–output type. They can be described by the following six-tuple $(T, Z, Y, U, \Psi, \mathscr{L})$.

Table 1 Interpretation of model parameters for different research domains

Research field	Input	Output	System state
Insurance	Premium	Indemnity	Surplus
Finance	Money inflow	Money outflow	Capital
Inventory	Supply	Demand	Inventory level
Storage	Water inflow	Water outflow	Water level in a dam
Reliability	New & repaired	Broken elements	Working elements
Queueing	Customers arrival	Served customers	Queue length
Population growth	Birth and immigration	Death and emigration	Population size

Here, T is the planning horizon, $Z = \{Z(t), t \in [0, T]\}$ and $Y = \{Y(t), t \in [0, T]\}$ being input and output processes, respectively. The next element $U = \{U(t), t \in [0, T]\}$ is a control, whereas Ψ represents the system configuration and operation mode. Hence, $X = \Psi(Z, Y, U)$ is the system state, so, $X = \{X(t), t \in [0, T]\}$. All the above-mentioned processes may be multidimensional, moreover, their dimensions may differ. Finally, $\mathscr{L}_T(U) = \mathscr{L}(Z, Y, U, X, T)$ is an objective function (target, valuation criterion, risk measure) evaluating the system performance quality.

Definition 1 A control $U_T^* = \{U^*(t), t \in [0, T]\}$ is called *optimal* if

$$\mathscr{L}_T(U_T^*) = \inf_{U_T \in \mathscr{U}_T} \mathscr{L}_T(U_T), \quad (\text{or} \quad \mathscr{L}_T(U_T^*) = \sup_{U_T \in \mathscr{U}_T} \mathscr{L}_T(U_T)), \tag{1}$$

where $\mathscr{U}_T$ is a class of all feasible controls. Furthermore, $U^* = \{U_T^*, T \geq 0\}$ is called an *optimal policy* (or strategy).

If the extremum in (1) cannot be attained, one has to use either the ε-optimal or asymptotic optimal policies.

Giving another interpretation to input and output processes, one can pass (see, e.g., [90]) from one research field to another as shown in Table 1.

3.1 Models Classification

Now, we turn to models classification according to parameters of their general description.

1. The planning horizon can be finite ($T < \infty$) or infinite ($T = \infty$). Furthermore, one can consider continuous or discrete time. In the first case, the system is observed at any time $t \in [0, T]$, in the second one, its behavior is known in a finite or countable set of points belonging to the planning horizon.

2. Input and output processes can be deterministic or stochastic. In the latter case, their distributions may be known completely, partly (unknown parameters), or

unknown at all. Thus, a system will be deterministic or stochastic if the same true for both (input and output) processes. It is called mixed if one process is deterministic while the other one is stochastic.

3. According to the set of feasible controls, the system can be static (control is applied only one time) or dynamic (control is applied many times or continuously). Moreover, one can control input or/and output processes, as well as the system initial state, configuration, and operation mode. Hence, dimensions of underlying processes (input, output, control, and system state) can differ and change in course of system functioning.

4. The last but not least element of systems description is an objective function (risk measure). At first, in many research fields, an objective function was not considered at all. Hence, there was no control and optimization. One can mention here queueing and dam theory. Nowadays, in all applied probability research fields, one is interested in the choice of optimal control providing extremum of some prescribed objective function. Multi-objective optimization (see, [318]) can also be studied.

The most widely used approaches in choosing the objective function are reliability and cost ones. It is clear that reliability approach has arisen in reliability theory. The researchers were always interested in survival time of the system under consideration, in other words, the time until the system failure, as well as, in survival probability. The reliability approach was also used in insurance. Since company solvency is very important for its existence, for a long time the primary task of actuarial sciences was investigation of ruin time and ruin probability.

On the other hand, the cost approach was applied from the beginning in finance and inventory theory. The expected (discounted) costs were typical for inventory models optimization. Mean variance principle was used for portfolio optimization and capital allocation since 1952 when the seminal paper [298] was published. Insurance application of this principle is presented, e.g., in [53, 210], whereas optimal portfolio choice for a loss averse insurer is treated in [192] (see also references therein). Other well-known financial risk measures, such as VaR (Value at Risk) or CVaR (Conditional Value at Risk), were widely used in insurance as well. Coherent risk measures (see, e.g., [22, 162]), deviation measures and expectation bounded risk measures (see, e.g., [360]) became very popular during the last two decades. Now, reliability and cost approaches (along with their various combinations) are used in any applied probability domain.

3.2 New Trends in Actuarial Sciences

Further on, the following characteristics of modern period of actuarial sciences are treated.

- Interplay of actuarial and finance methods, in particular, unification of reliability and cost approaches.

- Investigation of complex systems including dividend payment, reinsurance, investment, and bank loans, as well as taxes. Hence, the necessity of dealing with more intricate models and processes, application of sophisticated mathematical tools.
- Consideration of discrete-time models which turned out to be more appropriate for the description of some aspects of insurance company performance.

Historically, most insurance-related problems deal with jump processes due to the nature of insurance claims which occur at discrete-time points, whereas many classical models in financial mathematics rely on continuous processes to reflect fluctuations in the constantly changing financial markets. Although the two disciplines of applied probability have evolved rather independently, there is a common trend in recent years to incorporate stochastic models with both continuous and jump components, see, e.g., [385].

For example, on the ruin theory side, in addition to the random jumps which account for insurance claims, diffusion components have gained increasing popularity to describe investment returns in sophisticated risk models.

4   New Results for Continuous-Time Insurance Models

It was already mentioned that functioning of insurance company generates two cash flows. Namely, input $Z(t)$ describes the premiums acquired up to time t, whereas output $Y(t)$ represents the payments of company to policyholders in order to satisfy their claims. In other words, $Y(t)$ is the aggregate claim amount up to time t.

Thus, insurance company capital (surplus or reserve) at time t is given by

$$X(t) = x + Z(t) - Y(t), \tag{2}$$

where x is the initial capital.

Continuous-time models were used during the last century and still are very popular. The famous *Cramér–Lundberg model*, which appeared in 1903 (see [129]), has a mixed type. Its input is deterministic $Z(t) = ct$, $c > 0$ is the premium rate, whereas the output $Y(t)$ is a stochastic process

$$Y(t) = \sum_{i=1}^{N(t)} Y_i. \tag{3}$$

Here, the claim number $N(t)$ is a Poisson process with parameter λ, Y_i being the amount of the ith claim. The sequence $\{Y_i\}$ of i.i.d. r.v.'s and $N(t)$ are supposed independent. Thus, $Y(t)$ is a compound Poisson process with intensity λ. It is interesting to mention that $X(t)$ given by (2) and (3) is a particular case of spectral negative Lévy process.

4.1 Decision Problems and Objective Functions

The problems of interest for any insurance company are choice of underwriting procedure, premium principles (see, e.g., [114, 255, 274, 277, 288, 351, 440, 441]) and reserves (see, e.g., [1, 29, 84, 211, 303, 418]) to ensure the company solvency. Moreover, very important decisions are dividend payments, reinsurance, and investment. Hence, very popular research topics are

- calculation of ruin probabilities,
- estimation of ruin severity (Gerber–Shiu function),
- investigation of the rate of capital growth,

as well as, thorough study of models incorporating

- dividends, investment, reinsurance, tax.

4.1.1 Ruin Probability

From the beginning, the *ruin probability* attracted attention of actuaries occupied with company solvency. There exists a vast bibliography pertaining to this problem, see, e.g., [24, 25, 186] and references therein.

Denote by $\tau = \inf\{t > 0 : X(t) < 0\}$ the ruin time of the company. Then, finite-time ruin probability (ruin in interval [0, T]) is defined as follows:

$$\psi(x, T) = P(\tau \le T | X(0) = x) = P(\inf_{0 < t \le T} X(t) < 0),$$

whereas the probability of ultimate ruin is given by

$$\psi(x) = P(\tau < \infty | X(0) = x) = \lim_{T \to \infty} \psi(x, T).$$

Much of the literature on ruin theory is concentrated on classical risk model, in which the insurer starts with an initial surplus, and collects premiums continuously at a constant rate, while the aggregate claims process follows a compound Poisson process.

In 1957, Sparre Andersen (see, [19]) let claims occur according to a more general renewal process and derived an integral equation for the corresponding ruin probability. Since then, random walks and queuing theory have provided a more general framework, which has led to explicit results in the case where the interclaim times or the claim severities have distributions related to the Erlang or phase-type distributions.

Some *other generalizations of the basic model* will be outlined in the next subsubsection. Now, we only mention that ruin probability was investigated under various assumptions. Thus, the explicit formulas for ruin probability with dependence between risks, arising due to mixing over simple model parameters, were established in [13]. Archimedean dependence structure can be considered as a particular case of such procedure. Other classes of processes for which explicit expressions for ruin probability exist can be found in [25]. Estimates of ruin probabilities for Cramér–Lundberg model with stochastic premiums are established in [20]. Review of fluid methods in ruin theory is given in [40]. Generalization of De Vylder approximation for ruin probability is provided in [41].

The author of [80] deals with obtaining the optimal investment policy in a risky asset minimizing the ruin probability. The related objective of minimizing the expected discounted penalty paid at ruin is treated as well. Minimization of ruin probability by choosing the optimal investment is also the object of [57]. The authors consider an insurance company whose surplus is represented by the classical Cramér–Lundberg process. The company can invest its surplus in a risk-free asset and in a risky asset, governed by the Black–Scholes equation. There is a constraint that the insurance company can only invest in the risky asset at a limited leveraging level. The minimal ruin probability as a function of the initial surplus is characterized by a classical solution to the corresponding Hamilton–Jacobi–Bellman (HJB) equation. It is shown that the optimal investment policy significantly differs from those established in [203] for unrestricted case or in [35] for the case of no shortselling and no borrowing. Minimization of the ruin probability by investment and reinsurance is considered in [369].

Ruin probabilities with dependent rate interests are treated [99], whereas in [100] stochastic rates of interest and in [102] Markov Chain interests are assumed. The bounds for ruin probabilities in multivariate risk model are obtained in [103]. The ruin for the Erlang(n) risk process is tackled in [266]. Ruin probabilities for two classes of risk processes are studied in [269]. Ruin theoretical and financial applications of the first passage time for compound Poisson process perturbed by diffusion are given in [251]. Lundberg type bounds are obtained in [372] by investigation of renewal equations.

An important question in insurance is how to evaluate the probabilities of (non-) ruin of a company over any given horizon of finite length. The paper [261] aims to present some (not all) useful methods that have been proposed for computing, or approximating, these probabilities in the case of discrete claim severities. The starting model is the classical compound Poisson risk model with constant premium and independent and identically distributed claim severities. Two generalized versions of the model are then examined. The former incorporates a nonconstant premium function and a nonstationary claim process. The latter takes into account a possible interdependence between the successive claim severities. Special attention is paid to a recursive computational method that enables us to tackle, in a simple and unified way, the different models under consideration. The approach, still relatively little known, relies on the use of remarkable families of polynomials which are of Appell or generalized Appell (Sheffer) types.

Asymptotic behavior and estimates of ruin probabilities are given, e.g., in [26, 63, 123, 159, 187, 235]. Two papers, [321, 322], are devoted to investigation of ruin probabilities under capital injections. The paper [205] establishes the asymptotics of ruin probabilities for controlled risk processes in the small claims case.

A thorough survey of the ruin problem in risk models with investment income (until 2008) is presented in [333] (see also [331]). In addition to a general presentation of the problem, topics covered are a presentation of the relevant integro-differential equations, exact and numerical solutions, asymptotic results, bounds on the ruin probability and also the possibility of minimizing the ruin probability by investment and possibly reinsurance control. The main emphasis is on continuous-time models, but discrete-time models are also covered.

4.1.2 Gerber–Shiu Function

- *The ruin probability is a popular but not always a good risk measure.* To treat solvency problems, it is important to know the ruin time distribution and severity of ruin.

Already in 1988, Dufresne and Gerber (see [154]) in the classical compound Poisson model of the collective risk theory considered U, the surplus before the claim that causes ruin, and V, the deficit at the time of ruin. Let $f(x; u, v)$ be their joint density (x initial surplus) which is a defective probability density (since U and V are only defined, if ruin takes place). For an arbitrary claim amount distribution, they established that $f(0; u, v) = ap(u + v)$, where $p(z)$ is the probability density function of a claim amount and a is the ratio of the Poisson parameter and the rate of premium income. After that, the distribution of the surplus prior to ruin and that of the claim causing ruin were studied in [143, 144], respectively.

During 1997–1998, Gerber and Shiu (see [176, 177]) introduced the expected discounted penalty function (EDPF) taking into account the surpluses immediately before and at ruin. Since then, many researchers studied the following function

$$m(x) = \mathsf{E}(e^{-\delta\tau}w(X(\tau^-), |X(\tau)|)I(\tau < \infty)|X(0) = x),$$

where δ is the force of interest, $I(A)$ is indicator of event A and $w(x_1, x_2)$ is a nonnegative penalty function defined on $[0, \infty) \times [0, \infty)$.

- So one can see the unification of reliability and cost approaches. (The ruin probability is obtained for $\delta = 0$, $w(x_1, x_2) \equiv 1$.)

The joint analysis of these random variables, which had been traditionally studied separately, allowed to offer an elegant characterization of the ruin event in terms of a renewal equation.

The function $m(x)$ (called frequently EDPF) is useful whenever one wishes to place a value on cash flows triggered by the first passage of a process across a given barrier. Applications of the EDPF are natural not only in the context of solvency where it can be used to determine the initial capital required by a company to avoid insolvency with a minimum level of confidence, but in option pricing or dividends optimization as well. This is the case for credit risky securities, whose cash flows depend on a firm's assets falling below its liabilities, or for American options, whose exercise is triggered by the underlying security's market value crossing an exercise boundary.

By the end of the last century, Gerber and Landry (see [175]) and Gerber and Shiu (see [178]), for example, used the EDPF to price perpetual American options and reset guarantees.

The deficit at ruin and surplus before ruin were studied in [43] for a correlated risk process. Moments of the surplus before ruin and the deficit at ruin are obtained in [109] for Erlang-2 risk model. Approximations for moments of deficit at ruin for the case of exponential and sub-exponential claims are given in [110]. The distribution of the deficit at ruin when claims are phase-type is provided in [153]. The maximum surplus before ruin in an Erlang(n) risk process is treated in [265]. The moments of the time of ruin, the surplus before ruin, and the deficit at ruin are tackled in [281].

The ruin probability and the Gerber–Shiu function in a compound renewal (Sparre Andersen) risk process with interclaim times that have a K_n distribution (i.e., the Laplace transform of their density function is a ratio of two polynomials of degree at most $n \in N$) was studied in [267]. The Laplace transform of the expected discounted penalty function at ruin is derived. This leads to a generalization of the defective renewal equations given in [179, 410]. The explicit results are established for rationally distributed claim severities. The case of Erlang interclaim times has been studied in [179, 266].

By now, EDPF is usually called Gerber–Shiu function according to the names of its inventors. It was investigated in many papers under various assumptions about the underlying risk model. The almost universal approach of analysis is the derivation of some (defective) renewal equations, coming from a set of integro-differential equations which are obtained via Itô's formula or the infinitesimal generator of the risk reserve process. There exists already a special book [242] devoted to Gerber–Shiu risk theory.

Gerber–Shiu function is studied in [247] for the following generalization of Cramér–Lundberg model. The claim sizes are allowed to take positive as well as negative values. Depending on the sign of these amounts, they are interpreted either as claims made by insureds or as income from deceased annuitants, respectively. The classical risk model with a two-step premium rate is treated in [437]. Gerber–Shiu analysis in a perturbed risk model with dependence between claim sizes and interclaim times is implemented in [435]. A Sparre Andersen risk process perturbed by diffusion is dealt with in [268]. The Gerber–Shiu discounted penalty functions for a risk model with two classes of claims is investigated in [438].

In [116], a generalization of the usual penalty function is proposed, and a defective renewal equation is derived for the Gerber–Shiu discounted penalty function in the classical risk model. This is used to derive the trivariate distribution of the deficit at ruin, the surplus prior to ruin, and the surplus immediately following the second last claim before ruin. The marginal distribution of the last interclaim time before ruin is derived and studied, and its joint distribution with the claim causing ruin is derived. In [117], the results of previous paper are extended on the Sparre Andersen models allowing for possible dependence between claim sizes and interclaim times. The penalty function is assumed to depend on some or all of the surplus immediately prior to ruin, the deficit at ruin, the minimum surplus before ruin, and the surplus immediately after the second last claim before ruin. Defective joint and marginal distributions involving these quantities are derived. A discussion of Lundberg's fundamental equation and the generalized adjustment coefficient is given, and the connection to a defective renewal equation is considered.

The analysis of the Gerber–Shiu discounted penalty function for risk processes with Markovian arrivals is performed in [2]. The paper [32] concerns an optimal dividend distribution problem for an insurance company whose risk process evolves as a spectrally negative Lévy process (in the absence of dividend payments). The management of the company is assumed to control timing and size of dividend payments. The objective is to maximize the sum of the expected cumulative discounted dividend payments received until the moment of ruin and a penalty payment at the moment of ruin, which is an increasing function of the size of the shortfall at ruin. Compound geometric residual lifetime distributions and the deficit at ruin are studied in [411], whereas in [412] the author treats the discounted penalty function in the renewal risk model with general interclaim times.

The penalty delivered by the classical EDPF has local nature, in the sense that it only characterizes the surplus in a neighborhood of the ruin time. So, one can explore the possibility of introducing path-dependent variables in the EDPF such as the last minimum of the surplus before ruin (see [68]).

A generalized Gerber–Shiu measure for Markov additive risk processes with phase-type claims and capital injections is studied in [79]. It is supposed that the arrivals (either claims or capital injections) occur according to a Markovian point process. Both claim and capital injection sizes are phase-type distributed and the model allows for possible correlations between these and the interclaim times. The premium income is modeled by a Markov-modulated Brownian motion which may depend on the underlying phases of the point arrival process. For this risk reserve model, the authors derive a generalized Gerber–Shiu measure that is the joint distribution of the time to ruin, the surplus immediately before ruin, the deficit at ruin, the minimal risk reserve before ruin, and the time until this minimum is attained. The investigation is based on the results concerning the joint distribution of the space-time positions of overshoots and undershoots derived in [78] for Markov additive processes with phase-type jumps.

An explicit characterization of a generalized version of the Gerber–Shiu function in terms of scale functions is provided in [67] for spectrally negative Lévy insurance risk processes. The joint analysis of discounted aggregate claim costs until ruin is carried out in the recent thesis [282], the other ruin-related quantities are also examined.

- There arose the new research directions in actuarial sciences specific for modern period. They include, along with dividend payments, reinsurance, and investment problems.
- Thus, the treatment of complex models and consideration of new classes of processes, such as Markov-modulated processes, martingales, diffusion, Lévy processes or generalized renewal ones is needed.

- Several types of objective functions and various methods are used to implement the stochastic models optimization.

In order to understand the papers treating the modern actuarial problems, it is necessary to possess solid knowledge in the field of probability theory and stochastic processes. Let us mention Lévy processes (see, e.g., [21, 65, 241, 366]), point processes [215], Brownian motion and stochastic calculus [156, 227, 230], convergence of probability measures [69], limit theorems for stochastic processes [216] which are widely used nowadays by researchers. One has to be also acquainted with stochastic control and dynamic programming (see, e.g., [37, 327, 343, 370]), Markov decision processes [52] and controlled Markov processes [163]. Among the others, one finds in [40] fluid flow matrix analytic methods, in [238] Volterra integro-differential equations, in [309] renewal processes. It is necessary to be able to deal not only with ordinary differential equations (ODE), see, e.g., [197], but with SDE (stochastic differential equations), see, e.g. [328]. Very important area is risk management (see, e.g., [208, 300]). As previously, we stress that it is impossible to mention all the needed mathematical tools and sources to study them.

4.1.3 Dividends

- Now we turn to the decision problems arising in actuarial sciences.

We briefly recall that a *dividend* is a distribution of a portion of a company's earnings, decided by the board of directors, to a class of its shareholders. Dividends can be issued as cash payments, as shares of stock, or other property.

The study of dividends in insurance was proposed by B. de Finetti in 1957, see [139]. He argued that under net profit condition the company surplus could become infinitely large as time grows that is not realistic. So, it is necessary to decide when and how much to pay, in other words, to choose a dividend strategy.

There exist a lot of possible dividends strategies. The simplest one is a *barrier strategy* with barrier level b. Such a strategy means that there is no dividends payment if $X(t) < b$, whereas the payment intensity equals c (the premium rate), if $X(t) = b$.

Let $V(x, b) = \mathsf{E} \left[\int_0^\tau e^{-\delta t} \, dD(t) \right]$ be the expected discounted dividends until ruin time τ under barrier strategy with parameter b, whereas x denotes the initial company surplus, $0 \le x \le b$. Then, according to [181], $V(x, b)$, as a function of x, satisfies the following equation

$$cV'(x, b) - (\lambda + \delta)V(x, b) + \lambda \int_0^x V(y, b)p(x - y)dy = 0, \quad 0 < x < b, \quad (4)$$

with the boundary condition $V'(b, b) = 1$.

In [11], exact solutions for dividend strategies of threshold and linear barrier type in a Sparre Andersen model are established. Barrier strategies are studied in, e.g., [4, 9, 287, 291, 378, 429] under various assumptions.

The main drawback of a barrier strategy is that sooner or later the company surplus becomes negative bringing the ruin (or bankruptcy).

In a *threshold strategy*, no dividends are paid when the risk reserve is below a certain threshold, while above this threshold dividends are paid at a rate that is less than the rate of premium income, see, e.g., [38, 39, 44, 45, 121, 172, 279, 280, 284, 285, 311, 319, 400]. Such a strategy leads to probability of ruin less than 1.

It is necessary to mention multi-threshold (see, e.g., [6]) and band strategies (see, e.g., [36] or [370]) as well.

In insurance risk theory, dividend and aggregate claim amount are of great research interest as they represent the insurance company's payments to its shareholders and policyholders, respectively. Since the analyses of these two quantities are performed separately in the literature, the Gerber–Shiu expected discounted penalty function was generalized in [120] by further incorporating the moments of the aggregate discounted claims until ruin and the discounted dividends until ruin. While in [120], the authors considered the compound Poisson model with a dividend barrier in which ruin occurs almost surely, the paper [115] looks at this generalized Gerber–Shiu function under a threshold dividend strategy where the insurer has a positive survival probability. Because the Gerber–Shiu function is only defined for sample paths leading to ruin, the joint moments of the aggregate discounted claims and the discounted dividends without ruin occurring are also studied. Some explicit formulas are derived when the individual claim distribution follows a combination of exponentials. Numerical illustrations involving the correlation between aggregate discounted claims and discounted dividends are given.

Optimal dividend payments under a time of ruin constraint in case of exponential claims are considered by the authors of [199]. In [201], optimal dividend payment is studied under ruin constraint in three cases: de Finetti model in which time and space are discrete, continuous-time Brownian motion with drift model and Cramér–Lundberg model with exponential claims. Value function at each time point is supposed to depend on two variables (current surplus and current ruin probability). Dynamic equations are derived on the base of assumption that ruin probability does not exceed a given small α. They can be solved numerically in the discrete model and might be used to identify the optimal strategy in the other cases.

Dividend problems are also discussed in [8, 10, 15, 16, 28, 31, 32, 34, 36, 54, 55, 87, 89, 108, 124, 149, 160, 180, 181, 219, 220, 225, 239, 264, 270, 271, 275, 279, 287, 291, 292, 358, 376, 401, 431, 434, 439].

4.1.4 Investment

- Another notion we are going to use is *investment*.

To invest is to allocate money (or sometimes another resource, such as time) in the expectation of some benefit in the future. In finance, the expected future benefit from investment is a return. The return may consist of capital gain and/or investment income, including dividends, interest, rental income, etc.

Investment generally results in acquiring an asset, also called an investment. If the asset is available at a price worth investing, it is normally expected either to generate income, or to appreciate in value, so that it can be sold at a higher price (or both). It is worth mentioning that the Code of Hammurabi provided a legal framework for investment. Various aspects of investment role in company performance optimization are studied in many papers. We mention below only some recent results.

The optimal dividend problem for an insurance company whose uncontrolled reserve process evolves as a classical Cramér–Lundberg process is considered in [36]. The firm has the option of investing part of the surplus in a Black–Scholes financial market. The objective is to find a strategy consisting of both investment and dividend payment policies which maximizes the cumulative expected discounted dividend payouts until the time of bankruptcy. It is shown that the optimal value function is the smallest viscosity solution of the associated second-order integro-differential Hamilton–Jacobi–Bellman equation. The regularity of the optimal value function is studied. It is proved that the optimal dividend payment strategy has a band structure. A method is found to construct a candidate solution and obtain a verification result to check optimality. Finally, an example is given where the optimal dividend strategy is not barrier and the optimal value function is not twice continuously differentiable.

A combination of investment and reinsurance is treated in [66] under assumption of diffusion approximation. The aim is minimization of the absolute ruin risk (this notion will be discussed later). The paper [223] addresses the situation where the reserve of an insurance business is currently invested in an asset that may yield negative interest. Upper and lower bounds for the probability of ruin are obtained in the case where the cash flow of premiums less claims and the logarithm of the asset price are both Lévy processes. These bounds are in general power functions of the initial reserve. Thus, it is shown that risky investments may impair the insurer's solvency just as severely as do large claims. One can also find in this paper references on previous results concerning ruin problem and investment.

The paper [276] focuses on the optimal investment problem for an insurer and a reinsurer. The insurer's and reinsurer's surplus processes are both approximated by a Brownian motion with drift and the insurer can purchase proportional reinsurance from the reinsurer. In addition, both the insurer and the reinsurer are allowed to invest in a risk-free asset and a risky asset. First, the optimization problem of minimizing the ruin probability for the insurer is studied. Then according to the optimal reinsurance proportion chosen by the insurer, two optimal investment problems for the reinsurer are investigated, namely, the problem of maximizing the exponential utility and the problem of minimizing the ruin probability. By solving the corresponding Hamilton–Jacobi–Bellman (HJB) equations, optimal strategies for both the insurer and the reinsurer are derived explicitly. Furthermore, it is established that the reinsurer's optimal strategies in these two cases are equivalent for some special parameters. Finally, numerical simulations are presented to illustrate the effects of model parameters on the optimal strategies.

In [203], the ruin probability of the risk process, modeled as a compound Poisson process, is minimized by the choice of a suitable investment strategy in a risky asset (market index) that follows a geometric Brownian motion. The optimal strategy is computed using the Bellman equation. The existence of a smooth solution and a verification theorem are proved. The explicit solutions in some cases with exponential claim size distribution, as well as numerical results in a case with Pareto claim size, are given. For this last case, the optimal amount invested will not be bounded.

Optimal investment and proportional reinsurance in the Sparre Andersen model are treated in [278]. Optimal investment and risk control for an insurer under inside information are considered in [337]. Optimal investment, consumption, and proportional reinsurance under model uncertainty are studied in [338]. An extension of Paulsen–Gjessing's risk model with stochastic return on investments is dealt with in [430]. Expected utility maximization for insurer by optimal investment and risk control is provided in [445], see also [446].

Insurance models with stochastic return on investments are also considered in [57–62, 166, 169–171, 188, 189, 222, 332, 334, 340].

4.1.5   Reinsurance

- Now we have to answer what is *reinsurance*.

Reinsurance is the practice of insurers transferring portions of risk portfolios to other parties by some form of agreement in order to reduce the likelihood of having to pay a large obligation resulting from an insurance claim. The intent of reinsurance is for an insurance company to reduce the risks associated with underwritten policies by spreading risks across alternative institutions. It is well known as *insurance for insurers*. Legal rights of the policyholders (insureds) are in no way affected by reinsurance, and the insurer remains liable to the insureds for insurance policy benefits and claims.

The most popular approach is to minimize some measure of the first insurer's risk after reinsurance, although the interests of reinsurer are sometimes also taken into account. Thus, in [104] a "reciprocal reinsurance" was treated to consider the objectives of both companies, while in [213], portfolio selection problem for an insurer as well as a reinsurer aiming at maximizing the probability of survival is tackled. The authors of [48] propose a risk sharing approach in order to diversify the risk as much as possible, so as to make the "global market risk" (or systemic risk, in this paper) as close as possible to the total sum of partial risks. In other words, the paper deals with "reciprocal reinsurance contracts" involving n companies.

An optimal reinsurance strategy combining a proportional and an excess of loss reinsurance is obtained in [185] for a collective risk theory model with two classes of dependent risks. The aim is to maximize the expected utility of the terminal wealth. Using the control technique, the Hamilton–Jacobi–Bellman equation is written and, in the special case of the only excess of loss reinsurance, the optimal strategy and the corresponding value function are given in a closed form. In [315], more general case is studied, namely, optimal reinsurance in the model with several risks within one insurance policy.

A two-dimensional risk model with proportional reinsurance is treated in [47]. A review concerning optimal reinsurance up to year 2009 can be found in [106], whereas optimal reinsurance under ruin probability constraint is surveyed in [224]. In [49], the authors deal with optimization of reinsurance taking into account not only risk but uncertainty (or ambiguity) of statistical data possessed by insurer and reinsurer. The levels of uncertainty of insurer and reinsurer do not have to be identical. Furthermore, the decision variable is not the retained (or ceded) risk, but its sensitivity (mathematical derivative) with respect to the total claims. Thus, if one imposes strictly positive lower bounds for this variable, the reinsurer moral hazard is totally eliminated. Necessary and sufficient optimality conditions are given. The optimal reinsurance problem is shown to be equivalent to other linear programming problem (the double-dual problem), despite the fact that risk and uncertainty (and many pricing principles) cannot be represented by linear expressions. This fact explains why the nonlinear optimal reinsurance problem may be solved by a bang-bang reinsurance. Optimal investment, consumption, and proportional reinsurance under model uncertainty is treated in [338].

Optimal control of capital injections by reinsurance in a diffusion approximation is investigated in [157]. A correlated aggregate claims model with common Poisson shocks, which allows the dependence in n ($n \geq 2$) classes of business across m ($m \geq 1$) different types of stochastic events is presented in [209]. The dependence structure between different claim numbers is connected with the thinning procedure. Under combination of quota-share and excess of loss reinsurance arrangements, the properties of the proposed risk model are examined. An upper bound for the ruin probability determined by the adjustment coefficient is established through martingale approach. Optimal risk control and dividend policies under excess of loss reinsurance are considered in [313].

Optimal reinsurance under distortion risk measures is treated in [440, 441]. In the first paper, the authors impose a premium constraint, in the second one, expected value premium principle is applied for reinsurer. The paper [443] investigates optimal reinsurance strategies for an insurer with multiple lines of business under the criterion of minimizing its total capital requirement calculated based on the multivariate lower orthant Value at Risk. The reinsurance is purchased by the insurer for each line of business separately. The premium principles used to compute the reinsurance premiums are allowed to differ from one line of business to another, but they all satisfy three mild conditions: distribution invariance, risk loading and preserving the convex order, which are satisfied by many popular premium principles. It is shown that an optimal strategy for the insurer is to buy a two-layer reinsurance policy for each line of business, and it reduces to be a one-layer reinsurance contract for premium principles satisfying some additional mild conditions, which are met by the expected value principle, standard deviation principle, and Wang's principle among many others.

The risk models incorporating reinsurance can be also found in [34, 66, 72, 77, 86, 89, 96, 125, 206, 207, 225, 278, 295, 336, 390, 391].

4.1.6 Solvency

The *solvency problems* (see, e.g. [339, 365]), a company bankruptcy or liquidation gave rise to the introduction of new notions of ruin.

- *Absolute ruin*

Since its practical importance, the absolute ruin problem has attracted growing attention in risk theory. When the surplus is below zero or the insurer is on deficit, the insurer could borrow money at a debit interest rate to pay claims. Meanwhile, the insurer will repay the debts from the premium income. The negative surplus may return to a positive level. However, when the negative surplus is below a certain critical level, the surplus is no longer able to become positive. Absolute ruin occurs at this moment. One of the first papers in this direction is [174].

One of the latest is [167] where the dividend payments in a compound Poisson model with a constant debit interest r are considered. That is to say, the insurer can borrow an amount of money equal to the deficit at a debit interest force r when the surplus is negative. Meanwhile, the insurance company will repay the debts continuously from its premium income (acquired at rate c). Denoting the surplus of the insurer at time t with the debit interest r by $X(t)$, one easily gets the following equation satisfied

$$dX(t) = \begin{cases} cdt - dY(t), & X(t) \geq 0, \\ (c + rX(t))dt - dY(t), & -c/r \leq X(t) < 0, \end{cases} \tag{5}$$

where $Y(t)$ is given by (3). It is also assumed that dividends are paid to shareholders according to a barrier strategy with parameter $b > 0$. Under the barrier strategy, the premium incomes are paid out as dividends when the surplus reaches b, that is, when the value of the surplus hits b, dividends are paid continuously at rate c and the surplus remains at level b until the next claim occurs. Denote the aggregate dividends paid in the time interval $[0, t]$ by $D(t)$. So the modified surplus $X_b(t) = X(t) - D(t)$. The time of absolute ruin is defined as $T_b = \inf\{t > 0 : X_b(t) \leq -c/r\}$. Then $D_{x,b} = \int_0^{T_b} e^{-\delta t} dD(t)$ is the present value of all dividends payable to shareholders, till absolute ruin time T_b, calculated at a constant force of interest $\delta > 0$, whereas x is the initial surplus of insurer.

The authors investigate the moment generating function of $D_{x,b}$, that is, $M(x, y, b) = E \exp(y D_{x,b})$. They put $M(x, y, b) = M_1(x, y, b)$ for $0 \leq x \leq b$ and $M(x, y, b) = M_2(x, y, b)$ for $-c/r \leq x < 0$. Then, assuming the functions to be smooth in x and y and using the strong Markov property of the surplus process, they establish the following integro-differential equations. For $0 < x < b$

$$c(\partial/\partial x)M_1(x, y, b) = \delta y(\partial/\partial y)M_1(x, y, b) + \lambda M_1(x, y, b)$$

$$-\lambda \left[\int_0^x M_1(x - u, y, b)\, dF(u) + \int_x^{x+c/r} M_2(x - u, y, b)\, dF(u) + \bar{F}(x + c/r) \right]$$

and for $-c/r < x < 0$

$$(rx + c)(\partial/\partial x)M_2(x, y, b) = \delta y(\partial/\partial y)M_2(x, y, b) + \lambda M_2(x, y, b)$$

$$-\lambda \left[\int_0^{x+c/r} M_2(x - u, y, b)\, dF(u) + \bar{F}(x + c/r) \right].$$

Here, $\bar{F}(t) = 1 - F(t)$ and F is the distribution function of claim size. Additionally, $M(x, y, b)$ satisfies the following conditions

$$(\partial/\partial x)M_1(x, y, b) = yM_1(x, y, b), \quad x = b, \quad M_2(-c/r, y, b) = 1,$$

right and left limits of $M(x, y, b)$, as $x \to 0$, coincide.

This result allows to establish the equations for the moments of $D_{x,b}$ and calculate the explicit form of moments and $M(x, y, b)$ for the case of exponential claim distribution. Thus, it is possible to find the optimal dividend barrier for exponential claims.

Minimization of the risk of absolute ruin under a diffusion approximation model with reinsurance and investment is considered in [66]. On the contrary, in [101] it is assumed that the surplus of an insurer follows a compound Poisson surplus process. The expected discounted penalty function at absolute ruin is studied. Moreover, it is shown that when the initial surplus goes to infinity, the absolute ruin probability and the classical ruin probability are asymptotically equal for heavy-tailed claims, while the ratio of the absolute ruin probability to the classical ruin probability goes to a positive constant that is less than one for light-tailed claims. Explicit expressions for the function in exponential claims case are also given. Absolute ruin probability in a Markov risk model is treated in [286].

An Ornstein–Uhlenbeck type risk model is considered in [290]. The time value of absolute ruin in the compound Poisson process with tax is studied in [305]. First, a system of integro-differential equations satisfied by the expected discounted penalty function is derived. Second, closed-form expressions for the expected discounted total sum of tax payments until absolute ruin and the Laplace–Stieltjes transform (LST) of the total duration of negative surplus are obtained. Third, for exponential individual claims, closed-form expressions for the absolute ruin probability, the LST of the time to absolute ruin, the distribution function of the deficit at absolute ruin, and the expected accumulated discounted tax are given. Fourth, for general individual claim distributions, when the initial surplus goes to infinity, it is shown that the ratio of the absolute ruin probability with tax to that without tax goes to a positive constant which is greater than one. Finally, the asymptotic behavior of the absolute ruin probability is investigated for a modified risk model where the interest rate on a positive surplus is involved.

In [312], the absolute ruin in a Sparre Andersen risk model with constant interest is considered, whereas in [401, 402], the absolute ruin problems are treated for the classical risk model.

In the paper [296], it is assumed that the surplus process of an insurance entity is represented by a pure diffusion. The company can invest its surplus into a Black–Scholes risky asset and a risk-free asset. The following investment restrictions are imposed. Only a limited amount is allowed in the risky asset and no short-selling is allowed. When the surplus level becomes negative, the company can borrow to continue financing. The ultimate objective is to seek an optimal investment strategy that minimizes the probability of absolute ruin, i.e., the probability that the lim inf of the surplus process is $-\infty$. The corresponding Hamilton–Jacobi–Bellman (HJB) equation is analyzed and a verification theorem is proved. Applying the HJB method authors obtain explicit expressions for the S-shaped minimal absolute ruin function and its associated optimal investment strategy. In the second part of the paper, the optimization problem with both investment and proportional reinsurance control is studied. There, the minimal absolute ruin function and the feedback optimal investment-reinsurance control are found explicitly as well.

Absolute ruin probability for a multi-type-insurance risk model is treated in [422].

• *Parisian ruin*

In the last few years, the idea of Parisian ruin has attracted a lot of attention. The idea comes from Parisian options (see, e.g., [111]), the prices of which depend on the excursions of the underlying asset prices above or below a barrier. An example is a Parisian down-and-out option, the owner of which loses the option if the underlying asset price S reaches the level l and remains constantly below this level for a time interval longer than d.

In Parisian type ruin models, the insurance company is not immediately liquidated when it defaults: a grace period is granted before liquidation. More precisely, Parisian ruin occurs if the time spent below a predetermined critical level (red zone) is longer than the implementation delay, also called the clock. Originally, two types of Parisian ruin have been considered, one with deterministic delays (see, e.g., [132, 293]) and another one with stochastic delays ([253, 257]). These two types of Parisian ruin start a new clock each time the surplus enters the red zone, either deterministic or stochastic. A third definition of Parisian ruin, called cumulative Parisian ruin, has been proposed very recently in [191]; in that case, the race is between a single deterministic clock and the sum of the excursions below the critical level.

In the paper [289], the time of Parisian ruin with a deterministic delay is considered for a refracted Lévy insurance risk process.

In [293], for a spectrally negative Lévy process, a compact formula is given for the Parisian ruin probability, which is defined by the probability that the process exhibits an excursion below zero, with a length that exceeds a certain fixed period r. The formula involves only the scale function of the spectrally negative Lévy process and the distribution of the process at time r.

Another relevant paper is [257]. Here the authors study, for a spectrally negative Lévy process of bounded variation, a somewhat different type of Parisian stopping time, in which, loosely speaking, the deterministic, fixed delay r is replaced by an independent exponential random variable with a fixed parameter $p > 0$. To be a little bit more precise, each time the process starts a new excursion below zero, a new independent exponential random variable with parameter p is considered, and the stopping time of interest, let us denote it by $k_{exp}(p)$, is defined as the first time when the length of the excursion is bigger than the value of the accompanying exponential random variable. Although in insurance the stopping time $k_{exp}(p)$ is arguably less interesting than k_r (corresponding to a fixed delay r), working with exponentially distributed delays allowed the authors to obtain relatively simple expressions, for example, the Laplace transform of $k_{exp}(p)$ in terms of the so-called (q-)scale functions of X. In order to avoid a misunderstanding, we emphasize that, in the definition of $k_{exp}(p)$, by [257], there is not a single underlying exponential random variable, but a whole sequence (each attached to a separate excursion below zero); therefore $P_x(k_{exp}(p) \in dz)$ does not equal $\int_0^\infty pe^{-pr} P_x(k_r \in dz)\,dr$.

In the paper [137], a single barrier strategy is applied to optimize dividend payments in the situation where there is a time lag $d > 0$ between decision and implementation. Using a classical surplus process with exponentially distributed jumps, the optimal barrier b^* maximizing the expected present value of dividends is established.

Parisian-type ruin is treated in [357] for an insurance ruin model with an adaptive premium rate, referred to as restructuring/refraction, in which classical ruin and bankruptcy are distinguished. In this model, the premium rate is increased as soon as the wealth process falls into the red zone and is brought back to its regular level when the wealth process recovers. The analysis is focused mainly on the time a refracted Lévy risk process spends in the red zone (analogous to the duration of the negative surplus). Building on results from [243], the distribution of various functionals related to occupation times of refracted spectrally negative Lévy processes is obtained. For example, these results are used to compute both the probability of bankruptcy and the probability of Parisian ruin in this model with restructuring.

Other Parisian problems are treated in [414].

- *Omega model*

In classical risk theory, a company goes out of business as soon as ruin occurs, that is, when the surplus is negative for the first time. In the Omega model, there is a distinction between ruin (negative surplus) and bankruptcy (going out of business). It is assumed that even with a negative surplus, the company can do business as usual and continue until bankruptcy occurs. The probability for bankruptcy is quantified by a bankruptcy rate function $\omega(x)$, where x is the value of the negative surplus. The symbol for this function leads to the name Omega model. The idea of distinguishing ruin from bankruptcy comes from the impression that some companies and certain industries seem to be able to continue doing business even when they are technically ruined. This may especially be true for companies that are owned by governments or other companies. Such a model was introduced in [14]. Assuming that dividends can only be paid with a certain probability at each point of time, the authors derive closed-form formulas for the expected discounted dividends until bankruptcy under a barrier strategy. Subsequently, the optimal barrier is determined, and several explicit identities for the optimal value are found. The surplus process of the company is modeled by a Wiener process (Brownian motion). A similar model was also treated in [182] where the probability of bankruptcy and the expectation of a discounted penalty at the time of bankruptcy are determined. Explicit results are derived under assumption that the surplus process is described by the Brownian motion.

In [403], the Omega model with underlying Ornstein–Uhlenbeck type surplus process for an insurance company is considered. Explicit expressions for the expected discounted penalty function at bankruptcy with a constant bankruptcy rate and linear bankruptcy rate are derived. Based on random observations of the surplus process, the differentiability for the expected discounted penalty function at bankruptcy, especially at zero, is examined. Finally, the Laplace transforms for occupation times are given.

- *Drawdown analysis*

Another important research direction associated with solvency problems is drawdown analysis. The concept of drawdown is being used increasingly in risk analysis, as it provides surplus-related information similar to ruin-related quantities. For the insurer's surplus $\{X_t, t \geq 0\}$, the drawdown (or reflected) process Y_t is defined as the difference between its running maximum $M_t = \sup_{0 \leq s \leq t} X_s$ at time t and X_t.

A new drawdown-based regime-switching (DBRS) Lévy insurance model in which the underlying drawdown process is used to describe an insurer's level of financial distress over time, and to trigger regime-switching transitions is proposed in [259]. Explicit formulas are derived for a generalized two-sided exit problem. Conditions under which the survival probability is not trivially zero (which corresponds to the positive security loading conditions of the proposed model) are stated. The regime-dependent occupation time until ruin is later studied. As a special case of the general DBRS model, a regime-switching premium model is given further consideration. Connections with other existing risk models (such as the loss-carry-forward tax model of [7]) are established.

Some drawdown-related quantities in the context of the renewal insurance risk process with general interarrival times and phase-type distributed jump sizes are treated in [249]. Some recent results on the two-sided exit problem for the spectrally negative Markov additive process (see, e.g., [214]) and a fluid flow analogy between certain queues and risk processes (see, e.g., [4]) are used to solve the two-sided exit problem of the renewal insurance risk process. The two-sided exit quantities are later shown to be central to the analysis of such drawdown quantities as the drawdown time, the drawdown size, the running maximum (minimum) at the drawdown time, the last running maximum time prior to drawdown, the number of jumps before drawdown and the number of excursions from running maximum before drawdown. Finally, another application of this methodology is proposed for the study of the expected discounted dividend payments until ruin.

4.2   Generalization of the Classical Cramér–Lundberg Model

Generalization of the model has gone in the following directions.

- *Another type of counting process* for representation of claim number was introduced (instead of Poisson one).

A well known *Sparre Andersen model* appeared in 1957, see [19], and was studied in many papers afterwards. This model has also the mixed type, since the premium is supposed to be acquired continuously at a constant rate. Thus, the company surplus is described by (2) with $Y(t)$ given by (3) where $N(t)$ is assumed to be a renewal process. That means the intervals between the claims are nonnegative independent identically distributed random variables however their distribution is arbitrary (not exponential), see, e.g. [11, 146–148, 179, 254, 278, 312, 356, 388, 416].

Polya–Aeppli counting processes are treated in [306]. Generalized renewal process can be also considered as claim number, see, e.g., [88]. Two classes of claims were studied in [47, 184, 438], for multivariate case see, e.g., [103].

- *Dependence conditions*

In previous models, the counting process (number of events) and claim severities were supposed to be independent. Recently, this restriction was taken away. Various types of dependence exist between claim amounts and interarrival times.

In [33], a one-dimensional surplus process is considered with a certain Sparre Andersen type dependence structure under general interclaim times distribution and correlated phase-type claim sizes. The Laplace transform of the time to ruin is obtained as the solution of a fixed-point problem, under both the zero-delayed and the delayed cases. An efficient algorithm for solving the fixed-point problem is derived together with bounds that illustrate the quality of the approximation. A two-dimensional risk model is analyzed under a bailout-type strategy with both fixed and variable costs and a dependence structure of the proposed type.

In [46], the authors consider an extension of the Sparre Andersen insurance risk model by relaxing one of its independence assumptions. The newly proposed dependence structure is introduced through the assumption that the joint distribution of the interclaim time and the subsequent claim size is bivariate phase-type (see, e.g. [27, 240]). Relying on the existing connection between risk processes and fluid flows (see, e.g., [3, 4, 42, 44, 354]), an analytically tractable fluid flow is constructed. That leads to the analysis of various ruin-related quantities in the aforementioned risk model. Using matrix analytic methods, an explicit expression for the Gerber–Shiu discounted penalty function is obtained when the penalty function depends on the deficit at ruin only. It is investigated how some ruin-related quantities involving the surplus immediately prior to ruin can also be analyzed via the fluid flow methodology.

The discounted penalty function in a Markov-dependent risk model is considered in [5], whereas a correlated aggregate claims model with Poisson and Erlang risk processes is studied in [432]. Optimal dynamic proportional and excess of loss reinsurance under dependent risks are obtained in [185].

Other examples can be found in [13, 43, 74, 117, 128, 193, 198, 209, 252, 256, 258, 260, 274, 342, 350, 374, 389, 424, 432], as well as [119, 268, 283, 377, 423].

Several types of claims to treat heterogeneous insurance portfolios are considered in [438]. The authors obtain integro-differential equations for the Gerber–Shiu discounted penalty function, generalized Lundberg equation and Laplace transforms for the Gerber–Shiu discounted penalty function under assumption that the surplus process $X(t) = x + ct − Y(t)$, $t \geq 0$, is of the Cramér–Lundberg type where the aggregate claim process $Y(t)$ is generated by two classes of insurance risks, i.e.,

$$Y(t) = Y_1(t) + Y_2(t) = \sum_{i=1}^{N_1(t)} X_i + \sum_{i=1}^{N_2(t)} Y_i, \quad t \geq 0,$$

and $N_1(t)$ is a Poisson process and $N_2(t)$ is Erlang(n).

- *The Markovian claim arrivals, Markov additive processes (MAP), and Markov-modulated risk processes*

Beginning with [23, 355], researchers start consideration of risk processes in the Markovian environment.

Potential measures for spectrally negative Markov additive processes with applications in ruin theory are studied in [161]. Markovian arrivals were treated in [2, 112], where a unified analysis of claim costs up to ruin is given. In [118], a generalization of the risk model with Markovian claim arrivals is introduced. Moments of the discounted dividends in a threshold-type Markovian risk process are obtained in [38], whereas a multi-threshold Markovian risk model is analyzed in [45]. Analysis of a threshold dividend strategy for a MAP risk model is implemented in [44], while generalized penalty function with the maximum surplus prior to ruin in a MAP risk model is studied in [113], see also [252], where occupation times in the MAP risk model are treated.

For a Markov-modulated risk model, probability of ruin is obtained in [294], moments of the dividend payments and related problems are treated in [270], and decompositions of the discounted penalty functions and dividends-penalty identity are established in [271]. Bounds for the ruin probability in a Markovian modulated risk model are obtained in [417], while expected discounted penalty function is treated in [378], under additional assumption of constant barrier and stochastic income.

- *Spectrally negative Lévy processes* are considered in [31, 67, 132, 244, 253, 291, 293, 387, 429] and many other papers.

- *Perturbed and diffusion processes*

Ruin theory models incorporating a diffusion term aim to reflect small fluctuations in the insurance companies' surplus. Such fluctuations might be due to the uncertainty in the premium income or in the economic environment as a whole. Extensive research in this area has been carried out during the past 25 years.

We mention just a few papers. Thus, one of the first papers in this direction is [155] devoted to risk theory for the compound Poisson process perturbed by diffusion. In [400], dividend payments with a threshold strategy in the compound Poisson risk model perturbed by diffusion are considered. In [395], a generalized defective renewal equation for the surplus process perturbed by diffusion is studied, whereas in [264] the research focuses on the distribution of the dividend payments. The paper [251] treats the first passage times for compound Poisson processes with diffusion and provides actuarial and financial applications. The threshold dividend strategy is dealt with in [121] for a generalized jump-diffusion risk model. Gerber–Shiu function is investigated in [122] for a classical risk process perturbed by diffusion, while a linear barrier dividend strategy is a subject of [287]. The perturbed compound Poisson risk model with constant interest and a threshold dividend strategy is treated in [172]. The Gerber–Shiu function in a Sparre Andersen risk model perturbed by diffusion is studied in [268], whereas in [283] a generalized discounted penalty function is considered. A multi-threshold compound Poisson process perturbed by diffusion is investigated in [311]. Gerber–Shiu analysis in a perturbed risk model with dependence between claim sizes and interclaim times is provided in [435]. Absolute ruin minimization under a diffusion approximation model is carried out in [296]. The optimal dividend strategy in a regime-switching diffusion model is established in [405]. In contrast to classical case, it is assumed there that the dividends can be only paid at arrival times of a Poisson process. By solving an auxiliary optimization problem, it is shown that optimal is a modulated barrier strategy. The value function can be obtained by iteration or by solving a system of differential equations.

- *Stochastic premiums*

To reflect the cash flows of the insurance company more realistically, some papers assumed that the insurer earns random premium income. In the simplest case, the company surplus at time t is given by (2) where $Z(t)$ and $Y(t)$ are independent compound Poisson processes (with different intensities and jumps distributions). An interesting example is presented in the book [237] for modeling the speculative activity of money exchange point and optimization of its profit by using such a process.

In [308], the authors consider a generalization of the classical risk model when the premium intensity depends on the current surplus of an insurance company. All surplus is invested in the risky asset, the price of which follows a geometric Brownian motion. An exponential bound is established for the infinite-horizon ruin probability.

Models with stochastic premiums or income were also studied in [20, 76, 183, 195, 246, 288, 378, 393, 394, 444] and many others.

- *Dual processes*

In a model dual to classical Cramér–Lundberg one, see, e.g. [12], the surplus (without dividends) is described by the following equation

$$X(t) = x - ct + Y(t), \tag{6}$$

where c is now the rate of expenses, assumed to be deterministic and fixed. The process $Y(t)$ is compound Poisson. Such a model is natural for companies that have occasional gains whose amount and frequency can be modeled by the process $\{Y(t)\}$. For companies such as pharmaceutical or petroleum companies, the jump should be interpreted as the net present value of future gains from an invention or discovery. Other examples are commission-based businesses, such as real estate agent offices or brokerage firms that sell mutual funds of insurance products with a front-end load. Last but not least, a model of the form (6) might be appropriate for an annuity or pension fund. In this context, the probability of ruin has been calculated, see, e.g., [371]. The dividend problem for such a model is treated in [12]. A key tool is the method of Laplace transforms. A more general case where surplus is a skip-free downwards Lévy process is considered as well. The optimal strategy is of barrier type, the optimal barrier b^* is obtained. It is also shown that if the initial surplus is b^*, the expectation of the discounted dividends until ruin is the present value of a perpetuity with the payment rate being the drift of the surplus process.

A short proof of the optimality of barrier strategies for all spectrally positive Lévy processes of bounded or unbounded variation is given in [54]. Moreover, the optimal barrier is characterized using a functional inverse of the scale functions. A variant of the dividend payment problem in which the shareholders are expected to give capital injection in order to avoid ruin is also considered. The form of the value function for this problem is very similar to the problem in which the horizon is the time of ruin. The optimal dividend problem for a spectrally positive Lévy process is also considered in [428].

Optimal dividends in the dual model under transaction costs are treated in [55].

The time value of Parisian ruin in (dual) renewal risk processes with exponential jumps is considered in [415]. Other dual models are also considered in [108, 284, 319, 320].

- *Interest rates*

In recent years, the classical risk process has been extended to more practical and real situations. Thus, it is very important to deal with the risks that rise from monetary inflation in the insurance and finance market, and also to consider the operation uncertainties in administration of financial capital.

An optimal control problem is considered in [204] under assumption that a risky asset is used for investment, and this investment is financed by initial wealth as well as by a state dependent income. The objective function is accumulated discounted expected utility of wealth. Solution of this problem enables the authors to deal with the problem of optimal investment for an insurer with an insurance business modeled by a compound Poisson or a compound Cox process, under the presence of constant as well as (finite state space Markov) stochastic interest rate.

The aim of the paper [351] is to build recursive and integral equations for ruin probabilities of generalized risk processes under rates of interest with homogenous Markov chain claims and homogenous Markov chain premiums, while the interest rates follow a first-order autoregressive process. Generalized Lundberg inequalities for ruin probabilities of this process are derived by using recursive technique. Interest bearing surplus model with liquid reserves is considered in [373].

Asymptotic finite-time ruin probability for a two-dimensional renewal risk model with constant interest force and dependent sub-exponential claims is studied in [424]. The absolute ruin problems taking into account debit and credit interest rates are investigated, e.g., in [401, 402, 442] under some additional assumptions. A model with interest is studied in [310]. A multi-threshold compound Poisson surplus process is introduced there as follows. When the initial surplus is between any two consecutive thresholds, the insurer has the option to choose the respective premium rate and interest rate. Also, the model allows for borrowing the current amount of deficit whenever the surplus falls below zero. Explicit expressions for the Gerber–Shiu function are obtained if claim sizes are exponentially and phase-type(2) distributed.

5   Discrete-Time Models

A review [272] on discrete-time insurance models appeared in 2009. The authors underline that although most theoretical risk models use the concept of time continuity, the practical reality is discrete. Thus, dividend payment is usually based on results of financial year, whereas reinsurance treaties are discussed by the end of a year. It is important that recursive formulas for discrete-time models can be obtained without assuming a claim severity distribution and are readily programmable. The models, techniques used, and results for discrete-time risk models are of independent scientific interest. Moreover, results for discrete-time risk models can give, in addition, a simpler understanding of their continuous-time analog. For example, these results can serve as approximations or bounds for the corresponding results in continuous-time models. The expected discounted penalty functions and their special cases in the compound binomial model and its extensions are reviewed. In particular, the discrete-time Sparre Andersen models with K_m interclaim times and general interclaim times are treated, as well as other extensions to the compound binomial model including time-correlated claims and general premium rates, the compound Markov binomial risk model, and the compound binomial model defined in a Markovian environment.

Two papers [344, 345], not included in [272], deal with finite-time and ultimate ruin probability, respectively, for the following discrete-time model. It is supposed that the cumulative loss process has independent and stationary increments, the increments per unit of time take nonnegative integer values and their distribution $\{a_k\}_{k\geq 0}$ has a finite mean $\bar{a}$. The premium receipt process $\{c_k\}_{k\geq 0}$ is deterministic, nonnegative, and nonuniform. In addition, it is assumed that there exists a constant $c > \bar{a}$ such that the deviation $\sum_{k=0}^{t}(c_k - c)$ is bounded as the time t varies. In particular, $P(\tau = \infty)$, where τ is the ruin time, is obtained as $\lim_{t\to\infty} P(\tau > t)$, first, if $c = d^{-1}$ for some positive integer d, then general case if $a_0 > 0.5$.

A class of compound renewal (Sparre Andersen) risk processes with claim waiting times having a discrete K_m distribution is studied in [262, 263]. The classical compound binomial risk model is a special case when $m = 1$. A recursive formula is derived in the former paper for the expected discounted penalty (Gerber–Shiu) function, which can be used to analyze many quantities associated with the time of ruin. In the latter paper, an explicit formula for the Gerber–Shiu function is given in terms of a compound geometric distribution function. The finite-time ruin probability under the compound binomial model is treated in [273].

Discrete-time multi-risks insurance model is considered in [346]. The model describes the evolution in discrete time of an insurance portfolio covering several interdependent risks. The main problem under study is the determination of the probabilities of ruin over a finite horizon, for one or more risks. An underlying polynomial structure in the expression of these probabilities is exhibited. This result is then used to provide a simple recursive method for their numerical evaluation.

The discounted factorial moments of the deficit in discrete-time renewal risk model are treated in [50]. The discrete stationary renewal risk model and the Gerber–Shiu discounted penalty function were considered in [335].

We would also like to mention some papers considering other aspects of discrete-time models. Thus, two discrete-time risk models under rates of interest are dealt with in [98]. Stochastic inequalities for the ruin probabilities are derived by martingales and renewal recursive techniques.

In [149], the authors discuss a situation in which a surplus process is modified by the introduction of a constant dividend barrier. They extend some known results relating to the distribution of the present value of dividend payments until ruin in the classical risk model by allowing the process to continue after ruin. Moreover, they show how a discrete-time risk model can be used to provide approximations when analytic results are unavailable. Discrete-time financial surplus models for insurance companies are proposed in [218]. A generalization of the expected discounted penalty function in a discrete-time insurance risk model is introduced in [250].

Survival probabilities for compound binomial risk model with discrete phase-type claims are dealt with in [397]. Asymptotic ruin probabilities for a discrete-time risk model with dependent insurance and financial risks are obtained in [427], the ruin probability in a dependent discrete-time risk model with insurance and financial risks is studied in [426], whereas asymptotic results are established for a discrete-time risk model with Gamma-like insurance risks in [425]. Discrete-time insurance risk models with dependence structure are treated in the thesis [404]. A thorough analysis of the generalized Gerber–Shiu function in discrete-time dependent Sparre Andersen model is presented in the quite recent thesis [350].

Randomized observation periods were considered for compound Poisson risk model in [16] in connection with dividend payments. The authors study a modification of the horizontal dividend barrier strategy by introducing random observation times at which dividends can be paid and ruin can be observed. This model contains both the continuous-time and the discrete-time risk model as a limit and represents a certain type of bridge between them which still enables the explicit calculation of moments of total discounted dividend payments until ruin. In [17] for Erlang(n) distributed inter-observation times, explicit expressions for the discounted penalty function at ruin are derived. The resulting model contains both the usual continuous-time and the discrete-time risk model as limiting cases, and can be used as an effective approximation scheme for the latter. Optimal dividend payout in random discrete time is treated in [15].

In [434], a Markov additive insurance risk process under a randomized dividend strategy in the spirit of [16] is considered. Decisions on whether to pay dividends are only made at a sequence of dividend decision time points whose intervals are Erlang(n) distributed. At a dividend decision time, if the surplus level is larger than a predetermined dividend barrier, then the excess is paid as a dividend as long as ruin has not occurred. In contrast to [16], it is assumed that the event of ruin is monitored continuously (as in [30, 433]), i.e., the surplus process is stopped immediately once it drops below zero. The quantities of interest include the Gerber–Shiu expected discounted penalty function and the expected present value of dividends paid until ruin. Solutions are derived with the use of Markov renewal equations. Numerical examples are given, and the optimal dividend barrier is identified in some cases.

In [229], the authors focus on the development of a recursive computational procedure to calculate the finite-time ruin probabilities and expected total discounted dividends paid prior to ruin associated with a model which generalizes the single threshold-based risk model introduced in [152]. Namely, a discrete-time dependent Sparre Andersen risk model with multiple threshold levels is considered in an effort to characterize an insurer's minimal capital requirement, dividend paying scenarios, and external financial activities related to both investment and loan undertakings.

Computational aspects are also treated in [18]. A Sparre Andersen insurance risk model in discrete time was analyzed there as a doubly infinite Markov chain to establish a computational procedure for calculating the joint probability distribution of the time of ruin, the surplus immediately prior to ruin, and the deficit at ruin. Discounted factorial moments of the deficit in discrete-time renewal risk model are studied in [50].

Cost approach for solving discrete-time actuarial problems was introduced in [90], see also [89, 93–96].

The paper [70] deals with the discrete-time risk model with nonidentically distributed claims. The recursive formula of finite-time ruin probability is obtained, which enables one to evaluate the probability of ruin with desired accuracy. Rational valued claims and nonconstant premium payments are considered.

In [226], a discrete-time model of insurance company is considered. It is supposed that the company applies a dividend barrier strategy. The limit distribution for the time of ruin normalized by its expected value is found. It is assumed that shareholders cover the deficit at the time of ruin. The barrier strategies maximizing shareholders' dividends and profit accumulated until ruin are investigated. In case the additional capital is injected right after the ruin to enable infinite performance of the company, existence of optimal strategies is proved both for expected discounted dividends and net profit.

A discrete-time model for the cash flow of an insurance portfolio/business in which the net losses are random variables, while the return rates are fuzzy numbers was studied in [399]. The shape of these fuzzy numbers is assumed trapezoidal, Gaussian or lognormal, the last one having a more flexible shape than the previous ones. For the resulting fuzzy model, the fuzzy present value of its wealth is evaluated. The authors propose an approximation for the chance of ruin and a ranking criterion which could be used to compare different risk management strategies. A discrete-time insurance model with reinvested surplus and a fuzzy number interest rate is investigated in [307].

The discrete-time risk model with nonidentically distributed claims is studied in [70]. The recursive formula of finite-time ruin probability is obtained, which enables one to evaluate the probability of ruin with desired accuracy. Rational valued claims and nonconstant premium payments are considered. Some numerical examples of finite-time ruin probability calculation are presented. Ruin probability in the three-seasonal discrete-time risk model is obtained in [190]. It is also interesting to mention a discrete-time pricing model for individual insurance contracts studied in [325].

6 Examples

Below, we give three simple examples to demonstrate the problems and methods we did not discuss earlier and present some results of the author. At first, we deal with dividends optimization by reinsurance treaty with liability constraint, published in [87]. Then the stability of the periodic review model of insurance company performance with capital injections and reinsurance, introduced in [96], is studied. The full version of this results will be submitted for publication elsewhere. Finally, some limit theorems for generalized renewal processes introduced in [88] are provided.

6.1 Limited Liability of Reinsurer and Dividends

Below, we give some results proved in [87] concerning the dividend payments under barrier strategy and excess of loss reinsurance with limited liability of reinsurer in the framework of Cramér–Lundberg model.

Denote by d the retention level and by l the reinsurer's liability. Let Y be the initial claim size of direct insurer. Then, his payment under the above mentioned treaty is $Y_l = \min(d, Y) + \max(Y - l - d, 0)$, whereas the reinsurer's payment is equal to $Y_l' = \min(\max(Y - d, 0), l)$. We assume that $X(0) = x \le b$, hence, the insurer's surplus $X(t)$ never exceeds the dividend barrier b.

Let us suppose that direct insurer and reinsurer use for premiums calculation the expected value principle with loads θ and θ_1 respectively (and $\theta_1 > \theta > 0$). Then the insurer's premium net of reinsurance c_l has the form

$$c_l = \lambda(1 + \theta)p_1 - \lambda(1 + \theta_1) \int_d^{d+l} (1 - F(y)) \, dy$$

where λ is the intensity of the Poisson process describing claim arrivals, $F(y)$ is the claim distribution function with density $p(y)$ and the expected claim value $p_1 = \int_0^\infty yp(y)\,dy$.

Theorem 1 *The integro-differential equation for expected total discounted dividends until ruin, under reinsurance treaty, $V(x, b, d, l)$ can be written for $0 < x < d$ as follows*

$$\tilde{c}_l V'(x, b, d, l) - (1 + \alpha)V(x, b, d, l) + \int_0^x V(y, b, d, l)p(x - y)\,dy = 0$$

and for $d \leq x < b$

$$\tilde{c}_l V'(x, b, d, l) - (1 + \alpha)V(x, b, d, l) + \int_{x-d}^x V(y, b, d, l)p(x - y)\,dy$$

$$+V(x - d, b, d, l)(F(d + l) - F(d)) + \int_0^{x-d} V(y, b, d, l)p(l + x - y)\,dy = 0$$

with $\tilde{c}_l = c_l\lambda^{-1}$, $\alpha = \delta\lambda^{-1}$ and boundary condition $V'(b, b, d, l) = 1$.

Turning to exponential claim distribution with parameter β, one obtains the following results.

Theorem 2 *For $0 < x < d$, the function $V(x, b, d, l)$ satisfies the second-order differential equation*

$$\tilde{c}_l V''(x, b, d, l) + (\beta\tilde{c}_l - (1 + \alpha))V'(x, b, d, l) - \alpha\beta V(x, b, d, l) = 0,$$

whereas for $d \leq x < b$ one has

$$\tilde{c}_l V''(x, b, d, l) + (\beta\tilde{c}_l - (1 + \alpha))V'(x, b, d, l) - \alpha\beta V(x, b, d, l)$$
$$= -e^{-\beta d} F(l)V'(x - d, b, d, l).$$

Here, $\tilde{c}_l = \beta^{-1}\left((1 + \theta) + (1 + \theta_1)e^{-\beta d}(e^{-\beta l} - 1)\right)$.

Theorem 3 *For the exponential claim distribution, the optimal dividend barrier, under excess of loss reinsurance treaty with limited liability of reinsurer and assumption $0 < x \leq b < d$, is given by*

$$b_l^* = b^*(r_l, s_l) = \frac{1}{r_l - s_l} \ln \frac{s_l^2(s_l + \beta)}{r_l^2(r_l + \beta)}.$$

Here, $r_l > 0$, $s_l < 0$ are the roots of the characteristic equation

$$\tilde{c}_l \xi^2 + (\beta \tilde{c}_l - (1 + \alpha)) \xi - \alpha \beta = 0.$$

Assume the claims to be uniformly distributed on the interval $[0, h]$. It is reasonable to suppose that $d + l < h$.

Theorem 4 *For $0 < x < d$, the function $V(x, b, d, l)$ satisfies the second-order differential equation*

$$\tilde{c}_l V''(x, b, d, l) - (1 + \alpha) V'(x, b, d, l) + \frac{1}{h} V(x, b, d, l) = 0, \tag{7}$$

whereas for $d \le x < h - l$ one has

$$\tilde{c}_l V''(x, b, d, l) - (1 + \alpha) V'(x, b, d, l) + \frac{1}{h} V(x, b, d, l) + \frac{l}{h} V'(x - d, b, d, l) = 0 \tag{8}$$

and for $h - l \le x < b$

$$\tilde{c}_l V''(x, b, d, l) - (1 + \alpha) V'(x, b, d, l) + \frac{1}{h} V(x, b, d, l) \tag{9}$$

$$+ \frac{l}{h} V'(x - d, b, d, l) - \frac{1}{h} V(x - (h - l), b, d, l) = 0.$$

Here, $\tilde{c}_l = (1 + \theta)\frac{h}{2} - l(1 + \theta_1)(1 - \frac{2d+l}{2h})$.

Theorem 5 *If the claim distribution is uniform on interval $[0, h]$ and the roots of characteristic equation corresponding to differential equation (7) are real then the optimal dividend barrier b under assumption $0 < x \le b < d$ is equal to initial capital of insurance company x.*

To calculate $V(x, b, d, l)$ for $d \le x < b$ it is possible to use the following algorithm

1. Find expression of $V(x, b, d, l)$ on interval $(0, d)$.
2. Let $h - l \in (nd, (n + 1)d]$ for $n = 1, 2, \ldots$. The form of the function on half-interval $[kd, (k + 1)d)$ for $1 \le k \le n - 1$ can be obtained using its form on half-interval $[(k - 1)d, kd)$ and Eq. (8), the same is true for the last half-interval $[nd, h - l)$.
3. For $x \in [h - l, (n + 1)d)$ according to (9) the function $V(x, b, d, l)$ depends on $V'(x - d, b, d, l)$ and $V(x - (h - l), b, d, l)$. The same is true for $x \ge (n + 1)d$. Similarly, for $h - l \le x < b$, we use the expression of the function on two previous half-intervals.

Thus, for the exponential and uniform claim distributions, we have considered the barrier dividend strategy and obtained the form of optimal barrier level b_l^* for the model with limited reinsurer's liability l in the excess of loss reinsurance treaty having retention d.

Some results pertaining to the case of variable barriers which are changed after each claim arrival are obtained in [316], whereas a generalization of Lundberg inequality for the case of a joint-stock insurance company one can find in [314].

6.2 Discrete-Time Model with Reinsurance and Capital Injections

A periodic review insurance model is considered under the following assumptions. In order to avoid ruin, the insurer maintains the company surplus above a chosen level a by capital injections at the end of each period. One-period insurance claims form a sequence $\{\xi_n\}_{n\geq 1}$ of independent identically distributed nonnegative random variables with a known distribution function and finite mean. The company concludes at the end of each period the stop-loss reinsurance treaty. If the retention level is denoted by $z > 0$ then $c(z)$ is the insurer premium (net of reinsurance). It is necessary to choose the sequence of retention levels minimizing the total discounted injections during n periods.

Let x be the initial surplus of insurance company. One-period minimal capital injections are defined as follows

$$h_1(x) := \inf_{z>0} \mathsf{E}J(x, z), \quad \text{where} \quad J(x, z) = (\min(\xi, z) - (x - a) - c(z))^+.$$

For the n-step model, $n \geq 1$, the company surplus $X(n)$ at time n is given by the relation

$$X(n) = \max(X(n - 1) + c(z) - \min(\xi, z), a), \quad X(0) = x.$$

It was proved in [96] that the minimal expected discounted costs injected in company during n years satisfy the following Bellman equation

$$h_n(x) = \inf_{z>0}(\mathsf{E}J(x, z) + \alpha \mathsf{E}h_{n-1}(\max(x + c(z) - \min(\xi, z), a))), \quad h_0(x) = 0,$$
$$(10)$$

where $0 < \alpha < 1$ is the discount factor.

Under assumption that premiums of insurer and reinsurer are calculated according to mean value principle, the optimal reinsurance strategy was established. It turned out that its character depends on the relationship between the safety loading of insurer and reinsurer.

An important problem is investigation of the system asymptotic behavior and its stability with respect to parameters fluctuation and perturbation of underlying processes. It was established in [96] that $h_n(x) \to h(x)$ as $n \to \infty$ uniformly in x.

The analysis of the model sensitivity to cost parameters fluctuations is carried out, in the same way as in [95], using the results of [92, 324, 364, 386].

To study the perturbations of the processes one has to use the probability metrics, see, e.g., [353].

Definition 2 For random variables X and Y defined on some probability space $(\Omega, \mathscr{F}, P)$ and possessing finite expectations, it is possible to define their distance on the base of Kantorovich metric in the following way

$$\kappa(X, Y) = \int_{-\infty}^{+\infty} |F(t) - G(t)| dt,$$

where F and G are the distribution functions of X and Y respectively.

This metric coincides (see, e.g. [150] or [382]) with Wasserstein L_1 metric defined as $d_1(F, G) = \inf \mathsf{E}|X - Y|$ where infimum is taken over all jointly distributed X and Y having marginal distribution functions (d.f.'s) F and G. It is supposed that both d.f.'s belong to $\mathscr{B}_1$ consisting of all F such that $\int_{-\infty}^{+\infty} |x| \, dF(x) < \infty$.

Lemma 1 *The following statements are valid.*
1. Let $F^{-1}(t) = \inf\{x : F(x) \geq t\}$, then $d_1(F, G) = \int_0^1 |F^{-1}(t) - G^{-1}(t)| \, dt$.
2. $(\mathscr{B}_1, d_1)$ is a complete metric space.
3. For a sequence $\{F_n\}_{n \geq 1}$ from $\mathscr{B}_1$ one has $d_1(F_n, F) \to 0$ if and only if $F_n \overset{d}{\to}$
F_n and $\int_{-\infty}^{+\infty} |x| \, dF_n(x) \to \int_{-\infty}^{+\infty} |x| \, dF(x)$, as $n \to \infty$. Here $\overset{d}{\to}$ denotes, as usual, convergence in distribution.

The proof can be found in [150].

Lemma 2 *Let X, Y be nonnegative random variables possessing finite expected values and $\kappa(X, Y) \leq \rho$. Assume also that $g : R^+ \to R^+$ is a nondecreasing Lipschitz function. Then $\kappa(g(X), g(Y)) \leq C\rho$ where C is the Lipschitz constant.*

The next result enables us to estimate the difference between infimums of two functions.

Lemma 3 *Let functions $f_1(z)$, $f_2(z)$ be such that $|f_1(z) - f_2(z)| < \delta$ for some $\delta > 0$ and any $z > 0$. Then $|\inf_{z>0} f_1(z) - \inf_{z>0} f_2(z)| < \delta$.*

Note that we are going to add the label X to all functions depending on ξ if $\xi \sim law(X)$.

Putting $\Delta_1 := \sup_{u>a} |h_{1x}(u) - h_{1y}(u)|$, we prove the following result.

Theorem 6 *Let X, Y be nonnegative random variables possessing finite expectations, moreover $\kappa(X, Y) \leq \rho$. Then*

$$\Delta_1 \leq (1 + l + m)\rho$$

where l and m are the safety loading coefficients of insurer and reinsurer premiums, respectively. Both premiums are calculated according to expected value principle and $1 < l < m$.

For the multistep case, we get the following results.

Lemma 4 *Function $h_n(u)$ defined by (10) is non-increasing in u.*

Lemma 5 *For each $n \geq 0$ and any $u \geq a$, the following inequality is valid*

$$|h_n(u + \Delta u) - h_n(u)| \leq C_n \Delta u,$$

where $C_n = (1 - \alpha^n)(1 - \alpha)^{-1}$.

To establish the model stability, we put $\Delta_n = \sup_{u>a} |h_{nX}(u) - h_{nY}(u)|$ and formulate the following result.

Theorem 7 *Let X, Y be nonnegative random variables having finite means and $\kappa(X, Y) \leq \rho$. Then*

$$\Delta_n \leq \left(\sum_{i=0}^{n-1} \alpha^i C_{n-i} \right) (1 + l + m)\rho,$$

here $0 < \alpha < 1$ is the discount factor, $1 < l < m$ are the safety loadings of insurer and reinsurer and C_k, $k \leq n$, were defined in Lemma 5.

Furthermore, in practice neither the exact values of parameters nor the processes distributions are known. Thus, it is important to study the systems behavior under incomplete information. The estimates of distribution parameters are easily obtained on the base of previous observations.

If there is no a priori information, it may be useful to employ the empirical processes, see, e.g., [382].

For each fixed $t \in R$, the difference $H_n(\omega, t) =: F_n(\omega, t) - G_n(\omega, t)$ of two empirical distribution functions is a real-valued function of the random vector $(X_1, Y_1, \ldots, X_n, Y_n)$ defined on a probability space $(\Omega, \mathscr{F}, P)$, namely,

$$H_n(\omega, t) = \frac{1}{n} \sum_{i=1}^{n} I\{X_i \leq t\} - \frac{1}{n} \sum_{i=1}^{n} I\{Y_i \leq t\} = \frac{1}{n} \sum_{i=1}^{n} \zeta_i(t),$$

where $\zeta_i(t) = I\{X_i \leq t\} - I\{Y_i \leq t\}$, $i = \overline{1, n}$.

According to properties of convergence in distribution, we get immediately the following result

Lemma 6 *For any $t \in R$, as $n \to \infty$,*

$$\sqrt{n} |F_n(\omega, t) - G_n(\omega, t) - (F(t) - G(t))| \xrightarrow{d} \sqrt{F(t) + G(t) - (F^2(t) + G^2(t))} |N(0, 1)|.$$

We have also obtained a functional limit theorem. The established results are used to construct the empirical asymptotically optimal policies for the discrete-time model. The following three-step algorithm is proposed

1. Find the optimal control for known parameters and distributions.
2. Obtain stationary asymptotically optimal policy.
3. Calculate empirical asymptotically optimal policy using previous observations.

6.3 Generalized Renewal Processes

It is well known that ordinary renewal processes are widely used in various applications of probability theory not only in insurance, see, e.g., [309]. However, they are appropriate for the study of systems with time-homogeneous evolution.

In order to take into account the initial phase of a system functioning or its seasonal variations several generalizations of renewal processes are introduced, see, e.g., [88]. We focus here on delayed periodic processes and investigate their asymptotic behavior, in particular, state the strong law of large numbers and functional limit theorem. Some results concerning the reward-renewal processes are also provided.

Definition 3 Let $\{T_n\}_{n \geq 1}$ be a sequence of independent nonnegative random variables, F_j, $j = 1, \ldots, l$, being the distribution function of variable T_{ql+j} for some fixed integer $l \geq 1$, $q = 0, 1, \ldots$. Let $\{X_i\}_{i=0,\ldots,k-1}$ be another sequence of nonnegative independent r.v.'s with distribution functions G_i, respectively. The sequences $\{T_n\}$ and $\{X_i\}$ are also supposed to be independent.

The delayed periodical renewal process is formed in the following way: $S_n = X_0 + \cdots + X_n$, $0 \leq n \leq k - 1$, whereas $S_n = S_{k-1} + T_1 + \cdots + T_{n-k+1}$ for $n \geq k$. The partial sums S_n are called the renewals (or renewal epochs) and the summands X_j and T_i are the intervals between the renewals.

It is reasonable to call l the *process period* and k the *length of delay*, thus we have, say (k, l)-process. Taking $l = 1$, $k = 1$ and $X_0 = 0$, we obtain the ordinary renewal process. We can also consider the following types of generalized renewal processes

- generalized delayed process corresponds to $l = 1$, $k > 1$,
- putting $k = 1$, $X_0 = 0$ and leaving $l > 1$ we obtain a periodic renewal process;
- a special case of the periodic process with $l = 2$ is a well-known alternating process.

The asymptotic behavior of ordinary renewal process is thoroughly studied. Central limit theorem (CLT), strong law of large numbers (SLLN) and functional limit theorem (FCLT) are proved for them.

We have proved the same theorems for our generalized processes. In order to do this, we established that the delay length does not have any influence on the asymptotic behavior of a renewal process.

Lemma 7 *Let* $\{T_n\}_{n\geq 1}$ *and* $\{X_i\}_{i\geq 0}$ *be two independent sequences of independent r.v.'s. Put* $S_j = \sum_{i=1}^{j} T_i$, *the delayed sequence* $\{\Sigma_n\}_{n\geq 0}$ *is given by* $\Sigma_n = X_0 + \cdots + X_n$, $0 \leq n \leq k-1$, *while* $\Sigma_n = \Sigma_{k-1} + S_{n-k+1}$ *for* $n \geq k$.

If there exists an almost sure (a.s.) convergence $n^{-1}S_n \to \mu$, *then for any fixed* k *there exists the same limit for the delayed sequence:*

$$n^{-1}\Sigma_n \to \mu \quad a.s. \quad as \quad n \to \infty.$$

Lemma 8 *Let* $\{S_n\}$ *and* $\{\Sigma_n\}$ *be the sequences defined in Lemma 7. Assume that all random variables have finite mathematical expectations. If there exists a number* $\sigma > 0$ *such that*

$$\frac{S_n - \mathsf{E}S_n}{\sigma\sqrt{n}} \xrightarrow{d} \xi, \quad as \quad n \to \infty,$$

where ξ *has a standard Gaussian distribution, then for any fixed* k *the same statement is true for* Σ_n, *that is,*

$$\frac{\Sigma_n - \mathsf{E}\Sigma_n}{\sigma\sqrt{n}} \xrightarrow{d} \xi \quad as \quad n \to \infty.$$

Symbol $\xrightarrow{d}$ *denotes weak convergence of random variables.*

Lemma 9 *If there exists a finite number* μ *such that* $n^{-1}S_n \to \mu$ *a.s., then there is an a.s. convergence*

$$t^{-1}N_t \to \mu^{-1} \quad as \quad t \to \infty.$$

Lemma 10 *If there exist numbers* μ *and* σ *such that*

$$\frac{S_n - n\mu}{\sigma\sqrt{n}} \xrightarrow{d} \xi \quad as \quad n \to \infty,$$

where ξ *is a random variable having a standard Gaussian distribution, then*

$$\frac{N_t - t\mu^{-1}}{\sigma\sqrt{t\mu^{-3}}} \xrightarrow{d} \xi \quad as \quad t \to \infty.$$

Theorem 8 (SLLN) *Let* S_n *be a delayed periodical renewal process. Suppose that all the summands* T_{ql+i} *have finite mathematical expectation* $\mu_i < \infty$, $i = 1, \ldots, l$. *Then a.s.*

$$\frac{N_t}{t} \to \frac{l}{\mu} \quad as \quad t \to \infty.$$

Here, the counting process N_t *is defined as earlier,* $N_t = \min\{n \geq 0 : S_n > t\}$ *and* $\mu = \mu_1 + \cdots + \mu_l$.

Theorem 9 (CLT) *Suppose that r.v.'s* T_{lq+i} *have finite mathematical expectations* μ_i *and variances* $0 < \sigma_i^2 < \infty$ *respectively,* $i = 1, \ldots, l$, *and r.v.* X_j *has finite* *mathematical expectation v_j, $j \geq 1$. Then, as $t \to \infty$, we have*

$$\frac{N_t - tl\mu^{-1}}{\sigma l \sqrt{t\mu^{-3}}} \xrightarrow{d} \xi$$

where $\mu = \mu_1 + \cdots + \mu_l$, $\sigma^2 = \sigma_1^2 + \cdots + \sigma_l^2$ and r.v. ξ has the standard Gaussian distribution.

Next, we state the functional limit theorem for the generalized renewal process $\{S_n\}$ treated in Theorem 9.

Theorem 10 (FCLT) *Put $\mu = \mu_1 + \cdots + \mu_l$, $\sigma^2 = \sigma_1^2 + \cdots + \sigma_l^2$ and*

$$Z_n(t, \omega) = \frac{N_{nt}(\omega) - ntl\mu^{-1}}{\sigma l \sqrt{n\mu^{-3}}},$$

Then, $Z_n \xrightarrow{D} W$ as $n \to \infty$.

It is interesting to deal with controlled processes introduced in [236].

Definition 4 X_t is a controlled version of N_t if it is formed by the sequence of $S'_n = \sum_{i=0}^{n} T'_i$ where $T'_i = T_i/v(i)$, $0 < v(i) < \infty$. In other words, the ith inter-renewal time is scaled by a (deterministic) function of the number of previous times. The function v is called the speed of the process.

Note that for a constant speed $v(i) = c$ one gets $X_t = N_{tc}$.

For controlled versions of renewal processes, one can consider the so-called fluid (deterministic) and diffusion approximations. More precisely, consider a twice continuously differentiable function $c : (0, \infty) \to (0, \infty)$, and define the nth approximation X^n to N as the controlled renewal process with the speed $v^n(i) = nc(i/n)$.

Thus, X^n is a point process with points generated by $T_j^n = T_j/nc(j/n)$. We assume T_i to have finite mean and variance denoted by μ and σ^2, respectively.

Theorem 11 (Fluid approximation) *Consider the ODE $x'_t = \mu^{-1}c(x_t)$, $t \geq 0$, with $x_0 = 0$ and assume that c is such that x_t remains finite for all $t > 0$. Let $x_t^n = n^{-1}X_t^n$. Then, x^n converges to the solution x of the ODE, as $n \to \infty$, in the sense that for any $\varepsilon > 0$ and any $T > 0$,*

$$\lim_{n \to \infty} P(\sup_{0 \leq t \leq T} |x_t^n - x_t| > \varepsilon) = 0.$$

Theorem 12 (Diffusion approximation) *Consider the process $\xi_t^n = \sqrt{n}(x_t^n - x_t)$. Let $D[0, \infty)$ denote the space of càdlàg functions endowed with the Skorokhod topology. Then ξ^n converges weakly, as $n \to \infty$, to the solution of the following SDE*

$$d\xi_t = \mu^{-1}c'(x_t)\xi_t dt + \sqrt{\mu^{-3}\sigma^2 c(x_t)}dW_t, \quad t \geq 0,$$

$\xi_0 = 0$. *Here W_t is a Wiener process and x_t is the solution of ODE.*

At last, we turn to *reward-renewal* processes.

Definition 5 Let $(T_i, Y_i)_{i \geq 0}$ be a bivariate renewal sequence (vectors are i.i.d. for $i > 0$ and $T_i \geq 0$). Then, $Y_t = \sum_{i=0}^{N_t} Y_i$ is called a reward-renewal process.

Theorem 13 *If there exist* $\mathsf{E}T_i = \mu$ *and* $\mathsf{E}Y_i = \delta$, $i \geq 1$, *then almost surely*

$$\frac{Y_t}{t} \to \frac{\delta}{\mu}, \quad as \ t \to \infty.$$

Theorem 14 *If* $\{T_n\}_{n \geq 1}$ *and* $\{Y_n\}_{n \geq 1}$ *are periodic renewal sequences with periods* l_1 *and* l_2 *respectively and there exist* $\mathsf{E}T_i = \mu_i$, $\mathsf{E}Y_i = \delta_i$, *then almost surely*

$$\lim_{t \to \infty} \frac{Y_t}{t} = \frac{l_1}{l_2} \frac{\sum_{i=1}^{l_2} \delta_i}{\sum_{i=1}^{l_1} \mu_i}.$$

Note that $\lim_{t \to \infty} t^{-1} Y_t$ represents the long-run costs and widely used as objective function in various applications.

It is possible to consider purely stochastic model (difference of two reward-renewal processes) generalizing the model introduced in [247].

$$X(t) = x + Z(t) - Y(t)$$

where $Z(t) = \sum_{i=1}^{N_1(t)} Z_i$, $N_1(t)$ is generated by l_3 periodic process and $\{Z_i\}$ form a l_4 periodic process, the corresponding means being μ_i' and δ_i'. Then

$$\lim_{t \to \infty} \frac{X(t)}{t} = \frac{l_1}{l_2} \frac{\sum_{i=1}^{l_2} \delta_i}{\sum_{i=1}^{l_1} \mu_i} - \frac{l_3}{l_4} \frac{\sum_{i=1}^{l_4} \delta_i'}{\sum_{i=1}^{l_3} \mu_i'}. \tag{11}$$

The positivity of rhs in (11) is analog of classical net profit condition. Its fulfillment enables us to state that ultimate ruin probability is less than 1.

Diffusion approximation for insurance models was proposed for the first time by D.L. Iglehart in 1969, see [212]. It can be useful for estimation of ruin probabilities.

Denote by $W_{a,\sigma^2}(t)$ the Wiener process with the mean at and variance $\sigma^2 t$. This random process is stochastically equivalent to $at + \sigma W(t)$, where $W(t)$ is a standard Wiener process.

The process with stochastic premiums can be approximated (see, e.g., [444]) by $x + W_{a,\sigma^2}(t)$ where $\mathsf{E}R(t) = at$ and $\mathsf{Var} R(t) = \sigma^2 t$ for $R(t) = Z(t) - Y(t)$. So, parameters a and σ^2 can be easily calculated.

Hence, ultimate ruin probability is approximated as follows:

$$\psi(x) \approx P(\inf_{t > 0} W_{a,\sigma^2}(t) < -x) = \exp\{-2xa/\sigma^2\}$$

and ruin probability on finite interval

$$\psi(x, T) \approx P(\inf_{0 < t \leq T} W_{a,\sigma^2}(t) < -x)$$

$$= 1 - \Phi\left(\frac{aT + x}{\sigma\sqrt{T}}\right) + \exp\{-2xa/\sigma^2\}\Phi\left(\frac{aT - x}{\sigma\sqrt{T}}\right).$$

We have obtained the diffusion approximation and FLCT for the difference of two periodic renewal-reward processes to be published elsewhere.

7 Conclusion

Actuarial science is a fast growing research domain, so it turned out impossible even to include all recent publications. In this review, a classification of existing so far models is given, emphasizing the role of the new ones. Since some of the models possess several characteristics such as implementation of investment, reinsurance, capital injections, and so on, they can be mentioned not only in one group. Summing up, it is necessary to stress that three new notions of ruin (absolute, Parisian and Omega) were introduced for treating the solvency and bankruptcy problems. Many generalizations of Gerber–Shiu function, which unified reliability and cost approach, allow to investigate more precisely the company surplus behavior in order to control it avoiding bankruptcy. On the other hand, various extensions of classical Cramér–Lundberg and Sparre Andersen models aim at better description of reality, although they demand more profound knowledge of mathematics. So, hopefully, the review will be useful for the researcher in applied probability and professor teaching future actuaries, as well as, students themselves.

Acknowledgements The research was partially supported by RFBR grant No. 17-01-00468. The author would like to thank two anonymous referees for their helpful suggestions aimed at the paper improvement.

References

1. Abdallah, A., Boucher, J.P., Cossette, H.: Modeling dependence between loss triangles with hierarchical Archimedean copulas. ASTIN Bull. **45**, 577–599 (2015)
2. Ahn, S., Badescu, A.L.: On the analysis of the Gerber-Shiu discounted penalty function for risk processes with Markovian arrivals. Insur.: Math. Econ. **41**(2), 234–249 (2007)
3. Ahn, S., Ramaswami, V.: Efficient algorithms for transient analysis of stochastic fluid flow models. J. Appl. Probab. **42**, 531–549 (2005)
4. Ahn, S., Badescu, A.L., Ramaswami, V.: Time dependent analysis of finite buffer fluid flows and risk models with a dividend barrier. Queueing Syst. **55**, 207–222 (2007)
5. Albrecher, H., Boxma, O.J.: On the discounted penalty function in a Markov-dependent risk model. Insur.: Math. Econ. **37**, 650–672 (2005)
6. Albrecher, H., Hartinger, J.: A risk model with multi-layer dividend strategy. N. Am. Actuar. J. **11**, 43–64 (2007)

7. Albrecher, H., Hipp, C.: Lundberg's risk process with tax. Bl. DGVFM **28**(1), 13–28 (2007)
8. Albrecher, H., Thonhauser, S.: Optimal dividend strategies for a risk process under force of interest. Insur.: Math. Econ. **43**, 134–149 (2008)
9. Albrecher, H., Thonhauser, S.: Optimality results for dividend problems in insurance. Rev. R. Acad. Cien. Serie A Mat. **103**(2), 295–320 (2009)
10. Albrecher, H., Hartinger, J., Tichy, R.: On the distribution of dividend payments and the discounted penalty function in a risk model with linear dividend barrier. Scand. Actuar. J. **2005**(2), 103–126 (2005)
11. Albrecher, H., Hartinger, J., Thonhauser, S.: On exact solutions for dividend strategies of threshold and linear barrier type in a Sparre Andersen model. ASTIN Bull. **37**(2), 203–233 (2007)
12. Albrecher, H., Badescu, A.L., Landriault, D.: On the dual risk model with taxation. Insur.: Math. Econ. **42**(3), 1086–1094 (2008)
13. Albrecher, H., Constantinescu, C., Loisel, S.: Explicit ruin formulas for models with dependence among risks. Insur.: Math. Econ. **48**(2), 265–270 (2011)
14. Albrecher, H., Gerber, H.U., Shiu, E.S.W.: The optimal dividend barrier in the Gamma-Omega model. Eur. Actuar. J. **1**, 43–55 (2011)
15. Albrecher, H., Bäuerle, N., Thonhauser, S.: Optimal dividend pay-out in random discrete time. Stat. Risk Model. **28**, 251–276 (2011)
16. Albrecher, H., Cheung, E.C.K., Thonhauser, S.: Randomized observation periods for the compound Poisson risk model: dividends. ASTIN Bull. **41**(2), 645–672 (2011)
17. Albrecher, H., Cheung, E.C.K., Thonhauser, S.: Randomized observation periods for the compound Poisson risk model: the discounted penalty function. Scand. Actuar. J. **2013**(6), 224–252 (2013)
18. Alfa, A.S., Drekic, S.: Algorithmic analysis of the Sparre Andersen model in discrete time. ASTIN Bull. **37**, 293–317 (2007)
19. Andersen, S.: On the collective theory of risk in case of contagion between claims. Bull. Inst. Math. Appl. **12**, 275–279 (1957)
20. Andrusiv, A., Zinchenko, N.: Estimates for ruin probabilities and invariance principle for Cramér-Lundberg model with stochastic premiums. Prykladna Statist. Actuarna ta Financ. Matematyka. **2**, 5–17 (2004)
21. Applebaum, D.: Lévy Process and Stochastic Calculus. Cambridge University Press, Cambridge (2004)
22. Artzner, P., Delbaen, F., Eber, J.M., Heath, D.: Coherent measures of risk. Math. Financ. **9**, 203–228 (1999)
23. Asmussen, S.: Risk theory in a Markovian environment. Scand. Actuar. J. **1989**(2), 69–100 (1989)
24. Asmussen, S.: Ruin Probabilities. World Scientific, Singapore (2000)
25. Asmussen, S., Albrecher, H.: Ruin Probabilities, 2nd edn. World Scientific, New Jersey (2010)
26. Asmussen, S., Kluppelberg, C.: Large deviation results for subexponential tails, with applications to insurance risk. Stoch. Process. Appl. **64**, 105–125 (1996)
27. Assaf, D., Langberg, N.A., Savits, T.H., Shaked, M.: Multivariate phase-type distributions. Oper. Res. **32**, 688–702 (1984)
28. Avanzi, B.: Strategies for dividend distribution: a review. N. Am. Actuar. J. **13**(2), 217–251 (2009)
29. Avanzi, B., Cheung, E.C.K., Wong, B., Woo, J.-K.: On a periodic dividend barrier strategy in the dual model with continuous monitoring of solvency. Insur.: Math. Econ. **52**(1), 98–113 (2013)
30. Avanzi, B., Taylor, G., Vu, P.A., Wong, B.: Stochastic loss reserving with dependence: a flexible multivariate Tweedie approach (30 March 2016). UNSW Business School Research Paper No. 2016ACTL01. Available at SSRN. https://dx.doi.org/10.2139/ssrn.2753540
31. Avram, F., Palmowski, Z., Pistorius, M.R.: On the optimal dividend problem for a spectrally negative Lévy process. Ann. Appl. Probab. **17**, 156–180 (2007)

32. Avram, F., Palmowski, Z., Pistorius, M.R.: On Gerber-Shiu functions and optimal dividend distribution for a Lévy risk process in the presence of a penalty function. Ann. Appl. Probab. **25**(4), 1868–1935 (2015)
33. Avram, F., Badescu, A.L., Pistorius, M.R., Rabehasaina, L.: On a class of dependent Sparre Andersen risk models and a bailout application. Insur.: Math. Econ. **71**, 27–39 (2016)
34. Azcue, P., Muler, N.: Optimal reinsurance and dividend distribution policies in the Cramér-Lundberg model. Math. Financ. **15**, 261–308 (2005)
35. Azcue, P., Muler, N.: Optimal investment strategy to minimize the ruin probability of an insurance company under borrowing constraints. Insur.: Math. Econ. **44**(1), 26–34 (2009)
36. Azcue, P., Muler, N.: Optimal investment policy and dividend payment strategy in an insurance company. Ann. Appl. Probab. **20**, 1253–1302 (2010)
37. Azcue, P., Muler, N.: Stochastic Optimization in Insurance. A Dynamic Programming Approach. Springer, Berlin (2014)
38. Badescu, A.L., Landriault, D.: Moments of the discounted dividends in a threshold-type Markovian risk process. Braz. J. Probab. Stat. **21**, 13–25 (2007)
39. Badescu, A.L., Landriault, D.: Recursive calculation of the dividend moments in a multi-threshold risk model. N. Am. Actuar. J. **12**(1), 74–88 (2008)
40. Badescu, A.L., Landriault, D.: Applications of fluid flow matrix analytic methods in ruin theory - a review. Rev. R. Acad. Cien. Serie A Mat. **103**(2), 353–372 (2009)
41. Badescu, A.L., Stanford, D.A.: A generalization of the De Vylder approximation for the probability of ruin. Econ. Comput. Econ. Cybern. Stud. Res. **40**(3–4), 245–265 (2006)
42. Badescu, A., Breuer, L., da Silva Soares, A., Latouche, G., Remiche, M.-A., Stanford, D.: Risk processes analyzed as fluid queues. Scand. Actuar. J. **2005**(2), 127–141 (2005)
43. Badescu, A., Breuer, L., Drekic, S., Latouche, G., Stanford, D.: The surplus prior to ruin and the deficit at ruin for a correlated risk process. Scand. Actuar. J. **2005**, 433–445 (2005)
44. Badescu, A.L., Drekic, S., Landriault, D.: Analysis of a threshold dividend strategy for a MAP risk model. Scand. Actuar. J. **2007**(4), 227–247 (2007)
45. Badescu, A.L., Drekic, S., Landriault, D.: On the analysis of a multi-threshold Markovian risk model. Scand. Actuar. J. **2007**(4), 248–260 (2007)
46. Badescu, A.L., Cheung, E.C.K., Landriault, D.: Dependent risk models with bivariate phase-type distributions. J. Appl. Probab. **46**(1), 113–131 (2009)
47. Badescu, A.L., Cheung, E., Rabehasaina, L.: A two dimensional risk model with proportional reinsurance. J. Appl. Probab. **48**(3), 749–765 (2011)
48. Balbás, A., Balbás, B., Balbás, R.: Optimal reinsurance: a risk sharing approach. Risks **1**, 45–56 (2013)
49. Balbás, A., Balbás, B., Balbás, R., Heras, A.: Optimal reinsurance under risk and uncertainty. Insur.: Math. Econ. **60**(1), 61–74 (2015)
50. Bao, Zh., Liu, He.: On the discounted factorial moments of the deficit in discrete time renewal risk model. Int. J. Pure Appl. Math. **79**(2), 329–341 (2012)
51. Barton, T.L., Shenkir, W.G., Walker, P.L.: Making Enterprise Risk Management Pay Off: How Leading Companies Implement Risk Management. Prentice Hall, Upper Saddle River (2002)
52. Bäuerle, N., Rieder, U.: Markov Decision Processes with Applications to Finance. Springer, Berlin (2011)
53. Bäuerle, N.: Benchmark and mean-variance problems for insurers. Math. Methods Oper. Res. **62**(1), 159–165 (2005)
54. Bayraktar, E., Kyprianou, A.E., Yamazaki, K.: On optimal dividends in the dual model. ASTIN Bull. **43**(3), 359–372 (2013)
55. Bayraktar, E., Kyprianou, A.E., Yamazaki, K.: Optimal dividends in the dual model under transaction costs. Insur.: Math. Econ. **54**(1), 133–143 (2014)
56. Beard, R.E., Pentikäinen, T., Pesonen, E.: Risk Theory. The Stochastic Basis of Insurance, 3rd edn. Chapman and Hall, London (1984)
57. Belkina, T., Hipp, C., Luo, Sh., Taksar, M.: Optimal constrained investment in the Cramer-Lundberg model. Scand. Actuar. J. **2014**(5), 383–404 (2014)

58. Belkina, T., Kabanov, Yu.: Viscosity solutions of integro-differential equations for non-ruin probabilities. Theory Probab. Appl. **60**(4), 671–679 (2016)
59. Belkina, T., Konyukhova, N., Kurochkin, S.: Singular problems for integro-differential equations in dynamic insurance models. Springer Proceedings in Mathematics, Proceedings of the International Conference on Differential and Difference Equations and Applications (in honour of Prof. Ravi P. Agarval) (Azores University, Ponta Delgada, Portugal, 4–8 July 2011), vol. 47, pp. 27–44. Springer, Berlin (2013)
60. Belkina, T.: Risky investment for insurers and sufficiency theorems for the survival probability. Markov Process. Relat. Fields **20**(3), 505–525 (2014)
61. Belkina, T.A., Konyukhova, N.B., Kurochkin, S.V.: Dynamic insurance models with investment: constrained singular problems for integro-differential equations. Comput. Math. Math. Phys. **56**(1), 43–92 (2016)
62. Belkina, T.A., Konyukhova, N.B., Kurochkin, S.V.: Singular initial-value and boundary-value problems for integro-differential equations in dynamical insurance models with investments. J. Math. Sci. **218**(4), 369–394 (2016)
63. Bening, V.E., Korolev, V.Yu., Liu, L.X.: Asymptotic behavior of generalized risk processes. Acta Math. Sin. Engl. Ser. **20**(2), 349–356 (2004)
64. Bernstein, P.L.: Against the Gods: The Remarkable Story of Risk. Wiley, New York (1996)
65. Bertoin, J.: Lévy Processes. Cambridge Tracts in Mathematics, vol. 121. Cambridge University Press, Cambridge (1996)
66. Bi, X., Zhang, S.: Minimizing the risk of absolute ruin under a diffusion approximation model with reinsurance and investment. J. Syst. Sci. Complex. **28**(1), 144–155 (2015)
67. Biffis, E., Kyprianou, A.E.: A note on scale functions and the time value of ruin for Lévy insurance risk processes. Insur.: Math. Econ. **46**(1), 85–91 (2010)
68. Biffis, E., Morales, M.: On a generalization of the Gerber-Shiu function to path-dependent penalties. Insur.: Math. Econ. **46**, 92–97 (2010)
69. Billingsley, P.: Convergence of Probability Measures, 2nd edn. Wiley, New York (1999)
70. Blaževičius, K., Bieliauskienė, E., Šiaulys, J.: Finite-time ruin probability in the nonhomogeneous claim case. Lith. Math. J. **50**(3), 260–270 (2010)
71. Boland, P.J.: Statistical and Probabilistic Methods in Actuarial Science. Chapman and Hall, Boca Raton (2007)
72. Boonen, T.J., Tan, K.S., Zhuang, S.C.: The role of a representative reinsurer in optimal reinsurance. Insur.: Math. Econ. **70**, 196–204 (2016)
73. Booth, Ph., Chadburn, R., Haberman, S., James, D., Khorasanee, Z., Plumb, R.H., Rickayzen, B.: Modern Actuarial Theory and Practice, 2nd edn. Chapman and Hall/CRC, Boca Raton (2004)
74. Boudreault, M., Cossette, H., Landriault, D., Marceau, E.: On a risk model with dependence between interclaim arrivals and claim sizes. Scand. Actuar. J. **2005**, 265–285 (2006)
75. Bowers, N.L., Gerber, H.U., Hickman, J.C., Jones, D.A., Nesbitt, S.J.: Actuarial Mathematics, 2nd edn. Society of Actuaries, Schaumburg (1997)
76. Boykov, A.V.: Cramer-Lundberg model with stochastic premiums. Theory Probab. Appl. **47**(3), 549–553 (2002)
77. Brandtner, M., Kursten, W.: Solvency II, regulatory capital, and optimal reinsurance: how good are conditional value-at-risk and spectral risk measures? Insur.: Math. Econ. **59**, 156–167 (2014)
78. Breuer, L.: A quintuple law for Markov-additive processes with phase-type jumps. J. Appl. Probab. **47**(2), 441–458 (2010)
79. Breuer, L., Badescu, A.: A generalised Gerber-Shiu measure for Markov-additive risk processes with phase-type claims and capital injections. Scand. Actuar. J. **2014**(2), 93–115 (2014)
80. Browne, S.: Optimal investment policies for a firm with a random risk process: exponential utility and minimizing the probability of ruin. Math. Oper. Res. **20**(4), 937–958 (1995)
81. Bühlmann, H.: Mathematical Methods in Risk Theory. Grundlehrenband, vol. 172. Springer, Heidelberg (1970)

82. Bühlmann, H.: Actuaries of the third kind. ASTIN Bull. **17**(2), 137–138 (1987)
83. Bühlmann, H., Gisler, A.: A Course in Credibility Theory and Its Applications. Springer, Berlin (2005)
84. Bühlmann, H., Moriconi, F.: Credibility claims reserving with stochastic diagonal effects. ASTIN Bull. **45**, 309–353 (2015)
85. Bulinskaya, E.V., Chepurin, E.V.: Actuarial education at the Moscow State University. Transactions of the 26th International Congress of Actuaries, 7–12 June 1998, Birmingham, vol. 1, pp. 41–52 (1998)
86. Bulinskaya, E., Gromov, A.: New approach to dynamic XL reinsurance. In: Proceedings of SMTDA 2010, Chania, Greece, June 8–11, pp. 147–154 (2010)
87. Bulinskaya, E., Muromskaya, A.: Optimization of multi-component insurance system with dividend payments. In: Manca, R., McClean, S., Skiadas, Ch.H. (eds.) New Trends in Stochastic Modeling and Data Analysis. ISAST, Athens (2015)
88. Bulinskaya, E., Sokolova, A.: Asymptotic behaviour of stochastic storage systems. Mod. Probl. Math. Mech. **10**(3), 37–62 (2015) (in Russian)
89. Bulinskaya, E., Yartseva, D.: Discrete time models with dividends and reinsurance. In: Proceedings of SMTDA 2010, Chania, Greece, June 8–11, pp. 155–162 (2010)
90. Bulinskaya, E.: On the cost approach in insurance. Rev. Appl. Ind. Math. **10**(2), 276–286 (2003) (in Russian)
91. Bulinskaya, E.V.: Some aspects of decision making under uncertainty. J. Stat. Plan. Inference. **137**(8), 2613–2632 (2007)
92. Bulinskaya, E.V.: Sensitivity analysis of some applied models. Pliska Stud. Math. Bulg. **18**, 57–90 (2007)
93. Bulinskaya, E.: Asymptotic analysis of insurance models with bank loans. In: Bozeman, J.R., Girardin, V., Skiadas, C.H. (eds.) New Perspectives on Stochastic Modeling and Data Analysis, pp. 255–270. ISAST, Athens (2014)
94. Bulinskaya, E., Gromov, A.: Asymptotic behavior of the processes describing some insurance models. Commun. Stat. Theory Methods **45**, 1778–1793 (2016)
95. Bulinskaya, E., Gusak, J.: Optimal control and sensitivity analysis for two risk models. Commun. Stat. Simul. Comput. **44**, 1–17 (2015)
96. Bulinskaya, E., Gusak, J., Muromskaya, A.: Discrete-time insurance model with capital injections and reinsurance. Methodol. Comput. Appl. Probab. **17**(4), 899–914 (2015)
97. Bunyakovskij, V.Ya.: One empirical expression of the law of mortality. St. Petersburg (1869) (in Russian)
98. Cai, J.: Discrete time risk models under rates of interest. Probab. Eng. Inf. Sci. **16**, 309–324 (2002)
99. Cai, J.: Ruin probabilities with dependent rates of interest. J. Appl. Probab. **39**, 312–323 (2002)
100. Cai, J.: Ruin probabilities and penalty functions with stochastic rates of interest. Stoch. Process. Appl. **112**, 53–78 (2004)
101. Cai, J.: On the time value of absolute ruin with debit interest. Adv. Appl. Probab. **39**(2), 343–359 (2007)
102. Cai, J., Dickson, D.C.M.: Ruin probabilities with a Markov chain interest model. Insur.: Math. Econ. **35**(3), 513–525 (2004)
103. Cai, J., Li, H.: Dependence properties and bounds for ruin probabilities in multivariate compound risk models. J. Multivar. Anal. **98**, 757–773 (2007)
104. Cai, J., Fang, Y., Li, Z., Willmot, G.E.: Optimal reciprocal reinsurance treaties under the joint survival probability and the joint profitable probability. J. Risk Insur. **80**, 145–168 (2012)
105. Campolieti, G., Makarov, R.N.: Financial Mathematics: A Comprehensive Treatment. Chapman and Hall/CRC, Boca Raton (2014)
106. Centeno, M.L., Simoes, O.: Optimal reinsurance. Revista de la Real Academia de Ciencias, RACSAM **103**(2), 387–405 (2009)
107. Chapman, R.J.: Simple Tools and Techniques for Enterprise Risk Management. Wiley, New York (2011)

108. Chen, S., Wang, X., Deng, Y., Zeng, Y.: Optimal dividend-financing strategies in a dual risk model with time-inconsistent preferences. Insur.: Math. Econ. **70**, 196–204 (2016)
109. Cheng, Y., Tang, Q.: Moments of the surplus before ruin and the deficit at ruin in the Erlang(2) risk process. N. Am. Actuar. J. **7**, 1–12 (2003)
110. Cheng, Y.B., Tang, Q.H., Yang, H.L.: Approximations for moments of deficit at ruin with exponential and subexponential claims. Stat. Probab. Lett. **59**, 367–378 (2002)
111. Chesney, M., Jeanblanc-Picque, M., Yor, M.: Brownian excursions and Parisian barrier options. Adv. Appl. Probab. **29**(1), 165–184 (1997)
112. Cheung, E.C.K., Feng, R.: A unified analysis of claim costs up to ruin in a Markovian arrival risk model. Insur.: Math. Econ. **53**, 98–109 (2013)
113. Cheung, E.C.K., Landriault, D.: A generalized penalty function with the maximum surplus prior to ruin in a MAP risk model. Insur.: Math. Econ. **46**(1), 127–134 (2010)
114. Cheung, E.C.K., Landriault, D.: On a risk model with surplus-dependent premium and tax rates. Appl. Stoch. Models Bus. Ind. **14**(2), 233–251 (2012)
115. Cheung, E.C.K., Liu, H.: On the joint analysis of the total discounted payments to policyholders and shareholders: threshold dividend strategy. Ann. Actuar. Sci. **10**(2), 236–269 (2016)
116. Cheung, E.C.K., Landriault, D., Willmot, G.E., Woo, J.-K.: Gerber-Shiu analysis with a generalized penalty function. Scand. Actuar. J. **2010**(3), 185–199 (2010)
117. Cheung, E.C.K., Landriault, D., Willmot, G.E., Woo, J.-K.: Structural properties of Gerber-Shiu functions in dependent Sparre Andersen models. Insur.: Math. Econ. **46**(1), 117–126 (2010)
118. Cheung, E.C.K., Landriault, D., Badescu, A.L.: On a generalization of the risk model with Markovian claim arrivals. Stoch. Models **27**(3), 407–430 (2011)
119. Cheung, E.C.K., Landriault, D., Willmot, G.E., Woo, J.-K.: On ordering and bounds in a generalized Sparre Andersen risk model. Appl. Stoch. Models Bus. Ind. **27**(1), 51–60 (2011)
120. Cheung, E.C.K., Liu, H., Woo, J.-K.: On the joint analysis of the total discounted payments to policyholders and shareholders: dividend barrier strategy. Risks **3**(4), 491–514 (2015)
121. Chi, Y.C., Lin, X.S.: On the threshold dividend strategy for a generalized jump-diffusion risk model. Insur.: Math. Econ. **48**, 326–337 (2011)
122. Chiu, S.N., Yin, C.C.: The time of ruin, the surplus prior to ruin and the deficit at ruin for the classical risk process perturbed by diffusion. Insur.: Math. Econ. **33**, 59–66 (2003)
123. Chiu, S.N., Yin, C.C.: On the complete monotonicity of the compound geometric convolution with applications to risk theory. Scand. Actuar. J. **2014**, 116–124 (2014)
124. Choi, M.C.H., Cheung, E.C.K.: On the expected discounted dividends in the Cramér-Lundberg risk model with more frequent ruin monitoring than dividend decisions. Insur.: Math. Econ. **59**, 121–132 (2014)
125. Choulli, T., Taksar, M.: Excess-of-loss reinsurance under taxes and fixed costs. J. Risk Decis. Anal. **2**, 85–102 (2010)
126. Cizek, P., Härdle, W., Weron, R. (eds.): Statistical Tools for Finance and Insurance. Springer, Berlin (2005)
127. Corazza, M., Pizzi, Cl. (eds.): Mathematical and Statistical Methods for Actuarial Sciences and Finance. Springer International Publishing, Switzerland (2014)
128. Cossette, H., Marceau, E., Marri, F.: On the compound Poisson risk model with dependence based on a generalized Farlie-Gumbel-Morgenstern copula. Insur.: Math. Econ. **43**, 444–455 (2009)
129. Cramér, H.: Historical review of Filip Lundberg's works on risk theory. Scand. Actuar. J. **1969**, 6–9 (1969)
130. Cruz, M.G., Peters, G.W., Shevchenko, P.V.: Fundamental Aspects of Operational Risk and Insurance Analytics: A Handbook of Operational Risk. Wiley, New York (2015)
131. Cruz, M.G.: Modeling, Measuring and Hedging Operational Risk. Wiley, New York (2002)
132. Czarna, I., Palmowski, Z.: Ruin probability with Parisian delay for a spectrally negative Lévy risk process. J. Appl. Probab. **48**, 984–1002 (2011)
133. D'Arcy, S.P.: On becoming an actuary of the fourth kind. Proc. Casualty Actuar. Soc. **XCII**(177), 745–754 (2005). http://www.casact.org/pubs/proceed/proceed05/05755.pdf. Accessed 5 July 2007

134. D'Arcy, S.P.: On becoming an actuary of the third kind. Proc. Casualty Actuar. Soc. **LXXVI**, 45–76 (1989). https://www.casact.org/pubs/proceed/proceed89/89045.pdf
135. D'Arcy, S.: Enterprise risk management. J. Risk Manag. Korea **12**(1), 207–228 (2001)
136. D'Arcy, S.P.: Risk appetite. Risk Manag. **15**, 38–41 (2009)
137. Dassios, A., Wu, Sh.: On barrier strategy dividends with Parisian implementation delay for classical surplus processes. Insur.: Math. Econ. **45**(2), 195–202 (2009)
138. Daykin, C.D., Pentikainen, T., Pesonen, M.: Practical Risk Theory for Actuaries. Chapman and Hall/CRC Press, Boca Raton (1993)
139. De Finetti, B.: Su un'impostazione alternativa della teoria collettiva del rischio. In: Transactions of the XV-th International Congress of Actuaries, vol. 2, pp. 433–443 (1957)
140. Decker, A., Galer, D.: Enterprise Risk Management - Straight to the Point: An Implementation Guide Function by Function (Viewpoints on ERM). CreateSpace Independent Publishing Platform (2013)
141. Deelstra, G., Plantin, G.: Risk Theory and Reinsurance. Springer, Berlin (2013)
142. Denuit, M., Dhaene, J., Goovaerts, M., Kaas, R.: Actuarial Theory for Dependent Risks. Wiley, Chichester (2005)
143. Dickson, D.C.M.: On the distribution of the surplus prior to ruin. Insur.: Math. Econ. **11**, 191–207 (1992)
144. Dickson, D.C.M.: On the distribution of the claim causing ruin. Insur.: Math. Econ. **12**, 143–154 (1993)
145. Dickson, D.C.M.: Insurance Risk and Ruin. Cambridge University Press, Cambridge (2005)
146. Dickson, D.C.M., Drekic, S.: The joint distribution of the surplus prior to ruin and the deficit at ruin in some Sparre Andersen models. Insur.: Math. Econ. **34**, 97–107 (2004)
147. Dickson, D.C.M., Hipp, C.: Ruin problems for phase-type(2) risk processes. Scand. Actuar. J. **2000**, 147–167 (2000)
148. Dickson, D.C.M., Hipp, C.: On the time to ruin for Erlang(2) risk processes. Insur.: Math. Econ. **29**, 333–344 (2001)
149. Dickson, D.C.M., Waters, H.R.: Some optimal dividends problems. ASTIN Bull. **34**, 49–74 (2004)
150. Dobrushin, R.L.: Describing a system of random variables by conditional distributions. Theory Probab. Appl. **15**, 458–486 (1970)
151. Doherty, N.A.: Integrated Risk Management. McGraw-Hill, New York (2000)
152. Drekic, S., Mera, A.M.: Ruin analysis of a threshold strategy in a discrete-time Sparre Andersen model. Methodol. Comput. Appl. Probab. **13**, 723–747 (2011)
153. Drekic, S., Dickson, D.C.M., Stanford, D.A., Willmot, G.E.: On the distribution of the deficit at ruin when claims are phase-type. Scand. Actuar. J. **2004**, 105–120 (2004)
154. Dufresne, F., Gerber, H.U.: The surpluses immediately before and at ruin, and the amount of the claim causing ruin. Insur.: Math. Econ. **7**(3), 193–199 (1988)
155. Dufresne, F., Gerber, H.U.: Risk theory for the compound Poisson process that is perturbed by diffusion. Insur.: Math. Econ. **10**, 51–59 (1991)
156. Durrett, R.: Stochastic Calculus: A Practical Introduction. CRC Press, Boca Raton (1996)
157. Eisenberg, J., Schmidli, H.: Optimal control of capital injections by reinsurance in a diffusion approximation. Blätter der DGVFM **30**, 1–13 (2009)
158. Embrechts, P., Klüppelberg, C., Mikosch, T.: Modelling Extremal Events for Insurance and Finance. Springer, Berlin (2004)
159. Embrechts, P., Veraverbecke, N.: Estimates for the probability of ruin with special emphasis on the possibility of large claims. Insur.: Math. Econ. **1**, 55–72 (1982)
160. Fang, Y., Wu, R.: Optimal dividends in the Brownian motion risk model with interest. J. Comput. Appl. Math. **229**, 145–151 (2008)
161. Feng, R., Shimizu, Y.: Potential measures for spectrally negative Markov additive processes with applications in ruin theory. Insur.: Math. Econ. **59**, 11–26 (2014)
162. Feng, M.B., Tan, K.S.: Coherent distortion risk measures in portfolio selection. Syst. Eng. Procedia **4**, 25–34 (2012)

163. Fleming, W.H., Soner, H.M.: Controlled Markov Processes and Viscosity Solutions. Applications of Mathematics, vol. 25. Springer, New York (1993)
164. Fraser, J., Simkins, B., Narvaez, K.: Implementing Enterprise Risk Management: Case Studies and Best Practices (Robert W. Kolb Series). Wiley, New York (2014)
165. Frees, E.W.: Stochastic life contingencies with solvency considerations. Trans. Soc. Actuar. **42**, 91–148 (1990)
166. Frolova, A., Kabanov, Yu., Pergamenshchikov, S.: In the insurance business risky investments are dangerous. Financ. Stoch. **6**, 227–235 (2002)
167. Fu, D., Guo, Y.: On the compound Poisson model with debit interest under absolute ruin. Int. J. Sci. Res. (IJSR) **5**(6), 1872–1875 (2016)
168. Funston, F., Wagner, S.: Surviving and Thriving in Uncertainty: Creating the Risk Intelligent Enterprise. Wiley, New York (2010)
169. Gaier, J., Grandits, P.: Ruin probabilities in the presence of regularly varying tails and optimal investment. Insur.: Math. Econ. **30**, 211–217 (2002)
170. Gaier, J., Grandits, P.: Ruin probabilities and investment under interest force in the presence of regularly varying tails. Scand. Actuar. J. **2004**(4), 256–278 (2004)
171. Gaier, J., Grandits, P., Schachermayer, W.: Asymptotic ruin probabilities and optimal investment. Ann. Appl. Probab. **13**, 1054–1076 (2003)
172. Gao, S., Liu, Z.M.: The perturbed compound Poisson risk model with constant interest and a threshold dividend strategy. J. Comput. Appl. Math. **233**, 2181–2188 (2010)
173. Gerber, H.U.: An Introduction to Mathematical Risk Theory. Huebner, Philadelphia (1979)
174. Gerber, H.U.: Der Einfluss von Zins auf die Ruinwahrscheinlichkeit. Mitteilungen der Vereinigung schweizerischer Versicherungsmathematiker. **71**(1), 63–70 (1971)
175. Gerber, H.U., Landry, B.: On a discounted penalty at ruin in a jump-diffusion and the perpetual put option. Insur.: Math. Econ. **22**, 263–276 (1998)
176. Gerber, H.U., Shiu, E.S.W.: The joint distribution of the time of ruin, the surplus immediately before ruin, and the deficit at ruin. Insur.: Math. Econ. **21**(2), 129–137 (1997)
177. Gerber, H.U., Shiu, E.S.W.: On the time value of ruin. N. Am. Actuar. J. **2**(1), 48–78 (1998)
178. Gerber, H.U., Shiu, E.S.W.: From ruin theory to pricing reset guarantees and perpetual put options. Insur.: Math. Econ. **24**, 3–14 (1999)
179. Gerber, H.U., Shiu, E.S.W.: The time value of ruin in a Sparre Andersen model. N. Am. Actuar. J. **9**, 49–69 (2005)
180. Gerber, H., Shiu, E.: On optimal dividends: from reflection to refraction. J. Comput. Appl. Math. **186**, 4–22 (2006)
181. Gerber, H.U., Shiu, E.S.W., Smith, N.: Maximizing dividends without bankruptcy. ASTIN Bull. **36**(1), 5–23 (2006)
182. Gerber, H.U., Shiu, E.S.W., Yang, H.: The Omega model: from bankruptcy to occupation times in the red. Eur. Actuar. J. **2**, 259–272 (2012)
183. Gilina, L.C.: Estimation of ruin probability for some insurance model. Prykladna Statist. Actuarna ta Financ. Matematyka. **1**, 67–73 (2000)
184. Gong, L., Badescu, A.L., Cheung, E.: Recursive methods for a two-dimensional risk process with common shocks. Insur.: Math. Econ. **50**, 109–120 (2012)
185. Gosio, C., Lari, E., Ravera, M.: Optimal dynamic proportional and excess of loss reinsurance under dependent risks. Mod. Econ. **7**, 715–724 (2016)
186. Grandell, J.: Aspects of Risk Theory. Springer Series in Statistics: Probability and Its Applications. Springer, New York (1991)
187. Grandell, J.: Simple approximation of ruin probabilities. Insur.: Math. Econ. **26**, 157–173 (2000)
188. Grandits, P.: An analogue of the Cramér-Lundberg approximation in the optimal investment case. Appl. Math. Optim. **50**, 1–20 (2004)
189. Grandits, P.: Minimal ruin probabilities and investment under interest force for a class of subexponential distributions. Scand. Actuar. J. **2005**(6), 401–416 (2005)
190. Grigutis, A., Korvel, A., Šiaulys, J.: Ruin probability in the three-seasonal discrete-time risk model. Mod. Stoch.: Theory Appl. **2**, 421–441 (2015)

191. Guérin, H., Renaud, J.-F.: On distribution of cumulative Parisian ruin. arXiv:1509.06857v1 [math.PR]. 23 Sep 2015
192. Guo, W.: Optimal portfolio choice for an insurer with loss aversion. Insur.: Math. Econ. **58**, 217–222 (2014)
193. Guo, L., Landriault, D., Willmot, G.E.: On the analysis of a class of loss models incorporating time dependence. Eur. Actuar. J. **3**(1), 273–294 (2013)
194. Gup, B.E.: The Basics of Investing, 5th edn. Wiley, New York (1992)
195. Gusak, D.V.: Limit problems for processes with independent increments in risk theory. IM, Kyiv (2007)
196. Hampton, J.J.: Fundamentals of enterprise risk management: how top companies assess risk, manage exposure, and seize opportunity. In: AMACOM (2009)
197. Hartung, F., Pituk, M. (eds.): Recent Advances in Delay Differential and Difference Equations. Springer, Berlin (2014)
198. Heilpern, S.: Ruin measures for a compound Poisson risk model with dependence based on the Spearman copula and the exponential claim sizes. Insur.: Math. Econ. **59**, 251–257 (2014)
199. Hernandez, C., Junca, M.: Optimal dividend payments under a time of ruin constraint: exponential claims. Insur.: Math. Econ. **65**, 136–142 (2015)
200. Heywood, G.: Edmond Halley - actuary. Q. J. R. Astron. Soc. **35**(1), 151–154 (1994)
201. Hipp, C.: Dividend payment with ruin constraint: working paper (2016). https://www.researchgate.net/publication/291339576
202. Hipp, C.: Stochastic control for insurance: models, strategies and numerics (2016). https://www.researchgate.net/publication/308695862
203. Hipp, C., Plump, M.: Optimal investment for insurers. Insur.: Math. Econ. **27**(2), 215–228 (2000)
204. Hipp, C., Plump, M.: Optimal investment for investors with state dependent income, and for insurers. Financ. Stoch. **7**(3), 299–321 (2003)
205. Hipp, C., Schmidli, H.: Asymptotics of ruin probabilities for controlled risk processes in the small claims case. Scand. Actuar. J. **2004**(5), 321–335 (2004)
206. Hipp, C., Taksar, M.: Optimal non-proportional reinsurance control. Insur.: Math. Econ. **47**, 246–254 (2010)
207. Hipp, C., Vogt, M.: Optimal dynamic XL reinsurance. ASTIN Bull. **33**(2), 193–207 (2003)
208. Horcher, K.A.: Essentials of Financial Risk Management. Wiley, New York (2005)
209. Hu, X., Zhang, L.: Ruin probability in a correlated aggregate claims model with common Poisson shocks: application to reinsurance. Methodol. Comput. Appl. Probab. **18**(3), 675–689 (2016)
210. Hürlimann, W.: Mean-variance portfolio selection under portfolio insurance. In: Proceedings of the AFIR, Nürnberg, Germany, pp. 347–374 (1996)
211. Hürlimann, W.: A simple multi-state gamma claims reserving model. Int. J. Contemp. Math. Sci. **10**(2), 65–77 (2015)
212. Iglehart, D.L.: Diffusion approximations in collective risk theory. J. Appl. Probab. **6**, 285–292 (1969)
213. Ihedioha, S., Osu, B.: Optimal portfolios of an insurer and a reinsurer under proportional reinsurance and power utility preference. Open Access Libr. J. **2**(12), 1–11 (2015)
214. Ivanovs, J., Palmowski, Z.: Occupation densities in solving exit problems for Markov additive processes and their reflections. Stoch. Process. Appl. **122**(9), 3342–3360 (2012)
215. Jacobsen, M.: Point Processes, Theory and Applications. Birkhauser, Boston (2005)
216. Jacod, J., Shiryaev, A.: Limit Theorems for Stochastic Processes. Springer, Berlin (2003)
217. Janssen, J., Manca, R.: Semi-Markov Risk Models for Finance, Insurance and Reliability. Springer, Berlin (2007)
218. Jasiulewicz, H.: Discrete-time financial surplus models for insurance companies. Coll. Econ. Anal. Ann. **21**, 225–255 (2010)
219. Jeanblanc-Piqué, M., Shiryaev, A.N.: Optimization of the flow of dividends. Uspekhi Mat. Nauk. **50**(2(302)), 25–46 (1995)

220. Jiang, W.Y., Yang, Z.J., Li, X.P.: The discounted penalty function with multi-layer dividend strategy in the phase-type risk model. Insur.: Math. Econ. **82**, 1358–1366 (2012)
221. Kaas, R., Goovaerts, M., Dhaene, J., Denuit, M.: Modern Actuarial Risk Theory. Springer, Berlin (2008)
222. Kabanov, Yu., Pergamenshchikov, S.: In the insurance business risky investments are dangerous: the case of negative risk sums. Financ. Stoch. **20**(2), 355–379 (2016)
223. Kalashnikov, V., Norberg, R.: Power tailed ruin probabilities in the presence of risky investments. Stoch. Process. Appl. **98**, 221–228 (2002)
224. Karageyik, B.B., Şahin, Ş.: A review on optimal reinsurance under ruin probability constraint. J. Stat.: Stat. Actuar. Sci. **9**(1), 26–36 (2016)
225. Karapetyan, N.V.: Dividends and reinsurance. In: Proceedings of the 6th International Workshop on Simulation, VVM com.Ltd, pp. 47–52 (2009)
226. Karapetyan, N.V.: Optimization and limit distribution in a discrete insurance model. Mod. Probl. Math. Mech. **10**(3), 101–120 (2015) (in Russian)
227. Karatzas, I., Shreve, S.: Brownian Motion and Stochastic Calculus. Springer, New York (1998)
228. Kennedy, D.: Stochastic Financial Models. Chapman and Hall/CRC, Boca Raton (2010)
229. Kim, S.S., Drekic, S.: Ruin analysis of a discrete-time dependent Sparre Andersen model with external financial activities and randomized dividends. Risks **4**(2), 1–15 (2016)
230. Klebaner, F.: Introduction to Stochastic Calculus with Applications. World Scientific Publishing Company, Singapore (1999)
231. Klugman, S.A., Panjer, H.H., Willmot, G.E.: Student Solutions Manual to Accompany Loss Models: From Data to Decisions, 4th edn. Wiley, New York (2012)
232. Klugman, S.A., Panjer, H.H., Willmot, G.E.: Loss Models: From Data to Decisions, 3rd edn. Wiley, Hoboken (2008)
233. Koller, G.: Risk Assessment and Decision Making in Business and Industry: A Practical Guide, 2nd edn. Chapman and Hall/CRC, Boca Raton (2005)
234. Koller, M.: Stochastic Models in Life Insurance. Springer, Berlin (2012)
235. Konstantinides, D.G., Li, J.: Asymptotic ruin probabilities for a multidimensional renewal risk model with multivariate regularly varying claims. Insur.: Math. Econ. **69**, 38–44 (2016)
236. Konstantopoulos, T., Papadakis, S.N., Walrand, J.: Functional approximation theorems for controlled renewal processes. J. Appl. Probab. **31**, 765–776 (1994)
237. Korolev, V., Bening, V., Shorgin, S.: Mathematical Foundations of Risk Theory. Fizmatlit, Moscow (2007)
238. Kostić, M.: Abstract Volterra Integro-Differential Equations. CRC Press, Boca Raton (2015)
239. Kulenko, N., Schmidli, H.: Optimal dividend strategies in a Cramér-Lundberg model with capital injections. Insur.: Math. Econ. **43**, 270–278 (2008)
240. Kulkarni, V.G.: A new class of multivariate phase type distributions. Oper. Res. **37**, 151–158 (1989)
241. Kyprianou, A.E.: Introductory Lectures on Fluctuations of Lévy Processes with Applications. Springer, Berlin (2006)
242. Kyprianou, A.: Gerber-Shiu Risk Theory. Springer International Publishing, Switzerland (2013)
243. Kyprianou, A.E., Loeffen, R.L.: Refracted Lévy processes. Ann. Inst. H. Poincaré Probab. Stat. **46**(1), 24–44 (2010)
244. Kyprianou, A.E., Zhou, X.W.: General tax structures and the Lévy insurance risk model. J. Appl. Probab. **46**(4), 1146–1156 (2009)
245. Kyprianou, A.E., Loeffen, R., Perez, J.-L.: Optimal control with absolutely continuous strategies for spectrally negative Lévy processes (2010). arXiv:1008.2363
246. Labbé, C.D., Sendova, K.P.: The expected discounted penalty function under a risk model with stochastic income. Appl. Math. Comput. **215**, 1852–1867 (2009)
247. Labbé, C.D., Sendov, H.S., Sendova, K.P.: The Gerber-Shiu function and the generalized Cramér-Lundberg model. Appl. Math. Comput. **218**, 3035–3056 (2011)
248. Lam, J.: Enterprise Risk Management: From Incentives to Controls, 2nd edn. Wiley, New York (2014)

249. Landriault, D., Li, B., Li, S.: Drawdown analysis for the renewal insurance risk process. Scand. Actuar. J. **2016**, 1–19. doi:10.1080/03461238.2015.1123174

250. Landriault, D.: On a generalization of the expected discounted penalty function in a discrete-time insurance risk model. Appl. Stoch. Models Bus. Ind. **24**(6), 525–539 (2008)

251. Landriault, D., Shi, T.: First passage time for compound Poisson processes with diffusion: ruin theoretical and financial applications. Scand. Actuar. J. **2014**(4), 368–382 (2014)

252. Landriault, D., Shi, T.: Occupation times in the MAP risk model. Insur.: Math. Econ. **60**(1), 75–82 (2015)

253. Landriault, D., Renaud, J.-F., Zhou, X.: Occupation times of spectrally negative Lévy processes with applications. Stoch. Process. Appl. **212**(11), 2629–2641 (2011)

254. Landriault, D., Shi, T., Willmot, G.E.: Joint density involving the time to ruin in the Sparre Andersen risk model under the exponential assumption. Insur.: Math. Econ. **49**(3), 371–379 (2011)

255. Landriault, D., Lemieux, C., Willmot, G.E.: An adaptive premium policy with a Bayesian motivation in the classical risk model. Insur.: Math. Econ. **51**(2), 370–378 (2012)

256. Landriault, D., Lee, W.Y., Willmot, G.E., Woo, J.-K.: A note on deficit analysis in dependency models involving Coxian claim amounts. Scand. Actuar. J. **2014**(5), 405–423 (2014)

257. Landriault, D., Renaud, J.-F., Zhou, X.: An insurance risk model with Parisian implementation delays. Methodol. Comput. Appl. Probab. **16**(3), 583–607 (2014)

258. Landriault, D., Willmot, G.E., Xu, D.: On the analysis of time dependent claims in a class of birth process claim count models. Insur.: Math. Econ. **58**, 168–173 (2014)

259. Landriault, D., Li, B., Li, S.: Analysis of a drawdown-based regime-switching Lévy insurance model. Insur.: Math. Econ. **60**(1), 98–107 (2015)

260. Lee, W.Y., Willmot, G.E.: On the moments of the time to ruin in dependent Sparre Andersen models with emphasis on Coxian interclaim times. Insur.: Math. Econ. **59**, 1–10 (2014)

261. Lefèvre, C., Loisel, S.: Finite-time ruin probabilities for discrete, possibly dependent, claim severities. Methodol. Comput. Appl. Probab. **11**(3), 425–441 (2009)

262. Li, S.: On a class of discrete time renewal risk models. Scand. Actuar. J. **2005**(4), 241–260 (2005)

263. Li, S.: Distributions of the surplus before ruin, the deficit at ruin and the claim causing ruin in a class of discrete time risk models. Scand. Actuar. J. **2005**(4), 271–284 (2005)

264. Li, S.: The distribution of the dividend payments in the compound Poisson risk model perturbed by diffusion. Scand. Actuar. J. **2006**(2), 73–85 (2006)

265. Li, S., Dickson, D.C.M.: The maximum surplus before ruin in an Erlang(n) risk process and related problems. Insur.: Math. Econ. **38**(3), 529–539 (2006)

266. Li, S., Garrido, J.: On ruin for the Erlang(n) risk process. Insur.: Math. Econ. **34**, 391–408 (2004)

267. Li, S., Garrido, J.: On a general class of renewal risk process: analysis of the Gerber-Shiu function. Adv. Appl. Probab. **37**(3), 836–856 (2005)

268. Li, S., Garrido, J.: The Gerber-Shiu function in a Sparre Andersen risk process perturbed by diffusion. Scand. Actuar. J. **2005**(3), 161–186 (2005)

269. Li, S., Garrido, J.: Ruin probabilities for two classes of risk processes. ASTIN Bull. **35**, 61–77 (2005)

270. Li, S.M., Lu, Y.: Moments of the dividend payments and related problems in a Markov-modulated risk model. N. Am. Actuar. J. **11**(2), 65–76 (2007)

271. Li, S., Lu, Y.: The decompositions of the discounted penalty functions and dividends-penalty identity in a Markov-modulated risk model. ASTIN Bull. **38**(1), 53–71 (2008)

272. Li, S., Lu, Y., Garrido, J.: A review of discrete-time risk models. Rev. R. Acad. Cien. Serie A. Mat. **103**, 321–337 (2009)

273. Li, S., Sendova, K.P.: The finite-time ruin probability under the compound binomial model. Eur. Actuar. J. **3**(1), 249–271 (2013)

274. Li, Z., Sendova, K.P.: On a ruin model with both interclaim times and premiums depending on claim sizes. Scand. Actuar. J. **2015**(3), 245–265 (2015)

275. Li, P., Yin, C., Zhou, M.: Dividend payments with a hybrid strategy in the compound Poisson risk model. Appl. Math. **5**, 1933–1949 (2014)
276. Li, D., Rong, X., Zhao, H.: Optimal investment problem for an insurer and a reinsurer. J. Syst. Sci. Complex. **28**(6), 1326–1348 (2015)
277. Li, S., Landriault, D., Lemieux, C.: A risk model with varying premiums: its risk management implications. Insur.: Math. Econ. **60**(1), 38–46 (2015)
278. Liang, Zh., Guo, J.: Optimal investment and proportional reinsurance in the Sparre Andersen model. J. Syst. Sci. Complex. **25**(5), 926–941 (2012)
279. Lin, X.S., Pavlova, K.P.: The compound Poisson risk model with a threshold dividend strategy. Insur.: Math. Econ. **38**, 57–80 (2006)
280. Lin, X.S., Sendova, K.P.: The compound Poisson risk model with multiple thresholds. Insur.: Math. Econ. **42**, 617–627 (2008)
281. Lin, X.S., Willmot, G.E.: The moments of the time of ruin, the surplus before ruin, and the deficit at ruin. Insur.: Math. Econ. **27**, 19–44 (2000)
282. Liu, H.: On the joint analysis of discounted aggregate claim costs until ruin and other ruin-related quantities. Thesis. The University of Hong Kong Libraries, University of Hong Kong (2015)
283. Liu, Ch., Zhang, Zh.: A note on a generalized discounted penalty function in a Sparre Andersen risk model perturbed by diffusion. Abstr. Appl. Anal. **2013**, 6 p (2013)
284. Liu, Zh., Zhang, A., Li, C.: The expected discounted tax payments on dual risk model under a dividend threshold. Open J. Stat. **3**, 136–144 (2013)
285. Liu, J., Xu, J.C., Hu, H.C.: The Markov-dependent risk model with a threshold dividend strategy. Wuhan Univ. J. Nat. Sci. **16**(3), 193–198 (2011)
286. Liu, J., Xu, J.: A note on absolute ruin probability in a Markov risk model. In: 2011 International Conference on Electric Information and Control Engineering (ICEICE) (2011). doi:10.1109/ICEICE.2011.5777660
287. Liu, D.H., Liu, Z.M.: The perturbed compound Poisson risk model with linear dividend barrier. J. Comput. Appl. Math. **235**, 2357–2363 (2011)
288. Livshits, K., Yakimovich, K.: Cramér-Lundberg model with stochastic premiums and continuous non-insurance costs. In: Dudin, A., et al. (eds.) Information Technology and Mathematical Modelling, vol. 487, pp. 251–260. Springer, Berlin (2014)
289. Lkabous, M.A., Czarna, I., Renaud, J.-F.: Parisian ruin for a refracted Lévy process. arXiv:1603.09324v1 [math.PR]. Accessed 30 Mar 2016
290. Loeffen, R.L., Patie, P.: Absolute ruin in the Ornstein-Uhlenbeck type risk model (2010). arXiv:1006.2712
291. Loeffen, R.: On optimality of the barrier strategy in de Finetti's dividend problem for spectrally negative Lévy processes. Ann. Appl. Probab. **18**, 1669–1680 (2008)
292. Loeffen, R., Renaud, J.F.: De Finetti's optimal dividends problem with an affine penalty function at ruin. Insur.: Math. Econ. **46**, 98–108 (2010)
293. Loeffen, R., Czarna, I., Palmowski, Z.: Parisian ruin probability for spectrally negative Lévy processes. Bernoulli **19**(2), 599–609 (2013)
294. Lu, Y., Li, S.: On the probability of ruin in a Markov-modulated risk model. Insur.: Math. Econ. **37**(3), 522–532 (2005)
295. Luo, S., Taksar, M.: Optimal excess-of-loss reinsurance under borrowing constraints. J. Risk Decis. Anal. **2**, 103–123 (2010)
296. Luo, S., Taksar, M.: On absolute ruin minimization under a diffusion approximation model. Insur.: Math. Econ. **48**(1), 123–133 (2011)
297. Markov, A.A.: Calculus of Probability. St. Petersburg (1908) (in Russian)
298. Markowitz, H.: Portfolio selection. J. Financ. **7**(1), 77–91 (1952)
299. Martin-Löf, A.: Harald Cramér and insurance mathematics. Appl. Stoch. Models Data Anal. **11**, 271–276 (1995)
300. McNeil, A.J., Frey, R., Embrechts, P.: Quantitative Risk Management: Concepts, Techniques and Tools. Princeton University Press, Princeton (2005)

301. Mehr, R.I., Hedges, B.A.: Risk Management in the Business Enterprise. Richard D. Irwin, Inc., Homewood (1963)
302. Melnikov, A.: Risk Analysis in Finance and Insurance, 2nd edn. Chapman and Hall/CRC, Boca Raton (2011)
303. Meyers, G.G.: Stochastic Loss Reserving Using Bayesian MCMC Models. Casualty Actuarial Society, New York (2015)
304. Mikosch, T.: Non-life Insurance Mathematics. Springer, Berlin (2004)
305. Ming, R.X., Wang, W.Y., Xiao, L.Q.: On the time value of absolute ruin with tax. Insur.: Math. Econ. **46**(1), 67–84 (2010)
306. Minkova, L.D.: The Polya-Aeppli process and ruin problems. J. Appl. Math. Stoch. Anal. **3**, 221–234 (2004)
307. Mircea, I., Covrig, M.: A discrete time insurance model with reinvested surplus and a fuzzy number interest rate. Procedia Econ. Financ. **32**, 1005–1011 (2015)
308. Mishura, Yu., Perestyuk, M., Ragulina, O.: Ruin probability in a risk model with variable premium intensity and risky investments. Opusc. Math. **35**(3), 333–352 (2015)
309. Mitov, K.V., Omey, E.: Renewal Processes. Springer, Berlin (2014)
310. Mitric, I.-R., Sendova, K.P.: On a multi-threshold compound Poisson surplus process with interest. Scand. Actuar. J. **2011**(2), 75–95 (2011)
311. Mitric, I.-R., Sendova, K.P., Tsai, C.C.-L.: On a multi-threshold compound Poisson process perturbed by diffusion. Stat. Probab. Lett. **80**, 366–375 (2010)
312. Mitric, I.R., Badescu, A.L., Stanford, D.: On the absolute ruin in a Sparre Andersen risk model with constant interest. Insur.: Math. Econ. **50**, 167–178 (2012)
313. Mnif, M., Sulem, A.: Optimal risk control and dividend policies under excess of loss reinsurance. Stochastics **77**(5), 455–476 (2005)
314. Muromskaya, A.: A generalization of Lundberg inequality for the case of a joint-stock insurance company. Vestnik Moskovskogo Universiteta. Seriya 1: Matematica, Mekhanica. **72**(1), 32–36 (2017) (in Russian)
315. Muromskaya, A.A.: Optimal reinsurance in the model with several risks within one insurance policy. Vestnik TvGU. Seriya: Prikladnaya Matematika [Herald of Tver State University. Series: Applied Mathematics], vol. 2016(4), pp. 79–97 (2016) (in Russian)
316. Muromskaya, A.: Discounted dividends in a strategy with a step barrier function. Moscow Univ. Math. Bull. **71**(5), 200–203 (2016)
317. Murphy, D.: Understanding Risk: The Theory and Practice of Financial Risk Management. Chapman and Hall/CRC, Boca Raton (2008)
318. Nakayama, H., Sawaragi, Y., Tanino, T.: Theory of Multiobjective Optimization. Academic Press, Waltham (1985)
319. Ng, A.C.Y.: On a dual model with a dividend threshold. Insur.: Math. Econ. **44**, 315–324 (2009)
320. Ng, A.C.Y.: On the upcrossing and downcrossing probabilities of a dual risk model with phase-type gains. ASTIN Bull. **40**, 281–306 (2010)
321. Nie, C., Dickson, D.C.M., Li, Sh.: Minimizing the ruin probability through capital injections. Ann. Actuar. Sci. **5**, 195–209 (2011)
322. Nie, C., Dickson, D.C.M., Li, Sh.: The finite time ruin probability in a risk model with capital injections. Scand. Actuar. J. **2015**(4), 301–318 (2015)
323. Note on enterprise risk management for capital and solvency purposes in the insurance industry. http://www.actuaries.org. Accessed 31 Mar 2009
324. Oakley, J.E., O'Hagan, A.: Probabilistic sensitivity analysis of complex models: a Bayesian approach. J. R. Stat. Soc. B. **66**, Part 3, 751–769 (2004)
325. Oh, K., Kang, H.: A discrete time pricing model for individual insurance contracts. J. Insur. Issues **27**(1), 41–65 (2004)
326. Ohlsson, E., Johansson, B.: Non-life Insurance Pricing with Generalized Linear Models. Springer, Berlin (2010)
327. Oksendal, B., Sulem, A.: Applied Stochastic Control of Jump Diffusions. Springer, Universitext (2005)

328. Oksendal, B.: Stochastic Differential Equations. Springer Verlag, Universitext (2013)
329. Olivieri, A., Pitacco, E.: Introduction to Insurance Mathematics. Technical and Financial Features of Risk Transfers. Springer, Berlin (2015)
330. Outreville, J.F.: Theory and Practice of Insurance. Springer, Berlin (1998)
331. Paulsen, J.: Ruin theory with compounding assets - a survey. Insur.: Math. Econ. **22**, 3–16 (1998)
332. Paulsen, J.: On Cramér-like asymptotics for risk processes with stochastic return on investments. Ann. Appl. Probab. **12**, 1247–1260 (2002)
333. Paulsen, J.: Ruin models with investment income. Probab. Surv. **5**, 416–434 (2008)
334. Paulsen, J., Gjessing, H.K.: Ruin theory with stochastic return on investments. Adv. Appl. Probab. **29**, 965–985 (1997)
335. Pavlova, K.P., Willmot, G.E.: The discrete stationary renewal risk model and the Gerber-Shiu discounted penalty function. Insur.: Math. Econ. **35**, 267–277 (2004)
336. Peng, L.: Joint tail of ECOMOR and LCR reinsurance treaties. Insur.: Math. Econ. **59**, 116–120 (2014)
337. Peng, X., Wang, W.: Optimal investment and risk control for an insurer under inside information. Insur.: Math. Econ. **69**, 104–116 (2016)
338. Peng, X., Chen, F., Hu, Y.: Optimal investment, consumption and proportional reinsurance under model uncertainty. Insur.: Math. Econ. **59**, 222–234 (2014)
339. Pentikainen, T., Bornsdorff, H., Pesonen, M., Rantala, J., Ruohonen, M.: Insurance Solvency and Financial Strength. Finnish Insurance Training and Publishing Company Ltd., Helsinki (1989)
340. Pergamenshchikov, S., Zeitouny, O.: Ruin probability in the presence of risky investments. Stoch. Process. Appl. **116**(2), 267–278 (2006)
341. Perna, C., Sibillo, M. (eds.): Mathematical and Statistical Methods for Actuarial Sciences and Finance. Springer, Berlin (2014)
342. Peters, G.W., Dong, A.X.D., Kohn, R.: A copula based Bayesian approach for paid-incurred claims models for non-life insurance reserving. Insur.: Math. Econ. **59**, 258–278 (2014)
343. Pham, H.: Continuous-Time Stochastic Control and Optimization with Financial Applications. Springer, Berlin (2009)
344. Picard, P., Lefèvre, C.: Probabilité de ruine éventuelle dans un modèle de risque à temps discret. J. Appl. Probab. **40**(3), 543–556 (2003)
345. Picard, P., Lefèvre, C., Coulibaly, I.: Problèmes de ruine en théorie du risque à temps discret avec horizon fini. J. Appl. Probab. **40**, 527–542 (2003)
346. Picard, P., Lefèvre, C., Coulibaly, I.: Multirisks model and finite-time ruin probabilities. Methodol. Comput. Appl. Probab. **5**, 337–353 (2003)
347. Pitacco, E.: Health Insurance. Basic Actuarial Models. Springer, Switzerland (2014)
348. Prabhu, N.U.: Stochastic Storage Processes. Queues, Insurance Risk, Dams and Data Communications. Springer, New York (2012)
349. Promyslow, D.S.: Fundamentals of Actuarial Mathematics, 2nd edn. Wiley, New York (2011)
350. Qi, X.: Analysis of the generalized Gerber-Shiu function in discrete-time dependent Sparre Andersen model. Thesis. The University of Hong Kong Libraries, University of Hong Kong (2016)
351. Quang, P.D.: Ruin probability in a generalized risk process under interest force with homogenous Markov chain premiums. Int. J. Stat. Probab. **2**(4), 85–92 (2013)
352. Rachev, S.T., Stoyanov, S.V., Fabozzi, F.J.: Advanced Stochastic Models, Risk Assessment, Portfolio Optimization. Wiley, Hoboken (2008)
353. Rachev, S.T., Klebanov, L., Stoyanov, S.V., Fabozzi, F.: The Methods of Distances in the Theory of Probability and Statistics. Springer, New York (2013)
354. Ramaswami, V.: Passage times in fluid models with application to risk processes. Methodol. Comput. Appl. Probab. **8**, 497–515 (2006)
355. Reinhard, J.M.: On a class of semi-Markov risk models obtained as classical risk models in a Markovian enviroment. ASTIN Bull. **14**, 23–43 (1984)

356. Ren, J.: The discounted joint distribution of the surplus prior to ruin and the deficit at ruin in a Sparre Andersen model. N. Am. Actuar. J. **11**, 128–136 (2007)
357. Renaud, J.-F.: On the time spent in the red by a refracted Lévy risk process. J. Appl. Probab. **51**(4), 1171–1188 (2014)
358. Renaud, J.-F., Zhou, X.: Distribution of the dividend payments in a general Lévy risk model. J. Appl. Probab. **44**, 420–427 (2007)
359. Řezáč, M., Řezáč, F.: How to measure the quality of credit scoring models. Finance a úvěr (Czech J. Econ. Financ.) **61**(5), 486–507 (2011)
360. Rockafellar, R.T., Uryasev, S., Zabarankin, M.: Generalized deviations in risk analysis. Financ. Stoch. **10**, 51–74 (2006)
361. Rolski, T., Schmidli, H., Schmidt, V., Teugels, J.L.: Stochastic Processes for Insuarance and Finance. Wiley, Chichester (1999)
362. Şahin, Ş., Cairns, A.J.G., Kleinow, T., Wilkie, A.D.: Comparison of the Wilkie model and a "Yield-Macro Model" for UK data. http://www.actuaries.org/lyon2013/papers/AFIR-Sahin-Cairns-Kleinow-Wilkie.pdf
363. Şahin, Ş., Cairns, A.J.G., Kleinow, T., Wilkie, A.D.: Revisiting the Wilkie investment model. http://www.actuaries.org/AFIR/Colloquia/Rome2/Cairns-Kleinow-Sahin-Wilkie.pdf
364. Saltelli, A., Tarantola, S., Campolongo, F.: Sensitivity analysis as an ingredient of modeling. Stat. Sci. **15**, 377–395 (2000)
365. Sandström, A.: Handbook of Solvency for Actuaries and Risk Managers: Theory and Practice. Chapman and Hall/CRC Press, Boca Raton (2011)
366. Sato, K.: Lévy Process and Infinitely Divisible Distributions. Cambridge University Press, Cambridge (1999)
367. Savich, S.E.: Elementary Theory of Life Insurance and Disability. SPb., 1900 (3rd edn. Yanus-K 2003) (in Russian)
368. Savitsch, S. von: Der Einfluss der Dimensionen des Feuerrisikos auf den Prämiensatz. Zeitschrift für die gesamte Versicherungswissenschaft (1907)
369. Schmidli, H.: On minimizing the ruin probability by investment and reinsurance. Ann. Appl. Probab. **12**, 890–907 (2002)
370. Schmidli, H.: Stochastic Control in Insurance. Springer, New York (2008)
371. Seal, H.L.: The Stochastic Theory of a Risk Business. Wiley, New York (1969)
372. Sendova, K.P.: Discrete Lundberg-type bounds with actuarial applications. ESAIM: Probab. Stat. **11**, 217–235 (2007)
373. Sendova, K.P., Zang, Y.: Interest bearing surplus model with liquid reserves. J. Insur. Issues **33**(2), 178–196 (2010)
374. Sendova, K.P., Zitikis, R.: The order-statistic claim process with dependent claim frequencies and severities. J. Stat. Theory Pract. **6**, 597–620 (2012)
375. Shang, H. (ed.): Actuarial Science: Theory and Methodology. World Scientific, Singapore (2006)
376. Shen, Y., Yin, C.: Optimal dividend problem for a compound Poisson risk model. Appl. Math. **5**, 1496–1502 (2014)
377. Shi, T., Landriault, D.: Distribution of the time to ruin in some Sparre Andersen risk models. Astin Bull. **43**(1), 39–59 (2013)
378. Shija, G., Jacob, M.J.: Expected discounted penalty function of Markov-modulated, constant barrier and stochastic income model. IOSR J. Math. **9**(6), 34–42 (2014)
379. Shiraishi, H.: Review of statistical actuarial risk modelling. Cogent Math. **3**, 1123945 (2016). http://dx.doi.org/10.1080/23311835.2015.1123945
380. Shiryaev, A.N., Grossinho, M.D.R., Oliveira, P.E., Esquível, M.L. (eds.): Stochastic Finance. Springer, Berlin (2006)
381. Shiryaev, A.N.: Actuarial and financial business: current state of art and perspectives of development. Rev. Appl. Ind. Math. **1**(5), 684–697 (1994) (in Russian)
382. Shorack, G.R., Wellner, J.A.: Empirical Processes with Application to Statistics. Wiley, New York (1986)

383. Silvestrov, D., Martin-Löf, A. (eds.): Modern Problems in Insurance Mathematics. Springer, Berlin (2014)
384. Simkins, B., Fraser, J.: Enterprise Risk Management: Today's Leading Research and Best Practices for Tomorrow's Executives. Wiley, New York (2010)
385. Smith Jr., C.W.: On the convergence of insurance and finance research. J. Risk Insur. **53**(4), 693–717 (1986)
386. Sobol, I.M.: Sensitivity analysis for nonlinear mathematical models. Math. Model. Comput. Exp. **1**, 407–414 (1993)
387. Song, R., Vondracek, Z.: On suprema of Lévy processes and application in risk theory. Ann. Inst. H. Poincare Probab. Stat. **44**, 977–986 (2008)
388. Stanford, D.A., Avram, F., Badescu, A.L., Breuer, L., Da Silva Soares, A., Latouche, G.: Phase-type approximations to finite-time ruin probabilities in the Sparre Andersen and stationary renewal risk models. ASTIN Bull. **35**, 131–144 (2005)
389. Sun, Y., Wei, L.: The finite-time ruin probability with heavy-tailed and dependent insurance and financial risks. Insur.: Math. Econ. **59**, 178–183 (2014)
390. Taksar, M., Markussen, C.: Optimal dynamic reinsurance policies for large insurance portfolios. Financ. Stoch. **7**, 97–121 (2003)
391. Taksar, M., Zeng, X.: Optimal non-proportional reinsurance control and stochastic differential games. Insur.: Math. Econ. **48**, 64–71 (2011)
392. Tankov, P., Cont, R.: Financial modelling with jump processes. Chapman and Hall/CRC, Boca Raton (2003)
393. Temnov, G.: Risk process with random income. J. Math. Sci. **123**(1), 3780–3794 (2004)
394. Temnov, G.: Risk models with stochastic premium and ruin probability estimation. J. Math. Sci. **196**(1), 84–96 (2014)
395. Tsai, C.C.-L.: A generalized defective renewal equation for the surplus process perturbed by diffusion. Insur.: Math. Econ. **30**(1), 51–66 (2002)
396. Tsanakas, A., Beck, M.B., Thompson, M.: Taming uncertainty: the limits to quantification. ASTIN Bull. **46**, 1–7 (2016)
397. Tuncel, A.: Survival probabilities for compound binomial risk model with discrete phase-type claims. Commun. Fac. Sci. Univ. Ank. Ser. A1 Math. Stat. **65**(2), 11–22 (2016)
398. Turnbull, C.: A History of British Actuarial Thought. Springer, Berlin (2016)
399. Ungureanu, D., Vernic, R.: On a fuzzy cash flow model with insurance applications. Decis. Econ. Financ. **38**(1), 39–54 (2015)
400. Wan, N.: Dividend payments with a threshold strategy in the compound Poisson risk model perturbed by diffusion. Insur.: Math. Econ. **40**, 509–523 (2007)
401. Wang, C., Yin, C.: Dividend payments in the classical risk model under absolute ruin with debit interest. Appl. Stoch. Models Bus. Ind. **25**(3), 247–262 (2009)
402. Wang, C.W., Yin, C.C., Li, E.Q.: On the classical risk model with credit and debit interests under absolute ruin. Stat. Probab. Lett. **80**, 427–436 (2010)
403. Wang, X., Wang, W., Zhang, C.: Ornstein-Uhlenbeck type Omega model. Front. Math. China **11**(3), 735–751 (2016)
404. Wat, K.: Discrete-time insurance risk models with dependence structures. Thesis. The University of Hong Kong Libraries, University of Hong Kong (2012)
405. Wei, J., Wang, R., Yang, H.: On the optimal dividend strategy in a regime-switching diffusion model. Adv. Appl. Probab. **44**, 866–906 (2012)
406. Wilkie, A.D.: A stochastic investment model for actuarial use. Trans. Fac. Actuar. **39**, 341–403 (1986)
407. Wilkie, D.: Whither AFIR? Editorial. ASTIN Bull. **21**(1), 1–3 (1991)
408. Wilkie, A.D.: More on a stochastic asset model for actuarial use. Br. Actuar. J. **1**(5), 777–964 (1995)
409. Wilkie, A.D., Şahin, Ş., Cairns, A.J.G., Kleinow, T.: Yet more on a stochastic economic model: part 1: updating and refitting, 1995 to 2009. Ann. Actuar. Sci. **5**, 53–99 (2010)
410. Willmot, G.E.: A Laplace transform representation in a class of renewal queueing and risk process. J. Appl. Probab. **36**, 570–584 (1999)

411. Willmot, G.E.: Compound geometric residual lifetime distributions and the deficit at ruin. Insur.: Math. Econ. **30**, 421–438 (2002)
412. Willmot, G.E.: On the discounted penalty function in the renewal risk model with general interclaim times. Insur.: Math. Econ. **41**, 17–31 (2007)
413. Willmot, G.E., Lin, X.S.: Lundberg Approximations for Compound Distributions with Insurance Applications. Springer, New York (2001)
414. Wong, T.J.: On some Parisian problems in ruin theory. University of Hong Kong, Pokfulam, Hong Kong SAR (2014). http://dx.doi.org/10.5353/th-b5317068
415. Wong, J.T.Y., Cheung, E.C.K.: On the time value of Parisian ruin in (dual) renewal risk processes with exponential jumps. Insur.: Math. Econ. **65**, 280–290 (2015)
416. Wu, X., Li, S.: On a discrete-time Sparre Andersen model with phase-type claims. http://fbe.unimelb.edu.au/--data/assets/pdf-file/0005/806279/169.pdf
417. Wu, Y.: Bounds for the ruin probability under a Markovian modulated risk model. Commun. Stat. Stoch. Models **15**(1), 125–136 (1999)
418. Wüthrich, M.V., Merz, M.: Stochastic claims reserving manual: advances in dynamic modeling. Swiss Finance Institute Research Paper No. 15–34 (2015)
419. Wüthrich, M.V.: Market-Consistent Actuarial Valuation, 3rd edn. Springer, Berlin (2016)
420. Wüthrich, M.V., Merz, M.: Financial Modeling, Actuarial Valuation and Solvency in Insurance. Springer, Berlin (2013)
421. Wüthrich, M.V., Bühlmann, H., Furrer, H.: Market-Consistent Actuarial Valuation. Springer, Berlin (2010)
422. Xue, C.: Absolute ruin probability of a multi-type-insurance risk model. Int. J. Appl. Math. Stat. **53**(1), 74–81 (2015)
423. Yan, D.: Some results on a double compound Poisson-geometric risk model with interference. Theor. Econ. Lett. **2**(1), 45–49 (2012)
424. Yang, H., Li, J.: Asymptotic finite-time ruin probability for a bidimensional renewal risk model with constant interest force and dependent subexponential claims. Insur.: Math. Econ. **58**, 185–192 (2014)
425. Yang, Y., Yuen, K.C.: Asymptotics for a discrete-time risk model with gamma-like insurance risks. Scand. Actuar. J. **2016**(6), 565–579 (2016)
426. Yang, Y., Leipus, R., Siaulys, J.: On the ruin probability in a dependent discrete time risk model with insurance and financial risks. J. Comput. Appl. Math. **236**(13), 3286–3295 (2012)
427. Yang, H., Gao, W., Li, J.: Asymptotic ruin probabilities for a discrete-time risk model with dependent insurance and financial risks. Scand. Actuar. J. **2016**(1), 1–17 (2016)
428. Yin, C., Wen, Y., Zhao, Y.: On the optimal dividend problem for a spectrally positive Lévy process. arXiv:1302.2231v4 [q-fin.PM]. Accessed 10 Mar 2014
429. Yin, C.C., Wang, C.W.: Optimality of the barrier strategy in de Finetti's dividend problem for spectrally negative Lévy processes: an alternative approach. J. Comput. Appl. Math. **233**, 482–491 (2009)
430. Yin, C.C., Wen, Y.Z.: An extension of Paulsen-Gjessing's risk model with stochastic return on investments. Insur.: Math. Econ. **52**, 469–476 (2013)
431. Yu, W., Huang, Y.: Dividend payments and related problems in a Markov-dependent insurance risk model under absolute ruin. Am. J. Ind. Bus. Manag. **1**(1), 1–9 (2011)
432. Yuen, K.C., Guo, J., Wu, X.: On a correlated aggregate claims model with Poisson and Erlang risk processes. Insur.: Math. Econ. **31**, 205–214 (2002)
433. Zhang, Z.: On a risk model with randomized dividend-decision times. J. Ind. Manag. Optim. **10**(4), 1041–1058 (2014)
434. Zhang, Z., Cheung, E.C.K.: The Markov additive risk process under an Erlangized dividend barrier strategy. Methodol. Comput. Appl. Probab. **18**(2), 275–306 (2016)
435. Zhang, Z., Yang, H.: Gerber-Shiu analysis in a perturbed risk model with dependence between claim sizes and interclaim times. J. Comput. Appl. Math. **235**(5), 1189–1204 (2011)
436. Zhang, Z., Yang, H.: Nonparametric estimation for the ruin probability in a Lévy risk model under low-frequency observation. Insur.: Math. Econ. **59**, 168–177 (2014)

437. Zhang, H.Y., Zhou, M., Guo, J.Y.: The Gerber-Shiu discounted penalty function for classical risk model with a two-step premium rate. Stat. Probab. Lett. **76**, 1211–1218 (2006)
438. Zhang, Z., Li, S., Yang, H.: The Gerber-Shiu discounted penalty functions for a risk model with two classes of claims. J. Comput. Appl. Math. **230**, 643–655 (2009)
439. Zhao, Q., Wei, J., Wang, R.: On dividend strategies with non-exponential discounting. Insur.: Math. Econ. **58**(1), 1–13 (2014)
440. Zheng, Y., Cui, W.: Optimal reinsurance with premium constraint under distortion risk measures. Insur.: Math. Econ. **59**, 109–120 (2014)
441. Zheng, Y., Cui, W., Yang, J.: Optimal reinsurance under distortion risk measures and expected value premium principle for reinsurer. J. Syst. Sci. Complex. **28**(1), 122–143 (2015)
442. Zhu, J., Yang, H.: Estimates for the absolute ruin probability in the compound Poisson risk model with credit and debit interest. J. Appl. Probab. **45**(3), 818–830 (2008)
443. Zhu, Y., Chi, Y., Weng, C.: Multivariate reinsurance designs for minimizing an insurer's capital requirement. Insur.: Math. Econ. **59**, 144–155 (2014)
444. Zinchenko, N., Andrusiv, A.: Risk process with stochastic premiums. Theory Stoch. Process. **14**(30), 189–208 (2008)
445. Zou, B., Cadenillas, A.: Optimal investment and risk control policies for an insurer: expected utility maximization. Insur.: Math. Econ. **58**, 57–67 (2014)
446. Zou, B., Cadenillas, A.: Optimal investment and liability ratio policies in a multidimensional regime switching model. Risks **5**(1), 6 (2017)

Part IX
Population Dynamics

Population Processes with Immigration

Dan Han, Stanislav Molchanov and Joseph Whitmeyer

Abstract The paper contains a complete analysis of the Galton–Watson models with immigration, including the processes in the random environment, stationary or non-stationary ones. We also study the branching random walk on Z^d with immigration and prove the existence of the limits for the first two correlation functions.

Keywords Galton-Watson process · Branching process · Immigration
Random environment

1 Introduction

A problem with many single population models of population dynamics involving processes of birth, death, and migration is that the populations do not attain steady states or do so only under critical conditions. One solution is to allow immigration, which can stabilize the population when the birth rate is less than the mortality rate.

Here, we present analysis of several models that incorporate immigration. The first two are spatial Galton–Watson processes, the first with no migration and the second with finite Markov chain spatial dynamics (see Sects. 2 and 3 respectively). The third model allows migration on $\mathbb{Z}^d$ (see Sect. 4). The remaining models all involve random environments in some way (see Sect. 5). Two are again Galton–Watson processes, the first with a random environment based on population size and the second with

For the second author, this work has been funded by the Russian Academic Excellence Project '5-100'.

D. Han · S. Molchanov
University of North Carolina at Charlotte, Charlotte, NC 28223, USA

S. Molchanov
National Research University, Higher School of Economics, Moscow, Russian Federation

J. Whitmeyer (✉)
University of North Carolina at Charlotte, Charlotte, NC 28223, USA
e-mail: jwhitmey@uncc.edu

© Springer International Publishing AG 2017
V. Panov (ed.), *Modern Problems of Stochastic Analysis and Statistics*,
Springer Proceedings in Mathematics & Statistics 208,
DOI 10.1007/978-3-319-65313-6_16

411

a random environment given by a Markov chain. The last two models have birth, death, immigration, and migration in a random environment allowing in some way nonstationarity in both space and time. We study in this paper only first and second moments. We will return to the complete analysis of the models with immigration in another publication. It will include a theorem about the existence of steady states and an analysis of the stability of these states.

2 Spatial Galton–Watson Process with Immigration. No Migration and No Random Environment

2.1 Moments

Assume that at each site for each particle we have birth of one new particle with rate β and death of the particle with rate μ. Also, assume that regardless of the number of particles at the site we have immigration of one new particle with rate k (this is a simplified version of the process in [1]). Assume that $\beta < \mu$, for otherwise the population will grow exponentially. Assume we start with one particle at each site. In continuous time, for a given site $x, x \in Z^d$, we can obtain all moments recursively by means of the Laplace transform with respect to $n(t, x)$, where $n(t, x)$ is the population size at time t at x

$$\varphi_t(\lambda) = E\, e^{-\lambda n(t,x)} = \sum_{j=0}^{\infty} P\{n(t, x) = j\} e^{-\lambda j}.$$

Specifically, for the jth moment, m_j

$$m_j(t, x) = (-1)^j \frac{\partial^j \varphi}{\partial \lambda^j}\big|_{\lambda=0}. \tag{2.1}$$

A partial differential equation for $\varphi_t(\lambda)$ can be derived using the forward Kolmogorov equations

$$n(t + dt, x) = n(t, x) + \xi_{dt}(t, x) \tag{2.2}$$

where the r.v. ξ is defined

$$\xi_{dt}(t, x) = \begin{cases} +1 & \beta n(t, x)dt + kdt \\ -1 & \mu n(t, x)dt \\ 0 & 1 - ((\beta + \mu)n(t, x) + k)dt \end{cases} \tag{2.3}$$

In other words, our site (x) in a small time interval (dt) can gain a new particle at rate β for every particle at the site or through immigration with rate k; it can lose a particle at rate μ for every particle at the site; or no change at all can happen. Because our model is homogeneous in space, we can write $n(t)$ for $n(t, x)$. This leads to the general differential equation

$$\frac{\partial \varphi_t(\lambda)}{\partial t} = \varphi_t(\lambda) \left(\mu n(t)e^\lambda - ((\beta + \mu)n(t) + k) + (\beta n(t) + k)e^{-\lambda} \right)$$

$$\varphi_0(\lambda) = e^{-\lambda}$$

from which we can calculate the recursive set of differential equations

$$\frac{\partial \varphi_t(\lambda)^{(j)}}{\partial t} = \varphi_t(\lambda)^{(j)} \left(\mu n(t)e^\lambda - ((\beta + \mu)n(t) + k) + (\beta n(t) + k)e^{-\lambda} \right) +$$

$$+ \sum_{i=1}^{j} \binom{j}{i} \varphi_t(\lambda)^{(j-i)} \left(\mu n(t)e^\lambda + (-1)^i (\beta n(t) + k)e^{-\lambda} \right)$$

$$\varphi_0(\lambda)^{(j)} = (-1)^j e^{-\lambda}$$

Applying Eq. 2.1, we obtain a set of recursive differential equations for the moments

$$\frac{dm_j(t)}{dt} = \sum_{i=1}^{j} \binom{j}{i} \left((\beta + (-1)^i \mu)m_{j-i+1} + m_{j-i} \right)$$

$$= j(\beta - \mu)m_j + s_j \tag{2.4}$$

$$m_j(0) = 1$$

where s_j denotes a linear expression involving lower order moments and where we define $m_0 = 1$. For example, the differential equations for the first and second moments are

$$\frac{dm_1(t)}{dt} = (\beta - \mu)m_1(t) + k$$

$$m_1(0) = 1$$

and

$$\frac{dm_2(t)}{dt} = 2(\beta - \mu)m_2(t) + (\beta + \mu + 2k)m_1(t) + k$$

$$m_2(0) = 1$$

These have the solutions:

$$m_1(t) = \frac{k}{\mu - \beta} + \left(1 - \frac{k}{\mu - \beta} \right) e^{-(\mu - \beta)t}$$

and

$$m_2(t) = \frac{k(k+\mu)}{(\mu-\beta)^2} + \frac{\mu^2 - 2k^2 - \beta^2 + k\mu - 3k\beta}{(\mu-\beta)^2}e^{-(\mu-\beta)t} +$$
$$+ \frac{k^2 + 2\beta^2 + 3k\beta - 2\mu\beta - 2k\mu}{(\mu-\beta)^2}e^{-2(\mu-\beta)t}$$

Again, given that we have assumed that $\mu > \beta$, in other words, the birth rate is not high enough to maintain the population size, as $t \to \infty$

$$m_1(t) \xrightarrow[t\to\infty]{} \frac{k}{\mu-\beta}$$

$$m_2(t) \xrightarrow[t\to\infty]{} \frac{k(k+\mu)}{(\mu-\beta)^2}$$

and

$$\mathrm{Var}(n(t)) = m_2(t) - m_1^2(t) \xrightarrow[t\to\infty]{} \frac{\mu k}{(\mu-\beta)^2}.$$

Moreover, it is clear from Eq. 2.4 that all the moments are finite.

In other words, the population size will approach a finite limit, which can be regulated by controlling the immigration rate k, and this population size will be stable, as indicated by the fact that the limiting variance is finite. Without immigration, i.e., if $k = 0$, the population size will decay exponentially. Another possibility, because all sites are independent and there are no spatial dynamics, is for there to be immigration at some sites, which therefore reach stable population levels, and not at others, where the population thus decreases exponentially. Of course, if the birth rate exceeds the death rate, $\beta > \mu$, $m_1(t)$ increases exponentially and immigration has negligible effect, as shown by the solution for $m_1(t)$.

2.2 Local CLT

Setting $\lambda_n = n\beta + k$, $\mu_n = n\mu$, we see that the model given by Eqs. 2.2 and 2.3 is a particular case of the general random walk on $Z_+^1 = \{0, 1, 2, \ldots\}$ with generator

$$\mathcal{L}\psi(n) = \psi(n+1)\lambda_n - (\lambda_n + \mu_n)\psi(n) + \mu_n\psi(n-1), \quad n \geq 0 \quad (2.5)$$
$$\mathcal{L}\psi(0) = k\psi(1) - k\psi(0) \quad (2.6)$$

The theory of such chains has interesting connections to the theory of orthogonal polynomials, the moments problem, and related topics (see [2]). We recall several facts of this theory.

a. Equation $\mathcal{L}\psi = 0$, $x \geq 1$, (i.e., the equation for harmonic functions) has two linearly independent solutions:

$$\psi_1(n) \equiv 1$$

$$\psi_2(n) = \begin{cases} 0 & n = 0 \\ 1 & n = 1 \\ 1 + \frac{\mu_1}{\lambda_1} + \frac{\mu_1\mu_2}{\lambda_1\lambda_2} + \cdots + \frac{\mu_1\mu_2\cdots\mu_{n-1}}{\lambda_1\lambda_2\cdots\lambda_{n-1}} & n \geq 2 \end{cases} \tag{2.7}$$

b. Denoting the adjoint of $\mathcal{L}$ by $\mathcal{L}^*$, equation $\mathcal{L}^*\pi = 0$ (i.e., the equation for the stationary distribution, which can be infinite) has the positive solution

$$\pi(1) = \frac{\lambda_0}{\mu_1}\pi(0) \tag{2.8}$$

$$\pi(2) = \frac{\lambda_0\lambda_1}{\mu_1\mu_2}\pi(0) \tag{2.9}$$

$$\cdots \tag{2.10}$$

$$\pi(n) = \frac{\lambda_0\lambda_1\cdots\lambda_{n-1}}{\mu_1\mu_2\cdots\mu_n}\pi(0) \tag{2.11}$$

This random walk is ergodic (i.e., $n(t)$ converges to a statistical equilibrium, a steady state) if and only if the series $1 + \frac{\lambda_0}{\mu_1} + \cdots + \frac{\lambda_0\lambda_1}{\mu_1\mu_2} + \cdots + \frac{\lambda_0\lambda_1\cdots\lambda_{n-1}}{\mu_1\mu_2\cdots\mu_n}$ converges. In our case,

$$x_n = \frac{\lambda_0\cdots\lambda_{n-1}}{\mu_1\cdots\mu_n} = \frac{k(k+\beta)\cdots(k+(\mu-1))\beta}{\mu(2\mu)\cdots(n\mu)}.$$

If $\beta > \mu$, then, for $n > n_0$, for some fixed $\varepsilon > 0$, $\frac{k+(n-1)\beta}{n\mu} > 1 + \varepsilon$, that is, $x_n \geq C^n$, for $C > 1$ and $n \geq n_1(\varepsilon)$, and so $\sum x_n = \infty$. In contrast, if $\beta < \mu$, then, for some $0 < \varepsilon < 1$, $\frac{k+(n-1)\beta}{n\mu} < 1 - \varepsilon$, and $x_n \leq q^n$, for $0 < q < 1$ and $n > n_1(\varepsilon)$; thus, $\sum x_n < \infty$. In this ergodic case, the invariant distribution of the random walk $n(t)$ is given by the formula

$$\pi(n) = \frac{1}{S}\frac{\lambda_0\cdots\lambda_{n-1}}{\mu_1\cdots\mu_n},$$

where

$$\tilde{S} = 1 + \frac{k}{\mu} + \frac{k(\beta+k)}{\mu(2\mu)} + \cdots + \frac{k(k+\beta)\cdots(\beta(n-1)+k)}{\mu(2\mu)\cdots(n\mu)} + \cdots.$$

Theorem 2.1 (Local Central Limit theorem) *Let $\beta < \mu$. If $l = O(k^{2/3})$, then, for the invariant distribution $\pi(n)$*

$$\pi(n_0 + l) \sim \frac{e^{-\frac{l^2}{2\sigma^2}}}{\sqrt{2\pi\sigma^2}} \quad as \ k \to \infty \tag{2.12}$$

where $\sigma^2 = \frac{\mu k}{(\mu-\beta)^2}$, $n_0 \sim \frac{k}{\mu-\beta}$.

The proof, which we omit here, makes use of the fact that $\tilde{S}$ is a degenerate hypergeometric function and so $\tilde{S} = \left(1 - \frac{\beta}{\mu}\right)^{-\frac{k}{\beta}}$. If we define a_n by setting $\pi(n) = \frac{a_n}{\tilde{S}}$, then, $a_{n_0} \sim \frac{k}{\mu-\beta}$, and, setting $l = O(k^{2/3})$, straightforward computations yield $a_{n_0+l} \sim a_{n_0} e^{-\frac{l^2}{2\sigma^2}}$. Application of Stirling's formula leads to the result.

2.3 Global Limit Theorems

A functional Law of Large Numbers follows directly from Theorem 3.1 in Kurtz (1970 [3]). Likewise, a functional Central Limit Theorem follows from Theorems 3.1 and 3.5 in Kurtz (1971 [4]). We state these theorems here, therefore, without proof.

Write the population size as $n_k(t)$, a function of the immigration rate as well as time. Set $n_k^* = \frac{k}{\mu-\beta}$, the limit of the first moment as $t \to \infty$. Define a new stochastic process for the population size divided by the immigration rate, $Z_k(t) := \frac{n_k(t)}{k}$. Set $z^* = \frac{n_k^*}{k} = \frac{1}{\mu-\beta}$.

We define the transition function, $f_k(\frac{n_k}{k}, j) := \frac{1}{k} p(n_k, n_k + j)$. Thus,

$$
f_k(z, j) = \begin{cases} \frac{\beta n_k + k}{k} = \beta z + 1 & j = 1 \\ \frac{\mu n_k}{k} = \mu z & j = -1 \\ \text{(not needed)} & j = 0 \end{cases}
$$

Note that $f_k(z, j)$ does not, in fact, depend on k and we write simply $f(z, j)$.

Theorem 2.2 (Functional LLN) *Suppose* $\lim\limits_{k\to\infty} Z_k(0) = z_0$. *Then, as* $k \to \infty$, $Z_k(t) \to Z(t)$ *uniformly in probability, where* $Z(t)$ *is a deterministic process, the solution of*

$$
\frac{dZ(t)}{dt} = F(Z(t)), \quad Z(0) = z_0. \tag{2.13}
$$

where

$$
F(z) := \sum_j j f(z, j) = (\beta - \mu)z + 1.
$$

This has the solution

$$
Z(t, z) = \frac{1}{\mu - \beta} + \left(z_0 - \frac{1}{\mu - \beta}\right) e^{-(\mu-\beta)t} = z^* + (z_0 - z^*)e^{-(\mu-\beta)t}, \ t \geq 0.
$$

Next, define $G_k(z) := \sum_j j^2 f_k(z, j) = (b + \mu)z + 1$. This too does not depend on k and we simply write $G(z)$.

Theorem 2.3 (Functional CLT) *If* $\lim\limits_{k\to\infty} \sqrt{k}\,(Z_k(0) - z^*) = \zeta_0$, *the processes*

$$\zeta_k(t) := \sqrt{k}(Z_k(t) - Z(t))$$

converge weakly in the space of cadlag functions on any finite time interval $[0, T]$ *to a Gaussian diffusion* $\zeta(t)$ *with:*

(1) initial value $\zeta(0) = \zeta_0$,
(2) mean

$$E\zeta(s) = \zeta_0 L_s := \zeta_0 e^{\int_0^s F'(Z(u,z_0))du},$$

(3) variance

$$\mathrm{Var}(\zeta(s)) = L_s^2 \int_0^s L_u^{-2} G(Z(u, z_0))du.$$

Suppose, moreover, that $F(z_0) = 0$, i.e., $z_0 = z^*$, the equilibrium point. Then, $Z(t) \equiv z_0$ and $\zeta(t)$ is an Ornstein–Uhlenbeck process (OUP) with initial value ζ_0, infinitesimal drift

$$q := F'(z_0) = \beta - \mu$$

and infinitesimal variance

$$a := G(z_0) = \frac{2\mu}{\mu - \beta}.$$

Thus, $\zeta(t)$ is normally distributed with mean

$$\zeta_0 e^{qt} = \zeta_0 e^{-(\mu-\beta)t}$$

and variance

$$\frac{a}{-2q}\left(1 - e^{2qt}\right) = \frac{\mu}{(\mu - \beta)^2}\left(1 - e^{-2(\mu-\beta)t}\right).$$

3   Spatial Galton–Watson Process with Immigration and Finite Markov Chain Spatial Dynamics

Let $X = \{x, y, \ldots\}$ be a finite set, and define the following parameters.

$\beta(x)$ is the rate of duplication at $x \in X$.
$\mu(x)$ is the rate of annihilation at $x \in X$.
$a(x, y)$ is the rate of transition $x \to y$.
$k(x)$ is the rate of immigration into $x \in X$.

We define $\vec{n}(t) = \{n(t, x), x \in X\}$, the population at moment $t \geq 0$, with $n(t, x)$ the occupation number of site $x \in X$. Letting $\vec{\lambda} = \{\lambda_x \geq 0, x \in X\}$, we write the Laplace transform of the random vector $\vec{n}(t) \in \mathbb{R}^N$, $N = \text{Card}(X)$ as $u(t, \vec{\lambda}) = E\, e^{-(\vec{\lambda}, \vec{n}(t))}$.

Now, we derive the differential equation for $u(t, \vec{\lambda})$. Denote the σ-algebra of events before or including t by $\mathcal{F}_{\leq t}$. Setting $\vec{\varepsilon}(t, dt)) = \vec{n}(t + dt) - \vec{n}(t)$

$$u(t + dt, \vec{\lambda}) = E\, e^{-(\vec{\lambda}, \vec{n}(t+dt))} = E\, e^{-(\vec{\lambda}, \vec{n}(t))} E\,[e^{-(\vec{\lambda}, \vec{\varepsilon}(t,dt))}|\mathcal{F}_{\leq t}] \qquad (3.1)$$

The conditional distribution of $(\vec{\lambda}, \vec{\varepsilon})$ under $\mathcal{F}_{\leq t}$ is given by the formulas

(a) $P\{(\vec{\lambda}, \vec{\varepsilon}(t, dt)) = \lambda_x|\mathcal{F}_{\leq t}\} = n(t, x)\beta(x)dt + k(x)dt$
    (the birth of a new offspring at site x or the immigration of a new particle into $x \in X$)
(b) $P\{(\vec{\lambda}, \vec{\varepsilon}) = \lambda_y|\mathcal{F}_{\leq t}\} = n(t, y)\mu(y)dt$
    (the death of a particle at $y \in X$)
(c) $P\{(\vec{\lambda}, \vec{\varepsilon}) = \lambda_x - \lambda_z|\mathcal{F}_{\leq t}\} = n(t, x)a(x, z)dt; \ x, z \in X, \ x \neq z$
    (transition of a single particle from x to z. Then, $n(t + dt, x) = n(t, x) - 1$, $n(t + dt, z) = n(t, z) + 1$.)
(d) $P\{(\vec{\lambda}, \vec{\varepsilon}) = 0|\mathcal{F}_{\leq t}\} = 1 - \left(\sum_{x \in X} n(t, x)\beta(x)\right) dt - \left(\sum_{x \in X} k(x)\right) dt$
$$- \left(\sum_{y \in X} n(t, y)\mu(y)\right) dt - \left(\sum_{x \neq z} n(t, x)a(x, z)\right) dt$$

After substitution of these expressions into Eq. 3.1 and elementary transformations we obtain

$$\frac{\partial u(t, \vec{\lambda})}{\partial t} = E \sum_{x \in X} (e^{-\lambda_x} - 1)e^{-(\vec{\lambda}, \vec{n}(t))}(\beta(x)n(t, x) + k(x)) +$$
$$\sum_{y \in X} (e^{\lambda_y} - 1)e^{-(\vec{\lambda}, \vec{n}(t))}\mu(y)n(t, y)$$
$$+ \sum_{x,y;x \neq y} (e^{\lambda_x - \lambda_y} - 1)e^{-(\vec{\lambda}, \vec{n}(t))}a(x, y)n(t, x)$$

But

$$E\, e^{-(\vec{\lambda}, \vec{n}(t))}n(t, x) = -\frac{\partial u(t, \vec{\lambda})}{\partial \lambda_x}$$

I.e., finally

$$\frac{\partial u(t, \vec{\lambda})}{\partial t} = \sum_{x \in X} (e^{-\lambda_x} - 1)\left(-\frac{\partial u(t, \vec{\lambda})}{\partial \lambda_x}\beta(x) + u(t, \vec{\lambda})k(x)\right)$$

$$+ \sum_{y \in X} (e^{\lambda_y} - 1)\mu(y)\left(-\frac{\partial u(t, \vec{\lambda})}{\partial \lambda_y}\right) \tag{3.2}$$

$$+ \sum_{x,z; x \neq z} (e^{\lambda_x - \lambda_z} - 1)a(x, z)\left(-\frac{\partial u(t, \vec{\lambda})}{\partial \lambda_x}\right)$$

The initial condition is

$$u(0, \vec{\lambda}) = E\, e^{-(\vec{\lambda}, \vec{n}\,(0))}$$

(say, $u(0, \vec{\lambda}) = e^{-(\vec{\lambda}, 1)} = e^{\sum_{x \in X} \lambda_x}$ for $n(0, x) = 1$).

Differentiation of Eq. 3.2 and the substitution of $\vec{\lambda} = 0$ leads to the equations for the correlation functions (moments) of the field $n(t, x)$, $x \in X$. Put

$$m_1(t, v) = E\, n(t, v) = -\frac{\partial u(t, \vec{\lambda})}{\partial \lambda_v}\Big|_{\vec{\lambda}=0}, \qquad v \in X$$

Then

$$\frac{\partial m_1(t, v)}{\partial t} = k(v) + (\beta(v) - \mu(v))m_1(t, v) + \frac{\partial}{\partial \lambda_v}\left(\sum_{z: z \neq v} (e^{\lambda_v - \lambda_z} - 1)a(v, z)\frac{\partial u}{\partial \lambda_v}\right)\Big|_{\vec{\lambda}=0}$$

$$+ \frac{\partial}{\partial \lambda_v}\left(\sum_{z: z \neq v} (e^{\lambda_z - \lambda_v} - 1)a(z, v)\frac{\partial u}{\partial \lambda_z}\right)\Big|_{\vec{\lambda}=0}$$

$$= k(v) + \underbrace{(\beta(v) - \mu(v))}_{V(v)}m_1(t, v) + \sum a(z, v)m_1(t, z)$$

$$- \left(\sum_{z: z \neq v} a(v, z)\right)m_1(t, v)$$

If $a(x, z) = a(z, x)$ then finally

$$\frac{\partial m_1(t, x)}{\partial t} = Am_1 + Vm_1 + k(x), \qquad m_1(0, x) = n(0, x)$$

Here, A is the generator of a Markov chain $A = [a(x, y)] = A^*$.

By differentiating equation (3.2) over the variables λ_x, $x \in X$, one can get the equations for the correlation functions

$$k_{l_1 \dots l_m}(t, x_1, \dots, x_m) = E\, n^{l_1}(t, x_1) \cdots n^{l_m}(t, x_m)$$

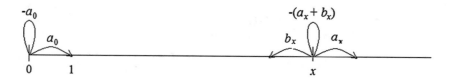

Fig. 1 General random walk with reflection at 0

where $x_1, \ldots, x_m$ are different points of X and $l_1, \ldots, l_m \geq 1$ are integers. Of course $k_{l_1 \ldots l_m}(t, x_1, \ldots, x_m) = (-1)^{l_1 + \cdots + l_m} \frac{\partial^{l_1 + \cdots + l_m} n(t, \vec{\lambda})}{\partial^{l_1} \lambda_{x_1} \ldots \partial^{l_m} \lambda_{x_m}} \big|_{\vec{\lambda} = 0}$. The corresponding equations will be linear. The central point here is that the factors $(e^{\lambda_x - \lambda_z} - 1)$, $(e^{\lambda_y} - 1)$, and $(e^{-\lambda_x} - 1)$ are equal to 0 for $\vec{\lambda} = 0$. As a result, the higher order $(n > l_1 + \cdots + l_m)$ correlation functions cannot appear in the equations for $\{k_{l_1 \ldots l_m}(\cdot), l_1 + \cdots + l_m = n\}$.

Consider, for instance, the correlation function (in fact, matrix- valued function)

$$k_2(t, x_1, x_2) = \begin{bmatrix} E\, n^2(t, x_1, x_1) & E\, n(t, x_1)\, n(t, x_2) \\ E\, n(t, x_1)\, n(t, x_2) & E\, n^2(t, x_2, x_2) \end{bmatrix}$$

The method based on generating functions is typical for the theory of branching processes. In the case of processes with immigration, another, Markovian approach gives new results. Let us start from the simplest case, when there is but one site, i.e., $X = \{x\}$. Then, the process $n(t), t \geq 0$ is a random walk with reflection on the half axis $n \geq 0$.

For a general random walk $y(t)$ on the half axis with reflection in continuous time, we have the following facts. Let the process be given by the generator $G = (g(w, z)), w, z \geq 0$, where $a_w = g(w, w + 1), w \geq 0$; $b_w = g(w, w - 1), w > 0$; $g(w, w) = -(a_w + b_w), w > 0$; and $g(0, 0) = -a_0$ (see Fig. 1).

The random walk is recurrent iff the series

$$S = 1 + \frac{b_1}{a_1} + \cdots + \frac{b_1 \cdots b_n}{a_1 \cdots a_n} + \cdots \tag{3.3}$$

diverges. It is ergodic (positively recurrent) iff the series

$$\tilde{S} = 1 + \frac{a_0}{b_1} + \cdots + \frac{a_0 \cdots a_{n-1}}{b_1 \cdots b_n} + \cdots \tag{3.4}$$

converges. In the ergodic case, the invariant distribution of the random walk $y(t)$ is given by the formula

$$\pi(n) = \frac{1}{\tilde{S}} \frac{a_0 \cdots a_{n-1}}{b_1 \cdots b_n} \tag{3.5}$$

(see [5]).

For our random walk, $n(t)$

$$g(0, 0) = -k, \qquad a_0 = g(0, 1) = k$$

and, for $n \geq 1$

$$b_n = g(n, n-1) = \mu n, \qquad g(n, n) = -(\mu n + \beta n + k), \qquad a_n = g(n, n+1) = \beta n + k.$$

Proposition 3.1   *1. If $\beta > \mu$ the process $n(t)$ is transient and the population $n(t)$ grows exponentially.*

2. If $\beta = \mu$, $k > 0$ the process is not ergodic but rather it is zero-recurrent for $\frac{k}{\beta} \leq 1$ and transient for $\frac{k}{\beta} > 1$.

3. If $\beta < \mu$ the process $n(t)$ is ergodic. The invariant distribution for $\beta < \mu$ is given by

$$\pi(n) = \frac{1}{\tilde{S}} \frac{k(k+\beta)\cdots(k+\beta(n-1))}{\mu \cdot 2\mu \cdots n\mu}$$

$$= \frac{1}{\tilde{S}} \left(\frac{\beta}{\mu}\right)^n \frac{\frac{k}{\beta}\left(\frac{k}{\beta}+1\right)\cdots\left(\frac{k}{\beta}+n-1\right)}{n!}$$

$$= \frac{1}{\tilde{S}} \left(\frac{\beta}{\mu}\right)^n (1+\alpha)\left(1+\frac{\alpha}{2}\right)\cdots\left(1+\frac{\alpha}{n}\right), \qquad \alpha = \frac{k}{\beta} - 1$$

$$= \frac{1}{\tilde{S}} \left(\frac{\beta}{\mu}\right)^n \exp\left(\sum_{j=1}^{n} \ln\left(1+\frac{\alpha}{j}\right)\right) \sim \frac{1}{\tilde{S}} \left(\frac{\beta}{\mu}\right)^n n^\alpha$$

where $\displaystyle \tilde{S} = \sum_{j=1}^{\infty} \frac{k(k+\beta)\cdots(k+\beta(j-1))}{\mu \cdot 2\mu \cdots j\mu}.$

Proof 1 and 3 follow from Eqs. 3.3–3.5. If $\beta = \mu$ (but $k > 0$), i.e., in the critical case, the process cannot be ergodic because, setting $\alpha = \frac{k}{\beta} - 1$, then $\alpha > -1$ and as $n \to \infty$ $\tilde{S} \sim \sum_n n^\alpha = +\infty$. The process is zero-recurrent, however, for $0 < \frac{k}{\beta} \leq 1$. In fact, for $\beta = \mu$

$$\frac{b_1 \cdots b_n}{a_1 \cdots a_n} = \frac{\beta \cdot 2\beta \cdots n\beta}{(k+\beta)\cdots(k+n\beta)} = \frac{1}{\displaystyle\prod_{i=1}^{n}\left(1+\frac{k}{i\beta}\right)} \asymp \frac{1}{n^{k/\beta}}$$

and the series in Eq. 3.4 diverges if $0 < \frac{k}{\beta} \leq 1$. If, however, $k > \beta$ the series converges and the process $n(t)$ is transient. $\square$

Consider, now, the general case of the finite space X. Let $N = \text{Card } X$ and $\overrightarrow{n}(t)$ be the vector of the occupation numbers. The process $\overrightarrow{n}(t)$, $t \geq 0$ is the random walk on $(\mathbb{Z}_+^1)^N = \{0, 1, ...\}^N$ with continuous time. The generator of this random walk was already described when we calculated the Laplace transform $u(t, \overrightarrow{\lambda}) = E\, e^{-(\overrightarrow{\lambda}, \overrightarrow{n}(t))}$. If at the moment t we have the configuration $\overrightarrow{n}(t) = \{n(t, x), x \in X\}$, then, for the interval $(t, t + dt)$ only the following events (up to terms of order$(dt)^2$) can happen:

(a) the birth of a new particle at the site $x_0 \in X$, with corresponding probability $n(t, x_0)\beta(x_0)dt + k(x_0)dt$. In this case we have the transition

$$\overrightarrow{n}(t) = \{n(t, x), x \in X\} \to \overrightarrow{n}(t + dt) = \begin{cases} n(t, x), x \neq x_0 \\ n(t, x_0) + 1, x = x_0 \end{cases}$$

(b) the death of one particle at the site $x_0 \in X$. This has corresponding probability $\mu(x_0)n(t, x_0)dt$ and the transition

$$\overrightarrow{n}(t) = \{n(t, x), x \in X\} \to \overrightarrow{n}(t + dt) = \begin{cases} n(t, x), x \neq x_0 \\ n(t, x_0) - 1, x = x_0 \end{cases}$$

(Of course, here $n(t, x_0) \geq 1$, otherwise $\mu(x_0)n(t, x_0)dt = 0$).

(c) the transfer of one particle from site x_0 to site $y_0 \in X$ (jump from x_0 to y_0), i.e., the transition

$$\overrightarrow{n}(t) = \{n(t, x), x \in X\} \to \overrightarrow{n}(t + dt) = \begin{cases} n(t, x), x \neq x_0, y_0 \\ n(t, x_0) - 1, x = x_0 \\ n(t, y_0) + 1, x = y_0 \end{cases}$$

with probability $n(t, x_0)a(x_0, y_0)dt$ for $n(t, x_0) \geq 1$.

The following theorem gives sufficient conditions for the ergodicity of the process $\overrightarrow{n}(t)$.

Theorem 3.2 *Assume that for some constants $\delta > 0$, $A > 0$ and any $x \in X$*

$$\mu(x) - \beta(x) \geq \delta, \quad k(x) \leq A.$$

Then, the process $\overrightarrow{n}(t)$ is an ergodic Markov chain and the invariant measure of this process has exponential moments, i.e., $E\, e^{(\overrightarrow{\lambda}, \overrightarrow{n}(t))} \leq c_0 < \infty$ if $|\overrightarrow{\lambda}| \leq \lambda_0$ for appropriate (small) $\lambda_0 > 0$.

Proof We take on $(\mathbb{Z}_+^1)^N = \{0, 1, ...\}^N$ as a Lyapunov function

$$f(\overrightarrow{n}) = (\overrightarrow{n}, \overrightarrow{1}) = \sum_{x \in X} n_x, \quad \overrightarrow{n} \in (\mathbb{Z}_+^1)^N,$$

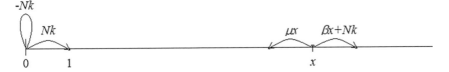

Fig. 2 Markov model for immigration process

Then, with G the generator of the process, $Gf(\overrightarrow{n}) \leq 0$ for large enough $(\overrightarrow{n}, \overrightarrow{1}) = \|\overrightarrow{n}\|_1$. In fact

$$Gf = \sum_{x \in X} ((\beta(x) - \mu(x))n_x + k(x)) < 0, \qquad \text{for large } \|\overrightarrow{n}\|_1.$$

(The terms concerning transitions of the particles between sites make no contribution: $1 - 1 = 0$.)   □

If $\beta(x) \equiv \beta < \mu \equiv \mu(x)$ and $k(x) \equiv k$ then $(\overrightarrow{n}, \overrightarrow{1})$, i.e., the total number of the particles in the phase space X is also a Galton–Watson process with immigration and the rates of transition shown in Fig. 2.

If $t \to \infty$ this process has a limiting distribution with invariant measure (in which Nk replaces k). That is

$$E(\overrightarrow{n}, \overrightarrow{1}) \xrightarrow[t \to \infty]{} \frac{Nk}{\mu - \beta}$$

4 Branching Process with Migration and Immigration

We now consider our process with birth, death, migration, and immigration on a countable space, specifically the lattice $\mathbb{Z}^d$. As in the other models, we have $\beta > 0$, the rate of duplication at $x \in \mathbb{Z}^d$; $\mu > 0$, the rate of death; and $k > 0$, the rate of immigration. Here, we add migration of the particles with rate $\kappa > 0$ and probability kernel $a(z)$, $z \in \mathbb{Z}^d$, $z \neq 0$, $a(z) = a(-z)$, $\sum_{z \neq 0} a(z) = 1$. That is, a particle jumps from site x to $x + z$ with probability $\kappa a(z)dt$. Here we put $\kappa = 1$ to simplify the notation.

For $n(t, x)$, the number of particles at x at time t, the forward equation for this process is given by $n(t + dt, x) = n(t, x) + \xi(dt, x)$, where

$$\xi(dt, x) = \begin{cases} 1 & \text{w. pr. } n(t, x)\beta dt + kdt + \sum_{z \neq 0} a(z)n(t, x + z)dt \\ -1 & \text{w. pr. } n(t, x)(\mu + 1)dt \\ 0 & \text{w. pr. } 1 - (\beta + \mu + 1)n(t, x)dt - \sum_{z \neq 0} a(z)n(t, x + z)dt - kdt \end{cases}$$

$$(4.1)$$

Note that $\xi(dt, x)$ is independent on $\mathcal{F}_{\leqslant t}$ (the σ-algebra of events before or including t) and

(a) $E[\xi(dt, x)|\mathcal{F}_{\leqslant t}] = n(t, x)(\beta - \mu - 1)dt + kdt + \sum_{z \neq 0} a(z)n(t, x + z)dt.$

(b) $E[\xi^2(dt, x)|\mathcal{F}_{\leqslant t}] = n(t, x)(\beta + \mu + 1)dt + kdt + \sum_{z \neq 0} a(z)n(t, x + z)dt.$

(c) $E[\xi(dt, x)\xi(dt, y)|\mathcal{F}_{\leqslant t}] = a(x - y)n(t, x)dt + a(y - x)n(t, y)dt.$
    A single particle jumps from x to y or from y to x. Other possibilities have probability $O((dt)^2) \approx 0$. Here, of course, $x \neq y$.

d) If $x \neq y$, $y \neq z$, and $x \neq z$, then $E[\xi(dt, x)\xi(dt, y)\xi(dt, z)] = 0$.
   We will not use property (d) in this paper, but it is crucial for the analysis of moments of order greater or equal to 3.

From here on, we concentrate on the first two moments.

4.1 First Moment

Due to the fact that $\beta < \mu$, the system has a short memory, and we can calculate all the moments under the condition that $n(0, x)$, $x \in \mathbb{Z}^d$, is a system of independent and identically distributed random variables with expectation $\frac{k}{\mu - \beta}$. We will select Poissonian random variables with parameter $\lambda = \frac{k}{\mu - \beta}$. Then, $m_1(t, x) = \frac{k}{\mu - \beta}, t \geqslant 0$, $x \in \mathbb{Z}^d$, and, as a result, $\mathcal{L}_a m_1(t, x) = 0$. Setting $m_1(t, x) = E[n(t, x)]$, we have

$$m_1(t + dt, x) = E[E[n(t + dt, x)|\mathcal{F}_t]] = E[E[n(t, x) + \xi(t, x)|\mathcal{F}_t]]$$

$$= m_1(t, x) + (\beta - \mu)m_1(t, x)dt + kdt + \sum_{z \neq 0} a(z)[m_1(t, x + z) - m_1(t, x)]dt$$

(4.2)

Defining the operator $\mathcal{L}_a(f(t, x)) = \sum_{z \neq 0} a(z)[f(t, x + z) - f(t, x)]$, then, from Eq. 4.2 we get the differential equation

$$\begin{cases} \dfrac{\partial m_1(t, x)}{\partial t} = (\beta - \mu)m_1(t, x) + k + \mathcal{L}_a m_1(t, x) \\ m_1(0, x) = 0 \end{cases}$$

Because of spatial homogeneity, $\mathcal{L}_a m_1(t, x) = 0$, giving

$$\begin{cases} \dfrac{\partial m_1(t, x)}{\partial t} = (\beta - \mu)m_1(t, x) + k \\ m_1(0, x) = 0 \end{cases}$$

which has the solution

$$m_1(t, x) = \frac{k}{\beta - \mu}(e^{(\beta - \mu)t} - 1).$$

Thus, if $\beta \geq \mu$, $m_1(t, x) \to \infty$, and if $\mu > \beta$,

$$\lim_{t \to \infty} m_1(t, x) = \frac{k}{\mu - \beta}.$$

4.2 Second Moment

We derive differential equations for the second correlation function $m_2(t, x, y)$ for $x = y$ and $x \neq y$ separately, then combine them and use a Fourier transform to prove a useful result concerning the covariance.

I. $x = y$

$$m_2(t + dt, x, x) = E[E[(n(t, x) + \xi(dt, x))^2 | \mathcal{F}_{\leqslant t}]]$$

$$= m_2(t, x, x) + 2E\left[n(t, x)[n(t, x)(\beta - \mu - 1)dt + kdt \right.$$

$$\left. + \sum_{z \neq 0} a(z)n(t, x + z)]dt \right]$$

$$+ E\left[n(t, x)(\beta + \mu + 1)dt + kdt + \sum_{z \neq 0} a(z)n(t, x + z)dt \right]$$

Denote $\mathcal{L}_{ax}m_2(t, x, y) = \sum_{z \neq 0} a(z)(m_2(t, x + z, y) - m_2(t, x, y))$.
From this follows the differential equation

$$\begin{cases} \dfrac{\partial m_2(t, x, x)}{\partial t} = 2(\beta - \mu)m_2(t, x, x) + 2\mathcal{L}_{ax}m_2(t, x, x) + \dfrac{2k^2}{\mu - \beta} + \dfrac{2k(\mu + 1)}{\mu - \beta} \\ m_2(0, x, x) = 0 \end{cases}$$

II. $x \neq y$
Because only one event can happen during dt

$$P\{\xi(dt, x) = 1, \xi(dt, y) = 1\} = P\{\xi(dt, x) = -1, \xi(dt, y) = -1\} = 0,$$

while the probability that one particle jumps from y to x is

$$P\{\xi(dt, x) = 1, \xi(dt, y) = -1\} = a(x - y)n(t, y)dt,$$

and the probability that one particle jumps from x to y is

$$P\{\xi(dt, x) = -1, \xi(dt, y) = 1\} = a(y - x)n(t, x)dt.$$

Then, similar to above

$$m_2(t + dt, x, y) = E[E[(n(t, x) + \xi(t, x))(n(t, y) + \xi(t, y))|\mathcal{F}_{\leqslant t}]]$$
$$= m_2(t, x, y) + (\beta - \mu)m_2(t, x, y)dt + km_1(t, y)dt$$
$$+ \sum_{z \neq 0} a(z)(m_2(t, x + z, y) - m_2(t, x, y))dt$$
$$+ (\beta - \mu)m_2(t, x, y)dt + km_1(t, x)dt$$
$$+ \sum_{z \neq 0} a(z)(m_2(t, x, y + z) - m_2(t, x, y))dt$$
$$+ a(x - y)m_1(t, y)dt + a(y - x)m_1(t, x)dt$$
$$= m_2(t, x, y) + 2(\beta - \mu)m_2(t, x, y)dt + k(m_1(t, y) + m_1(t, x))dt$$
$$+ (\mathcal{L}_{ax} + \mathcal{L}_{ay})m_2(t, x, y)dt$$
$$+ a(x - y)(m_1(t, x) + m_1(t, y))dt$$

The resulting differential equation is

$$\frac{\partial m_2(t, x, y)}{\partial t} = 2(\beta - \mu)m_2(t, x, y) + (\mathcal{L}_{ax} + \mathcal{L}_{ay})m_2(t, x, y) + k(m_1(t, x)$$
$$+ m_1(t, y)) + a(x - y)[m_1(t, x) + m_1(t, y)]$$

(4.3)

That is

$$\frac{\partial m_2(t, x, y)}{\partial t} = 2(\beta - \mu)m_2(t, x, y) + (\mathcal{L}_{ax} + \mathcal{L}_{ay})m_2(t, x, y)$$
$$+ \frac{2k^2}{\mu - \beta} + 2a(x - y)\frac{k}{\mu - \beta}$$

Because, for fixed t, $n(t, x)$ is homogeneous in space, we can write $m_2(t, x, y) = m_2(t, x - y) = m_2(t, u)$. Then, we can condense the two cases into a single differential equation

$$\begin{cases} \dfrac{\partial m_2(t, u)}{\partial t} = 2(\beta - \mu)m_2(t, u) + 2\mathcal{L}_{au}m_2(t, u) + \frac{2k^2}{\mu - \beta} + 2a(u)\frac{k}{\mu - \beta} + \delta_0(u)\frac{2k(\mu + 1)}{\mu - \beta} \\ m_2(0, u) = En^2(0, x) \end{cases}$$

Here $u = x - y \neq 0$ and $a(0) = 0$.

We can partition $m_2(t, u)$ into $m_2(t, u) = m_{21} + m_{22}$, where the solution for m_{21} depends on time but not position and the solution for m_{22} depends on position but not time. Thus, $\mathcal{L}_{au} m_{21} = 0$ and m_{21} corresponds to the source $\frac{2k^2}{\mu - \beta}$, which gives

$$\frac{\partial m_{21}(t, u)}{\partial t} = 2(\beta - \mu) m_{21}(t, u) + \frac{2k^2}{\mu - \beta}$$

As $t \to \infty$, $m_{21} \to \bar{M}_2 = m_1^2(t, x) = \frac{k^2}{(\mu - \beta)^2}$.

For the second part, m_{22}, $\frac{\partial m_{22}}{\partial t} = 0$, i.e.,

$$\frac{\partial m_{22}(t, u)}{\partial t} = 2(\beta - \mu) m_{22}(t, u) + 2\mathcal{L}_{au} m_{22}(t, u) + 2a(u) \frac{k}{\mu - \beta}$$
$$+ \delta_0(u) \frac{2k(\mu + 1)}{\mu - \beta} = 0$$

As $t \to \infty$, $m_{22} \to \tilde{M}_2$. $\tilde{M}_2$ is the limiting correlation function for the particle field $n(t, x)$, $t \to \infty$. It is the solution of the "elliptic" problem

$$2\mathcal{L}_{au} \tilde{M}_2(u) - 2(\mu - \beta) \tilde{M}_2(u) + \delta_0(u) \frac{2k(\mu + 1)}{\mu - \beta} + 2a(u) \frac{k}{\mu - \beta} = 0$$

Applying the Fourier transform $\widehat{\tilde{M}_2}(\theta) = \sum_{u \in Z^d} \tilde{M}_2(u) e^{i(\theta, u)}$, $\theta \in T^d = [-\pi, \pi]^d$,

we obtain

$$\widehat{\tilde{M}_2}(\theta) = \frac{\frac{k}{\mu - \beta} + \frac{k\hat{a}(\theta)}{\mu - \beta}}{(\mu - \beta) + (1 - \hat{a}(\theta))}.$$

We have proved the following result.

Theorem 4.1 If $t \to \infty$, then $\mathrm{Cov}(n(t, x), n(t, y)) = E[n(t, x)n(t, y)] - E[n(t, x)]E[n(t, y)] = m_2(t, x, y) - m_1(t, x)m_1(t, y)$, tends to $\tilde{M}_2(x - y) = \tilde{M}_2(u) \in L^2(Z^d)$

The Fourier transform of $\tilde{M}_2(\cdot)$ *is equal to*

$$\widehat{\tilde{M}_2}(\theta) = \frac{c_1 + c_2 \hat{a}(\theta)}{c_3 + (1 - \hat{a}(\theta))} \in C(T^d)$$

where $c_1 = \frac{k}{\mu - \beta}$, $c_2 = \frac{k}{\mu - \beta}$, $c_3 = \mu - \beta$

Let us compare our results with the corresponding results for the critical contact model [6] (where $k = 0$, $\mu = \beta$). In the last case, the limiting distribution for the field $n(t, x)$, $t \geq 0$, $x \in \mathbb{Z}^d$, exists if and only if the underlying random walk with generator $\mathcal{L}_a$ is transient. In the recurrent case, we have the phenomenon of clusterization. The limiting correlation function is always slowly decreasing (like the Green kernel of $\mathcal{L}_a$).

In the presence of immigration, the situation is much better: the limiting correlation function always exists and we believe that the same is true for all moments.
The decay of $\tilde{M}_2(u)$ depends on the smoothness of $\hat{a}(\theta)$. Under minimal regularity
conditions, correlations have the same order of decay as $a(z)$, $z \to \infty$. For instance,
if $a(z)$ is finitely supported or exponentially decreasing, the correlation also has an
exponential decay. If $a(z)$ has power decay, then the same is true for correlation
$\tilde{M}_2(u)$, $u \to \infty$.

5   Processes in a Random Environment

The final four models involve a random environment. Two are Galton–Watson models
with immigration and lack a spatial component. In the first, the parameters are random
functions of the population size; in the second, they are random functions of a Markov
chain on a finite space. The last two models are spatial and feature immigration,
migration, and, most importantly, a random environment in space, still stationary in
time for the third but not stationary in time for the fourth.

5.1   Galton–Watson Processes with Immigration in Random Environments

5.1.1   Galton–Watson Process with Immigration in Random Environment Based on Population Size

Assume that rates of mortality $\mu(\cdot)$, duplication $\beta(\cdot)$, and immigration $k(\cdot)$ are random functions of the volume of the population $x \geq 0$. Namely, the random vectors
$(\mu, \beta, k)(x, \omega)$ are i.i.d on the underlying probability space $(\Omega_e, \mathcal{F}_e, P_e)$ (e: environment).

The Galton–Watson Process is ergodic (P_e-a.s) if and only if the random series

$$S = \sum_{n=1}^{\infty} \frac{k(0)(\beta(1) + k(1))(2\beta(2) + k(2)) \cdots ((n-1)\beta(n-1) + k(n-1))}{\mu(1)(2\mu(2)) \cdots (n\mu(n))} < \infty, \quad P_e\text{-a.s.}$$

Theorem 5.1 *Assume that the random variables* $\beta(x, \omega)$, $\mu(x, \omega)$, $k(x, \omega)$ *are
bounded from above and below by the positive constants* $C^{\pm}$: $0 < C^- \leq \beta(x, \omega) \leq
C^+ < \infty$. *Then, the process* $n(t, \omega_e)$ *is ergodic* P_e-*a.s. if and only if* $\langle \ln \frac{\beta(x,\omega)}{\mu(x,\omega)} \rangle =
\langle \ln \beta(\cdot) \rangle - \langle \ln(\mu(\cdot)) \rangle < 0$

Proof It is sufficient to note that

$$\frac{k(n-1,\omega) + (n-1)\beta(n-1,\omega)}{n\mu(x,\omega)} = \frac{\frac{k(n-1,\omega)-\beta(n-1,\omega))}{n} + \beta(n-1,\omega)}{\mu(n,\omega)}$$

$$= e^{\ln\beta(n-1)-\ln\mu(n)+o(\frac{1}{n})}.$$

□

It follows from the strong LLN that the series diverges exponentially fast for $\langle \ln\beta(\cdot)\rangle - \langle \ln\mu(\cdot)\rangle > 0$; it converges like a decreasing geometric progression for $\langle \ln\beta(\cdot)\rangle - \langle \ln\mu(\cdot)\rangle < 0$; and it is divergent if $\langle \ln\beta(\cdot)\rangle = \langle \ln\mu(\cdot)\rangle$. It diverges even when $\beta(x,\omega_e) = \mu(x,\omega_e)$ due to the presence of $k^- \geq C^- > 0$.

Note that $ES < \infty$ if and only if $\langle \frac{\lambda(x-1)}{\mu(x)}\rangle = \langle\lambda\rangle\langle\frac{1}{\mu}\rangle < \infty$, i.e., the fluctuations of S, even in the case of convergence, can be very high.

5.1.2   Random Nonstationary (Time Dependent) Environment

Assume that $k(t)$ and $\Delta = (\mu - \beta)(t)$ are stationary random processes on (Ω_m, P_m) and that $k(t)$ is independent of Δ. For a fixed environment, i.e., fixed $k(\cdot)$ and $\Delta(\cdot)$, the equation for the first moment takes the form

$$\frac{dm_1(t,\omega_m)}{dt} = -\Delta(t,\omega_m)m_1 + k(t,\omega_m)$$

$$m_1(0,\omega_m) = m_1(0)$$

Then

$$m_1(t,\omega_m) = m_1(0)e^{-\int_0^t \Delta(u,\omega_m)du} + \int_0^t k(s,\omega_m)e^{-\int_s^t \Delta(u,\omega_m)du}ds$$

Assume that $\frac{1}{\delta} \geq \Delta(\cdot) \geq \delta > 0$, $\frac{1}{\delta} \geq k(\cdot) \geq \delta > 0$. Then

$$m_1(t,\omega_m) = \int_{-\infty}^t k(s,\omega_m)e^{-\int_s^t \Delta(u,\omega_m)du}ds + O(e^{-\delta t}).$$

Thus, for large t, the process $m_1(t,\omega_m)$ is exponentially close to the stationary process

$$\tilde{m}_1(t,\omega) = \int_\infty^t k(s,\omega_m)e^{-\int_s^t \Delta(u,\omega_m)du}ds$$

Assume now that $k(t)$ and $\Delta(s)$ are independent stationary processes and $-\Delta(t) = V(x(t))$, where $x(t)$, $t \geq 0$, is a Markov Chain with continuous time and symmetric geometry on the finite set X. (One can also consider $x(t)$, $t \geq 0$, as a diffusion process on a compact Riemannian manifold with Laplace–Beltrami generator Δ.) Let

$$u(t, x) = E_x e^{\int_0^t V(x_s)dx} f(x_t)$$
$$= E_x e^{\int_0^t -\Delta(x_s)dx} f(x_t)$$

Then

$$\begin{cases} \dfrac{\partial u}{\partial t} = \mathcal{L}u + Vu = Hu \\[2mm] u(0, x) = f(x) \end{cases} \tag{5.1}$$

The operator $\mathcal{L}$ is symmetric in $L^2(x)$ with dot product $(f, g) = \sum_{x \in X} f(x)\bar{g}(x)$. Thus, $H = \mathcal{L} + V$ is also symmetric and has real spectrum $0 > -\delta \geqslant \lambda_0 > \lambda_1 \geqslant \cdots$ with orthonormal eigenfunctions $\psi_0(x) > 0, \psi_1(x) > 0, \dots$ Inequality $\lambda_0 \leqslant \delta < 0$ follows from our assumption on $\Delta(\cdot)$.

The solution of Eq. 5.1 is given by

$$u(t, x) = \sum_{n=1}^{N} e^{\lambda_k t} \psi_k(x)(t, \psi_k).$$

Now, we can calculate $< \tilde{m}_1(t, x, \omega_m) >$.

$$< \tilde{m} > = \int_{-\infty}^{t} < k(\cdot) > < E_\pi e^{\int_s^t V(x_u)du} > ds \tag{5.2}$$

Here, $\pi(x) = \frac{1}{N} = \frac{\mathbb{1}(x)}{N}$ is the invariant distribution of x_s. Then

$$< \tilde{m} > = \int_{-\infty}^{t} < k > \sum_{k=0}^{k=N} e^{\lambda_k(t-s)}(\psi_k \pi)(\mathbb{1}\psi_k)ds$$

$$= - < k > \sum_{k=0}^{k=N} \frac{1}{\lambda_k}(\psi_k \mathbb{1})^2 \frac{1}{N}$$

$$= -\frac{< k >}{N} \sum_{k=0}^{N} \frac{(\psi_k \mathbb{1})^2}{\lambda_k}$$

5.1.3 Galton–Watson Process with Immigration in Random Environment Given by Markov Chain

Let $x(t)$ be an ergodic MCh on the finite space X and let $\beta(x), \mu(x), k(x)$, the rates of duplication, annihilation, and immigration, be functions from X to R^+, and, therefore, functions of t and ω_e. The process $(n(t), x(t))$ is a Markov chain on $\mathbb{Z}_+^1 \times X$.

Let $a(x, y), x, y \in X, a(x, y) \geq 0, \sum_{y \in X} a(x, y) = 1$ for all $x \in X$, be the transition function for $x(t)$. Consider $E_{(n,x)} f(n(t), x(t)) = u(t, (n, x))$. Then

$$
\begin{aligned}
u(t + dt, (n, x)) = {} & (1 - (n\beta(x) + n\mu(x) + k(x) - a(x, x))dt)u(t, x) \\
& + n\beta(x)u(t, (n + 1, x))dt + k(x)u(t, (n + 1, x))dt \\
& + n\mu(x)u(t, (n - 1, x))dt + \sum_{y:y \neq x} a(x, y)u(t, (n, y))dt
\end{aligned}
$$

We obtain the backward Kolmogorov equation

$$
\frac{\partial u}{\partial t} = \sum_{y:y \neq z} a(t, y)(u(t, (n, y)) - u(t, (n, x))) + (n\beta(x) + k(x))(u(t, (n + 1, x))
$$
$$
- u(t, (n, x))) + n\mu(x)(u(t, (n - 1, x)) - u(t, (n, x)))
$$
$$
u(0, (n, x)) = 0
$$

Example. Two-state random environment.
Here, $x(t)$ indicates which one of two possible states, $\{1, 2\}$ the process is in at time t. The birth, mortality, and immigration rates are different for each state: β_1 and β_2, μ_1 and μ_2, and k_1 and k_2. For a process in state 1, at any time the rate of switching to state 2 is α_1, with α_2 the rate of the reverse switch. This creates the two-state random environment. Let G be the generator for the process, as shown in Fig. 3.

The following theorem gives sufficient conditions for the ergodicity of the process $(n(t), x(t))$.

Theorem 5.2 *Assume that for some constants $\delta > 0$ and $A > 0$*

$$
\mu_i - \beta_i \geq \delta, \; k_i \leq A, \; i = 1, 2
$$

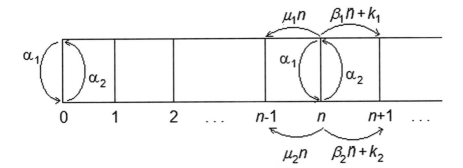

Fig. 3 GW process with immigration with random environment as two states

*Then, the process $(n(t), x(t))$ is an ergodic Markov chain and the invariant mea-
sure of this process has exponential moments, i.e., $E\, e^{\lambda n(t)} \leq c_0 < \infty$ if $\lambda \leq \lambda_0$ for
appropriate (small) $\lambda_0 > 0$.*

Proof We take as a Lyapunov function $f(n, x) = n$.

Then, $Gf(n(t), x(t)) = (\beta_x - \mu_x)n + k_x$. So for sufficiently large n, specifically
$n > \frac{A}{\delta}$, we have $Gf \leq 0$. $\square$

5.2 Models with Immigration and Migration in a Random Environment

For this most general case, we have migration and a nonstationary environment in
space and time. The rates of duplication, mortality, and immigration at time t and
position $x \in \mathbb{Z}^d$ are given by $\beta(t, x)$, $\mu(t, x)$, and $k(t, x)$. As in the above models,
immigration is uninfluenced by the presence of other particles; also set $\delta_1 \leq k(t, x) \leq
\delta_2, 0 < \delta_1 < \delta_2 < \infty$. The rate of migration is given by κ, with the process governed
by the probability kernel $a(z)$, the rate of transition from x to $x + z, z \in \mathbb{Z}^d$.

If $n(t, x)$ is the number of particles at $x \in \mathbb{Z}^d$ at time $t, n(t + dt, x) = n(t, x) +
\xi(t, x)$, where

$$
\xi(t, x) = \begin{cases}
1 & \text{w. pr. } n(t, x)\beta(t, x)dt + k(t, x)dt + \sum_{z \neq 0} a(-z)n(t, x + z)dt \\
-1 & \text{w. pr. } n(t, x)\mu(t, x)dt + \sum_{z \neq 0} a(z)n(t, x)dt \\
0 & \text{w. pr. } 1 - (\beta(t, x) + \mu(t, x))n(t, x)dt - \sum_{z \neq 0} a(z)n(t, x + z)dt \\
& \qquad\qquad - \sum_{z \neq 0} a(z)n(t, x)dt - k(t, x)dt
\end{cases}
$$

For the first moment, $m_1(t, x) = E[n(t, x)]$, we can write

$$
\begin{aligned}
m_1(t + dt, x) &= E[E[n(t + dt, x)|\mathcal{F}_t]] = E[E[n(t, x) + \epsilon(t, x)|\mathcal{F}_t]] \\
&= m_1(t, x) + (\beta(t, x) - \mu(t, x))m_1(t, x)dt + k(t, x)dt \\
&\quad + \sum_{z \neq 0} a(z)[m_1(t, x + z) - m_1(t, x)]dt
\end{aligned}
$$

and so, defining, as above, $\mathcal{L}_a(f(t, x)) = \sum_{z \neq 0} a(z)[f(t, x + z) - f(t, x)]$, we obtain

$$
\begin{cases}
\dfrac{\partial m_1(t, x)}{\partial t} = (\beta(t, x) - \mu(t, x))m_1(t, x) + k(t, x) + \mathcal{L}_a m_1(t, x) \\
m_1(0, x) = 0
\end{cases}
\tag{5.3}
$$

We consider two cases. The first is where the duplication and mortality rates are equal, $\beta(t, x) = \mu(t, x)$. Because of the immigration rate bounded above 0, we find that the expected population size at each site tends to infinity. In the second case, to simplify, we consider $\beta(t, x)$ and $\mu(t, x)$ to be stationary in time, and assume the mortality rate to be greater than the duplication rate everywhere by at least a minimal amount. Here, we show that the interplay between the excess mortality and the positive immigration results in a finite positive expected population size at each site.

5.2.1 Case I

If $\beta(t, x) = \mu(t, x)$

$$\begin{cases} \dfrac{\partial m_1(t, x)}{\partial t} = k(t, x) + \mathcal{L}_a m_1(t, x) \\ m_1(0, x) = 0 \end{cases}$$

By taking the Fourier and, then, inverse Fourier transforms, we obtain

$$m_1(t, x) = \int_0^t ds \sum_{y \in \mathbb{Z}^d} k(s, y) p(t - s, x - y, 0) \geq \int_0^t \delta_1 ds = \delta_1 t$$

where

$$p(t, x, y) = \frac{1}{(2\pi)^d} \int_{T^d} e^{-t \sum_{j=1}^d (\cos(v_j) - 1) - i(v, x - y)} \, dv \qquad (5.4)$$

As $t \to \infty$, $\delta_1 t \to \infty$. Thus, when the birth rate equals the death rate, the expected population at each site $x \in \mathbb{Z}^d$ will go to infinity as $t \to \infty$.

5.2.2 Case II

Here, $\beta(t, x) \neq \mu(t, x)$. For simplification we assume that only immigration, $k(t, x)$, is not stationary in time. In other words, we assume that the duplication and mortality rates *are* stationary in time and depend only on position: $\beta(t, x) = \beta(x)$, $\mu(t, x) = \mu(x)$ and $\mu(x) - \beta(x) \geq \delta_1 > 0$. From Eq. 5.3, we get

$$\begin{cases} \dfrac{\partial m_1(t, x)}{\partial t} = k(t, x) + \mathcal{L}_a m_1(t, x) + (\beta(t, x) - \mu(t, x)) m_1(t, x) \\ m_1(0, x) = 0 \end{cases}$$

This has the solution

$$m_1(t, x) = \int_0^t ds \sum_{y \in Z^d} k(s, y) q(t - s, x, y)$$

where $q(t - s, x, y)$ is the solution for

$$\begin{cases} \dfrac{\partial q}{\partial t} = \mathcal{L}_a q + (\beta(t, x) - \mu(t, x)) q \\ q(0, x, y) = \delta(x - y) = \begin{cases} 1 & y = x \\ 0 & y \neq x \end{cases} \end{cases}$$

Using the Feynman–Kac formula, we obtain

$$q(t, x, y) = p(t, x, y) E_{x \to y} [e^{\int_0^t (\beta(x_u) - \mu(x_u)) du}]$$

with $p(t, x, y)$ as in Eq. 5.4.

Finally

$$\lim_{t \to \infty} m_1(t, x) = \lim_{t \to \infty} \int_0^t ds \sum_{y \in Z^d} k(s, y) E_{x \to y} [e^{\int_0^{t-s} (\beta(x_u) - \mu(x_u)) du}] p(t - s, x, y)$$

$$\leq \|k\|_\infty \int_0^\infty e^{-\delta_1 w} dw$$

$$= \frac{\|k\|_\infty}{\delta_1}.$$

Thus, when $\mu(x) - \beta(x)$ is bounded above 0, then $\lim_{t \to \infty} m_1(t, x)$ is bounded by 0 and $\frac{\|k\|_\infty}{\delta_1}$, so this limit exists and is finite.

References

1. Sevast'yanov, R.A.: Limit theorems for branching stochastic processes of special form. Theory Probab. Appl. **3**, 321–331 (1957)
2. Karlin, S., McGregor, J.: Ehrenfest urn models. J. Appl. Probab. **2**, 352–376 (1965)
3. Kurtz, T.G.: Solutions of ordinary differential equations as limits of pure jump Markov processes. J. Appl. Prob **7**, 49–58 (1970)
4. Kurtz, T.G.: Limit theorems for sequences of jump Markov processes approximating ordinary differential equations. J. Appl. Prob **8**, 344–356 (1971)
5. Feller, W.: An Introduction to Probability Theory and Its Applications, vol. I, 3rd edn. Wiley, New York (1968)
6. Feng, Y., Molchanov, S.A., Whitmeyer, J.: Random walks with heavy tails and limit theorems for branching processes with migration and immigration. Stoch. Dyn. **12**(1), 1150007 (2012). 23 pages

Spatial Models of Population Processes

Stanislav Molchanov and Joseph Whitmeyer

Abstract Recent progress has been made on spatial mathematical models of population processes. We review a few of these: the spatial Galton–Watson model, modern versions that add migration and immigration and thereby may avoid the increasing concentration of population into an ever smaller space (clusterization), models involving a random environment, and two versions of the Bolker–Pakala model, in which mortality (or birth rate) is affected by competition.

Keywords Population process · Galton–Watson model · Mean-field model Bolker–Pacala model · Random environment

1 Introduction

Recent advances have been made in developing mathematical models for population processes over a large spatial scale, with application primarily to biological populations other than humans (e.g., [2, 3, 15]). Here, we discuss some of this work and its possible application to human populations. This work may be seen as the development of baseline models, which show the processes and patterns that emerge from basic regenerative and migration processes, prior to economic political, and social considerations. Note that in keeping with the universality of these models as

For the first author, this work has been funded by the Russian Academic Excellence Project '5-100'.

S. Molchanov
Department of Mathematics and Statistics, University of North Carolina at Charlotte, Charlotte, NC 28223, USA

S. Molchanov
National Research University, Higher School of Economics, Moscow, Russian Federation

J. Whitmeyer (✉)
Department of Sociology, University of North Carolina at Charlotte, Charlotte, NC 28223, USA
e-mail: jwhitmey@uncc.edu

© Springer International Publishing AG 2017
V. Panov (ed.), *Modern Problems of Stochastic Analysis and Statistics*,
Springer Proceedings in Mathematics & Statistics 208,
DOI 10.1007/978-3-319-65313-6_17

well as their simplicity, we will use the neutral terminology of "particles" for population members. These models are in the spirit of a general approach to population dynamics as part of statistical physics (e.g., work carried out by Y. Kondratiev and his group [15, 16]).

We use these models to focus on two questions: the long-run spatial distribution and the temporal fluctuations of a population. We are particularly interested in models that describe two common features of empirical populations, stationarity in space and time and strong deviations from the classical Poissonian picture, i.e., spatial intermittency in the distribution of species (clusterization or "patches"). Let us elaborate. By stationarity, we mean roughly that the stochastic process in question depends neither on the time we begin observing it nor on the place where we observe it. Mathematically, we will take this to mean that the mean and the variance of the number of particles at a given location do not depend on either the location or the time. Empirically, this is unlikely to be completely true, for there will be ecological features that make some places more favorable to population growth than others, and events such as climatic change occur that make some stretches of time more propitious than others for population growth. Nevertheless, variation in such conditions may not be very great and stationarity is often a reasonable first approximation for many populations. Stationarity also may be a goal in some modern human societies. As for clusterization, we note that random spatial placement of population members will result in a spatial Poisson distribution, which we might describe as mild clumping of the population. Nevertheless, a variety of empirical populations, from humans to other biological populations (e.g., tropical arboreal ants [21]) to even stars, display a higher degree of clusterization than that; in the extreme, situations where there are relatively sparse locations with high population concentrations isolated by vast unpopulated regions.

Again, these are baseline, simple models. We assume an isolated population that is not involved in complex multipopulation interaction (such as a predator–prey scheme). Most of the models we discuss are branching processes or developments of branching processes and, as is typical for these processes, exclude direct interaction between particles, although in some the birth–death mechanism can create a kind of mean-field attractive potential. We discuss a model that allows inhibition or stimulation to particle reproduction due to the presence of existing particles. Both kinds of models satisfy the Markov property, namely, that evolution of the system from time t depends only on the state of the system at time t and not additionally on its state before time t.

The organization of this paper is as follows. We begin with the background to these models, the simple nonspatial Galton–Watson process. We then present nine models, roughly in order of increasing complexity. The first three lack spatial dynamics: the spatial Galton–Watson process, which produces a high level of clusterization, the same model but with immigration added, and a mean-field approximation to the Bolker–Pacala model, which is characterized by intra-population competition. The second set of six models allow migration in various ways, including one with immigration as well, two involving something of a random environment, and a multilayered Bolker–Pacala model with migration between layers.

2   Mean-Field Models

2.1   Galton–Watson Model

Recent applications of these models have been to organisms such as trees, crabgrass, and butterflies. This line of work began, however, with humans. In 1873, Francis Galton posed a problem [7] concerning the extinction of surnames, i.e., the extinction of male lines of descendants. He wanted to know, given the probability of a given number of male offspring per male, what proportion of surnames would disappear and how many people would hold a surname that survived. In 1874, Galton and the Reverend Henry William Watson published the first mathematical treatment of what has become known as the Galton–Watson process [8].

The Galton–Watson (GW) process is a simple example of a branching process [13], a term for stochastic processes arising from incorporating probability theory into population processes [12]. Both continuous- and discrete-time versions of this model exist. In the continuous-time version of the GW process, a particle in an infinitesimal period of time dt produces one offspring with probability $\beta\,dt$ and disappears (dies) with probability $\mu\,dt$. If it produced an offspring, then there are two particles, each of which can produce an offspring or die, and the process continues in the same fashion. It is well known that the entire population, encompassing all lines, becomes extinct with probability 1 for $\mu \geq \beta$. Equal birth and death rates, $\beta = \mu$, are known as the critical case. Only when $\beta > \mu$ (the supercritical case), there is a positive probability that extinction does not occur. In fact, in this case the population follows the predictions of the Reverend Malthus [19] and grows exponentially: $En(t) = N_0 e^{(\beta-\mu)t}$, where E means to take the expectation, $n(t)$ denotes the population at time t, and N_0 is the initial population [11].

A model of population processes in space may be obtained by extending the Galton–Watson process by considering independent GW processes occurring in space. Specifically, we can consider a random point field $n(t, x)$ in the d-dimensional lattice $\mathbb{Z}^d$, with a critical GW process at each occupied point and no interaction or movement in space. It is possible also to consider the branching process models in d-dimensional Euclidean space $\mathbb{R}^d$, but in this paper we treat only the lattice; results are similar for the two settings. For our applications, generally, $d = 2$. Assume that $n(0, x)$ is the initial point field on $\mathbb{Z}^d$, given by the Bernoulli law: for any independent $x \in \mathbb{Z}^d$, $P\{n(0, x) = 1\} = \rho_0$, $P\{n(0, x) = 0\} = 1 - \rho_0$, where ρ_0 is the initial density of the population members. Assume now that each initial population member (located at x for $n(0, x) = 1$) generates its own family, concentrated at the same location $x \in \mathbb{Z}^d$. Assume that the corresponding Galton–Watson processes $n(t, x)$, $t \geq 0$, $x \in \mathbb{Z}^d$, are critical, i.e., $\beta = \mu$. The result is a field $n(t, x)$ with independent values and constant density: $En(t, x) \equiv \rho_0$.

For large t, in this model, the majority of the cells $x \in \mathbb{Z}^d$ will be empty because $P\{n(t, x) = 0\} = \frac{\beta t}{1+\beta t} = 1 - \frac{1}{\beta t} + O(\frac{1}{t^2})$ (which gives the formula $P\{n(t, x) = 0 \mid n(0, x) = N_0\} \sim e^{-N_0/\beta t}$) [9]. The populated points, moreover, are increasingly sparse (of order $\frac{1}{\beta t}$) and contain increasingly large families (of order βt). This is the phenomenon of clusterization: the population consists of large dense groups of particles separated by large distances (the distances will be of order $t^{1/d}$, so the square root of t in two dimensions). As $t \to \infty$, the clusterization becomes stronger and stronger. Figure 1 illustrates this phenomenon by showing three progressive moments of a simulated critical spatial Galton–Watson process in discrete time on a 10×10 lattice. The initial distribution is a spatial Poisson distribution (and so at $t = 1$, the distribution is still close to spatially Poissonian). Again, being critical, the birth and death rates are equal: $\beta = \mu = \frac{1}{2}$.

2.2   Spatial Galton–Watson Process with Immigration

One simple addition to the spatial GW process is to allow immigration, that is, the appearance of a new particle at a site, uninfluenced by the presence of particles at that site or other sites. Adding immigration has two advantages. First, it increases the realism of the model. Second, it helps to alleviate the concern that the total population size is stable only in the critical case, that is, if the birth rate and death rate are precisely and, in many situations, improbably equal ($\beta = \mu$). An analysis of this model may be found in Sect. 2.1 of the preceding chapter in this volume, by Han et al. We refer the reader to that section.

2.3   Bolker–Pakala Model in Mean-Field Approximation

The fact that in the preceding branching process models the population is stable only in a narrow critical condition, e.g., that $b = \mu$ in the Galton–Watson model, or simply due to immigration in the model with independent immigration, may not be entirely satisfactory. In the first case, there is no obvious reason why the critical condition should hold; in the second, the results seem to rest on the extreme simplicity of the model of immigration.

One alternative model that yields a stable distribution more robustly is the Bolker–Pacala model [2, 3]. The Bolker–Pacala model, well known in the theory of population dynamics, is a stochastic spatial model that incorporates both spatial dynamics and competition. The general Bolker–Pacala model can be formulated as follows.

At time $t = 0$, we have an initial homogeneous population, that is, a locally finite point process

$$n_0(\Gamma) = \#(\text{individuals in } \Gamma \text{ at time } t = 0),$$

where Γ denotes a bounded and connected region in $\mathbb{R}^d$. The simplest option is for $n_0(\Gamma)$ to be a Poissonian point field with intensity $\rho > 0$, i.e.,

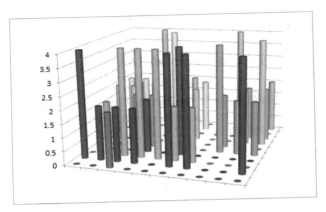

a) After 1 time step.

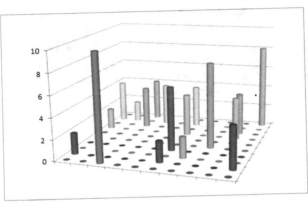

b) After 5 time steps.

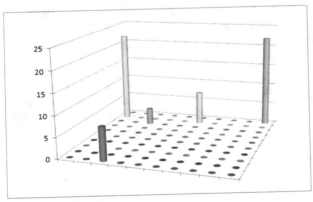

c) After 20 time steps.

Fig. 1 Critical ($\beta = \mu = 1/2$) spatial Galton–Watson process at three times

$$P\{n_0(\Gamma) = k\} = \exp(-\rho|\Gamma|)\frac{(\rho|\Gamma|)^k}{k!}, \quad k = 0, 1, 2, \ldots$$

where $|\Gamma|$ is the finite Lebesgue measure of Γ. The following rules dictate the evolution of the field:

(i) Each population member, independent of the others, during time interval $(t, t + dt)$ can produce a new population member(offspring) with probability $bdt = A^+dt$, $A^+ > 0$. The initial individual remains at its initial position x but the offspring jumps to $x + z + dz$ with probability

$$a^+(z)dz, \quad A^+ = \int_{\mathbb{R}^d} a^+(x)dx.$$

In the mean-field approximation, the spatial aspect is averaged and so the jump of the offspring becomes irrelevant.

(ii) Each population member at point x during the time interval $(t, t + dt)$ dies with probability $\mu\,dt$, where μ is the mortality rate.

(iii) Most important is the competition factor. If two population members are located at the points $x, y \in \mathbb{R}^d$, then each of them dies with probability $a^-(x - y)dt$ during the time interval $(t, t + dt)$ (we may assume that both do not die). This requires that $a^-(\cdot)$ be integrable; set

$$A^- = \int_{\mathbb{R}^d} a^-(z)dz.$$

The total effect of competition on a individual is the sum of the effects of competition with all population members. For modern human populations, it is probably more appropriate to include the suppressive effect of competition in the birth parameter b than to add it to mortality. The probability of production of a new population member at x, then, will become $b(x - y)$, for it will depend on the presence of individuals at points y.

In the Bolker–Pacala model, we have interacting individuals, in contrast to the usual branching process. One can expect physically that for arbitrary nontrivial competition ($a^- \in C(\mathbb{R}^d)$, $A^- > 0$), there will exist a limiting distribution of the population. At each site x, with population at time t given by $n(t, x)$, three rates are relevant, the birth rate b and mortality rate μ, each proportional to $n(t, x)$, and the death rate due to competition, proportional to $n(t, x)^2$. Heuristically, when $n(t, x)$ is small, the linear effects will dominate, which means that if $b > \mu$ the population will grow. As $n(t, x)$ becomes large, however, the quadratic effect will become increasingly dominant, which will prevent unlimited growth.

This can be seen in the mean-field approximation. We assume all particles on the lattice in fact are contained in a large but finite box of size L. The total population inside the box is described by a continuous-time random walk, the transition rates for which are

$$P\left(N_L(t+dt) = j | N_L(t) = n\right) = \begin{cases} n\kappa b\, dt + o(dt^2) & \text{if } j = n+1 \\ n\kappa\mu\, dt + \kappa\gamma n^2/L\, dt + o(dt^2) & \text{if } j = n-1 \\ o(dt^2) & \text{if } |j-n| > 1 \end{cases}$$

In [1], we prove a set of limit theorems for this random walk and show that, appropriately normalized, as $L \to \infty$, the process approaches an Ornstein–Uhlenbeck process, a well-known stochastic process that may be loosely described as fluctuations around an evolving central tendency, which may be a fixed equilibrium, or may be characterized by drift.

3 Models with Spatial Dynamics

3.1 KPP Model on $\mathbb{Z}^d$ with Migration (Heavy Tails)

In order to avoid clusterization, the process must fill out empty space to compensate for the degenerating families. One simple alternative to immigration is to add to the branching process a simple random walk to nearest neighbors. Given that we are on the lattice, this move is to one of two places in dimension 1, one of four places in dimension 2, and so on. In mathematical terms, the model includes diffusion with generator Δ, where Δ is the discrete or lattice Laplacian

$$\Delta f(x) = \sum_{x':|x'-x|=1} (f(x') - f(x)).$$

In high dimensions ($d \geq 3$), this simple random walk (diffusion) with generator Δ is sufficient to eliminate clusterization. For $d \leq 2$, which is after all the appropriate setting for most demographic or ecological applications, such local diffusion is not sufficient and the clusterization still increases infinitely. If, however, we modify the simple random walk to allow for "long jumps," that is, moves an indefinitely long distance, with sufficiently heavy tails and other conditions, then we can eliminate clusterization even in two or fewer dimensions. This modified random walk may be called "migration."

We are interested in the evolution of the configuration $N(t, x)$, $x \in \mathbb{Z}^d$, meaning the total number of individuals at position x in the d-dimensional lattice at time t. The following models are similar to the Kolmogorov–Petrovskii–Piskunov (KPP) model [14], a well-known and influential model from the 1930s. Two rather technical differences that do not have much effect on the conclusions are that in the KPP model the phase (or state) space is continuous ($\mathbb{R}^d$ instead of $\mathbb{Z}^d$) and the underlying process is Brownian motion instead of a random walk, but these are rather technical points. More essential is that in the KPP model the initial population $N(0, \cdot)$ contains but a single individual. Under the condition of supercriticality, $\beta > \mu$, think of a novel, superior gene that may spread through a species or a seed that may propagate in space. We consider, in contrast, the critical case where $\beta = \mu$ with an initial population that is stationary in the phase space $\mathbb{Z}^d$ with positive finite density, and, thus, is infinite.

The central simplifying assumption of these models is the absence of interaction between individuals. As a result, we can write the total population at point y, $N(t, y)$, as the sum of subpopulations as follows. Let $n(t, y; x)$ be the particle field generated by the initial $n(0, x)$ particles at the site $x \in \mathbb{Z}^d$. Then

$$N(t, y) = \sum_{x \in \mathbb{Z}^d} n(t, y; x).$$

Each subpopulation, in turn, is the sum of the contribution (the progeny) of each individual initially at the given site x, which we can write

$$n(t, y; x) = \sum_{i=1}^{n(0,x)} n(t, y; x_i).$$

The dynamics of the process includes three components, the familiar *birth rate* β and *death rate* μ, and the *migration* of population members. Migration depends on the probability kernel $a(z)$, $z \in \mathbb{Z}^d$, $z \neq 0$, $\sum_{z \neq 0} a(z) = 1$ and a rate of migration, which we can set to 1 by scaling time appropriately. An individual located at time t in some site $x \in \mathbb{Z}^d$, therefore, jumps to the point $(x + z) \in \mathbb{Z}^d$ with probability $a(z)dt$, independently of the other population members.

To implement the heavy tails assumption for migration, we assume that $a(z)$ takes the form:

$$a(z) = \frac{h_1(\theta)}{|z|^{2+\alpha}} \left(1 + O\left(\frac{1}{|z|^2}\right)\right), \quad z \neq 0$$

with $0 < \alpha < 2$, $\theta = \arg \frac{z}{|z|} \in (-\pi, \pi] = T^1$, $h_1 \in C^2(T^1)$, $h_1 > 0$. The second moment of the spatial distribution $a(z)$ is infinite. The stipulation that $\sum_{z \neq 0} a(z) = 1$ may be met by appropriate scaling of the bounded function h_1. The heaviness of the tails is controlled by α.

The generator for the migration process $\mathcal{L}$ is a generalization of the discrete Laplacian. The operator $\mathcal{L}$ is defined:

$$\mathcal{L}f(x) := \sum_{z \neq 0} a(z)(f(x + z) - f(x))$$

For the study of subpopulation $n(t, y; x)$, $x, y \in \mathbb{Z}^d$, let us define the generating function $u_z(t, x; y) = E_x z^{n(t,y;x)} = \sum_{j=0}^{\infty} P\{n(t, y; x) = j\}z^j$. This is a polynomial that is especially useful in generating moments. The nonlinear differential equation for $u_z(t, x; y)$ is [14]

$$\frac{\partial u_z}{\partial t} = \mathcal{L}u_z + \beta u_z^2 - (\beta + \mu)u_z + \mu \tag{3.1}$$

$$u(0, x; y) = \begin{cases} z, & x = y \\ 1, & x \neq y \end{cases}$$

Repeated differentiation over z and the substitution $z = 1$ leads to the sequence of moment equations for the factorial moments, given by

$$m_1(t, x; y) = E_x n(t, y; x)$$
$$m_2(t, x; y) = E_x n(t, y; x)(n(t, y; x) - 1)$$
$$m_3(t, x; y) = E_x n(t, y; x)(n(t, y; x) - 1)(n(t, y; x) - 2)$$
etc.

Then, for the critical case $\beta = \mu$

$$\frac{\partial m_1}{\partial t} = \mathcal{L}m_1, \qquad m_1(0, x; y) = \delta_y(x),$$

where $\delta_i(j) = 1$ for $i = j$ and 0 for $i \neq j$. This means $m_1(t, x; y) = p(t, x, y)$, where $p(t, x, y)$ is the transition probability from x to y in time t, i.e., $p(t, x, y) = P_x\{x(t) = y\}$ where $x(t)$ is the trajectory of the random walk (random jump!) with generator $\mathcal{L}$.

From here, we can obtain a theorem using what is known as the "method of moments" to establish the existence of a stable distribution as $t \to \infty$—in other words, no exponential decay, no exponential growth, and no clusterization. We state and explain the theorem here, but do not give the proof.

Let us note a well-known distinction concerning stochastic processes. A random walk $x(t)$ is called "recurrent" if $P\{x(t)$ returns to i infinitely often $|x(0) = i\} = 1$ and "transient" if $P\{x(t)$ returns to i infinitely often $|x(0) = i\} = 0$. An equivalent way of expressing this is $x(t)$ is transient if and only if $\int_0^\infty p(t, x, x)dt < \infty$.

Theorem 3.1 *Suppose $x(t)$ is transient, i.e., $\int_0^\infty p(t, x, x)dt < \infty$. Then,*

$$E N(t, x) \leq c_0^n n!$$

for some constant c_0 (Carleman conditions). For our model

$$E N(t, x)(N(t, x) - 1) \cdots (N(t, x) - l + 1) = m_l(t) \xrightarrow[t \to \infty]{} m_l(\infty)$$

and, therefore

$$N(t, x) \xrightarrow[t \to \infty]{\text{law}} N(\infty, x)$$

where $N(\infty, x)$ is a steady state, that is, a random variable with a finite distribution.

Let us elaborate two points. The Carleman conditions are time-independent bounds on the moments which, when satisfied as they are here, mean that the moments uniquely define the distribution. In other words, it is possible to construct the field $N(t, \cdot)$ and study its limiting behaviors $t \to \infty$ using the moments. The last conclusion gives us the desired result that we will have a stable population, without exponential growth or decay and without clusterization.

In the KPP case, a similar result goes back to [4, 18], who developed ideas by R.L. Dobrushin [5] using a technique involving partial differential equations. For branching random walks in $\mathbb{R}^d$, the case of so-called contact processes, [17] used what are called the "forward Kolmogorov equations" to prove the existence of the steady state $N(\infty, \infty)$. Equation 3.1, in contrast, is constructed using the related "backward" Kolmogorov equations. We proved the above theorem by using this method for individual subpopulations $n(t, y; x)$, $y \in \mathbb{Z}^d$ and then combining the results, which we were able to do because of the *independence* of these subpopulations.

The most convenient way to calculate the moments is by using the Fourier transform. In Fourier representation

$$\hat{m}_l(t, k; y) = \sum_{x \in \mathbb{Z}^d} e^{i(k, x)} m_l(t, x; y).$$

Note that, therefore

$$\sum_{x \in \mathbb{Z}^d} m_l(t, x; y) = \hat{m}_l(t, k; y)|_{k=0}.$$

It is straightforward to show that $\widehat{\mathcal{L}f(x)} = \hat{\mathcal{L}}(k)\hat{f}(k)$, where $\hat{\mathcal{L}} = \hat{a}(k) - 1$; note, also, $\hat{a}(0) = 1$. As a result

$$\hat{m}_1(t, k; y) = e^{\hat{\mathcal{L}}t}$$

and so

$$m_1(t, y) = \sum_{x \in \mathbb{Z}^d} m_1(t, x; y) = \hat{m}_1(t, k; y)|_{k=0} = 1.$$

For the second factorial moment, Eq. 3.1 gives

$$\frac{\partial m_2(t, x; y)}{\partial t} = \mathcal{L}m_2(t, x; y) + 2\beta m_1(t, x; y)^2.$$

Again, we use the Fourier transform to obtain

$$\sum_{x \in \mathbb{Z}^d} m_2(t, x; y) = \hat{m}_2(t, k; y)|_{k=0} = \beta \int_{T^d} \frac{d\theta}{1 - \hat{a}(\theta)} \left(1 - e^{-2t(1-\hat{a}(\theta))} \right).$$

By using cumulants and their properties, it can be shown that $m_2(t, y) = \sum_{x \in \mathbb{Z}^d} m_2$ $(t, x; y) + o(1) + 1$.

Intermittency or full clusterization is identified by the property

$$\frac{m_2}{m_1^2} \xrightarrow[t \to \infty]{} \infty.$$

In fact, clusterization is evident if $m_2 \gg m_1^2$. In our situation, $x(t)$ is transient if $\int_{T^d} \frac{d\theta}{1-\hat{a}(\theta)} < \infty$, but the limiting distribution of particles will show some clusterization if $\int_{T^d} \frac{d\theta}{1-\hat{a}(\theta)} \gg 1$.

3.2   KKP Model on $\mathbb{Z}^d$ with Multiple Offspring (Contact Process)

This introduces only one complication of the previous model. Namely, the number of offspring is no longer limited to two. When a particle splits, it may do so into j particles, $j = 2, 3, \dots, \infty$, with rates b_j. We need only the assumption, setting

$$\beta := \sum_{j=2}^{\infty} b_j \quad \text{and} \quad \beta_1 := \sum_{j=2}^{\infty} j b_j,$$

that $\beta < \infty$, $\beta_1 < \infty$.

With, as before, $u_z(t, x; y) = E_x z^{n(t, y; x)}$,

$$\frac{\partial u_z}{\partial t} = \mathcal{L} u_z + \sum_{j=2}^{\infty} b_j u_z^j - (\beta + \mu) u_z + \mu$$

$$u(0, x; y) = \begin{cases} z^{\rho_0}, & x = y \\ 1, & x \neq y \end{cases}$$

where ρ_0 is the initial population density.

For the first moment

$$\frac{\partial m_1(t, x; y)}{\partial t} = \mathcal{L} m_1(t, x; y) + \sum_{j=2}^{\infty} j b_j m_1(t, x; y) - (\beta + \mu) m_1(t, x; y),$$

$$m_1(0, x; y) = \rho_0 \delta_y(x).$$

As before, this is easily solved using the Fourier transform

$$\hat{m}_1(t, k; y) = \rho_0 e^{(\beta_1 - \beta - \mu)t} e^{\hat{\mathcal{L}}(k)t}$$

and

$$m_1(t, y) = \hat{m}_1(t, k; y)|_{k=0} = 1 = \rho_0 e^{(\beta_1 - \beta - \mu)t}.$$

This establishes $\beta_1 - \beta - \mu = 0$ as the critical setting of parameters for this process.

For the second factorial moment, we need to assume that $\beta_2 < \infty$, where $\beta_2 = \sum_{j=2}^{\infty} j(j-1)b_j$. Using the Fourier transform

$$\sum_{x \in \mathbb{Z}^d} m_2(t, x; y) = \hat{m}_2(t, k; y)|_{k=0} = \frac{\beta_2}{2} \int_{T^d} \frac{d\theta}{1 - \hat{a}(\theta)} \left(1 - e^{-2t(1-\hat{a}(\theta))}\right).$$

Then, as above, because $m_2(t, y) = \sum_{x \in \mathbb{Z}^d} m_2(t, x; y) + o(1) + 1$, the population will be unstable due to intermittency, be stable with some clusterization, or be stable without clusterization, depending on the evaluation of $\int_{T^d} \frac{d\theta}{1-\hat{a}(\theta)}$.

3.3 Stability Under a Single Point Perturbation

A natural next step is to probe the effect of perturbations on the stability created by the critical condition of the KPP-type model of the previous section. We consider, here, the same model with the critical condition that $\beta = \mu$ everywhere on the lattice $\mathbb{Z}^d$ except at a single point 0, that is,

$$\beta(x) - \mu(x) = \sigma \delta_0(x), \quad x \in \mathbb{Z}^d$$

with $\sigma > 0$. This model is due to Yarovaya (e.g., [20]).

The PDE for the first moment is then

$$\frac{\partial m_1}{\partial t} = \mathcal{L}m_1 + \sigma \delta_0(x)m_1$$

$$m_1(0, x) \equiv 1.$$

The stability of this model hinges on the value of σ. Specifically, there is a critical σ_{cr} such that if $\sigma < \sigma_{cr}$ the population attains a stable state but if $\sigma > \sigma_{cr}$ the population does not stabilize but grows indefinitely.

This follows from spectral analysis, using Fourier transforms. The spectrum of $\mathcal{L}$, $\mathrm{Sp}(\mathcal{L}) = [\min(\hat{\mathcal{L}}), 0]$. We define the Hamiltonian $H = \mathcal{L} + \sigma \delta_0(x)$. If H has discrete eigenvalue λ_0 with eigenvector ψ_0, then, $\hat{H}\hat{\psi}_0 = \lambda_0\hat{\psi}_0$. Thus, $\hat{\mathcal{L}}(\theta)\hat{\psi}_0(\theta) + \sigma\psi_0(0) = \lambda_0\hat{\psi}_0(\theta)$. Rearranging, we obtain

$$\hat{\psi}_0(\theta) = \frac{\sigma\psi_0(0)}{\lambda_0 - \hat{\mathcal{L}}(\theta)}$$

Taking the inverse Fourier transform

$$\psi_0(x) = \frac{\sigma\psi_0(0)}{(2\pi)^d} \int_{T^d} \frac{d\theta\, e^{-i(\theta,x)}}{\lambda_0 - \hat{\mathcal{L}}(\theta)}$$

$\psi_0(0) \neq 0$, otherwise $\psi_0(x) \equiv 0$, which means

$$\frac{1}{\sigma} = \frac{1}{(2\pi)^d} \int_{T^d} \frac{d\theta\, e^{-i(\theta,x)}}{\lambda_0 - \hat{\mathcal{L}}(\theta)} =: I(\lambda_0)$$

$I(0) > 0$ and as λ_0 increases from 0, $I(\lambda_0)$ decreases monotonically. Consequently, if $\frac{1}{\sigma} > I(0)$, there is no $\lambda_0 > 0$. Put otherwise, we set $\sigma_{\mathrm{cr}} = \frac{1}{I(0)}$. Then there is a simple $\lambda_0(\sigma) > 0$ iff $\sigma > \sigma_{\mathrm{cr}}$.

The corresponding eigenfunction, up to a constant factor, is

$$\psi_0(x) = \frac{1}{(2\pi)^d} \int_{T^d} \frac{d\theta\, e^{-i(\theta,x)}}{\lambda_0 - \hat{\mathcal{L}}(\theta)} = G_{\lambda_0}(0, x)$$

where $G_\lambda(0, x) = \int_0^\infty e^{-\lambda t} p(t, 0, x)\,dt$ is the Green function of the underlying random walk, which is given by

$$\frac{\partial p(t, x, y)}{\partial t} = \mathcal{L}p(t, x, y)$$
$$p(0, x, y) = \delta_x(y).$$

Because of translation invariance, we may write $p(t, y - x) = p(t, x, y)$

Set $\mu_1(t, x) = m_1(t, x) - 1$.

$$\frac{\partial \mu_1(t, x)}{\partial t} = H m_1(t, x) = \mathcal{L}\mu_1 + \sigma\delta_0(x)\mu_1 + \sigma\delta_0(x)$$
$$\mu_1(0, x) \equiv 0.$$

We now have two cases:

(1) If $\lambda_0(\sigma) > 0$, then $\mu_1 = O(1) + e^{\lambda_0 t} \sigma \psi_0(0) \psi_0(x)$, and because $\|\psi_0\| = 1$ it follows that the population size is unstable and increases exponentially; there is no steady-state population.
(2) If $\lambda_0(\sigma) < 0$, we may apply Duhamel's principle to obtain

$$\mu_1(t, x) = \sigma \int_0^t ds \sum_z p(t - s, x - z)(\delta_0(z)\mu_1(s, z) + \delta_0(z))$$

$$= \sigma \int_0^t p(t - s, x)(\mu_1(s, 0) + 1)ds$$

$$m_1(t, x) = 1 + \sigma \int_0^t p(t - s, x)m_1(s, 0)ds$$

$$= 1 + \sigma \int_0^t p(t - s, x)ds + \sigma^2 \int_0^t \int_0^s p(t - s, x)p(s - u, 0)m_1(u, 0)du\,ds$$

$$= 1 + \sigma \int_0^t p(s, x)ds + \sigma^2 \int_0^t p(t - s, x) \int_0^s p(u, 0)du\,ds + \dots$$

For $\sigma < \sigma_{cr}$, $\sigma \int_0^\infty p(s, 0)ds < 1$, and so the above series converges for all t and as $t \to \infty$.

Turning to the second moment, the PDE for the second factorial moment is

$$\frac{\partial m_2(t, x)}{\partial t} = \mathcal{L}m_2(t, x) + \sigma \delta_0(x)(m_2(t, x) + 2m_1^2(t, x))$$

$$m_2(0, x) \equiv 0.$$

An analysis parallel to that for the first moment shows that $m_2(\infty, x) < \infty$. Consequently, for $\sigma < \sigma_{cr}$ the population stabilizes.

3.4   Spatial Galton–Watson Process with Immigration and Finite Markov Chain Spatial Dynamics

We return to the spatial Galton–Watson process with immigration, but here with the possibility of migration between sites and allowing birth, death, and immigration rates to vary across sites. The number of sites is finite, which facilitates calculations.

We present the main results, here, and sketch their rationale; for full analysis, see [10] in this volume.

Let $X = \{x, y, \ldots\}$ be a finite set. Define the following parameters. At x in X, let $\beta(x)$ be the rate of duplication, $\mu(x)$ be the rate of annihilation, and $k(x)$ be the rate of immigration. For x and y in X, let $a(x, y)$ be the rate of transition $x \to y$.

Define $\vec{n}(t) = \{n(t, x), x \in X\}$ to be the population at moment $t \geq 0$, with $n(t, x)$ the occupation number of site $x \in X$. Letting $\vec{\lambda} = \{\lambda_x \geq 0, x \in X\}$, we write the Laplace transform of the random vector $\vec{n}(t) \in \mathbb{R}^N$, $N = \text{Card}(X)$ as $u(t, \vec{\lambda}) = E\, e^{-(\vec{\lambda}, \vec{n}(t))}$.

The differential equation for $u(t, \vec{\lambda})$ is

$$
\begin{cases}
\dfrac{\partial u(t,\vec{\lambda})}{\partial t} = \sum_{x \in X}(e^{-\lambda_x} - 1)(-\dfrac{\partial u(t,\vec{\lambda})}{\partial \lambda_x})\beta(x) + u(t,\vec{\lambda})k(x)) + \sum_{y \in X}(e^{\lambda_y} - 1)\mu(y)(-\dfrac{\partial u(t,\vec{\lambda})}{\partial \lambda_y}) \\[3mm]
\qquad + \sum_{x,z;x \neq z}(e^{\lambda_x - \lambda_z} - 1)a(x,z)(-\dfrac{\partial u(t,\vec{\lambda})}{\partial \lambda_x}) \\[3mm]
u(0, \vec{\lambda}) = E\, e^{-(\vec{\lambda}, \vec{n}(0))}
\end{cases}
$$

$$(3.2)$$

By differentiating Eq. 3.2 over the variables λ_x, $x \in X$, one can get the equations for the correlation functions

$$
k_{l_1 \ldots l_m}(t, x_1, \ldots, x_m) = E\, n^{l_1}(t, x_1) \cdots n^{l_m}(t, x_m),
$$

where $x_1, \ldots, x_m$ are different points of X and $l_1, \ldots, l_m \geq 1$ are integers. Specifically

$$
k_{l_1 \ldots l_m}(t, x_1, \ldots, x_m) = (-1)^{l_1 + \cdots + l_m} \frac{\partial^{l_1 + \cdots + l_m} n(t, \vec{\lambda})}{\partial^{l_1} \lambda_{x_1} \cdots \partial^{l_m} \lambda_{x_m}}\Big|_{\vec{\lambda}=0}.
$$

The corresponding equations will be linear. The central point here is that the factors $(e^{\lambda_x - \lambda_z} - 1)$, $(e^{\lambda_y} - 1)$, and $(e^{-\lambda_x} - 1)$ are equal to 0 for $\vec{\lambda} = 0$. As a result, the higher order $(n > l_1 + \ldots + l_m)$ correlation functions cannot appear in the equations for $\{k_{l_1 \ldots l_m}(\cdot), l_1 + \ldots + l_m = n\}$.

For the first moment, for example, if we assume the symmetry $a(x, z) = a(z, x)$ and define $V(v) = \beta(v) - \mu(v)$, we obtain

$$
\frac{\partial m_1(t, x)}{\partial t} = A m_1 + V m_1 + k(x), \qquad m_1(0, x) = n(0, x)
$$

where $A = [a(x, y)] = A^*$ is the generator of a Markov chain.

An alternative approach to the generating function method is to treat the birth and death process with immigration as a random walk with reflection on the half axis $n \geq 0$.. If we start from the simplest case, when there is one site, i.e., $X = \{x\}$, then application of known facts concerning random walks (see [6]) yields the following result.

Proposition 3.2

1. *If $\beta > \mu$, the process $n(t)$ is transient and the population $n(t)$ grows exponentially.*
2. *If $\beta = \mu$, $k > 0$, the process is not ergodic but rather it is zero-recurrent for $\frac{k}{\beta} \leq 1$ and transient for $\frac{k}{\beta} > 1$.*
3. *If $\beta < \mu$, the process $n(t)$ is ergodic. The invariant distribution for $\beta < \mu$ is given by*

$$\pi(n) = \frac{1}{\tilde{S}} \frac{k(k+\beta)\cdots(k+\beta(n-1))}{n!\mu^n}$$

where $\tilde{S} = \displaystyle\sum_{j=1}^{\infty} \frac{k(k+\beta)\cdots(k+\beta(j-1))}{\mu \cdot 2\mu \cdots j\mu}$.

Let us turn to the general case of the finite space X. Let $N = \text{Card } X$ and $\overrightarrow{n}(t)$ be the vector of the occupation numbers. The process $\overrightarrow{n}(t)$, $t \geq 0$ is a random walk on $(\mathbb{Z}_+^1)^N = \{0, 1, \ldots\}^N$ with continuous time. If at the moment t we have the configuration $\overrightarrow{n}(t) = \{n(t, x), x \in X\}$, then, for the interval $(t, t+dt)$, only the following events (up to terms of order$(dt)^2$) can happen:

(a) the appearance of a new particle at the site $x_0 \in X$, due to birth or immigration, with probability $n(t, x_0)\beta(x_0)dt + k(x_0)dt$.
(b) the death of one particle at the site $x_0 \in X$, with probability $\mu(x_0)n(t, x_0)dt$, for $n(t, x_0) \geq 1$.
(c) the transfer of one particle from site x_0 to $y_0 \in X$ (jump from x_0 to y_0), with probability $n(t, x_0)a(x_0, y_0)dt$, for $n(t, x_0) \geq 1$.

Theorem 3.2 in the preceding chapter in this volume, by Han et al., gives sufficient conditions for the ergodicity of the process $\overrightarrow{n}(t)$. We refer the reader to that analysis.

3.5 Branching Process with Stationary Random Environment

The last of our models without interaction between particles is a recently developed one that relaxes the artificiality of uniform birth and death rates, at β and μ, for the entire phase space. Working now in continuous space $\mathbb{R}^d$, [16] stipulates a random environment ω_m for the process with birth rate and death rates given by $b(x, \omega_m)$ and $m(x, \omega_m)$. Define the potential $V(x, \omega_m) = b(x, \omega_m) - m(x, \omega_m)$. In addition, there is migration but no immigration. Let the generator of the underlying migration $\mathcal{L}$ be the continuous version of our usual one with long jumps

$$\mathcal{L}f(x) = \int_{\mathbb{R}^d} a(z)(f(x+z) - f(x))dz.$$

The population density $\rho(t, x)$ satisfies

$$\frac{\partial \rho(t, x)}{\partial t} = \mathcal{L}\rho(t, x) + V(x, \omega_m)\rho(t, x)$$

$$\rho(0, x) \equiv \rho_0.$$

Suppose that $b(x, \omega_m)$ and $m(x, \omega_m)$ are continuous, ergodic, homogeneous, and nonnegative fields. Suppose also that $\langle e^{tb(0,\omega_m)} \rangle < \infty$, where $\langle \cdot \rangle$ indicates the expectation over ω_m. Then, if $V(x, \omega_m)$ satisfies the condition that there exists a (small) $\epsilon_0 > 0$ such that for any $L > 0$

$$P\{V(z, \omega_m) \geq \epsilon_0, |z| \leq L\} > 0$$

Reference [16] show that for any open domain $D \in \mathbb{R}^d$, with the measure of the domain $|D| < \infty$, $n(t, D) \xrightarrow[t \to \infty]{} \infty$ with probability 1.

This is true, moreover, even if $\langle V \rangle < 0$, in other words, if on average the death rate exceeds the birth rate. The reason is that, despite the fact that most places the death rate prevails and the population decays to 0, there are an infinite number of places where the birth rate exceeds the death rate so that the population grows exponentially. This is sufficient for the population as a whole to grow without limit.

3.6   Multilayer Bolker–Pacala Model

Some of the most intriguing population questions involve the interplay between multiple populations. A model that can capture some of this is a generalization of the mean-field approximation to the Bolker–Pacala model. We take the idea of a mean field over a box of size L and extend that to a set of N boxes, each of size L.

As always, there are birth rates and death rates. With multiple boxes, they can vary by box, although in simpler models we may keep them uniform across boxes. Migration (the "jump of the offspring"), which was irrelevant in the one-box mean-field approximation, here, can occur between boxes and so cannot be ignored as in the simpler Bolker–Pacala model. Migration can be seen equivalently as two random events, the birth of a individual and its dispersal, as in Bolker and Pacala's presentation [2], or as a single random event, as in our model. (We stress that this differs from the classical branching process, in which the "parental" individual and its offspring commence independent motion from the same point.) We assume, of course, that all offspring evolve independently according to the same rules.

Most interesting is the competition or suppression effect, which now can occur both internally, the population in a given box suppressing its own population, and externally, the population in one box suppressing the population of other boxes. The migration and suppression parameters can vary across boxes, or, again, in the simplest models, can be kept uniform across boxes.

Different general configurations of the parameters may be more appropriate for different modeling scenarios. For example, if the multiple populations are geographical regions, migration rates and internal suppression or competition rates may be relatively high, while external suppression rates would be low. Whereas if the populations are human social classes, migration rates are likely to be low, while external suppression rates, one class's population constraining the growth of another class's population, might be relatively high. Moreover, these last rates might well be nonuniform, with not all classes affecting other social classes equally.

The N-box Bolker–Pacala model gives rise to a random walk on

$$(\mathbb{Z}_+)^N = \{(n_1, n_2, \ldots, n_N) : n_i \in \mathbb{Z}_+, 1 \leq i \leq N\}.$$

Consider a system of N disjoint rectangles $Q_{i,L} \subset \mathbb{R}^2$, $i = 1, 2, \ldots, N$, N fixed, with

$$|Q_{i,L} \cap \mathbb{Z}^2| = L.$$

Parameters β_i, $\mu_i > 0$ represent the natural (biological) birth and death rates of particles in box i, $i = 1, \ldots, N$, respectively. The migration potential a^+ and the competition potential a^- also are constant on each $Q_{i,L}$. For $\mathbf{x} \in Q_{i,L}, \mathbf{y} \in Q_{j,L}$,

$$a_L^-(\mathbf{x}, \mathbf{y}) = a_{ij}^-/L^2, \qquad\qquad i, j = 1, 2, \ldots, N, \qquad (3.3)$$

and

$$a_L^+(\mathbf{x}, \mathbf{y}) = a_{ij}^+/L, \qquad\qquad i, j = 1, 2, \ldots, N. \qquad (3.4)$$

Specifically, a_{ij}^- indicates the supressive effect on the population in box i due to the population in box j (such as due to competition between boxes i and j), while $a_L^+(\mathbf{x}, \mathbf{y})$ is the rate of migration from $\mathbf{x} \in Q_{i,L}$ to $\mathbf{y} \in Q_{j,L}$.

Let $\bigcup_{i=1}^N Q_{i,L} = Q_L$. Then set

$$A_i^+ := \sum_{\mathbf{y} \in Q_L} a^+(\mathbf{x}, \mathbf{y}) = \sum_{j=1}^N a_{ij}^+, \quad A_i^- := \sum_{\mathbf{y} \in Q_L} a^-(\mathbf{x}, \mathbf{y}) = \sum_{j=1}^N a_{ij}^-$$

Assume that

$$A_i^+, A_i^- \leq A < \infty$$

uniformly in L.

The population in each square $Q_{i,L}, i = 1, \ldots, N$, at time t is represented by

$$\mathbf{n}(t) = \{n_1(t), n_2(t), \ldots, n_N(t)\}, \qquad (3.5)$$

a continuous-time random walk on $(\mathbb{Z}_+)^N$ with transition rates, for $i, j = 1, 2, \ldots, N$

$$\boldsymbol{n}(t + dt | \boldsymbol{n}(t)) \tag{3.6}$$

$$= \boldsymbol{n}(t) + \begin{cases} e_i & \text{w. pr. } \beta_i n_i(t)dt + o(dt^2) \\ -e_i & \text{w. pr. } \mu_i n_i(t)dt + \frac{n_i(t)}{L}\sum_{j=1}^{N} a_{ij}^- n_j(t)dt + o(dt^2) \\ e_j - e_i & \text{w. pr. } n_i(t)a_{ij}^+ dt + o(dt^2), \quad j \neq i \\ 0 & \text{w. pr. } 1 - \sum_{i=1}^{N}(\beta_i + \mu_i)n_i(t)dt \\ & \qquad - \frac{1}{L}\sum_{i,j} n_i(t)n_j(t)a_{ij}^- dt + \sum_{i,j} n_i(t)a_{ij}^+ + o(dt^2) \\ \text{other} & \text{w. pr. } o(dt^2) \end{cases}$$

where e_i is the vector with 1 in the ith position and 0 everywhere else.

This more general model exhibits some of the same characteristics of the simple mean-field approximation but reveals some new effects as well. Once again, there is convergence, as the size of the boxes L increases, to an Ornstein–Uhlenbeck process. The N-dimensional random walk is geometrically ergodic, meaning that it shows exponential convergence to a stable distribution. New, however, is that, for at least $N = 2$ and 3 (solutions become increasingly difficult to find as N increases), the population level may have multiple nontrivial equilibria. This is true only for some rate values, however. In particular, at least some of the values of the a_{ij}^-, $i \neq j$, the suppression of population across boxes, must be high enough.

This creates intriguing possibilities. For example, given the perpetual probabilistic fluctuations in population size, there is a certain chance that a population fluctuating about one equilibrium could swing wildly enough to put it into the attractive basin of a different equilibrium. This phenomenon should be amenable to analysis although it has not yet been done. Research into these models is ongoing.

References

1. Bessonov, M., Molchanov, S., Whitmeyer, J.: A mean field approximation of the Bolker–Pacala population model. Markov Process. Relat. Fields **20**, 329–348 (2014)
2. Bolker, B.M., Pacala, S.W.: Spatial moment equations for plant competition: understanding spatial strategies and the advantages of short dispersal. Am. Nat. **153**, 575–602 (1999)
3. Bolker, B.M., Pacala, S.W., Neuhauser, C.: Spatial dynamics in model plant communities: what do we really know? Am. Nat. **162**, 135–148 (2003)
4. Debes, H., Kerstan, J., Liemant, A., Matthes, K.: Verallgemeinerungen eines Satzes von Dobruschin I. Math. Nachr. **47**, 183–244 (1970)
5. Dobrushin, R.L., Siegmund-Schultze, R.: The hydrodynamic limit for systems of particles with independent evolution. Math. Nachr. **105**, 199–224 (1982)
6. Feller, W.: An Introduction to Probability Theory and Its Applications, 3rd edn. Wiley, New York (1968)
7. Galton, F.: Problem 4001. Educational Times **1**(17) (April 1873)
8. Galton, F., Watson, H.W.: On the probability of the extinction of families. J. R. Anthr. Inst. **4**, 138–144 (1874)
9. Gikhman, I.I., Skorokhod, A.V.: The Theory of Stochastic Processes. Springer, Berlin (1974)
10. Han, D., Molchanov, S., Whitmeyer, J.: Population Processes with Immigration
11. Harris, T.E.: The Theory of Branching Processes. Springer, Berlin (1963)
12. Kendall, D.G.: Branching processes since 1873. J. Lond. Math. Soc. **41**, 385–406 (1966)

13. Kolmogorov, A.N., Dmitriev, N.A.: Branching stochastic processes. Dokl. Akad. Nauk U.S.S.R. **56**, 5–8 (1947)
14. Kolmogorov, A.N., Petrovskii, I.G., Piskunov, N.S.: A study of the diffusion equation with increase in the quantity of matter, and its application to a biological problem. Bull. Moscow Univ. Math. Ser. A **1**, 1–25 (1937)
15. Kondratiev, Y.G., Skorokhod, A.V.: On contact processes in continuum. Infin. Dimens. Anal. Quantum Probab. Relat. Top. **9**(2), 187–198 (2006)
16. Kondratiev, Y., Kutoviy, O., Molchanov. S.: On population dynamics in a stationary random environment, U. of Bielefeld preprint
17. Kondratiev, Y., Kutovyi, O., Pirogov, S.: Correlation functions and invariant measures in continuous contact model. Infin. Dimens. Anal. Quantum Probab. Relat. Top. **11**, 231–258 (2008)
18. Liemant, A.: Invariante zufallige Punktfolgen. Wiss. Z. Friedrich-Schiller-Univ. Jena **19**, 361–372 (1969)
19. Malthus, T.R.: An Essay on the Principle of Population. John Murray, London (1826)
20. Molchanov, S.A., Yarovaya, E.B.: Branching processes with lattice spatial dynamics and a finite set of particle generation centers. Dokl. Akad. Nauk **446**, 259–262 (2012)
21. Vandermeer, J., Perfecto, I., Philpott, S.M.: Clusters of ant colonies and robust criticality in a tropical agroecosystem. Nature **451**, 457–459 (2008)

Part X
Ergodic Markov Processes

Ergodic Markov Processes and Poisson Equations (Lecture Notes)

Alexander Veretennikov

Abstract These are lecture notes on the subject defined in the title. As such, they do not pretend to be really new, perhaps, except for the Sect. 10 about Poisson equations with potentials; also, the convergence rate shown in (83)–(84) is possibly less known. Yet, the hope of the author is that these notes may serve as a bridge to the important area of Poisson equations 'in the whole space' and with a parameter, the latter theme not being presented here. Why this area is so important was explained in many papers and books including (Ethier and Kurtz, Markov Processes: Characterization and Convergence, New Jersey, 2005) [12], (Papanicolaou et al. Statistical Mechanics, Dynamical Systems and the Duke Turbulence Conference, vol. 3. Durham, N.C., 1977) [34], (Pardoux and Veretennikov, Ann. Prob. 31(3), 1166–1192, 2003) [35]: it provides one of the main tools in diffusion approximation in the area stochastic averaging. Hence, the aim of these lectures is to prepare the reader to 'real' Poisson equations—i.e. for differential operators instead of difference operators—and, indeed, to diffusion approximation. Among other presented topics, we mention coupling method and convergence rates in the Ergodic theorem.

Keywords Markov chains · Ergodic theorem · Limit theorems · Coupling Discrete poisson equations

This work has been funded by the Russian Academic Excellence Project '5-100', and supported by the Russian Foundation for Basic Research grant 17-01-00633-a. The author is also grateful to two anonymous referees for many valuable remarks.

A. Veretennikov (✉)
University of Leeds, Leeds, UK
e-mail: a.veretennikov@leeds.ac.uk

A. Veretennikov
National Research University Higher School of Economics, Moscow, Russian Federation

A. Veretennikov
Institute for Information Transmission Problems, Moscow, Russian Federation

© Springer International Publishing AG 2017
V. Panov (ed.), *Modern Problems of Stochastic Analysis and Statistics*,
Springer Proceedings in Mathematics & Statistics 208,
DOI 10.1007/978-3-319-65313-6_18

1   Introduction

In these lecture notes we will consider the following issues: Ergodic theorem (in some textbooks called Convergence theorem, while Ergodic would be reserved for what we call Law of Large Numbers—see below), Law of Large Numbers (LLN), Central Limit Theorem (CLT), Large Deviations (LDs) for Markov chains (MC), and as one of the most important applications, a Poisson equation. LLN, CLT and LDs are the basis of most of statistical applications. Everything is presented on the simplest model of a Markov chain with positive transition probabilities on a finite state space, and in some cases we show a few more general results where it does not require too much of additional efforts. This simplified version may be regarded as a preparation to more advanced situations of Markov chains on a more general state space, including non-compact ones and including Markov diffusions. A special place in this plan is occupied by coupling method, a famous idea, which is not necessary for any result in these lecture notes; yet, it is a rather convenient tool 'for thinking', although sometimes not very easy for a rigorous presentation. We show the Ergodic theorem firstly without and then with coupling method. Poisson equations in this paper are discrete analogues of 'real' Poisson equations for elliptic differential operators of the second order in mathematical physics. We consider equations *without* a potential—the most useful tool in diffusion approximations, cf. [12, 34, 35]—and also *with* a potential. The problem of smoothness of solutions with respect to a parameter—which makes this stuff so important in diffusion approximations and which is one of the main motivations of the whole theory—is not presented; however, these notes may be regarded as a bridge to this smoothness issue.

These notes are based on several different courses delivered by the author at various universities in various years, including Moscow State University, Helsinki Technical University (now Aalto University), University of Leeds and Magic consortium (http://maths-magic.ac.uk/index.php), and National Research University Higher School of Economics—Moscow. The author thanks all participants—not only students—for their interest and patience and for many useful remarks.

The initial plan involved non-compact cases with problems related to stability or recurrence properties of processes in such spaces. However, this would require significantly more time and many more pages. Hence, this more ambitious task is postponed for some future.

Some classical results are given without proofs although they were proved in the courses delivered. The references on all such 'missing' proofs are straightforward.

Finally, let us mention that the following numeration system is accepted here: all items such as Theorem, Lemma, Remark, Definition and some others are numbered by a unique sequence of natural numbers. This method was accepted in some well-known textbooks and the author shares the view about its convenience.

The following notations will be used for a process $(X_n, \; n \geq 0)$:

$$\mathcal{F}_n^X = \sigma(X_k : k \leq n); \quad \mathcal{F}_{(n)}^X = \sigma(X_n).$$

The following notations from the theory of Markov processes will be accepted (cf. [11]): the index x in $\mathbb{E}_x$ or $\mathbb{P}_x$ signifies the expectation or the probability measure related to the non-random initial state of the process X_0. This initial state may be also random with some distribution μ, in which case notations $\mathbb{E}_\mu$ or $\mathbb{P}_\mu$ may be used.

If state space S is finite, then $|S|$ denotes the number of its elements. In the sequel $\mathcal{P}$ denotes the transition matrix $(p_{ij})_{1 \le i, j \le |S|}$ of the process in the cases where state space of the process is finite.

Since this is a course about ergodic properties, we do not recall the definitions of what are Markov, strong Markov, homogeneous Markov processes (MP) which are assumed to be known to the reader: consult any of the textbooks [4, 10–12, 20, 27, 38, 49] if in doubt.

2 Ergodic Theorem – 1

In this section, we state and prove a simple ergodic theorem for Markov chains on a finite state space. However, we start with a more general setting because later in the end of these lecture notes a more general setting will be addressed. Ergodic Theorem for Markov chains in a simple situation of finite state spaces is due to Markov, although sometimes it is attributed to Kolmogorov with a reference to Gnedenko's textbook, and sometimes to Doeblin (see [9, 15]). We emphasize that this approach was introduced by Markov himself (see [30, 38, 39]). Kolmogorov, indeed, has contributed to this area: see, in particular, [23].

Let us consider a homogeneous Markov chain $X = (X_n)$, $n = 0, 1, 2, \ldots$ with a general topological state space $(S, \mathcal{S})$ where $\mathcal{S}$ is the family of all Borel sets in S assuming that $\mathcal{S}$ contains all single point subsets. Let $P_x(A)$ be the transition kernel, that is, $P_x(A) = \mathbb{P}(X_1 \in A | X_0 = x) \equiv \mathbb{P}_x(X_1 \in A)$; recall that for any $A \in \mathcal{S}$ this function is assumed Borel measurable in x (see [11]) and a measure in A (of course, for a finite S this is not a restriction). Denote by $P_x(n, A)$ the n-step transition kernel, i.e. $P_x(n, A) = \mathbb{P}_x(X_n \in A)$; for a finite Markov chain and if $A = j$, the notation $p_{ij}^{(n)}$ will be used, too. If initial state is random with distribution μ, we will be using a similar notation $P_\mu(n, A)$ for the probability $\mathbb{P}_\mu(X_n \in A)$. Repeat that $\mathbb{P}_{inv}(X_n \in A)$ signifies $P_\mu(X_n \in A)$ with the (unique) invariant measure μ; naturally, this value does not depend on n.

Recall the definition of ergodicity for Markov chains (MC).

Definition 1 An MC (X_n) is called Markov ergodic iff the sequence of transition measures $(\mathbb{P}_x(n, \cdot))$ has a limit in total variation metric, which is a probability measure and if, in addition, this limiting measure does not depend on x,

$$\lim_{n \to \infty} \mathbb{P}_x(n, A) = \mu(A), \quad \forall A \in \mathcal{S}. \tag{1}$$

Recall that the total variation distance or metric between two probability measures may be defined as

$$\|\mu - \nu\|_{TV} := 2 \sup_{A \in \mathcal{S}} (\mu(A) - \nu(A)).$$

Definition 2 An MC (X_n) is called irreducible iff for any $x \in S$ and $A \in \mathcal{S}$, $A \neq \emptyset$, there exists n such that

$$\mathbb{P}_x(X_n \in A) > 0.$$

An MC (X_n) is called ν-irreducible for a given measure ν on $(S, \mathcal{S})$ iff for any $x \in S$ and $A \in \mathcal{S}$, $\nu(A) > 0$ there exists n such that

$$\mathbb{P}_x(X_n \in A) > 0.$$

Of course, weaker or stronger ergodicity properties (definitions) may be stated with weaker, or, respectively, stronger metrics. Yet, in the finite state space case all of them are equivalent.

Exercise 3 *In the case of a finite state space S with $\mathcal{S} = 2^S$ (all subsets of S) and a counting measure ν such that $\nu(A) = |A| :=$ the number of elements in $A \subset S$, show that ν-irreducibility of a MC is equivalent to the claim that there exists $n > 0$ such that the n-step transition probability matrix $\mathcal{P}^n$ is* **positive***, that is, all elements of it are strictly positive.*

The most standard is the notion of ν-irreducibility of an MC where ν is the unique invariant measure of the process.

Definition 4 Stationary or invariant probability measure μ for a Markov process X is a measure on $\mathcal{S}$ such that for each $A \in \mathcal{S}$ and any n,

$$\mu(A) = \sum_{x \in S} \mu(x) P_x(n, A).$$

Lemma 5 *A probability measure μ is stationary for X iff*

$$\mu \mathcal{P} = \mu,$$

where $\mathcal{P}$ is the transition probability matrix of X.

Proof is straightforward by induction.

Lemma 6 *For any (homogeneous) Markov chain in a finite state space S there exists at least one stationary measure.*

Proof of the Lemma 6. The method is due to Krylov and Bogoliubov (Kryloff and Bogoliuboff, [26]). Let us fix some (any) $i_0 \in S$, and consider Cesàro averages

$$\frac{1}{n+1} \sum_{k=0}^{n} p_{i_0,j}^{(k)}, \quad 1 \leq j \leq N, \quad n \geq 1,$$

where $N = |S|$. Due to the boundedness, this sequence of vectors as $n \to \infty$ has a limit over some subsequence, say, $n' \to \infty$,

$$\frac{1}{n'+1} \sum_{k=0}^{n'} p_{i_0,j}^{(k)} \to \pi_j, \quad 1 \le j \le N, \quad n' \to 1,$$

where by the standard convention, $p_{ij}^{(0)} = \delta_{ij}$ (Kronecker's symbol). Since S is finite, it follows that $(\pi_j, 1 \le j \le N)$ is a probability distribution on S. Finally, stationarity follows from the following calculus based on Chapman–Kolmogorov's equations,

$$\frac{1}{n'+1} \sum_{k=0}^{n'} p_{i_0,j}^{(k)} = \frac{1}{n'+1} \sum_{k=0}^{n'} \sum_{\ell=1}^{N} p_{i_0,\ell}^{(k-1)} p_{\ell,j} + \frac{1}{n'+1} p_{i_0,j}^{(0)}$$

$$= \sum_{\ell=1}^{N} \frac{1}{n'+1} \sum_{k=0}^{n'-1} p_{i_0,\ell}^{(k)} p_{\ell,j} + \frac{1}{n'+1} p_{i_0,j}^{(0)}$$

$$= \sum_{\ell=1}^{N} \frac{1}{n'+1} \sum_{k=0}^{n'} p_{i_0,\ell}^{(k)} p_{\ell,j} + \frac{1}{n'+1} p_{i_0,j}^{(0)} - \frac{1}{n'+1} \sum_{\ell=1}^{N} p_{i_0,\ell}^{(n')} p_{\ell,j}.$$

It follows,

$$\lim_{n' \to \infty} \frac{1}{n'+1} \sum_{k=0}^{n'} p_{i_0,j}^{(k)} = \sum_{\ell=1}^{N} \pi_\ell p_{\ell,j}.$$

Hence,

$$\pi_j = \sum_{\ell=1}^{N} \pi_j p_{\ell,j} \quad \sim \quad \pi = \pi P.$$

Hence, the distribution (π_j) is stationary due to the Lemma 5. The Lemma 6 is proved.

Remark 7 Note that for a finite S the statement of the Lemma, actually, may be proved much faster by applying the Brouwer fixed-point theorem, as it is done, for example, in [41]. Yet, the method used in the proof seems deeper, and it can be used in a much more general situation including 'non-compact' cases. (However, we are not saying that the use of Brouwer's fixed-point theorem is restricted to finite state spaces.)

From now on, in this and several following sections we consider the case of a finite state space S; a more general case will be addressed in the last sections. The next condition suggested by Markov himself plays a very important role in the analysis of asymptotic behaviour of a (homogeneous) Markov chain (MC in the sequel). Let there exist n_0 such that

$$\kappa_{n_0} := \inf_{i,i'} \sum_j \min(P_i(n_0, j), P_{i'}(n_0, j)) \equiv \inf_{i,i'} \sum_j \min(p_{i,j}^{n_0}, p_{i',j}^{n_0}) > 0. \qquad (2)$$

By the suggestion of S. Seneta, this coefficient κ_{n_0} (as well as κ in (3) and in (52)) is properly called Markov–Dobrushin's.

Unlike in the continuous time case, in discrete-time situation there are potential complications related to possible *cycles*, that is, to a *periodic structure* of the process. A typical example of such a periodic structure is a situation where the state space is split into two parts, $S = S_1 \cup S_2$, which do not intersect, and $X_{2n} \in S_1$, while $X_{2n+1} \in S_2$ for each n. Then ergodic properties is reasonable to study separately for $Y_n := X_{2n}$ and for $Z_n := X_{2n+1}$. In other words, this complication due to periodicity does not introduce any real news, and by this reason there is a tradition to avoid this situation. Hence, in the sequel we will study our ergodic process under the assumption $n_0 = 1$ in the condition (2). Similar results could be obtained under a more general assumption of *aperiodicity*.

So, here is the simplified version of (2), which will be accepted in the sequel:

$$\kappa := \inf_{i,i'} \sum_j \min(P_i(1, j), P_{i'}(1, j)) \equiv \inf_{i,i'} \sum_j \min(p_{ij}, p_{i'j}) > 0. \qquad (3)$$

Also, to clarify the ideas we will be using in some cases the following stronger assumption,

$$\kappa_0 := \inf_{ij} p_{ij} > 0. \qquad (4)$$

However, eventually, the assumption (4) will be dropped and only (3) will remain in use.

Theorem 8 *Let the assumption (3) hold true. Then the process (X_n) is ergodic, i.e. there exists a limiting probability measure μ such that (1) holds true. Moreover, the uniform bound is satisfied for every n,*

$$\sup_x \sup_{A \in S} |P_x(n, A) - \mu(A)| \le (1 - \kappa)^n, \qquad (5)$$

and the measure μ is a unique invariant one.

Proof of Theorem 8 is classical and may be found in many places, for example, in [15].

(A) Denote for any A,

$$m^{(n)}(A) := \min_i P_i(n, A), \quad M^{(n)}(A) := \max_i P_i(n, A).$$

By Chapman–Kolmogorov's equation,

$$m^{(n+1)}(A) = \min_i P_i(n+1, A) = \min_i \sum_j p_{ij} P_j(n, A)$$

$$\geq \min_i \sum_j p_{ij} \min_{j'} P_{j'}(n, A) = m^{(n)}(A),$$

which signifies that the sequence $m^{(n)}(A)$ does not decrease in n. Similarly, the sequence $M^{(n)}(A)$ does not increase in n. Hence, it suffices to show that

$$M^{(n)}(A) - m^{(n)}(A) \leq (1 - \kappa)^n. \tag{6}$$

(B) Again by Chapman–Kolmogorov's equation,

$$M^{(n)}(A) - m^{(n)}(A) = \max_i P_i(n, A) - \min_{i'} P_{i'}(n, A)$$

$$= \max_i \sum_j p_{ij} P_j(n-1, A) - \min_{i'} \sum_j p_{i'j} P_j(n-1, A).$$

Let maximum here be attained at i_+ while minimum at i_-. Then,

$$M^{(n)}(A) - m^{(n)}(A) = \sum_j p_{i_+ j} P_j(n-1, A) - \sum_j p_{i_- j} P_j(n-1, A)$$

$$= \sum_j (p_{i_+ j} - p_{i_- j}) P_j(n-1, A). \tag{7}$$

(C) Denote by S^+ the part of the sum in the right hand side of (7) with just $(p_{i_+ j} - p_{i_- j}) \geq 0$, and by S^- the part of the sum with $(p_{i_+ j} - p_{i_- j}) < 0$. Using notations $a_+ = a \vee 0$ and $a_- = a \wedge 0$ (where $a \vee b = \max(a, b)$ and $a \wedge b = \min(a, b)$), we estimate,

$$S^+ \leq \sum_j (p_{i_+ j} - p_{i_- j})_+ M^{(n-1)}(A) = M^{(n-1)}(A) \sum_j (p_{i_+ j} - p_{i_- j})_+,$$

and

$$S^- \leq \sum_j (p_{i_+ j} - p_{i_- j})_- m^{(n-1)}(A).$$

Therefore,

$$M^{(n)}(A) - m^{(n)}(A) = S^+ + S^-$$

$$\leq M^{(n-1)}(A) \sum_j (p_{i_+j} - p_{i_-j})_+ + m^{(n-1)}(A) \sum_j (p_{i_+j} - p_{i_-j})_-.$$

(D) It remains to notice that

$$\sum_j (p_{i_+j} - p_{i_-j})_- = -\sum_j (p_{i_+j} - p_{i_-j})_+,$$

and

$$\sum_j (p_{i_+j} - p_{i_-j})_+ \leq 1 - \kappa. \tag{8}$$

The first follows from the normalization condition

$$\sum_j p_{i_+j} = \sum_j p_{i_-j} = 1,$$

while the second from (recall that $(a - b)_+ = a - a \wedge b \equiv a - \min(a, b)$ for any real values a, b)

$$\sum_j (p_{i_+j} - p_{i_-j})_+ = \sum_j (p_{i_+j} - \min(p_{i_-j}, p_{i_+j}))$$

$$= 1 - \sum_j \min(p_{i_-j}, p_{i_+j}) \leq 1 - \kappa$$

(see the definition of κ in (3)). So, we find that

$$M^{(n)}(A) - m^{(n)}(A) \leq (1 - \kappa)(M^{(n-1)}(A) - m^{(n-1)}(A)).$$

By induction this implies (6). So, (5) and uniqueness of the limits $\pi_j = \lim_{n \to \infty} p_{ij}^{(n)}$ follow.

(E) The invariance of the measure μ and uniqueness of the invariant measure follow, in turn, from (5). Indeed, let us start the process from any invariant distribution μ—which exists due to the Lemma 6—then $\mu_j \equiv \mathbb{P}_\mu(X_n = j) = \sum_\ell \mu_\ell p_{ij}^{(n)} \to \pi_j$, $n \to \infty$. However, the left hand side here does not depend on n. Hence, $\mu_j = \pi_j$. The Theorem 8 is proved.

Recall that the **total variation distance** or metric between two probability measures may be defined as
$$\|\mu - \nu\|_{TV} := 2 \sup_A (\mu(A) - \nu(A)).$$

Hence, the inequality (5) may be rewritten as

$$\sup_x \| P_x(n, \cdot) - \mu(\cdot) \|_{TV} \le 2(1 - \kappa)^n. \qquad (9)$$

Corollary 9 *Under the assumption of the Theorem 8, for any bounded Borel function f and for any $0 \le s < t$,*

$$\sup_x |\mathbb{E}_x(f(X_t)|X_s) - \mathbb{E}_{inv} f(X_t)| \equiv \sup_x |\mathbb{E}_x(f(X_t) - \mathbb{E}_{inv} f(X_t)|X_s)| \le C_f (1 - \kappa)^{t-s},$$

or, equivalently,

$$\sup_x |\mathbb{E}_x(f(X_t)|\mathcal{F}_s^X) - \mathbb{E}_{inv} f(X_t)| \le C_f (1 - \kappa)^{t-s},$$

where $C_f = \max_j |f(j)| \equiv \|f\|_{B(S)}$.

This useful Corollary follows from the Theorem 8.

It is worth noting that in a general case there is a significantly weaker condition than (2) (or, in the general case weaker than (52)—see below in the Sect. 11), which also guarantees an exponential convergence rate to a unique invariant measure. We will show this condition—called Doeblin-Doob's one—and state the corresponding famous Doeblin–Doob's theorem on convergence, but for the proof we refer the reader to [10].

Definition 10 (DD-condition) There exist a finite (sigma-additive) measure $\nu \ge 0$ and $\epsilon > 0$, $s > 0$ such that $\nu(A) \le \epsilon$ implies

$$\sup_x P_x(s, A) \le 1 - \epsilon.$$

Theorem 11 (Doeblin–Doob, without proof) *If the DD-condition is satisfied for an aperiodic MP with a unique class of ergodicity (see [10]) on the state space S, then there exist $C, c > 0$ such that*

$$\sup_x \sup_{A \in S} |P_x(n, A) - \mu(A)| \le C \exp(-cn), \quad n \ge 0. \qquad (10)$$

It turns out that under the assumption (DD), the constants in the upper bound (10) *cannot be effectively computed*, i.e. they may be arbitrary even for the same ϵ and ν, say. This situation dramatically differs from the case of conditions (4) and (3), where both constants in the upper bound are effectively and explicitly evaluated.

Open Question 12 *It is interesting whether or not there may exist any intermediate situation with a bound like (10)—in particular, it should be uniform in the initial state—with computable constants C, c under an assumption lying somewhere in 'between' Markov–Dobrushin's and Doeblin–Doob's. Apparently, such a condition* *may be artificially constructed from a 'non-compact' theory with an exponential recurrence, but then the bounds would not be uniform in the initial data. In fact, some relatively simple version of a desired condition will be shown in the end of this text, see the Theorem 47. However, it does not totally close the problem, e.g. for non-compact spaces.*

3 LLN for Homogeneous MC, Finite S

It may seem as if the Ergodic Theorem with uniform exponential convergence rate in total variation metric were all we could wish about ergodic features of the process. Yet, the statement of this theorem itself even does not include the Law of Large Numbers (LLN), which is not emphasized in most of the textbooks. However, the situation with LLN (as well as with Central Limit Theorem – CLT) is good enough, which is demonstrated below. The Theorem 13 under the assumption (4) belongs to A.A. Markov, see [30, 38].

Theorem 13 (Weak LLN) *Under the assumptions of the Theorem 8, for any function f on a finite state space S,*

$$\frac{1}{n}\sum_{k=0}^{n-1} f(X_k) \xrightarrow{\mathbb{P}} \mathbb{E}_{inv} f(X_0),\tag{11}$$

where $\mathbb{E}_{inv}$ stands for the expectation of $f(X_0)$ with respect to the invariant probability measure of the process, while $\mathbb{P}$ denotes the measure, which corresponds to the initial value or distribution of X_0: the latter may be, or may be not stationary.

NB. Note that a simultaneous use of stationary and non-stationary measures is not a contradiction here. The initial state could be either non-random, or it may have some distribution. At the same time, the process has a unique invariant measure, and the writing $\mathbb{E}_{inv} f(X_0) = 0$ signifies the mere fact that $\sum_{y \in S} f(y)\mu(y) = 0$, but it is in no way in a conflict with a non-stationary initial distribution. In the next proof we use $\mathbb{P}$ and, respectively, $\mathbb{E}$ without specifying the initial state or distribution. However, this initial distribution (possibly concentrated at one single state) exists and it is fixed throughout the proof.

Proof of the Theorem 13. **1**. First of all, note that (11) is equivalent to

$$\frac{1}{n}\sum_{k=0}^{n-1}(f(X_k) - \mathbb{E}_{inv} f(X_0)) \xrightarrow{\mathbb{P}} 0,$$

so, without loss of generality we may and will assume that $\mathbb{E}_{inv} f(X_0) = 0$. Now we estimate with any $\epsilon > 0$ by the Bienaymé–Chebyshev–Markov inequality,

$$\mathbb{P}\left(|\frac{1}{n}\sum_{k=0}^{n-1} f(X_k)| > \epsilon\right) \le \epsilon^{-2} n^{-2} \mathbb{E}|\sum_{k=0}^{n-1} f(X_k)|^2$$

(12)

$$= \epsilon^{-2} n^{-2} \mathbb{E} \sum_{k=0}^{n-1} f^2(X_k) + 2\epsilon^{-2} n^{-2} \mathbb{E} \sum_{0 \le k < j \le n-1} f(X_k) f(X_j).$$

Here the first term, clearly (as f is bounded), satisfies,

$$\epsilon^{-2} n^{-2} \mathbb{E} \sum_{k=0}^{n-1} f^2(X_k) \to 0, \quad n \to \infty.$$

Let us transform the second term as follows for $k < j$:

$$\mathbb{E} f(X_k) f(X_j) = \mathbb{E}(f(X_k)\mathbb{E}(f(X_j)|X_k)),$$

and recall that due to the Corollary 9 to the Ergodic theorem,

$$|\mathbb{E}(f(X_j)|X_k) - \mathbb{E}_{inv} f(X_j)| \le C_f (1 - \kappa)^{j-k},$$

where due to our convention $\mathbb{E}_{inv} f(X_j) = 0$. Therefore, we have,

$$|\mathbb{E} \sum_{k<j} f(X_k) f(X_j)| = |\mathbb{E} \sum_{k<j} f(X_k)\mathbb{E}(f(X_j)|X_k)|$$

$$\le C_f \sum_{k,j:0\le k<j<n} (1-\kappa)^{j-k} \le Cn, \quad \text{with } C = C_f \kappa^{-1}.$$

Thus, the second term in (12) also goes to zero as $n \to \infty$. The Theorem 13 is proved.

Remark 14 Recall that f is bounded and exponential rate of convergence is guaranteed by the assumptions. This suffices for a strong LLN via higher moments for sums. However, it will not be used in the sequel, so we do not show it here.

4   CLT, Finite S

In this section, state space S is also finite. For the function f on S, let

$$\sigma^2 := \mathbb{E}_{inv}(f(X_0) - \mathbb{E}_{inv} f(X_0))^2 + 2\sum_{k=1}^{\infty} \mathbb{E}_{inv}(f(X_0)$$

$$- \mathbb{E}_{inv} f(X_0))(f(X_k) - \mathbb{E}_{inv} f(X_k)).$$

(13)

It is known that this definition provides a non-negative value (for completeness, see the two lemmata below).

Lemma 15 *Under our standing assumptions (S is finite and $\min\limits_{ij} p_{ij} > 0$),*

$$\sigma^2 \geq 0, \tag{14}$$

and, moreover,

$$n^{-1}\mathbb{E}_{inv}\left(\sum_{r=0}^{n-1}(f(X_r) - \mathbb{E}_{inv}f(X_0))\right)^2 \to \sigma^2, \quad n \to \infty, \tag{15}$$

where the latter convergence is irrespectively of whether $\sigma^2 > 0$, or $\sigma^2 = 0$.

Proof Without loss of generality, we may and will assume now that $\mathbb{E}_{inv}f(X_0) = 0$ (otherwise, this mean value can be subtracted from f as in the formula (15)). Note also that in this case the variance of the random variable $n^{-1/2}\sum_{r=0}^{n-1}f(X_r)$ computed **with respect to the invariant measure** coincides in this case with its second moment. Since $\mathbb{E}_{inv}f(X_i) = 0$ for any i, this second moment may be evaluated as follows,

$$n^{-1}\mathbb{E}_{inv}(\sum_{r=0}^{n-1}f(X_r))^2 = \mathbb{E}_{inv}f^2(X_0) + 2n^{-1}\sum_{0 \leq i < j \leq n-1}\mathbb{E}_{inv}f(X_i)f(X_j)$$

$$= \mathbb{E}_{inv}f^2(X_0) + 2n^{-1}\sum_{r=1}^{n-1}(n-r)\mathbb{E}_{inv}f(X_0)f(X_r)$$

$$\stackrel{clearly}{\to} \mathbb{E}_{inv}f^2(X_0) + 2\sum_{r=1}^{\infty}\mathbb{E}_{inv}f(X_0)f(X_k) = \sigma^2, \quad n \to \infty.$$

Here the left hand side is non-negative, so σ^2 is non-negative, too. The Lemma 15 is proved.

Lemma 16 *Under the same assumptions as in the previous Lemma, $\sigma^2 < \infty$.*

Proof Again, without loss of generality, we may and will assume $\bar{f} := \mathbb{E}_{inv}f(X_0) = 0$, and $\|f\|_B \leq 1$. We have, due to the Corollary 9 applied with $\bar{f} = 0$,

$$|\mathbb{E}_{inv}f(X_0)f(X_k)| = |\mathbb{E}_{inv}f(X_0)\mathbb{E}_{inv}(f(X_k)|X_0)| \leq C_f\mathbb{E}_{inv}|f(X_0)|q^k,$$

with some $0 \leq q < 1$ and $C_f = \|f\|_B \leq 1$. So, the series in (13) does converge and the Lemma 16 is proved.

Theorem 17 *Let the assumption (3) hold true. Then for any function f on S,*

$$\frac{1}{\sqrt{n}}\sum_{k=0}^{n-1}(f(X_k) - \mathbb{E}_{inv}f(X_0)) \xRightarrow{\mathbb{P}} \eta \sim \mathcal{N}(0, \sigma^2), \qquad (16)$$

where $\Longrightarrow$ stands for the weak convergence with respect to the original probability measure (i.e. generally speaking, non-invariant).

Emphasize that we subtract the expectation with respect to the invariant measure, while weak convergence holds true with respect to the initial measure, which is not necessarily invariant. (We could have subtracted the actual expectation instead; the difference would have been negligible due to the Corollary 9.)

Remark 18 About Markov's method in CLT the reader may consult the textbook [41]. Various approaches can be found in [1, 2, 10, 23, 31, 32, 38], et al. For a historical review see [39]. A nontrivial issue of distinguishing the cases $\sigma^2 > 0$ and $\sigma^2 = 0$ for stationary Markov chains is under discussion in [3] for finite MC where a criterion has been established for $\sigma^2 = 0$; this criterion was extended to more general cases in [24]. A simple example of irreducible aperiodic MC (with $\min_{ij} p_{ij} = 0$) and a non-constant function f where $\sigma^2 = 0$ can be found in [41, ch. 6]. Nevertheless, there is a general belief that 'normally' in 'most of cases' $\sigma^2 > 0$. (Recall that zero (a constant) is regarded as a degenerate Gaussian random variable $\mathcal{N}(0, 0)$.) On using weaker norms in CLT for Markov chains see [28].

Proof of the Theorem 17. Without loss of generality, assume that $\| f \|_B \leq 1$, and that

$$\mathbb{E}_{inv}f(X_0) = 0.$$

I. Firstly, consider the case $\sigma^2 > 0$. We want to check the assertion,

$$\mathbb{E} \exp\left(i\frac{\lambda}{\sqrt{n}}\sum_{r=0}^{n}f(X_r)\right) \to \exp(-\lambda^2\sigma^2/2), \quad n \to \infty.$$

In the calculus below there will be expectations with respect to the measure $\mathbb{P}$ (denoted by $\mathbb{E}$) and some other expectations $\mathbb{E}_{inv}$. Note that they are different: the second one means expectation of a function of a random variable X_k computed with respect to the invariant measure of this process.

We are going to use Bernstein's method of 'corridors and windows' (cf. [1, 2]). Let us split the interval $[0, n]$ into partitions of two types: larger ones called 'corridors' and smaller ones called 'windows'. Their sizes will increase with n as follows. Let $k := [n/[n^{3/4}]]$ be the total number of long corridors of equal length (here $[a]$ is the integer part of $a \in \mathbb{R}$); this length will be chosen shortly as equivalent to $n^{3/4}$. The length of each window is $w := [n^{1/5}]$. Now, the length of each corridor except the last one is $c := [n/k] - w \equiv [n/k] - [n^{1/5}]$; the last complementary corridor has the length $c_L := n - k[n/k]$; note that $c_L \leq [n/k] \sim n^{3/4}$, $k \sim n^{1/4}$ (i.e. $k/n^{1/4} \to 1$, $n \to \infty$), and $c \sim n^{3/4}$.

The total length of all windows is then equivalent to $w \times k \sim n^{1/5+1/4} = n^{9/20}$; note for the sequel that $n^{9/20} \ll n^{1/2}$. As was mentioned earlier, the length of the last corridor does not exceed k, and, hence, asymptotically is no more than $n^{1/4}$ (which is much less than the length of any other corridor).

Now, denote all partial sums $\sum_{r=0}^{n} f(X_r)$ over the first k corridors by η_j, $1 \leq j \leq k$. In particular,

$$\eta_1 = \sum_{r=0}^{c-1} f(X_r), \quad \eta_2 = \sum_{r=c+w}^{2c+w-1} f(X_r), \quad \text{etc.}$$

Note that

$$\frac{1}{\sqrt{n}} |\sum_{r=0}^{n} f(X_r) - \sum_{j=1}^{k} \eta_j| \leq C_f \frac{(wk+k)}{\sqrt{n}} \sim C_f \frac{n^{9/20} + n^{1/4}}{\sqrt{n}} \to 0, \quad n \to \infty,$$

uniformly in $\omega \in \Omega$. Hence, it suffices to show that

$$\frac{1}{\sqrt{n}} \sum_{j=1}^{k} \eta_j \Longrightarrow \eta' \sim \mathcal{N}(0, \sigma^2).$$

Note that

$$n^{-1} \mathbb{E}_{inv} \eta_1^2 \sim \frac{c}{n} \sigma^2, \quad n \to \infty,$$

or,

$$n^{-3/4} \mathbb{E}_{inv} \eta_1^2 \to \sigma^2, \quad n \to \infty, \tag{17}$$

and the latter convergence is irrespectively of whether $\sigma^2 > 0$, or $\sigma^2 = 0$.

Now, to show the desired weak convergence, let us check the behaviour of the characteristic functions. Due to the Corollary 9, we estimate for any $\lambda \in \mathbb{R}$,

$$|\mathbb{E}(\exp(i\lambda\eta_j)|\mathcal{F}^X_{(j-1)[n/k]}) - \mathbb{E}_{inv} \exp(i\lambda\eta_j)| \leq C(1 - \kappa)^{[n^{1/5}]}.$$

So, by induction,

$$\mathbb{E}\exp\left(i\frac{\lambda}{\sqrt{n}}\sum_{j=1}^{k+1}\eta_j\right) = \mathbb{E}\exp\left(i\frac{\lambda}{\sqrt{n}}\sum_{j=1}^{k}\eta_j\right)\mathbb{E}\left(\exp\left(i\frac{\lambda}{\sqrt{n}}\eta_{k+1}\right)|\mathcal{F}_{k[n/k]}^X\right)$$

$$= \mathbb{E}\exp\left(i\frac{\lambda}{\sqrt{n}}\sum_{j=1}^{k}\eta_j\right)\left(\mathbb{E}_{inv}\left(\exp(i\frac{\lambda}{\sqrt{n}}\eta_{k+1}\right)+O((1-\kappa)^{n^{1/5}}))\right) = \dots$$

$$= \mathbb{E}_{inv}\left(\exp\left(i\frac{\lambda}{\sqrt{n}}\eta_{k+1}+O((1-\kappa)^{n^{1/5}})\right)\right)\left(\mathbb{E}_{inv}\left(\exp\left(i\frac{\lambda}{\sqrt{n}}\eta_1\right)\right)^k + O(k(1-\kappa)^{n^{1/5}})\right).$$

$$(18)$$

Here $O(k(1-\kappa)^{n^{1/5}})$ is, generally speaking, random and it is a function of $X_{k[n/k]}$, but the modulus of this random variable does not exceed a nonrandom constant multiplied by $k(1-\kappa)^{n^{1/5}}$. We replaced $[n^{1/5}]$ by $n^{1/5}$, which does not change the asymptotic (in)equality. Note that

$$O(k(1-\kappa)^{n^{1/5}})) = O(n^{3/4}(1-\kappa)^{n^{1/5}})) \to 0, \quad n \to \infty.$$

Now the idea is to use Taylor's expansion

$$\mathbb{E}_{inv}\exp\left(i\frac{\lambda}{\sqrt{n}}\eta_1\right) = 1 - \frac{\lambda^2}{2n}n^{3/4}\sigma^2 + R_n = 1 - \frac{\lambda^2}{2n^{1/4}}\sigma^2 + R_n. \quad (19)$$

Here, to prove the desired statement it suffices to estimate accurately the remainder term R_n, that is, to show that $R_n = o(n^{-1/4})$, $n \to \infty$.

Since we, actually, transferred the problem to studying an array scheme (as η_1 itself changes with n), we have to inspect carefully this remainder R_n. Due to the Taylor expansion we have,

$$\mathrm{Re}\,\varphi\left(\frac{\lambda}{\sqrt{n}}\right) = \mathbb{E}_{inv}\cos\left(\frac{\lambda\eta_1}{\sqrt{n}}\right) = 1 - \frac{\lambda^2}{2n}\mathbb{E}_{inv}\eta_1^2 + \frac{\hat{\lambda}^3}{6\sqrt{n^3}}\mathbb{E}_{inv}\eta_1^3\sin(\hat{\lambda}\eta_1),$$

with some $\hat{\lambda}$ between 0 and λ, and similarly, with some $\tilde{\lambda}$ between 0 and λ,

$$\mathrm{Im}\,\varphi\left(\frac{\lambda}{\sqrt{n}}\right) = \mathbb{E}_{inv}\sin\left(\frac{\lambda\eta_1}{\sqrt{n}}\right) = -\frac{\tilde{\lambda}^3}{6\sqrt{n^3}}\mathbb{E}_{inv}\eta_1^3\cos(\tilde{\lambda}\eta_1).$$

Here in general $\hat{\lambda}$ and $\tilde{\lambda}$ may differ. However, this is not important in our calculus because in any case $|\tilde{\lambda}| \leq |\lambda|$ and $|\hat{\lambda}| \leq |\lambda|$. All we need to do now is to justify a bound

$$|\mathbb{E}_{inv}\eta_1^3| \leq Kc, \quad (20)$$

with some non-random constant K. This is a rather standard estimation and we show the details only for completeness. (See similar in [14, 18, 22], et al.) It suffices to consider the case $C_f \leq 1$, which restriction we assume without loss of generality.

(a) Consider the case $\mathbb{E} f(X_k)^3$. We have, clearly,

$$\left| \sum_{k=1}^{c} \mathbb{E} f(X_k)^3 \right| \leq c.$$

(b) For simplicity, denote $f_k = f(X_k)$ and consider the case $\mathbb{E} f_j f_k f_\ell$, $\ell > k > j$. We have,

$$\sum_{j=0}^{c-2} \sum_{k=j+1}^{c-1} \sum_{\ell=k+1}^{c} \mathbb{E} f_j f_k f_\ell = \sum_{j=0}^{c-2} \sum_{k=j+1}^{c-1} \sum_{\ell=k+1}^{c} \mathbb{E} f_j f_k \mathbb{E}(f_\ell | X_k)$$

$$= \sum_{j=0}^{c-2} \sum_{k=j+1}^{c-1} \sum_{\ell=k+1}^{c} \mathbb{E} f_j f_k \psi_{k,\ell} q^{\ell-k} \quad (\text{here } \psi_{k,\ell} \in \mathcal{F}_{(k)}^X \equiv \sigma(X_k) \text{ and } |\psi_{k,\ell}| \leq 1).$$

Note that, with a $0 \leq q < 1$, the expression

$$\zeta_k := \sum_{\ell=k+1}^{c-1} \psi_{k,\ell} q^{\ell-k}$$

is a random variable, which modulus is bounded by the absolute constant $(1-q)^{-1}$ and which is $\mathcal{F}_{(k)}^X$-measurable, i.e. it may be represented as some Borel function of X_k. So, we continue the calculus,

$$\sum_{j=0}^{c-2} \sum_{k=j+1}^{c-1} \sum_{\ell=k+1}^{c} \mathbb{E} f_j f_k f_\ell = \sum_{j=0}^{c-2} \sum_{k=j+1}^{c-1} \sum_{\ell=k+1}^{c} \mathbb{E} f_j f_k \zeta_k$$

$$= \sum_{j=0}^{c-2} \sum_{k=j+1}^{c-1} \sum_{\ell=k+1}^{c} \mathbb{E} f_j E(f_k \zeta_k | X_j) = \sum_{j=0}^{c-2} \sum_{k=j+1}^{c-1} \mathbb{E} f_j (\mathbb{E} f_k \zeta_k + \zeta'_{k,j} q^{k-j})$$

$$= \sum_{j=0}^{c-2} \sum_{k=j+1}^{c-1} \mathbb{E} f_j \sum_{k=j+1}^{c-1} \zeta'_{k,j} q^{k-j} = \sum_{j=0}^{c-2} \mathbb{E} f_j \sum_{k=j+1}^{c-1} \zeta'_{k,j} q^{k-j},$$

due to $\mathbb{E} f_j \mathbb{E} f_k \zeta_k = 0$, since $\mathbb{E} f_j = 0$. Here $\zeta'_{k,j}$, in turn, for each k does not exceed by modulus the value $(1-q)^{-1}$ and is $\mathcal{F}_{(j)}^X$-measurable. Therefore, the inner sum in the last expression satisfies,

$$\left| \sum_{k=j+1}^{c-1} \zeta'_{k,j} q^{k-j} \right| \leq \sum_{k=j+1}^{c-1} |\zeta'_{k,j}| q^{k-j} \leq (1-q)^{-1} \sum_{k=j+1}^{c-1} q^{k-j} \leq (1-q)^{-2}.$$

Thus,

$$\left| \sum_{j=0}^{c-2} \sum_{k=j+1}^{c-1} \sum_{\ell=k+1}^{c} \mathbb{E} f_j f_k f_\ell \right| \leq (1-q)^{-2} \sum_{j=0}^{c-2} \mathbb{E}|f_j| \leq c(1-q)^{-2},$$

as required.

(c) Consider the terms with $\mathbb{E} f(X_k)^2 f(X_\ell)$, $\ell > k$. We estimate, with some (random) $|\psi'_{\ell,k}| \leq 1$ and $0 \leq q < 1$,

$$\left| \sum_{k<\ell}^{c-1} \mathbb{E} f(X_k)^2 \mathbb{E}(f(X_\ell)|X_k) \right| = \left| \sum_{k<\ell<c} \mathbb{E} f(X_k)^2 \psi'_{\ell,k} q^{\ell-k} \right| \leq \frac{c}{1-q}.$$

(d) Consider the case $\mathbb{E} f(X_k)^2 f(X_\ell)$, $\ell < k$. We have similarly, for $\ell < k$,

$$\mathbb{E} f_k^2 f_\ell = \mathbb{E} f_\ell \mathbb{E}(f_k^2|X_\ell) = \mathbb{E} f_\ell (\mathbb{E} f_k^2 + \psi''_{\ell,k} q^{k-\ell}), \quad |\psi_{\ell,k}| \leq 1,$$

with some (random) $|\psi''_{\ell,k}| \leq 1$. So, again,

$$\left| \sum_{\ell<k}^{c-1} \mathbb{E} f_\ell \mathbb{E}(f_k^2|X_\ell) \right| = \left| \sum_{\ell<k<c} \mathbb{E} f_k^2 \psi''_{\ell,k} q^{k-\ell} \right| \leq \frac{c}{1-q}.$$

(e) Finally, collecting all intermediate bounds we obtain the bound (20), as required:

$$|\mathbb{E} \eta_1^3| \leq Kc.$$

This implies the estimate for the remainder term R_n in (19) of the form

$$|R_n| \leq \frac{c}{n^{3/2}} \sim n^{3/4-3/2} = n^{-3/4} = o(n^{-1/4}),$$

as required. The last detail is to consider the term $\mathbb{E}_{inv} \exp(i \frac{\lambda}{\sqrt{n}} \eta_{k+1})$ in (18), for which we have $\sigma_{k+1}^2 := \mathbb{E} \eta_{k+1}^2$ satisfying

$$\mathbb{E}_{inv} \eta_{k+1}^2 = O(n^{3/4} \sigma^2), \quad n \to \infty. \tag{21}$$

This term may be tackled similarly to all others, and, in any case, we get the estimate

$$\mathbb{E}_{inv} \exp\left(i \frac{\lambda}{\sqrt{n}} \eta_{k+1}\right) = 1 + o(1), \quad n \to \infty.$$

Hence, we eventually get (recall that $c \sim n^{3/4}$),

$$\mathbb{E} \exp\left(i \frac{\lambda}{\sqrt{n}} \sum_{r=0}^{n} f(X_r) \right) = \left(1 - \frac{\lambda^2 \sigma^2 c}{2n} + O(\frac{c}{n^{3/2}}) \right)^{n^{1/4}}$$

$$= \left(1 - \frac{\lambda^2 \sigma^2}{2n^{1/4}} + O\left(\frac{1}{n^{3/4}} \right) \right)^{n^{1/4}} \to \exp(-\lambda^2 \sigma^2 / 2),$$

which is the characteristic function for the Gaussian distribution $\mathcal{N}(0, \sigma^2)$, as required.

(II) The case $\sigma^2 = 0$ is considered absolutely similarly. Namely, with a practically identical arguments we get, now with $\sigma^2 = 0$,

$$\mathbb{E} \exp\left(i \frac{\lambda}{\sqrt{n}} \sum_{r=0}^{n} f(X_r) \right) = \left(1 - \frac{\lambda^2 \sigma^2 c}{2n} + O\left(\frac{c}{n^{3/2}} \right) \right)^{n^{1/4}}$$

$$= \left(1 + O\left(\frac{1}{n^{3/4}} \right) \right)^{n^{1/4}} \to 1,$$

which is the characteristic function for the degenerate Gaussian distribution $\mathcal{N}(0, 0)$, as required. Hence, the Theorem 17 is proved.

5 Coupling Method for Markov Chain: Simple Version

Concerning coupling method, it is difficult to say who exactly invented this method. The common view—shared by the author of these lecture notes—is that it was introduced by W. Doeblin [9], even though he himself refers to some ideas of Kolmogorov with relation to the study of ergodic properties of Markov chains. Leaving this subject to the historians of mathematics, let us just mention that there are quite a few articles and monographs where this method is presented [16, 29, 33, 40], et al. Also there are many papers and books where this or close method is used for further investigations without being explicitly named, see, e.g. [4]. This method itself provides 'another way' to establish geometric convergence in the Ergodic theorem. In the simple form as in this section, this method has limited applications; however, in a more elaborated version—see the Sect. 13 below—it is most useful, and applicable to a large variety of Markov processes including rather general diffusions, providing not necessarily geometric rates of convergence but also much weaker rates in non-compact spaces.

By simple coupling for two random variables X^1, X^2 we understand the situation where both X^1, X^2 are defined on the same probability space and

$$\mathbb{P}(X^1 = X^2) > 0.$$

Consider a Markov chain $(X_n, n = 0, 1, \ldots)$. In fact, this simple 'Doeblin's' version of coupling provides bounds of convergence which are far from optimal in most cases. (By 'far from optimal' we understand that the constant under the exponential is too rough.) Yet, its advantage is its simplicity and, in particular, no change of the initial probability space. From the beginning we need two 'independent' probability spaces, $(\Omega^1, \mathcal{F}^1, \mathbb{P}^1)$, and $(\Omega^2, \mathcal{F}^2, \mathbb{P}^2)$, and the whole construction runs on the direct product of those two:

$$(\Omega, \mathcal{F}, \mathbb{P}) := (\Omega^1, \mathcal{F}^1, \mathbb{P}^1) \times (\Omega^2, \mathcal{F}^2, \mathbb{P}^2).$$

This space $(\Omega, \mathcal{F}, \mathbb{P})$ will remain unchanged in this section. We assume that there are two Markov processes (X_n^1) on $(\Omega^1, \mathcal{F}^1, \mathbb{P}^1)$ and (X_n^2) on $(\Omega^2, \mathcal{F}^2, \mathbb{P}^2)$, correspondingly, with the same transition probability matrix $\mathcal{P} = (p_{ij})_{i,j \in S}$ satisfying the 'simple ergodic assumption',

$$\kappa_0 := \min_{i,j} p_{ij} > 0. \tag{22}$$

Naturally, both processes are defined on $(\Omega, \mathcal{F}, \mathbb{P})$ as follows,

$$X_n^1(\omega) = X_n^1(\omega^1, \omega^2) := X_n^1(\omega^1), \quad \& \quad X_n^2(\omega) = X_n^2(\omega^1, \omega^2) := X_n^2(\omega^2).$$

We will need some (well-known) auxiliary results. Recall that given a filtration $(\mathcal{F}_n)$, stopping time is any random variable $\tau < \infty$ a.s. with values in $\mathbb{Z}_+$ such that for any $n \in \mathbb{Z}_+$,

$$(\omega : \tau > n) \in \mathcal{F}_n.$$

In most of textbooks on Markov chains the following Lemma may be found (see, e.g. [49]).

Lemma 19 *Any Markov chain (i.e. a Markov process with discrete time) is strong Markov.*

Consider a new process composed of two, $X_n := (X_n^1, X_n^2)$, evidently, with two independent coordinates. Due to this independence, the following Lemma holds true.

Lemma 20 *The (vector-valued) process (X_n) is a (homogeneous) Markov chain; hence, this chain is also strong Markov.*

In the following main result of this section, μ stands for the (unique) stationary distribution of our Markov chain (X_n^1) (as well as of (X_n^2)).

Theorem 21 *For any initial distribution μ_0,*

$$\sup_A |P_\mu(n, A) - \mu(A)| \leq (1 - \kappa_0)^n. \tag{23}$$

Let us emphasize again that the bound may be not optimal; however, the advantage is that the construction of coupling here does not require any change of the probability space.

Proof of Theorem 21. Recall that a new Markov chain $X_n := (X_n^1, X_n^2)$ with two independent coordinates is strong Markov. Let

$$\tau := \inf(n \geq 0 : X_n^1 = X_n^2).$$

We have seen that $\mathbb{P}(\tau < \infty) = 1$. More than that, from Markov property it follows for any n by induction (with a random variable called *indicator*, $1(A)(\omega) = 1$ if $\omega \in A$ and $1(A)(\omega) = 0$ if $\omega \notin A$),

$$\mathbb{P}(\tau > n) = \mathbb{E}1(\tau > n) = \mathbb{E}\prod_{k=1}^{n} 1(\tau > k)$$

$$= \mathbb{E}\left(\mathbb{E}(\prod_{k=1}^{n} 1(\tau > k)|\mathcal{F}_{n-1})\right) = \mathbb{E}\left(\prod_{k=1}^{n-1} 1(\tau > k)\mathbb{E}(1(\tau > n)|\mathcal{F}_{n-1})\right)$$

$$\leq \mathbb{E}\prod_{k=1}^{n-1} 1(\tau > k)(1 - \kappa_0) = (1 - \kappa_0)\mathbb{E}\prod_{k=1}^{n-1} 1(\tau > k) \leq \overset{\text{(induction)}}{\cdots} \leq (1 - \kappa_0)^n.$$

$$(24)$$

Define

$$X_n^3 := X_n^1 1(n < \tau) + X_n^2 1(n \geq \tau).$$

Due to the strong Markov property, (X^3) is also a *Markov chain* and it is *equivalent* to (X^1)—that is, they both have the same distribution in the space of trajectories. This follows from the fact that at τ which is a stopping time the process follows X^3, so that it uses the same transition probabilities while choosing the next state at $\tau + 1$ and further.

Now, here is the most standard and most frequent calculus in most of works on coupling method, or where this method is used (recall that all the processes X^1, X^2, X^3 are defined on the same probability space): for any $A \in \mathcal{S}$,

$$|\mathbb{P}(X_n^1 \in A) - \mathbb{P}(X_n^2 \in A)| = |\mathbb{P}(X_n^3 \in A) - \mathbb{P}(X_n^2 \in A)|$$

$$= |\mathbb{E}1(X_n^1 \in A) - \mathbb{E}1(X_n^2 \in A)| = |\mathbb{E}(1(X_n^3 \in A) - 1(X_n^2 \in A))|$$

$$= |\mathbb{E}(1(X_n^3 \in A) - 1(X_n^2 \in A))1(\tau > n) + \mathbb{E}(1(X_n^3 \in A) - 1(X_n^2 \in A))1(\tau \le n)|$$

$$\overset{(*)}{=} |\mathbb{E}(1(X_n^3 \in A) - 1(X_n^2 \in A))1(\tau > n)| \le |\mathbb{E}(1(X_n^3 \in A) - 1(X_n^2 \in A))1(\tau > n)|$$

$$\le \mathbb{E}|1(X_n^3 \in A) - 1(X_n^2 \in A)|1(\tau > n) \le \mathbb{E}1(\tau > n) = \mathbb{P}(\tau > n) \overset{(24)}{\le} (1 - \kappa_0)^n.$$

Note that the final bound is uniform in A. Here the equality $(*)$ is due to the trivial fact that since $n \ge \tau$, the values of X_n^3 and X_n^2 coincide, so either $1(X_n^3 \in A) = 1(X_n^2 \in A) = 0$, or $1(X_n^3 \in A) = 1(X_n^2 \in A) = 1$ simultaneously on each ω, which immediately implies that $(1(X_n^3 \in A) - 1(X_n^2 \in A))1(\tau \le n) = 0$. So, the Theorem 21 is proved.

6   A Bit of Large Deviations

In this section, assume

$$\mathbb{E}_{inv} f(X_0) = 0.$$

We will be interested in the existence and properties of the limit,

$$\lim_{n \to \infty} \frac{1}{n} \ln \mathbb{E}_x \exp\left(\beta \sum_{k=0}^{n-1} f(X_k)\right) =: H(\beta). \tag{25}$$

Note that we do not use x in the right hand side because in 'good cases'—as below— the limit does not depend on the initial state. Denote

$$H_n(\beta, x) := \frac{1}{n} \ln \mathbb{E}_x \exp\left(\beta \sum_{k=0}^{n-1} f(X_k)\right),$$

and define the operator $T = T^\beta$ acting on functions on S as follows,

$$T^\beta h(x) := \exp(\beta f(x)) \mathbb{E}_x h(X_1),$$

for any function h defined on S. Note that

$$\mathbb{E}_x \exp\left(\beta \sum_{k=0}^{n-1} f(X_k)\right) = (T^\beta)^n h(x),$$

with $h(x) \equiv 1$. Indeed, for $n = 1$ this coincides with the definition of T^β. Further, for $n > 1$ due to the Markov property by induction,

$$\mathbb{E}_x \exp\left(\beta \sum_{k=0}^{n-1} f(X_k)\right) = \mathbb{E}_x \mathbb{E}_x \left(\exp\left(\beta \sum_{k=0}^{n-1} f(X_k)\right) | X_1\right)$$

$$= \exp(\beta f(x)) \mathbb{E}_x \mathbb{E}_x \left(\exp\left(\beta \sum_{k=1}^{n-1} f(X_k)\right) | X_1\right)$$

$$= \exp(\beta f(x)) \mathbb{E}_x (T^\beta)^n h(x) = T^\beta (T^\beta)^{n-1} h(x) = (T^\beta)^n h(x),$$

as required. So, the function H_n can be rewritten as

$$H_n(\beta, x) = \frac{1}{n} \ln(T^\beta)^n h(x),$$

($h(x) \equiv 1$). It is an easy exercise to check that the function $H_n(\beta, x)$ is convex in β. Hence, if the limit exists, then the limiting function H is also convex. Now recall the following classical and basic result about positive matrices.

Theorem 22 (Perron–Frobenius) *Any positive quadratic matrix (i.e. with all entries positive) has a positive eigenvalue r called its spectral radius, which is strictly greater than the moduli of the rest of the spectrum, this eigenvalue is simple, and its corresponding eigenfunction (eigenvector) has all positive coordinates.*

In fact, this result under the specified conditions is due to Perron, while Frobenius extended it to non-negative matrices. We do not discuss the details of this difference and how it can be used. Various presentations may be found, in particular, in [20, 25, 38]. As an easy corollary, the Theorem 22 implies the existence of the limit in (25)—which, as was promised, does not depend on x—with,

$$H(\beta) = \ln r(\beta), \tag{26}$$

where $r(\beta)$ is the spectral radius of the operator T^β, see, for example, [14, Theorem 7.4.2]. (Emphasize that in the proof of this theorem it is important that the eigenvector corresponding to the spectral radius is strictly positive, i.e. it has all positive components.) More than that, in our case it follows from the theorem about analytic properties of simple eigenvalues that $r(\beta)$ is analytic, see, e.g. [21]. Therefore, $H(\beta)$ is analytic, too. Also, clearly, analytic is H_n as a function of the variable β. Then it follows from the properties of analytic (or convex) functions that convergence $H_n(\beta, x) \to H(\beta)$ implies that also

$$H_n'(0, x) \to H'(0), \quad n \to \infty,$$

where by H_n' we understand the derivative with respect to β. On the other hand, we have,

$$H_n'(0, x) = \frac{\partial}{\partial \beta} \left(\frac{1}{n} \ln \mathbb{E}_x \exp(\beta \sum_{k=0}^{n-1} f(X_k)) \right) |_{\beta=0}$$

$$= \frac{1}{n} \frac{\mathbb{E}_x \left(\sum_{k=0}^{n-1} f(X_k) \exp(\beta \sum_{k=0}^{n-1} f(X_k)) \right)}{\mathbb{E}_x \exp(\beta \sum_{k=0}^{n-1} f(X_k))} |_{\beta=0} = \frac{1}{n} \mathbb{E}_x \sum_{k=0}^{n-1} f(X_k).$$

So, due to the Law of Large Numbers,

$$H_n'(0, x) = \frac{1}{n} \mathbb{E}_x \sum_{k=0}^{n-1} f(X_k) \to \mathbb{E}_{inv} f(X_0) = 0.$$

Hence,

$$H'(0) = \mathbb{E}_{inv} f(X_0) = 0.$$

Also, again due to the analyticity,

$$H_n''(0, x) \to H''(0), \quad n \to \infty.$$

On the other hand, due to (17),

$$H_n''(0) = \frac{1}{n} \mathbb{E}_x \left(\sum_{k=0}^{n-1} f(X_k) \right)^2 \to \sigma^2, \quad n \to \infty.$$

Hence,

$$H''(0) = \sigma^2.$$

This last assertion will not be used in the sequel.
Let us state it all as a lemma.

Lemma 23 *There exists a limit $H(\beta)$ in (25). This function H is convex and differentiable, and, in particular,*

$$H'(0) = 0, \quad H''(0) = \sigma^2.$$

Actually, we will not use *large deviations* (LDs) in these lecture notes, except for the Lemma 23, which is often regarded as a preliminary auxiliary result in large deviation theory. Yet, once the title of the section uses this term, let us state one simple inequality of LD type. Recall that $\mathbb{E}_{inv} f(X_0) = 0$ in this section.

Proposition 24 *Let*

$$L(\alpha) := \sup_{\beta}(\alpha\beta - H(\beta)), \quad \tilde{L}(\alpha) := \limsup_{\delta \to 0} L(\alpha + \delta). \tag{27}$$

Then under the assumptions of the Ergodic Theorem 8 for any $\epsilon > 0$,

$$\limsup_{n \to \infty} \frac{1}{n} \ln \mathbb{P}_x\left(\frac{1}{n}\sum_{k=0}^{n-1} f(X_k) \geq \epsilon\right) \leq -\tilde{L}(\epsilon). \tag{28}$$

The function L is called Legendre transformation of the function H. It is convex and lower semicontinuous; see [37] about this and more general transformations (e.g. where H is convex but not necessarily smooth—in which case L is called Fenchel–Legendre's transformation). Notice that 'usually' in (28) there is a limit instead of lim sup, and this limit equals the right hand side, and both $\tilde{L}(\epsilon) = L(\epsilon) > 0$; the latter is certainly true, at least, for small $\epsilon > 0$ if $\sigma^2 > 0$. However, this simple result does not pretend to be even an introduction to large deviations, about which theory see [5, 7, 13, 14, 17, 36, 42], et al. In the next sections the Proposition 24 will not be used: all we will need is the limit in (25) due to the Lemma 23 and some its properties, which will be specified.

Proof of Proposition 24. We have for any $0 < \delta < \epsilon$, by Chebyshev–Markov's exponential inequality with any $\lambda > 0$,

$$\mathbb{P}_x\left(\frac{1}{n}\sum_{k=0}^{n-1} f(X_k) \geq \epsilon\right) = \mathbb{P}_x\left(\exp\left(\lambda\sum_{k=0}^{n-1} f(X_k)\right) \geq \exp(n\lambda\epsilon)\right)$$

$$\leq \exp(-n\lambda\epsilon)\mathbb{E}_x \exp\left(\lambda\sum_{k=0}^{n-1} f(X_k)\right) \overset{(25)}{\leq} \exp(-n(\lambda(\epsilon - \delta) + H(\lambda))),$$

if n is large enough. The first and the last terms here with the inequality between them can be rewritten equivalently as

$$\frac{1}{n} \ln \mathbb{P}_x\left(\frac{1}{n}\sum_{k=0}^{n-1} f(X_k) \geq \epsilon\right) \leq -\lambda(\epsilon - \delta) + H(\lambda),$$

for n large enough. So, we have,

$$\limsup_{n \to \infty} \frac{1}{n} \ln \mathbb{P}_x\left(\frac{1}{n}\sum_{k=0}^{n-1} f(X_k) \geq \epsilon\right) \leq -(\lambda(\epsilon - \delta) - H(\lambda)).$$

Since this is true for any $\lambda > 0$, we also get,

$$\limsup_{n \to \infty} \frac{1}{n} \ln \mathbb{P}_x \left(\frac{1}{n} \sum_{k=0}^{n-1} f(X_k) \geq \epsilon \right) \leq -\sup_{\lambda > 0}(\lambda(\epsilon - \delta) - H(\lambda)),$$

However, since $H(0) = 0$ and $H'(0) = 0$ and due to the convexity of H, the supremum on *all* $\lambda \in \mathbb{R}$ here on positive $\epsilon - \delta$ is attained at $\lambda > 0$, i.e.

$$\sup_{\lambda > 0}(\lambda(\epsilon - \delta) - H(\lambda)) = \sup_{\lambda \in \mathbb{R}}(\lambda(\epsilon - \delta) - H(\lambda)) \equiv L(\epsilon - \delta).$$

Thus, the left hand side in (28) does not exceed the value $-\limsup_{\delta \downarrow 0} L(\epsilon - \delta) \leq$

$-\tilde{L}(\epsilon)$, as required. The Proposition 24 is proved.

7   Dynkin's Formulae

Let L be a generator of some Markov chain on a finite state space S, that is, for any function u on S,

$$Lu := \mathbb{E}_x u(X_1) - u(x) \equiv \mathcal{P}u(x) - u(x). \qquad (29)$$

Recall that here $\mathcal{P}$ is the transition probability matrix of the corresponding Markov chain (X_n), a function u on S is considered as a column-vector, $\mathcal{P}u$ is this matrix multiplied by this vector, and $\mathcal{P}u(x)$ is the x-component of the resulting vector. Note that such difference operators are discrete analogues of elliptic differential operators of the second order studied extensively, in particular, in mathematical physics. What makes them the analogues is that both are generators of Markov processes, either in discrete or in continuous time; also, it may be argued about limiting procedures approximating continuous time processes by discrete ones. Yet, the level of this comparison here is, of course, intuitive and we will not try to justify in any way, or to explain it further.

As usual in these lecture notes, we will assume that the corresponding process (X_n) satisfies the Ergodic Theorem 8. The Poisson equation for the operator L from (29) is as follows:

$$Lu(x) = -f(x), \quad x \in S. \qquad (30)$$

This equation may be studied *with* or *without* some boundary and certain boundary conditions. The goal of this chapter is to present how such equations may be solved probabilistically. This simple study may be also considered as an introduction to the Poisson equations for elliptic differential operators. We start with **Dynkin's formula** or Dynkin's identity.

Theorem 25 (Dynkin's formula 1) *On the finite state space S, for any function h and any n = 1, 2, ...,*

$$\mathbb{E}_x h(X_n) = h(x) + \sum_{k=0}^{n-1} \mathbb{E}_x L h(X_k), \quad n \geq 0. \tag{31}$$

Proof **1.** For $n = 1$ the formula (31) reads,

$$\mathbb{E}_x h(X_1) = h(x) + L h(x),$$

where x is a non-random initial value of the process. Hence, by inspection, the desired identity for $n = 1$ is equivalent to the definition of the generator in (29).

2. For the general case n, the desired formula follows by induction. Indeed, assume that the formula (31) holds true for some $n = k$ and check it for $n = k + 1$. We have,

$$\mathbb{E}_x h(X_{n+1}) = \mathbb{E}_x h(X_{n+1}) - \mathbb{E}_x h(X_n) + \mathbb{E}_x h(X_n)$$

$$= \mathbb{E}_x \mathbb{E}_x (h(X_{n+1}) - h(X_n)|X_n) + \mathbb{E}_x h(X_n)$$

$$= \mathbb{E}_x \mathbb{E}_x (L h(X_n)|X_n) + h(x) + \sum_{k=0}^{n-1} \mathbb{E}_x L h(X_k)$$

$$= \mathbb{E}_x L h(X_n) + h(x) + \sum_{k=0}^{n-1} \mathbb{E}_x L h(X_k) = h(x) + \sum_{k=0}^{n} \mathbb{E}_x L h(X_k).$$

So, the formula (31) for all values of n follows by induction. The Theorem 25 is proved.

8 Stopping Times and Martingales: Reminder

Definition 26 Filtration $(\mathcal{F}_n, n = 0, 1, \ldots)$ is a family of increasing sigma-fields on a probability space $(\Omega, \mathcal{F}, \mathbb{P})$ completed with respect to the measure $\mathbb{P}$ (that is, each $\mathcal{F}_n$ contains each subset of all $\mathbb{P}$-zero sets from $\mathcal{F}$). The process (M_n) is called a martingale with respect to a filtration $(\mathcal{F}_n)$ iff $\mathbb{E} M_n < \infty$ and $\mathbb{E}(M_{n+1}|\mathcal{F}_n) = M_n$ (a.s.).

Definition 27 A random variable $\tau < \infty$ a.s. with values in $\mathbb{Z}_+$ is called a stopping time with respect to a filtration $(\mathcal{F}_n)$ iff for each $n \in \mathbb{Z}_+$ the event $(\tau > n)$ is measurable with respect to $\mathcal{F}_n$.

It is recommended to read about simple properties of martingales and stopping times in one of the textbooks on stochastic processes, e.g. [27]. We will only need the following classical result about stopped martingales given here without proof.

Theorem 28 (Doob) *Let (M_n) be a martingale and let τ be a stopping time with respect to a filtration $(\mathcal{F}_n)$. Then $(\tilde{M}_n := M_{n \wedge \tau})$ is also a martingale.*

In terms of martingales, the first Dynkin's formula may be re-phrased as follows.

Theorem 29 (Dynkin's formula 2) *On the finite state space S, for any function h and any $n = 1, 2, \ldots$, the process*

$$M_n := h(X_n) - h(x) - \sum_{k=0}^{n-1} Lh(X_k), \quad n \geq 0, \tag{32}$$

is a martingales with respect to the natural filtration $\mathcal{F}_n^X$ 'generated' by the process X. Vice versa, if the process M_n from (32) is a martingale then (31) holds true.

Proof The inverse statement is trivial. The main part follows due to the Markov property,

$$\mathbb{E}(M_n | \mathcal{F}_{n-1}) = \mathbb{E}(h(X_n) | X_{n-1}) - h(x) - \sum_{k=0}^{n-1} Lh(X_k)$$

$$= Ph(X_{n-1}) - Lh(X_{n-1}) - h(x) - \sum_{k=0}^{n-2} Lh(X_k)$$

$$= h(X_{n-1}) - h(x) - \sum_{k=0}^{n-2} Lh(X_k) = M_{n-1}.$$

The Theorem 29 is thus proved.

Lemma 30 (Dynkin's formula 3) *Let τ be a stopping time with*

$$\mathbb{E}_x \tau < \infty, \quad \forall x \in S.$$

Then for any function h on S,

$$\mathbb{E}_x h(X_\tau) = h(x) + \mathbb{E}_x \sum_{k=0}^{\tau-1} Lh(X_k).$$

Proof Follows straightforward from the Theorem 29.

9   Poisson Equation Without a Potential

9.1   Introduction

Here we consider the following discrete Poisson equation *without a potential,*

$$Lu(x) \equiv \mathcal{P}u(x) - u(x) = -f(x). \tag{33}$$

In the next section a similar discrete equation *with a potential* $c = c(x)$, $x \in S$, will be studied,

$$L^c u(x) := \exp(-c(x))\mathcal{P}u(x) - u(x) = -f(x), \tag{34}$$

firstly because it is natural for PDEs—and here we present an easier but similar discrete-time theory—and secondly with a hope that it may be also useful for some further extensions, as it already happened with equations without a potential. Let μ be, as usual, the (unique) invariant probability measure of the process $(X_n, n \geq 0)$.

9.2   Poisson Equation (33) with a Boundary

Firstly, we consider Poisson equation with a non-empty boundary,

$$Lu(x) = -f(x), \quad x \in S \setminus \Gamma, \quad u(x) = g(x), \quad x \in \Gamma, \tag{35}$$

where $\Gamma \subset S$, $\Gamma \neq \emptyset$. If the right hand side equals zero, this equation is called the Laplace equation with Dirichlet boundary conditions:

$$Lu(x) = 0, \quad x \in S \setminus \Gamma, \quad u(x) = g(x), \quad x \in \Gamma. \tag{36}$$

Let

$$\tau := \inf(n \geq 0 : X_n \in \Gamma),$$

and denote

$$v(x) := \mathbb{E}_x \left(\sum_{k=0}^{\tau-1} f(X_k) + g(X_\tau) \right). \tag{37}$$

Recall that under our assumptions on the process, necessarily $\mathbb{E}_x \tau < \infty$.

For the uniqueness, we would need a **maximum principle**, which holds true for the Laplace equation (recall that we always assume $\min_{i,j} p_{ij} > 0$):

Lemma 31 (Maximum principle) *If the function u satisfies the Eq.(36), then the maximal value (as well as minimal) of this function is necessarily attained at the boundary* Γ.

Proof Since $Lu(x) = 0$ for any $x \notin \Gamma$, we have

$$u(x) = \mathcal{P}u(x), \tag{38}$$

for such x. In other words, the value $u(x)$ is equal to the average of the values $u(y)$ at **all** other $y \in S$ with some positive weights, due to the assumption $\min_{ij} p_{ij} > 0$.

However, if a maximal value, say, M, is attained by u *not* at the boundary, say, $u(x_0) = M$, $x_0 \notin \Gamma$, and if at least one value on Γ (or, actually, anywhere else) is strictly less than M, then we get a contradiction, as the equality $\sum_{y \in S} p_{xy} v(y) = M$ with all $v(y) \le M$ and with at least one $v(y) < M$ is impossible. Similar arguments apply to the minimal value of u. This proves the Lemma 31.

Theorem 32 *The function v(x) given by the formula (37) is a unique solution of the Poisson equation (35).*

Proof 1. The boundary condition $v(x) = g(x)$ on $x \in \Gamma$ is trivial because $\tau = 0$ in this case.
2. Let $x \notin \Gamma$. Then $\tau \ge 1$. We have, due to the Markov property,

$$v(x) = f(x) + \sum_{y} \mathbb{E}_x 1(X_1 = y)\mathbb{E}_y \left(\sum_{k=0}^{\tau-1} f(X_k) + g(X_\tau) \right)$$

$$= f(x) + \sum_{y} p_{xy} v(y) = f(x) + \mathbb{E}_x v(X_1).$$

From this, it follows clearly the statement about solving the equation,

$$Lv(x) = \mathbb{E}_x v(X_1) - v(x) = -f(x).$$

3. Uniqueness follows from the maximum principle. Indeed, let v^1 and v^2 be two solutions. Then

$$u(x) := v^1(x) - v^2(x) = 0, \quad \forall \ x \in \Gamma.$$

Also, at any $x \notin \Gamma$,

$$Lu(x) = Lv^1(x) - Lv^2(x) = 0.$$

Hence, by virtue of the Lemma 31, both maximal and minimal values of the function u are attained at the boundary Γ. However, at the boundary both these values are equal to zero. Therefore,

$$u(x) = 0, \quad \forall x \in S,$$

that is, $v^1 - v^2 \equiv 0$, as required. This completes the proof of the Theorem 32.

9.3   Poisson Equation (33) without a Boundary

Consider the equation on the whole S,

$$Lu(x) = -f(x), \quad x \in S. \tag{39}$$

We will need an additional assumption on f called 'centering'. This condition is a close analogue of the subtraction in the standardization for a CLT.

Assumption 33 (Centering) It is assumed that the function f satisfies the condition,

$$\mathbb{E}_{inv} f(X_0) \equiv \sum_x f(x)\mu(x) = 0, \tag{40}$$

where μ is the (unique) invariant measure of the process X.

Theorem 34 *Under the assumption (40), the Eq. (39) has a solution u, which is unique up to an additive constant. This solution is given by the formula*

$$u(x) = \sum_{k=0}^{\infty} \mathbb{E}_x f(X_k). \tag{41}$$

The solution u from (41) itself satisfies the centering condition,

$$\sum u(x)\mu(x) = 0. \tag{42}$$

Note that the 'educated guess' about a solution represented by the formula (41) may be deduced from the comparison with (37) where, so to say, we want to drop the terminal summand g as there is no boundary and to replace τ by infinity; naturally, expectation and summation should be interchanged. Also, in the present setting the idea based on considering the series for $(I - \mathcal{P})^{-1}$ on centred functions may be applied. Yet, we would like to avoid this way because in a more general 'non-compact' situation a *polynomial* convergence of the series in (41) would also suffice, and, hence, this approach looks more general.

Proof of Theorem 34. **1. Convergence**. Follows straightforward from the Corollary 9. This shows that the function $u(x)$ defined in (41) is everywhere finite.
2. Satisfying the equation. From the Markov property,

$$u(x) = f(x) + \sum_y \mathbb{E}_x 1(X_1 = y)\mathbb{E}_y \sum_{k=0}^{\infty} f(X_k)$$

$$= f(x) + \sum_y p_{xy} v(y) = f(x) + \mathbb{E}_x u(X_1).$$

From this, it follows clearly the statement,

$$Lu(x) = \mathbb{E}_x u(X_1) - u(x) = -f(x).$$

3. Uniqueness. Let u^1 and u^2 be two solutions both satisfying the moderate growth and centering. Denote $v = u^1 - u^2$. Then

$$Lv = 0.$$

By virtue of Dynkin's formula (31),

$$\mathbb{E}v(X_n) - v(x) = 0.$$

However, due to the Corollary 9,

$$\mathbb{E}_x v(X_n) \to \mathbb{E}_{inv} v(X_0) = 0.$$

Hence,
$$v(x) \equiv 0,$$

as required.

4. Centering. We have, due to a good convergence—see the Corollary 9—and Fubini's theorem, and since measure μ is stationary, and finally because f is centered,

$$\sum_x u(x)\mu(x) = \sum_x \mu(x) \sum_{k=0}^{\infty} \mathbb{E}_x f(X_k)$$

$$= \sum_{k=0}^{\infty} \sum_x \mu(x)\mathbb{E}_x f(X_k) = \sum_{k=0}^{\infty} \mathbb{E}_{inv} f(X_k) = 0.$$

The Theorem 34 is proved.

10 Poisson Equation with a Potential

Let us remind the reader that the case $|S| < \infty$ is under consideration.

10.1 Equation (34)

Recall the Eq. (34),

$$\exp(-c(x))\mathcal{P}u(x) - u(x) = -f(x).$$

A natural candidate for the solution is the function

$$u(x) := \sum_{n=0}^{\infty} \mathbb{E}_x \exp\left(-\sum_{k=0}^{n-1} c(X_k)\right) f(X_k), \tag{43}$$

provided that this expression is well-defined. Naturally on our finite state space S both f and c bounded. Denote

$$\varphi_n := \sum_{k=0}^{n} c(X_k), \quad \varphi_{-1} = 0,$$

and

$$L^c := \exp(-c(x))\mathcal{P} - I,$$

that is,

$$L^c u(x) := \exp(-c(x))\mathcal{P}u(x) - u(x).$$

We can tackle several cases, and the most interesting one in our view is where $c(x) = \varepsilon c_1(x)$, $\varepsilon > 0$ *small* and $\bar{c}_1 := \sum_x c_1(x)\mu(x) > 0$. Denote also $\bar{c} = \sum_x c(x)\mu(x)$.

10.2 Further Dynkin's Formulae

Lemma 35 (Dynkin's formula 4)

$$\mathbb{E}_x \exp(-\varphi_{n-1}) h(X_n) = h(x) + \sum_{k=0}^{n-1} \mathbb{E}_x \exp(-\varphi_{k-1}) L^c h(X_k). \tag{44}$$

In other words, the process

$$M_n := \exp(-\varphi_{n-1}) h(X_n) - h(x) - \sum_{k=0}^{n-1} \exp(-\varphi_{k-1}) L^c h(X_k), \quad n \geq 0, \tag{45}$$

is a martingale.

Proof Let the initial state x be fixed. Let us check the base, $n = 0$. Note that $\varphi_0 = c(x)$, $\varphi_{-1} = 0$, and $L^c h(x) = \exp(-\varphi_0)\mathcal{P}h(x) - h(x)$. So, for $n = 0$ the formula (44) reads,

$$h(x) = h(x) + \sum_{k=0}^{-1} \mathbb{E}_x L^c h(X_k),$$

which is true due to the standard convention that $\sum_{k=0}^{-1} \cdots = 0$.

Let us check the first step, $n = 1$:

$$\mathbb{E}_x \exp(-c(x))\, h(X_1) = h(x) + \sum_{k=0}^{0} \mathbb{E}_x \exp(-\varphi_{-1}) L^c h(X_k) \equiv h(x)$$
$$+ \exp(-c(x))\mathcal{P}h(x) - h(x),$$

or, equivalently,

$$\mathbb{E}_x \exp(-c(x))\, h(X_1) = \exp(-c(x))\mathcal{P}h(x),$$

which is also true.

The induction step with a general $n \geq 1$ follows similarly, using the Markov property. Indeed, assume that the formula (44) is true for some $n \geq 0$. Then, for $n + 1$ we have,

$$\mathbb{E}_x \exp(-\varphi_n)\, h(X_{n+1}) - h(x) - \sum_{k=0}^{n} \mathbb{E}_x \exp(-\varphi_{k-1}) L^c h(X_k)$$

$$= \mathbb{E}_x \exp(-\varphi_n)\, h(X_{n+1}) - \mathbb{E}_x \exp(-\varphi_{n-1})\, h(X_n) + \mathbb{E}_x \exp(-\varphi_{n-1})\, h(X_n)$$

$$- h(x) - \sum_{k=0}^{n-1} \mathbb{E}_x \exp(-\varphi_{k-1}) L^c h(X_k) - \mathbb{E}_x \exp(-\varphi_{n-1}) L^c h(X_n)$$

$$= \mathbb{E}_x \exp(-\varphi_n)\, h(X_{n+1}) - \mathbb{E}_x \exp(-\varphi_{n-1})\, h(X_n) - \mathbb{E}_x \exp(-\varphi_{n-1}) L^c h(X_n)$$

$$= \mathbb{E}_x \big[\mathbb{E}_x \big(\exp(-\varphi_n)\, h(X_{n+1}) - \exp(-\varphi_{n-1})\, h(X_n) - \exp(-\varphi_{n-1}) L^c h(X_n) | \mathcal{F}_n \big) \big]$$

$$= \mathbb{E}_x \exp(-\varphi_{n-1}) \big[\mathbb{E}_x \big(\exp(-c(X_n))\, h(X_{n+1}) - h(X_n) - L^c h(X_n) | X_n \big) \big] = 0,$$

by definition of L^c. This completes the induction step, so the Lemma 44 is proved.

Lemma 36 (Dynkin's formula 5) *Let τ be a stopping time with*

$$\mathbb{E}_x e^{\alpha \tau} < \infty, \quad \forall\, x \in S,$$

for some $\alpha > 0$. Then for any function h on S and if $c = \epsilon c_1$ and ϵ is small enough,

$$\mathbb{E}_x e^{-\varphi_{\tau-1}} h(X_\tau) = h(x) + \mathbb{E}_x \sum_{k=0}^{\tau-1} e^{-\varphi_{k-1}} L^c h(X_k).$$

Recall that for an irreducible Markov chain with values in a finite state space any hitting time has *some* finite exponential moment. This will be used in the next subsection.

Proof We conclude from (44), or (45), due to Doob's theorem about stopped martingales,

$$\mathbb{E}_x e^{-\varphi_{(\tau-1)\wedge n}} h(X_{\tau\wedge n}) = h(x) + \mathbb{E}_x \sum_{k=0}^{(\tau-1)\wedge n} e^{-\varphi_{k-1}} L^c h(X_k).$$

Now if ϵ is small enough, then we may pass to the limit as $n \to \infty$, due to the Lebesgue theorem about a limit under the uniform integrability condition. We have,

$$\mathbb{E}_x e^{-\varphi_{(\tau-1)\wedge n}} h(X_{\tau\wedge n}) \to \mathbb{E}_x e^{-\varphi_{\tau-1}} h(X_\tau),$$

and

$$h(x) + \mathbb{E}_x \sum_{k=0}^{(\tau-1)\wedge n} e^{-\varphi_{k-1}} L^c h(X_k) \to h(x) + \mathbb{E}_x \sum_{k=0}^{\tau-1} e^{-\varphi_{k-1}} L^c h(X_k), \quad n \to \infty,$$

as required. The Lemma 36 is proved.

10.3   Poisson Equation with a Potential with a Boundary

Recall the equation *with the boundary*:

$$\exp(-c(x)) \mathcal{P} u(x) - u(x) = -f(x), \quad x \in S \setminus \Gamma, \quad u(x) = g(x), \quad x \in \Gamma, \quad (46)$$

with a boundary $\Gamma \neq \emptyset$. The natural candidate for the solution is the function

$$u(x) := \mathbb{E}_x \left(\sum_{n=0}^{\tau-1} \exp\left(-\varphi_{n-1}\right) f(X_n) + \exp\left(-\varphi_{\tau-1}\right) g(X_\tau) \right), \quad (47)$$

$\tau = \inf(n \geq 0: X_n \in \Gamma)$. If $x \in \Gamma$, then $\tau = 0$, and we agree that the term $\sum_{k=0}^{-1}$ equals zero.

Theorem 37 *If the expectation in (47) is finite then the function $u(x)$ is a unique solution of the equation (46).*

Recall that τ does have some exponential moment, so if $c = \epsilon c_1$ as in the statement of the Lemma 36, and if ϵ is small enough, then the expression in (47), **indeed, converges**.

The proof of the Theorem 37 can be established similarly to the proof of the Theorem 32. Firstly, if $x \in \Gamma$, then clearly $\tau = 0$, so that $u(x) = g(x)$. Secondly, if $x \notin \Gamma$, then clearly $\tau \geq 1$. Then, due to the Markov property and by splitting the sum, i.e. taking a sum $\sum_{k=1}^{\tau-1}$ and separately considering the term corresponding to $n = 0$ which is just $f(x)$, we have,

$$u(x) = f(x) + \mathbb{E}_x \left(\sum_{n=1}^{\tau-1} \exp\left(-\sum_{k=0}^{n-1} c(X_k) \right) f(X_k) + \exp\left(-\sum_{k=0}^{\tau-1} c(X_k) \right) g(X_\tau) \right)$$

$$= f(x) + \mathbb{E}_x \mathbb{E}_x \left[\sum_{n=1}^{\tau-1} \exp\left(-\sum_{k=0}^{n-1} c(X_k) \right) f(X_k) + \exp\left(-\sum_{k=0}^{\tau-1} c(X_k) \right) g(X_\tau) | X_1 \right]$$

$$= f(x) + \mathbb{E}_x \exp(-c(x)) \mathbb{E}_{X_1} \left(\sum_{n=0}^{\tau-1} \exp\left(-\sum_{k=0}^{n-1} c(X_k) \right) f(X_k) + \exp\left(-\sum_{k=0}^{\tau-1} c(X_k) \right) g(X_\tau) \right)$$

$$= f(x) + \exp(-c(x)) \mathbb{E}_x u(X_1) = f(x) + \exp(-c(x)) \mathcal{P}u(x),$$

which shows exactly the Eq. (46), as required. The Theorem 37 is proved.

10.4   Poisson Equation with a Potential Without a Boundary

Recall the Eq. (34):

$$\exp(-c(x))\mathcal{P}u(x) - u(x) = -f(x),$$

and the natural candidate for the solution 'in the whole space' is the function

$$u(x) := \sum_{n=0}^{\infty} \mathbb{E}_x \exp\left(-\sum_{k=0}^{n-1} c(X_k) \right) f(X_k), \tag{48}$$

The main question here is the question of convergence. As was mentioned earlier, we are interested in the following case: $c(x) = \epsilon c_1(x)$, $\epsilon > 0$ small, and $\sum c_1(x)\mu(x) > 0$, where μ is the unique invariant measure of the Markov chain X.

10.5   Convergence

The first goal is to justify that u is well-defined. Recall that we want to show convergence of the series,

$$u(x) = \sum_{n=0}^{\infty} \mathbb{E}_x \exp\left(-\sum_{k=0}^{n-1} c(X_k)\right) f(X_n),$$

with $c(x) = \epsilon c_1(x)$, $\bar{c}_1 = \sum c_1(x)\mu(x) > 0$, with $\epsilon > 0$ small. Denote

$$H_n(\beta, x) := n^{-1} \ln \mathbb{E}_x \exp\left(\beta \sum_{k=0}^{n-1} c_1(X_k)\right), \quad \beta \in \mathbb{R}^1,$$

or, equivalently,

$$\mathbb{E}_x \exp\left(\beta \sum_{k=0}^{n-1} c_1(X_k)\right) = \mathbb{E}_x \exp(n\, H_n(\beta, x)).$$

(Note that this notation just slightly differs from how the function H_n—and in the next formula also H—was defined in the Sect. 6: now it is constructed via the 'additive functional' related to another function c_1. Yet, the meaning is similar, so that there is no need to change this standard notation.) Let

$$H(\beta) := \lim_{T \to \infty} H_T(\beta, x), \quad \beta \in \mathbb{R}^1.$$

As we have seen in the Sect. 6, this limit does exist **for all values of** β. (The fact that in the Sect. 6 this was shown for another function and under the centering condition for that function is of no importance because the average may be always subtracted.)

Also, it may be proved—*left as an exercise to the reader (here some Lemma from [25] about estimating the spectral radius may be useful)*—that if $\delta > 0$ then there exists $n(\delta)$ such that uniformly in x

$$\sup_{|\beta| \leq B} |H(\beta) - H_n(\beta, x)| \leq \delta, \quad n \geq n(\delta). \tag{49}$$

Unlike in the Sect. 6 where it was assumed that $\bar{f} = 0$, here we compute,

$$H_n'(0, x) = n^{-1} \mathbb{E}_x \sum_{k=0}^{n-1} c_1(X_k),$$

where, as usual, the notation $H_n'(0, x)$ stands for $\partial H_n'(\beta, x)/\partial \beta|_{\beta=0}$. Now, due to the Corollary 9 it follows,

$$\lim_{n\to\infty} n^{-1}\mathbb{E}_x \sum_{k=0}^{n-1} c_1(X_k) = \bar{c}_1 = \langle c_1, \mu \rangle > 0.$$

This means that in our case

$$H'(0) = \bar{c}_1 > 0,$$

and that, at least, in some neighbourhood of zero,

$$H(\beta) > 0, \quad \beta > 0, \quad \& \quad H(\beta) < 0, \quad \beta < 0. \tag{50}$$

Now, convergence of the sum defining u for each x for $\epsilon > 0$ small enough and uniformly in x—recall that $|S| < \infty$—follows from (50). Indeed, choose $\epsilon > 0$ so that $H(-\epsilon) < 0$ and for a fixed $\delta = -H(-\epsilon)/2$ also choose n_0 such that $|H_n(-\epsilon, x) - H(-\epsilon)| < \delta$, for all $n \geq n_0$ and any x. We estimate, for ϵ small and any x (and with ϵ independent of x),

$$|u(x)| \leq \|f\|_B \sum_{n=0}^{\infty} \mathbb{E}_x \exp\left(-\epsilon \sum_{k=0}^{n-1} c_1(X_k)\right) = \|f\|_B \sum_{n=0}^{\infty} \exp(n H_n(-\epsilon, x))$$

$$\leq \|f\|_B \sum_{n=0}^{\infty} \exp(n(H(-\epsilon) + \delta)) \leq \|f\|_B \exp(\delta) \sum_{n=0}^{\infty} \exp(n H(-\epsilon)) < \infty.$$

10.6   u Solves the Equation

Let us argue why the function u solves the Poisson equation (34). By the Markov property,

$$u(x) = f(x) + \exp(-c(x)) \sum_y \mathbb{E}_x 1(X_1 = y) \mathbb{E}_y \sum_{k=0}^{\infty} \exp(-\varphi_{k-1}) f(X_k)$$

$$= f(x) + \exp(-c(x)) \sum_y p_{xy} v(y) = f(x) + \exp(-c(x)) \mathbb{E}_x u(X_1).$$

From this, it follows clearly that, as required,

$$L^c u(x) = \exp(-c(x)) \mathbb{E}_x u(X_1) - u(x) = -f(x).$$

10.7 Uniqueness of Solution

Uniqueness may be shown in a standard manner. For the difference of two solutions $v = u^1 - u^2$ we have $L^c v = 0$. Therefore, we get,

$$v(x) = \exp(-c(x))\mathbb{E}_x v(X_1).$$

After iterating this formula by induction n times, we obtain,

$$v(x) = \mathbb{E}_x \exp\left(-\sum_{k=0}^{n-1} c(X_k)\right) v(X_n).$$

Recall that the function v is necessarily bounded on a finite state space S. Hence, it follows that $v(x) \equiv 0$. Indeed, we estimate,

$$|v(x)| = |\mathbb{E}_x \exp\left(-\sum_{k=0}^{n-1} c(X_k)\right) v(X_n)| \le C\mathbb{E}_x \exp\left(-\sum_{k=0}^{n-1} c(X_k)\right).$$

Hence, we get, for *any* $n \ge 0$,

$$|v(x)| \le C\mathbb{E}_x \exp\left(-\epsilon \sum_{k=0}^{n-1} c_1(X_k)\right) = C \exp(n H_n(-\epsilon, x)). \tag{51}$$

Recall that $H_n(\beta, x) \to H(\beta)$, $n \to \infty$, and that $H(-\epsilon) < 0$ for $\epsilon > 0$ small enough. So, the right hand side in (51) converges to zero exponentially fast with $n \to \infty$. Since the left hand side does not depend on n, we get $|v(x)| = 0$, i.e. $u^1 \equiv u^2$, as required.

11 Ergodic Theorem, General Case

Now let us consider a more general construction on a **more general state space**. It is assumed that

$$\kappa := \inf_{x,x'} \int \left(\frac{P_{x'}(1, dy)}{P_x(1, dy)} \wedge 1\right) P_x(1, dy) > 0. \tag{52}$$

Note that here $\dfrac{P_{x'}(1, dy)}{P_x(1, dy)}$ is understood in the sense of the density of the absolute continuous components. For brevity we will be using a simplified notation $P_x(dz)$ for $P_x(1, dz)$. Another slightly less general condition will be accepted in the next section but it is convenient to introduce it here: **suppose** that there exists a measure

Λ with respect to which each measure $P_x(1, dz)$ for any x is absolutely continuous,

$$P_x(1, dz) \ll \Lambda(dz), \qquad \forall x \in S. \tag{53}$$

Under the assumption (53) we have another representation of the constant κ from (52).

Lemma 38 *Under the assumption (53), we have the following representation for the constant from (52),*

$$\kappa = \inf_{x,x'} \int \left(\frac{P_{x'}(1, dy)}{\Lambda(dy)} \wedge \frac{P_x(1, dy)}{\Lambda(dy)} \right) \Lambda(dy). \tag{54}$$

Proof Firstly, note that clearly the right hand side in (38) does not depend on any particular measure Λ, i.e. for any other measure with respect to which both $P_{x'}(1, dy)$ and $P_x(1, dy)$ are absolutely continuous the formula (52) gives the same result. Indeed, it follows straightforward from the fact that if, say, $d\Lambda \ll d\tilde{\Lambda}$ and $d\Lambda = f d\tilde{\Lambda}$, then we get,

$$\int \left(\frac{P_{x'}(1, dy)}{\Lambda(dy)} \wedge \frac{P_x(1, dy)}{\Lambda(dy)} \right) \Lambda(dy)$$

$$= \int \left(\frac{P_{x'}(1, dy)}{f\tilde{\Lambda}(dy)} \wedge \frac{P_x(1, dy)}{f\tilde{\Lambda}(dy)} \right) f(y) 1(f(y) > 0) \tilde{\Lambda}(dy)$$

$$= \int \left(\frac{P_{x'}(1, dy)}{\tilde{\Lambda}(dy)} \wedge \frac{P_x(1, dy)}{\tilde{\Lambda}(dy)} \right) 1(f(y) > 0) \tilde{\Lambda}(dy).$$

However, $P_{x'}(1, dy) \ll \Lambda(dy) = f(y)\tilde{\Lambda}(dy)$, so for any measurable A we have $\int_A P_{x'}(1, dy) 1(f(y) = 0) = 0$ and the same for $P_x(1, dy)$, which means that, actually,

$$\int \left(\frac{P_{x'}(1, dy)}{\tilde{\Lambda}(dy)} \wedge \frac{P_x(1, dy)}{\tilde{\Lambda}(dy)} \right) 1(f(y) > 0) \tilde{\Lambda}(dy)$$

$$= \int \left(\frac{P_{x'}(1, dy)}{\tilde{\Lambda}(dy)} \wedge \frac{P_x(1, dy)}{\tilde{\Lambda}(dy)} \right) \tilde{\Lambda}(dy).$$

Respectively, if there are two reference measure Λ and, say, Λ', then we may take $\tilde{\Lambda} = \Lambda + \Lambda'$, and the coefficients computed by using each of the two—Λ and Λ'—will be represented via $\tilde{\Lambda}$ in the same way.

Secondly, let $f_x(y) = \dfrac{P_x(1, dy)}{\Lambda(dy)}(y)$. Then,

$$\kappa = \inf_{x,x'} \int \left(\frac{P_{x'}(1, dy)}{P_x(1, dy)} \wedge \frac{P_x(1, dy)}{P_x(1, dy)} \right) P_x(1, dy)$$

$$= \inf_{x,x'} \int \left(\frac{P_{x'}(1, dy)}{f_x(y) \Lambda(dy)} \wedge \frac{P_x(1, dy)}{f_x(y) \Lambda(dy)} \right) f_x(y) \Lambda(dy)$$

$$= \inf_{x,x'} \int \left(\frac{P_{x'}(1, dy)}{\Lambda(dy)} \wedge \frac{P_x(1, dy)}{\Lambda(dy)} \right) \Lambda(dy),$$

as required. The Lemma 38 is proved.

Denote

$$\kappa(x, x') := \int \left(\frac{P_{x'}(1, dy)}{P_x(1, dy)} \wedge 1 \right) P_x(1, dy)$$

Clearly, for any $x, x' \in S$,

$$\kappa(x, x') \ge \kappa. \tag{55}$$

Lemma 39 *For any $x, x' \in S$,*

$$\kappa(x, x') = \kappa(x', x).$$

Proof Under the more restrictive assumption (54) we have,

$$\kappa(x', x) = \int \left(\frac{P_{x'}(1, dy)}{P_x(1, dy)} \wedge 1 \right) P_x(dy) = \int \left(\frac{P_{x'}(1, dy)}{\Lambda(dy)} \wedge \frac{P_x(1, dy)}{\Lambda(dy)} \right) \Lambda(dy),$$

which expression is, apparently, symmetric with respect to x and x', as required. Without assuming (54) we can argue as follows. Denote $\Lambda_{x,x'}(dz) = P_x(1, dz) + P_{x'}(1, dz)$. Note that by definition, $\Lambda_{x,x'} = \Lambda_{x',x}$. Then we have,

$$\kappa(x', x) = \int \left(\frac{P_{x'}(1, dy)}{P_x(1, dy)} \wedge 1 \right) P_x(1, dy)$$

$$= \int \left(\frac{P_{x'}(1, dy)}{P_x(1, dy)} \wedge 1 \right) \frac{P_x(1, dy)}{\Lambda_{x,x'}(dy)} \Lambda_{x,x'}(dy)$$

$$= \int \left(\frac{P_{x'}(1, dy)}{\Lambda_{x,x'}(dy)} \wedge \frac{P_x(1, dy)}{\Lambda_{x,x'}(dy)} \right) \Lambda_{x,x'}(dy). \tag{56}$$

The latter expression is symmetric with respect to x and x', which proves the Lemma 39.

Definition 40 If an MC (X_n) satisfies the condition (52)—we call it **MD-condition** in the sequel—then we call this process *Markov–Dobrushin's or* **MD-process.**

This condition in an easier situation of finite chains was introduced by Markov himself [30]; later on, for non-homogeneous Markov processes its analogue was suggested and used by Dobrushin [8]. So, we call it Markov–Dobrushin's condition, as already suggested earlier by Seneta. Note that in all cases $\kappa \leq 1$. The case $\kappa = 1$ corresponds to the i.i.d. sequence (X_n). In the opposite extreme situation where the transition kernels are singular for different x and x', we have $\kappa = 0$. The MD-condition (52)—as well as (54)—is most useful because it provides an **effective** quantitative upper bound for convergence rate of a Markov chain towards its (unique) invariant measure in total variation metric.

Theorem 41 *Let the assumption (52) hold true. Then the process (X_n) is ergodic, i.e. there exists a limiting probability measure μ, which is stationary and such that (1) holds true. Moreover, the uniform bound is satisfied for every n,*

$$\sup_{x} \sup_{A \in \mathcal{S}} |P_x(n, A) - \mu(A)| \leq (1 - \kappa)^n. \tag{57}$$

Recall that the **total variation distance** or metric between two probability measures may be defined as

$$\|\mu - \nu\|_{TV} := 2 \sup_{A}(\mu(A) - \nu(A)).$$

Hence, the inequality (57) may be rewritten as

$$\sup_{x} \|P_x(n, \cdot) - \mu(\cdot)\|_{TV} \leq 2(1 - \kappa)^n, \tag{58}$$

Proof **1**. Denote for any measurable $A \in \mathcal{S}$,

$$M^{(n)}(A) := \sup_{x} P_x(n, A), \quad m^{(n)}(A) := \inf_{x} P_x(n, A).$$

Due to the Chapman–Kolmogorov equation we have,

$$m^{(n+1)}(A) = \inf_{x} P_x(n + 1, A) = \inf_{x} \int P_x(dz) P_z(n, A)$$

$$\geq \inf_{x} \int P_x(dz) m^{(n)}(A) = m^{(n)}(A).$$

So, the sequence $(m^{(n)}(A))$ does not decrease. Similarly, $(M^{(n)}(A))$ does not increase. We are going to show the estimate

$$(0 \leq) \ M^{(n)}(A) - m^{(n)}(A) \leq (1 - \kappa)^n. \tag{59}$$

In particular, it follows that for any $x, y \in S$ we have,

$$|P_x(n, A) - P_y(n, A)| \leq (1 - \kappa)^n. \tag{60}$$

More than that, by virtue of (59) and due to the monotonicity ($M^{(n)}(A)$ decreases, while $m^{(n)}(A)$ increases) both sequences $M^{(n)}(A)$ and $m^{(n)}(A)$ have limits, which limits coincide and are uniform in A:

$$\lim_{n\to\infty} M^{(n)}(A) = \lim_{n\to\infty} m^{(n)}(A) =: m(A), \tag{61}$$

and

$$\sup_A |M^{(n)}(A) - m(A)| \vee \sup_A |m^{(n)}(A) - m(A)| \le (1-\kappa)^n. \tag{62}$$

2. Let $x, x' \in S$, and let $\Lambda_{x,x'}$ be some reference measure for both $P_x(1, dz)$ and $P_{x'}(1, dz)$. Again by virtue of Chapman–Kolmogorov's equation we have for any $n > 1$ (recall that we accept the notations, $a_+ = a \vee 0 \equiv \max(a, 0)$, and $a_- = a \wedge 0 \equiv \min(a, 0)$),

$$P_x(n, A) - P_{x'}(n, A) = \int [P_x(1, dz) - P_{x'}(1, dz)] P_z(n-1, A)$$

$$= \int \left(\frac{P_x(1, dz)}{\Lambda_{x,x'}(dz)} - \frac{P_{x'}(1, dz)}{\Lambda_{x,x'}(dz)} \right) \Lambda_{x,x'}(dz) P_z(n-1, A)$$

$$= \int \left(\frac{P_x(1, dz)}{\Lambda_{x,x'}(dz)} - \frac{P_{x'}(1, dz)}{\Lambda_{x,x'}(dz)} \right)_+ \Lambda_{x,x'}(dz) P_z(n-1, A)$$

$$+ \int \left(\frac{P_x(1, dz)}{\Lambda_{x,x'}(dz)} - \frac{P_{x'}(1, dz)}{\Lambda_{x,x'}(dz)} \right)_- \Lambda_{x,x'}(dz) P_z(n-1, A). \tag{63}$$

Further, we have,

$$\int \left(\frac{P_x(1, dz)}{\Lambda_{x,x'}(dz)} - \frac{P_{x'}(1, dz)}{\Lambda_{x,x'}(dz)} \right)_+ \Lambda_{x,x'}(dz) P_z(n-1, A)$$

$$\le \int \left(\frac{P_x(1, dz)}{\Lambda_{x,x'}(dz)} - \frac{P_{x'}(1, dz)}{\Lambda_{x,x'}(dz)} \right)_+ \Lambda_{x,x'}(dz) M^{(n-1)}(A),$$

and similarly,

$$\int \left(\frac{P_x(1, dz)}{\Lambda_{x,x'}(dz)} - \frac{P_{x'}(1, dz)}{\Lambda_{x,x'}(dz)} \right)_- \Lambda_{x,x'}(dz) P_z(n-1, A)$$

$$\le \int \left(\frac{P_x(1, dz)}{\Lambda_{x,x'}(dz)} - \frac{P_{x'}(1, dz)}{\Lambda_{x,x'}(dz)} \right)_- \Lambda_{x,x'}(dz) m^{(n-1)}(A),$$

On the other hand,

$$\int \left(\frac{P_x(1, dz)}{\Lambda_{x,x'}(dz)} - \frac{P_{x'}(1, dz)}{\Lambda_{x,x'}(dz)} \right)_+ \Lambda_{x,x'}(dz) + \int \left(\frac{P_x(1, dz)}{\Lambda_{x,x'}(dz)} - \frac{P_{x'}(1, dz)}{\Lambda_{x,x'}(dz)} \right)_- \Lambda_{x,x'}(dz)$$

$$= \int \left(\frac{P_x(1, dz)}{\Lambda_{x,x'}(dz)} - \frac{P_{x'}(1, dz)}{\Lambda_{x,x'}(dz)} \right) \Lambda_{x,x'}(dz) = 1 - 1 = 0.$$

Thus, we get,

$$M^{(n)}(A) - m^{(n)}(A) = \sup_x P_x(n, A) - \inf_{x'} P_{x'}(n, A)$$

$$\leq \sup_{x,x'} \int \left(\frac{P_x(1, dz)}{\Lambda_{x,x'}(dz)} - \frac{P_{x'}(1, dz)}{\Lambda_{x,x'}(dz)} \right)_+ \Lambda_{x,x'}(dz) \, (M^{(n-1)}(A) - m^{(n)}(A)).$$

It remains to notice that (recall that $(a - b)_+ = a - a \wedge b \equiv a - \min(a, b)$)

$$\int \left(\frac{P_x(1, dz)}{\Lambda_{x,x'}(dz)} - \frac{P_{x'}(1, dz)}{\Lambda_{x,x'}(dz)} \right)_+ \Lambda_{x,x'}(dz)$$

$$= \int \left(\frac{P_x(1, dz)}{\Lambda_{x,x'}(dz)} - \frac{P_{x'}(1, dz)}{\Lambda_{x,x'}(dz)} \wedge \frac{P_x(1, dz)}{\Lambda_{x,x'}(dz)} \right) \Lambda_{x,x'}(dz) = 1 - \kappa(x, x') \leq 1 - \kappa.$$

Now the bound (59) follows by induction.

3. Let us establish the existence of at least one stationary distribution. For any $x \in S$ and any measurable A,

$$m^{(n)}(A) \leq P_x(n, A) \leq M^{(n)}(A). \tag{64}$$

Due to (61) and (62), $(P_x(n, A))$ is a Cauchy sequence which converges exponentially fast and uniformly with respect to A. Denote

$$q(A) := \lim_{n \to \infty} P_x(n, A). \tag{65}$$

Clearly, due to this uniform convergence, $q(\cdot) \geq 0$, $q(S) = 1$, and the function q is additive in A. More than that, by virtue of the same uniform convergence in A in (65), the function $q(\cdot)$ is also 'continuous at zero', i.e. it is, actually, a sigma-additive measure. More than that, the uniform convergence implies that

$$\|P_x(n, \cdot) - q(\cdot)\|_{TV} \to 0, \quad n \to \infty. \tag{66}$$

4. Now, let us show stationarity. We have,

$$q(A) = \lim_{n \to \infty} P_{x_0}(n, A) = \lim_{n \to \infty} \int P_{x_0}(n - 1, dz) P_z(A)$$

$$= \int q(dz) P_z(A) + \lim_{n \to \infty} \int (P_{x_0}(n - 1, dz) - q(dz)) P_z(A).$$

Here, in fact, the second term equals zero. Indeed,

$$\left| \int (P_{x_0}(n-1, dz) - q(dz)) P_z(A) \right| \leq \int |P_{x_0}(n-1, dz) - q(dz)| P_z(A)$$

$$\leq \int |P_{x_0}(n-1, dz) - q(dz)| = \|P_{x_0}(n-1, \cdot) - q(\cdot)\|_{TV} \to 0, \quad n \to \infty.$$

Thus, we find that

$$q(A) = \int q(dz) P_z(A),$$

which is the definition of stationarity. This completes the proof of the Theorem 41.

Corollary 42 *For any bounded Borel function f and any $0 \leq s < t$,*

$$\sup_x |\mathbb{E}_x(f(X_t)|X_s) - \mathbb{E}_{inv} f(X_t)| \equiv \sup_x |\mathbb{E}_x(f(X_t) - \mathbb{E}_{inv} f(X_t)|X_s)| \leq C_f (1-\kappa)^{t-s},$$

or, equivalently,

$$\sup_x |\mathbb{E}_x(f(X_t)|\mathcal{F}_s^X) - \mathbb{E}_{inv} f(X_t)| \leq C_f (1-\kappa)^{t-s},$$

12 Coupling Method: General Version

This more general version requires a change of probability space so as to construct coupling. Results themselves in no way pretend to be new: we just suggest a presentation convenient for the author. In particular, all newly arising probability spaces on each step (i.e. at each time n) are explicitly shown. By 'general' we do not mean that it is the most general possible: this issue is not addressed here. Just it is more general that in the Sect. 5, and it is more involved because of the more complicated probability space, and it provides a better constant in the convergence bound. It turns out that the general version requires a bit of preparation; hence, we start with the section devoted to a couple of random variables, while the case of Markov chains will be considered separately in the next section.

The following folklore yet important lemma answers the following question: suppose we have two distributions, which are not singular, and the 'common area' equals some positive constant κ. Is it possible to realize these two distributions on the same probability space so that the two corresponding random variables *coincide* exactly with probability κ? We call one version of this result 'the lemma about three random variables', and another one 'the lemma about two random variables'.

Lemma 43 ('Of three random variables') *Let ξ^1 and ξ^2 be two random variables on their (without loss of generality different, and they will be made independent after we take their direct product!) probability spaces $(\Omega^1, \mathcal{F}^1, \mathbb{P}^1)$ and $(\Omega^2, \mathcal{F}^2, \mathbb{P}^2)$ and* *with densities p^1 and p^2 with respect to some reference measure Λ, correspondingly. Then, if Markov–Dobrushin's condition holds true,*

$$\kappa := \int \left(p^1(x) \wedge p^2(x)\right) \Lambda(dx) > 0, \tag{67}$$

then there exists one more probability space $(\Omega, \mathcal{F}, \mathbb{P})$ and a random variable on it ξ^3 (and ξ^2 also lives on $(\Omega, \mathcal{F}, \mathbb{P})$, clearly, with the same distribution) such that

$$\mathcal{L}(\xi^3) = \mathcal{L}(\xi^1), \quad \& \quad \mathbb{P}(\xi^3 = \xi^2) = \kappa. \tag{68}$$

Here $\mathcal{L}$ denotes the distribution of a random variable under consideration. Note that in the case $\kappa = 1$ we have $p^1 = p^2$, so we can just assign $\xi^3 := \xi^2$, and then immediately both assertions of (68) hold. Mention that even if κ were equal to zero (excluded by the assumption (67)), i.e. the two distributions were singular, we could have posed $\xi^3 := \xi^1$, and again both claims in (68) would have been satisfied trivially. Hence, in the proof below it suffices to assume

$$0 < \kappa < 1.$$

Proof of the Lemma 43. **1: Construction.** Let

$$A_1 := \{x : \ p^1(x) \geq p^2(x)\}, \quad A_2 := \{x : \ p^1(x) < p^2(x)\},$$

We will need two new independent random variables, $\zeta \sim U[0, 1]$ (uniformly distributed random variable on $[0, 1]$) and η with the density

$$p^\eta(x) := \frac{p^1 - p^1 \wedge p^2}{\int (p^1 - p^1 \wedge p^2)(y)\Lambda(dy)}(x) \equiv \frac{p^1 - p^1 \wedge p^2}{\int_{A_1} (p^1 - p^1 \wedge p^2)(y)\Lambda(dy)}(x).$$

Both ζ and η are assumed to be defined on *their own* probability spaces. Now let **(on the direct product of all these probability spaces**, i.e. of the probability spaces where the random variables $\xi^1, \xi^2, \zeta, \eta$ are defined)

$$\xi^3 := \xi^2 1(\frac{p^1}{p^1 \vee p^2}(\xi^2) \geq \zeta) + \eta 1(\frac{p^1}{p^1 \vee p^2}(\xi^2) < \zeta).$$

We shall see that ξ^3 admits all the desired properties. Denote

$$C := \{\omega : \ \frac{p^1}{p^1 \vee p^2}(\xi^2) \geq \zeta\}.$$

Then ξ^3 may be rewritten as

$$\xi^3 = \xi^2 1(C) + \eta 1(\bar{C}). \tag{69}$$

2: Verification. Below $\mathbb{P}$ is understood as the probability arising on the direct product of the probability spaces mentioned earlier. Let

$$c := \int_{A_1} (p^1(x) - p^2(x)) \Lambda(dx) \equiv \int_{A_2} (p^2(x) - p^1(x)) \Lambda(dx).$$

Due to our assumptions we have,

$$c + \kappa = \int_{A_1} (p^1(x) - p^2(x)) \Lambda(dx) + \int \left(p^1(x) \wedge p^2(x) \right) \Lambda(dx)$$

$$= \int_{A_1} (p^1(x) - p^2(x)) \Lambda(dx) + \int_{A_1} \left(p^1(x) \wedge p^2(x) \right) \Lambda(dx) + \int_{A_2} \left(p^1(x) \wedge p^2(x) \right) \Lambda(dx)$$

$$= \int_{A_1} p^1(x) \Lambda(dx) + \int_{A_2} p^1(x) \Lambda(dx) = \int_{A_1 \cup A_2} p^1(x) \Lambda(dx) = 1.$$

So,

$$c = 1 - \kappa \in (0, 1).$$

Also,

$$p^\eta(x) = \frac{p^1 - p^1 \wedge p^2}{c}(x).$$

Also notice that

$$\mathbb{P}(C|\xi^2) = \frac{p^1}{p^1 \vee p^2}(\xi^2),$$

and recall that on C, $\xi^3 = \xi^2$, while on its complement $\bar{C}$, $\xi^3 = \eta$. Now, for any bounded Borel measurable function g we have,

$$\mathbb{E}g(\xi^3) = \mathbb{E}g(\xi^3)1(C) + \mathbb{E}g(\xi^3)1(\bar{C}) = \mathbb{E}g(\xi^2)1(C) + \mathbb{E}g(\eta)1(\bar{C})$$

$$= \mathbb{E}g(\xi^2)\frac{p^1}{p^1 \vee p^2}(\xi^2) + \mathbb{E}g(\eta)(1 - \frac{p^1}{p^1 \vee p^2}(\xi^2))$$

$$= \mathbb{E}g(\xi^2)\frac{p^1}{p^1 \vee p^2}(\xi^2) + \mathbb{E}g(\eta)\mathbb{E}(1 - \frac{p^1}{p^1 \vee p^2}(\xi^2))$$

$$= \int_{A_1 \cup A_2} g(x)\frac{p^1}{p^1 \vee p^2}(x)p^2(x)\Lambda(dx) + \int_{(A_1)} g(x)p^\eta(x)\Lambda(dx)$$

$$\times \int_{(A_2)} (1 - \frac{p^1}{p^1 \vee p^2}(y))p^2(y)\Lambda(dy)$$

$$= \int_{A_1} g(x)p^2(x)\Lambda(dx) + \int_{A_2} g(x)p^1(x)\Lambda(dx) + \int_{A_1} g(x)\frac{p^1 - p^2}{c}(x)\Lambda(dx)$$

$$\times \int_{A_2} (p^2 - p^1)(y)\Lambda(dy)$$

$$= \int_{A_1 \cup A_2} g(x)p^1(x)\Lambda(dx) = \mathbb{E}g(\xi^1).$$

Here (A_1) in brackets in $\int_{(A_1)} g(x)p^\eta(x)\Lambda(dx)$ is used with the following meaning: the integral is originally taken over the whole domain, but integration outside the set A_1 gives zero; hence, only the integral over this domain remains. The established equality $\mathbb{E}g(\xi^3) = \mathbb{E}g(\xi^1)$ means that $\mathcal{L}(\xi^3) = \mathcal{L}(\xi^1)$, as required. Finally, from the definition of ξ^3 it is straightforward that

$$\mathbb{P}(\xi^3 = \xi^2) \geq \mathbb{P}(C).$$

So,

$$\mathbb{P}(\xi^3 = \xi^2) \geq P(C) = \mathbb{E}\frac{p^1}{p^1 \vee p^2}(\xi^2) = \int \frac{p^1}{p^1 \vee p^2}(x)p^2(x)\Lambda(dx)$$

$$= \int_{A_1} \frac{p^1}{p^1 \vee p^2}(x)p^2(x)\Lambda(dx) + \int_{A_2} \frac{p^1}{p^1 \vee p^2}(x)p^2(x)\Lambda(dx)$$

$$= \int_{A_1} p^2(x)\Lambda(dx) + \int_{A_2} \frac{p^1}{p^1 \vee p^2}(x)p^1(x)\Lambda(dx) = \int (p^1 \wedge p^2)\Lambda(dx) = \kappa.$$

Let us argue why, actually,

$$\mathbb{P}(\xi^3 = \xi^2) = \mathbb{P}(C) = \kappa,$$

i.e. why the inequality $\mathbb{P}(\xi^3 = \xi^2) \geq \mathbb{P}(C)$ may not be strict. Indeed, $\mathbb{P}(\xi^3 = \xi^2) > \mathbb{P}(C)$ may only occur if $\mathbb{P}(\eta 1(\bar{C}) = \xi^2) > 0$ (cf. with (69)), or, equivalently, if $\mathbb{P}\left(\eta 1(\dfrac{p^1}{p^1 \vee p^2}(\xi^2) < \zeta) = \xi^2\right) > 0$. However,

$$\omega \in \bar{C} = \{\omega : \frac{p^1}{p^1 \vee p^2}(\xi^2) < \zeta\}.$$

implies $p^1(\xi_2) < p^2(\xi_2)$, that is, $\xi_2 \in A_2$. But on this set the density of η equals zero. Hence, $\mathbb{P}(\xi^3 = \xi^2) > \mathbb{P}(C)$ is not possible, which means that, in fact, we have proved that $\mathbb{P}(\xi^3 = \xi^2) = \mathbb{P}(C) = \kappa$, as required. The Lemma 43 is proved.

Here is another, 'symmetric' version of the latter lemma.

Lemma 44 ('Of two random variables') *Let ξ^1 and ξ^2 be two random variables on their (without loss of generality different, which will be made independent after we take their direct product!) probability spaces $(\Omega^1, \mathcal{F}^1, \mathbb{P}^1)$ and $(\Omega^2, \mathcal{F}^2, \mathbb{P}^2)$ and with densities p^1 and p^2 with respect to some reference measure Λ, correspondingly. Then, if*

$$\kappa := \int \left(p^1(x) \wedge p^2(x)\right) \Lambda(dx) > 0, \tag{70}$$

then there exists one more probability space $(\Omega, \mathcal{F}, \mathbb{P})$ and two random variables on it η^1, η^2 such that

$$\mathcal{L}(\eta^j) = \mathcal{L}(\xi^j), \quad j = 1, 2, \quad \& \quad \mathbb{P}(\eta^1 = \eta^2) = \kappa. \tag{71}$$

Proof of the Lemma 44. **1: Construction.** We will need now *four* new independent random variables, Bernoulli random variable γ with $\mathbb{P}(\gamma = 0) = \kappa$ and $\zeta^{0,1,2}$ with the densities

$$p^{\zeta^1}(x) := \frac{p^1 - p^1 \wedge p^2}{\int (p^1 - p^1 \wedge p^2)(y)\Lambda(dy)}(x),$$

$$p^{\zeta^2}(x) := \frac{p^2 - p^1 \wedge p^2}{\int (p^2 - p^1 \wedge p^2)(y)\Lambda(dy)}(x),$$

$$p^{\zeta^0}(x) := \frac{p^1 \wedge p^2}{\int (p^1 \wedge p^2)(y)\Lambda(dy)}(x).$$

We may assume that they are all defined on their own probability spaces and eventually we consider the **direct product** of these probability spaces denoted as $(\Omega, \mathcal{F}, \mathbb{P})$. As a result, they are all defined on one unique probability space and they are independent there. Now, on the same product of all probability spaces just mentioned, let

$$\eta^1 := \zeta^0 1(\gamma = 0) + \zeta^1 1(\gamma \neq 0), \quad \& \quad \eta^2 := \zeta^0 1(\gamma = 0) + \zeta^2 1(\gamma \neq 0). \quad (72)$$

We shall see that $\eta^{1,2}$ admit all the desired properties claimed in the Lemma.

2: Verification. From (72), clearly,

$$\mathbb{P}(\eta^1 = \eta^2) \geq \mathbb{P}(\gamma = 0) = \kappa.$$

Yet, we already saw earlier (in slightly different terms) that this may be only an equality, that is, $\mathbb{P}(\eta^1 = \eta^2) = \mathbb{P}(\gamma = 0) = \kappa$.

Next, since γ, ζ^0 and ζ^1 are independent on $(\Omega, \mathcal{F}, \mathbb{P})$, for any bounded measurable function g we have,

$$\mathbb{E}g(\eta^1) = \mathbb{E}g(\eta^1)1(\gamma = 0) + \mathbb{E}g(\eta^1)1(\gamma \neq 0)$$

$$= \mathbb{E}g(\zeta^0)1(\gamma = 0) + \mathbb{E}g(\zeta^1)1(\gamma \neq 0) = \mathbb{E}g(\zeta^0)\mathbb{E}1(\gamma = 0) + \mathbb{E}g(\zeta^1)\mathbb{E}1(\gamma \neq 0)$$

$$= \kappa \int g(y) p^{\zeta^0}(y)\,\Lambda(dy) + (1-\kappa) \int g(y) p^{\zeta^1}(y)\,\Lambda(dy)$$

$$= \kappa \int \frac{p^1 \wedge p^2}{\int (p^1 \wedge p^2)\Lambda(dy)}(x)\Lambda(dx) + (1-\kappa)\int g(x)\frac{p^1 - p^1 \wedge p^2}{\int (p^1 - p^1 \wedge p^2)(y)\Lambda(dy)}(x)\Lambda(dx)$$

$$= \int p^1 \wedge p^2(x)\Lambda(dx) + \int g(x)(p^1 - p^1 \wedge p^2)(x)\Lambda(dx) = \int g(y)p^1(y)\,dy = \mathbb{E}g(\xi^1).$$

For η^2 the arguments are similar, so also $\mathbb{E}g(\eta^2) = \mathbb{E}g(\xi^2)$. The Lemma 44 is proved.

Remark 45 Note that the extended probability space in the proof of the Lemma 44 has the form,

$$(\Omega, \mathcal{F}, \mathbb{P}) = (\Omega^1, \mathcal{F}^1, \mathbb{P}^1) \times (\Omega^2, \mathcal{F}^2, \mathbb{P}^2) \times (\Omega^\gamma, \mathcal{F}^\gamma, \mathbb{P}^\gamma) \times \prod_{k=0}^{2} (\Omega^{\zeta_k}, \mathcal{F}^{\zeta_k}, \mathbb{P}^{\zeta_k}).$$

13 General Coupling Method for Markov Chains

Throughout this section the assumption (54) is assumed. In this section, it is explained how to apply general coupling method as in the Sect. 12 to Markov chains in general state spaces $(S, \mathcal{S})$. Various presentations of this method may be found in [19, 29, 33, 40, 43], et al. This section follows the lines from [6], which, in turn, is based on [43]. Note that in [6] the state space was $\mathbb{R}^1$; however, in $\mathbb{R}^d$ all formulae remain the same. Clearly, this may be further extended to more general state spaces, although, we will not pursue this goal here.

Let us generalize the Lemma 44 to a sequence of random variables and present our coupling construction for Markov chains based on [43]. Assume that the process has a transition density $p(x, y)$ with respect to some reference measure Λ and consider two versions (X_n^1), (X_n^2) of the same Markov process with two initial distributions, respectively, which also have densities with respect to this Λ denoted by $p_{X_0^1}$ and $p_{X_0^2}$ (of course, this does not exclude the case of non-random initial states). Let

$$\kappa(u, v) := \int p(u, t) \wedge p(v, t) \, \Lambda(dt), \quad \kappa = \inf_{u, v} \kappa(u, v), \qquad (73)$$

and

$$\kappa(0) := \int p_{X_0^1}(t) \wedge p_{X_0^2}(t) \, \Lambda(dt). \qquad (74)$$

It is clear that $0 \le \kappa(u, v) \le 1$ for all u, v. Note that $\kappa(0)$ is not the same as κ_0 in the previous sections. We assume that X_0^1 and X_0^2 have different distributions, so $\kappa(0) < 1$. Otherwise we obviously have $X_n^1 \overset{d}{=} X_n^2$ (equality in distribution) for all n, and the coupling can be made trivially, for example, by letting $\widetilde{X}_n^1 = \widetilde{X}_n^2 := X_n^1$.

Let us introduce a new, vector-valued **Markov process** $\left(\eta_n^1, \eta_n^2, \xi_n, \zeta_n\right)$. If $\kappa_0 = 0$ then we set

$$\eta_0^1 := X_0^1, \quad \eta_0^2 := X_0^2, \quad \xi_0 := 0, \quad \zeta_0 := 1.$$

Otherwise, if $0 < \kappa(0) < 1$, then we apply the Lemma 44 to the random variables X_0^1 and X_0^2 so as to create the random variables $\eta_0^1, \eta_0^2, \xi_0$ and ζ_0 (they correspond to η^1, η^2, ξ, and ζ in the Lemma). Now, assuming that the random variables $\left(\eta_n^1, \eta_n^2, \xi_n, \zeta_n\right)$ have been determined for some n, let us show how to construct them for $n + 1$. For this aim, we define the transition probability density φ with respect to the same measure Λ for this (vector-valued) process as follows,

$$\varphi(x, y) := \varphi_1(x, y^1)\varphi_2(x, y^2)\varphi_3(x, y^3)\varphi_4(x, y^4), \tag{75}$$

where $x = (x^1, x^2, x^3, x^4)$, $y = (y^1, y^2, y^3, y^4)$, and if $0 < \kappa(x^1, x^2) < 1$, then

$$\varphi_1(x, u) := \frac{p(x^1, u) - p(x^1, u) \wedge p(x^2, u)}{1 - \kappa(x^1, x^2)}, \quad \varphi_2(x, u) := \frac{p(x^2, u) - p(x^1, u) \wedge p(x^2, u)}{1 - \kappa(x^1, x^2)},$$

$$\varphi_3(x, u) := 1(x^4 = 1)\frac{p(x^1, u) \wedge p(x^2, u)}{\kappa(x^1, x^2)} + 1(x^4 = 0)p(x^3, u),$$

$$\varphi_4(x, u) := 1(x^4 = 1)\left(\delta_1(u)(1 - \kappa(x^1, x^2)) + \delta_0(u)\kappa(x^1, x^2)\right) + 1(x^4 = 0)\delta_0(u), \tag{76}$$

where $\delta_i(u)$ is the Kronecker symbol, $\delta_i(u) = 1(u = i)$, or, in other words, the delta measure concentrated at state i. The case $x^4 = 0$ signifies coupling already realized at the previous step, and $u = 0$ means successful coupling at the transition. In the degenerate cases, if $\kappa(x^1, x^2) = 0$ (coupling at the transition is impossible), then we may set, e.g.

$$\varphi_3(x, u) := 1(x^4 = 1)1(0 < u < 1) + 1(x^4 = 0)p(x^3, u),$$

and if $\kappa(x^1, x^2) = 1$, then we may set

$$\varphi_1(x, u) = \varphi_2(x, u) := 1(0 < u < 1).$$

In fact, in both degenerate cases $\kappa(x^1, x^2) = 0$ or $\kappa(x^1, x^2) = 1$, the functions $\varphi_3(x, u)1(x^4 = 1)$ (or, respectively, $\varphi_1(x, u)$ and $\varphi_2(x, u)$) can be defined more or less arbitrarily, only so as to keep the property of conditional independence of the four random variables $\left(\eta_{n+1}^1, \eta_{n+1}^2, \xi_{n+1}, \zeta_{n+1}\right)$ given $\left(\eta_n^1, \eta_n^2, \xi_n, \zeta_n\right)$.

Lemma 46 *Let the random variables $\tilde{X}_n^1$ and $\tilde{X}_n^2$, for $n \in \mathbb{Z}_+$ be defined by the following formulae:*

$$\tilde{X}_n^1 := \eta_n^1 1(\zeta_n = 1) + \xi_n 1(\zeta_n = 0), \quad \tilde{X}_n^2 := \eta_n^2 1(\zeta_n = 1) + \xi_n 1(\zeta_n = 0).$$

Then

$$\tilde{X}_n^1 \stackrel{d}{=} X_n^1, \quad \tilde{X}_n^2 \stackrel{d}{=} X_n^2, \quad \textit{for all } n \geq 0.$$

Moreover,

$$\tilde{X}_n^1 = \tilde{X}_n^2, \quad \forall\, n \geq n_0(\omega) := \inf\{k \geq 0 : \zeta_k = 0\},$$

and

$$\mathbb{P}(\tilde{X}_n^1 \neq \tilde{X}_n^2) \leq (1 - \kappa(0))\,\mathbb{E}\prod_{i=0}^{n-1}(1 - \kappa(\eta_i^1, \eta_i^2)). \tag{77}$$

Moreover, $\left(\tilde{X}_n^1\right)_{n\geq 0}$ *and* $\left(\tilde{X}_n^2\right)_{n\geq 0}$ *are both homogeneous Markov processes, and*

$$\left(\tilde{X}_n^1\right)_{n\geq 0} \stackrel{d}{=} \left(X_n^1\right)_{n\geq 0}, \quad \& \quad \left(\tilde{X}_n^2\right)_{n\geq 0} \stackrel{d}{=} \left(X_n^2\right)_{n\geq 0}. \tag{78}$$

Informally, the processes η_n^1 and η_n^2 represent X_n^1 and X_n^2, correspondingly, under condition that the coupling was not successful until time n, while the process ξ_n represents both X_n^1 and X_n^2 if the coupling does occur no later than at time n. The process ζ_n represents the moment of coupling: the event $\zeta_n = 0$ is equivalent to the event that coupling occurs no later than at time n. As it follows from (75) and (76),

$$\mathbb{P}(\zeta_{n+1} = 0|\zeta_n = 0) = 1,$$

$$\mathbb{P}(\zeta_{n+1} = 0|\zeta_n = 1, \eta_n^1 = x^1, \eta_n^2 = x^2) = \kappa(x^1, x^2).$$

Hence, if two processes were coupled at time n, then they remain coupled at time $n + 1$, and if they were not coupled, then the coupling occurs with the probability $\kappa(\eta_n^1, \eta_n^2)$. At each time the probability of coupling at the next step is as large as possible, given the current states.

For the proof of Lemma 46 see [6].

From the last lemma a new version of the exponential bound in the Ergodic Theorem may be derived. In general, it *may* somehow improve the estimate based on the constant κ from Markov–Dobrushin's condition (52) or (54). In the remaining paragraphs we do not pursue the most general situation **restricting ourselves again to a simple setting** of $|S| < \infty$. Introduce the operator V acting on a (bounded continuous) function h on the space $S \times S$ as follows: for $x = (x^1, x^2) \in S \times S$ and $X_n := (\tilde{X}_n^1, \tilde{X}_n^2)$,

$$Vh(x) := (1 - \kappa(x^1, x^2))\mathbb{E}_{x^1, x^2}h(X_1) \equiv \exp(\psi(x))\mathbb{E}_{x^1, x^2}h(X_1), \tag{79}$$

where in the last expression $\psi(x) := \ln(1 - \kappa(x^1, x^2))$. The aim is now to find out whether the geometric bound $(1 - \kappa)^n$ in (5) under the assumption (3) is the optimal one, or it could be further improved, let under some additional assumptions. Let us rewrite the estimate (77) as follows:

$$\mathbb{P}(\tilde{X}_n^1 \neq \tilde{X}_n^2) \leq (1 - \kappa(0))V^n 1(x). \tag{80}$$

Note that by definition (79), for the **non-negative** matrix V its sup-norm $\|V\| = \|V\|_{B,B} := \sup_{|h|_B \leq 1} |Vh|_B$ equals $\sup_x V1(x)$, where $|h|_B := \max_x |h(x)|$ and $1 = 1(x)$ is considered as a function on $S \times S$ identically equal to one. Note that $\sup_x V1(x) = 1 - \kappa$.

Now the well-known inequality (see, for example, [25, §8]) reads,

$$r(V) \leq \|V\| = (1 - \kappa). \tag{81}$$

Further, from the Perron–Frobenius Theorem it follows (see, e.g. [14, (7.4.10)]),

$$\lim_n \frac{1}{n} \ln V^n 1(x) = \ln r(V). \tag{82}$$

The assertions (80) and (82) together lead to the following result.

Theorem 47 *Let state space S be finite and let the Markov condition (3) be satisfied. Then*

$$\limsup_{n \to \infty} \frac{1}{n} \ln \|P_x(n, \cdot) - \mu(\cdot)\|_{TV} \leq \ln r(V). \tag{83}$$

In other words, for any $\epsilon > 0$ and n large enough,

$$\|P_x(n, \cdot) - \mu(\cdot)\|_{TV} \leq (r(V) + \epsilon)^n, \tag{84}$$

which is strictly better than (5) if $r(V) < \|V\| = 1 - \kappa$ and $\epsilon > 0$ is chosen small enough, i.e. so that $r(V) + \epsilon < 1 - \kappa$. It is also likely to be true in more general cases for compact operators V where $r(V) + \epsilon < 1 - \kappa$. However, the full problem remains open.

References

1. Bernstein, S.: Sur les sommes de quantités dépendantes, Izv. AN SSSR, ser. VI, **20**, 15–17, 1459–1478 (1926)
2. Bernstein, S.N.: Extension of a limit theorem of probability theory to sums of dependent random variables. Russian Math. Surv. **10**, 65–114 (1944). (in Russian)
3. Bezhaeva, Z.I., Oseledets, V.I.: On the variance of sums for functions of a stationary Markov process. Theory Prob. Appl. **41**(3), 537–541 (1997)
4. Borovkov, A.A.: Ergodicity and Stability of Stochastic Processes. Wiley, Chichester (1998)
5. Borovkov, A.A., Mogul'skii, A.A.: Large deviation principles for sums of random vectors and the corresponding renewal functions in the inhomogeneous case. Siberian Adv. Math. **25**(4), 255–267 (2015)
6. Butkovsky, O.A., Veretennikov, A.Yu.: On asymptotics for Vaserstein coupling of Markov chains. Stoch. Process. Appl. **123**(9), 3518–3541 (2013)
7. Dembo, A., Zeitouni, O.: Large Deviations Techniques and Applications, 2nd edn. Springer, Berlin (1998)

8. Dobrushin, R.L.: Central limit theorem for non-stationary Markov chains. I II Theory Prob. Appl. **1**, 65–80, 329–383 (1956). [English translation]
9. Doeblin, W.: Exposé de la théorie des chaines simples constantes de Markov à un nombre fini d'états. Mathématique de l'Union Interbalkanique **2**, 77–105 & 78–80 (1938)
10. Doob, J.L.: Stochastic Processes. Wiley, New Jersey (1953)
11. Dynkin, E.B.: Markov Processes, vol. 1. Springer, Berlin (2012). (paperback)
12. Ethier, S.N., Kurtz, T.G.: Markov Processes: Characterization and Convergence, Wiley Series in Probability and Statistics, New Jersey (2005). (paperback)
13. Feng, J., Kurtz, T.G.: Large Deviations for Stochastic Processes. AMS (2006)
14. Freidlin, M.I., Wentzell, A.D.: Random Perturbations of Dynamical Systems. Springer, Berlin (1984)
15. Gnedenko, B.V.: Theory of Probability, 6th edn. Gordon and Breach Sci. Publ., Amsterdam (1997)
16. Griffeath, D.Z.: A maximal coupling for Markov chains. Wahrscheinlichkeitstheorie verw. Gebiete **31**(2), 95–106 (1975)
17. Gulinsky, O.V., Veretennikov, AYu.: Large Deviations for Discrete - Time Processes with Averaging. VSP, Utrecht, The Netherlands (1993)
18. Ibragimov, IbragimovLinnik I.A., Yu, V.: Linnik, Independent and Stationary Sequences of Random Variables. Wolters-Noordhoff Publishing, Groningen (1971)
19. Kalashnikov, V.V.: Coupling Method, its Development and Applications. In the Russian translation of E, Nummelin, General Irreducible Markov Chains and Non-negative Operators (1984)
20. Karlin, S.: A First Course in Stochastic Processes. Academic press, Cambridge (2014)
21. Kato, T.: Perturbation Theory for Linear Operators. Springer Science & Business Media, Berlin (2013)
22. Khasminsky, R.Z.: Stochastic Stability of Differential Equations, 2nd edn. Springer, Berlin (2012). https://dx.doi.org/10.1007/978-3-642-23280-0
23. Kolmogorov, A.N.: A local limit theorem for classical Markov chains. (Russian) Izvestiya Akad. Nauk SSSR. Ser. Mat. **13**, 281–300 (1949)
24. Kontoyiannis, I., Meyn, S.P.: Spectral theory and limit theorems for geometrically ergodic Markov processes. Ann. Appl. Probab. **13**(1), 304–362 (2003)
25. Krasnosel'skii, M.A., Lifshits, E.A., Sobolev, A.V.: Positive Linear Systems: The method of positive operators. Helderman Verlag, Berlin (1989)
26. Krylov, N.M., Bogolyubov, N.N.: Les propriétés ergodiques des suites des probabilités en chaîne. CR Math. Acad. Sci. Paris **204**, 1454–1546 (1937)
27. Krylov, N.V.: Introduction to the Theory of Random Processes. AMS, Providence (2002)
28. Kulik, A.: Introduction to Ergodic Rates for Markov Chains and Processes. Potsdam University Press, Potsdam (2015)
29. Lindvall, T.: Lectures on the Coupling Method (Dover Books on Mathematics) (paperback) (2002)
30. Markov, A.A.: Extension of the limit theorems of probability theory to a sum of variables connected in a chain (1906, in Russian), reprinted in Appendix B of: R. Howard. Dynamic Probabilistic Systems, volume 1: Markov Chains. Wiley, New Jersey (1971)
31. Nagaev, S.V.: A central limit theorem for discrete-time Markov processes. Selected Translations in Math. Stat. and Probab. **7**, 156–164 (1968)
32. Nagaev, S.V.: The spectral method and the central limit theorem for general Markov chains. Dokl. Math. **91**(1), 56–59 (2015)
33. Nummelin, E.: General Irreducible Markov Chains (Cambridge Tracts in Mathematics) (paperback). CUP, Cambridge (2008)
34. Papanicolaou, S.V., Stroock, D., Varadhan, S.R.S.: Martingale approach to some limit theorems. In: Ruelle, D.: (ed.) Statistical Mechanics, Dynamical Systems and the Duke Turbulence Conference. Duke Univ. Math. Series, vol. 3. Durham, N.C. (1977). ftp://171.64.38.20/pub/papers/papanicolaou/pubs_old/martingale_duke_77.pdf
35. Pardoux, E., Veretennikov, Yu, A.: On Poisson equation and diffusion approximation 2. Ann. Prob. **31**(3), 1166–1192 (2003)

36. Puhalskii, A.: Large Deviations and Idempotent Probability. Chapman & Hall/CRC, Boca Raton (2001)
37. Rockafellar, R.T.: Convex Analysis, Princeton Landmarks in Mathematics and Physics (paperback) (1997)
38. Seneta, E.: Non-negative Matrices and Markov Chains, 2nd edn. Springer, New York (1981)
39. Seneta, E.: Markov and the Birth of Chain dependence theory. Int. Stat. Rev./Revue Internationale de Statistique **64**(3), 255–263 (1996)
40. Thorisson, H.: Coupling, Stationarity, and Regeneration. Springer, New York (2000)
41. Tutubalin, V.N.: Theory of Probability and Random Processes. MSU, Moscow (in Russian) (1992)
42. Varadhan, S.R.S.: Large Deviations and Applications. SIAM, Philadelphia (1984)
43. Vaserstein, L.N.: Markov processes over denumerable products of spaces. Describ. Large Syst. Automata Probl. Inf. Trans. **5**(3), 47–52 (1969)
44. Veretennikov, Yu, A.: Bounds for the mixing rate in the theory of stochastic equations. Theory Probab. Appl. **32**, 273–281 (1987)
45. Veretennikov, Yu, A.: On large deviations for systems of Itô stochastic equations. Theory Probab. Appl. **36**(4), 772–782 (1991)
46. Veretennikov, Yu, A.: On polynomial mixing bounds for stochastic differential equations. Stoch. Process. Appl. **70**, 115–127 (1997)
47. Veretennikov, Yu, A.: On polynomial mixing and convergence rate for stochastic difference and differential equations. Theory Probab. Appl. **45**(1), 160–163 (2001)
48. Veretennikov, Yu, A.: Parameter and Non-parametric Estimation for Markov Chains. Publ, House of Applied Studies, Mechanics and Mathematics Faculty, Mocow State University (2000). (in Russian)
49. Wentzell, A.D.: A Course in the Theory of Random Processes. McGraw-Hill, New York (1981)

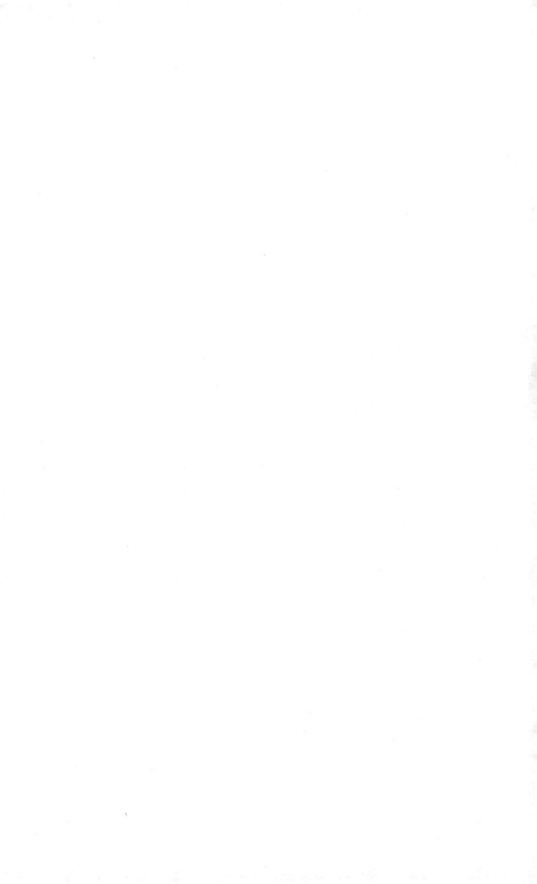

Printed in the United States
By Bookmasters